T0134437

Management of Urology

Series Editors

Sanchia S. Goonewardene
Southend University Hospital NHS Foundation Trust
Southend, UK

Raj Persad
North Bristol NHS Trust
Bristol, UK

This series addresses the need for an increase in the quantity of literature focused upon the management in urology. Books within it will draw attention to the management of subtype specific urology. Therefore, it is of interest to a range of trainee and practicing physicians in a range of disciplines including urology, oncology, specialist nurse and general practitioners.

More information about this series at http://www.springer.com/series/16626

Sanchia S. Goonewardene • Karen Ventii
Amit Bahl • Raj Persad • Hanif Motiwala
David Albala

Management of Muscle Invasive Bladder Cancer

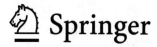

Sanchia S. Goonewardene
Southend University Hospital NHS
Foundation Trust
Southend
UK

Amit Bahl
North Bristol NHS Trust
Bristol
UK

Hanif Motiwala
Southend University Hospital
Westcliff-on-Sea
UK

Karen Ventii
Harvard University
Boston, MA
USA

Raj Persad
North Bristol NHS Trust
Bristol
UK

David Albala
Fayetteville, NY
USA

ISSN 2730-6372 ISSN 2730-6380 (electronic)
Management of Urology
ISBN 978-3-030-57917-3 ISBN 978-3-030-57915-9 (eBook)
https://doi.org/10.1007/978-3-030-57915-9

This Springer imprint is published by the registered company Springer Nature Switzerland AG
The registered company address is: Gewerbestrasse 11, 6330 Cham, Switzerland

Preface

Welcome to Management of Muscle Invasive Bladder Cancer (NMIBC). The concept of this book first came to me as a young trainee, whilst assisting with cystectomies. I had often read papers, but very rarely understood controversies in management of muscle invasive bladder cancer.

Bladder cancer has considerable impact on patients. It presents aggressively, very often, already having advanced into muscle. The patient pathway is very often prolonged and, due to the nature of disease, has poor outcomes.

Bladder cancer is often considered the 'Cinderella' of all the cancers—underfunded for research. The aim of this book is to use the knowledge to further develop your practice and improve patient care. It has been a pleasure to put this together for you.

Southend, UK   Sanchia S. Goonewardene

Acknowledgements

For my family and friends—always supporting me in what I do.

For all the superheroes in my life—you are truly inspirational.

For my team at Springer Nature, for always giving me a chance to get published.

For Dr. Ventii, a true friend and colleague.

For Prof Persad—my mentor for the past 7 years, thank you.

For Prof Motiwala—former TPD and Chief Examiner, FRCS Urol, a visionary in the urology field.

For Prof Albala—My Editor In Chief, friend and mentor—generally awesome.

For my TPD, Ms Georgina Wilson, for always supporting me and my academic endeavours.

Contents

Abbreviations

+LN	Positive lymph nodes
BC/BCa	Bladder cancer
BCG	Bacille Calmette Guerin
BMI	Basal metabolic index
BNA	Beta-naphthylamine
BP	Blood pressure
BZ	Benzidine
CK	Creatinine kinase
CK	CytoKeratin
CPD	Cigarettes per day
CS	Carcinosarcoma
DCB	Dichlorobenzidine
DFS	Disease-free survival
DNA	Deoxyribonucleic acid
EAU	European Association of Urology
EBRT	External beam radiotherapy
EMA	Epithelial membrane antigen
GSCC	Genitourinary SCC
HR	Hazard ratio
HSP	Heat shock protein
LDH	Lactic dehydrogenase
MeSH	Medical Subject Headings
MIBC	Muscle invasive bladder cancer
MPC/MPUC/MPV	Micropapillary
MSA	Muscle specific actin
NCDB	National Cancer Database
NMI	Non-muscle invasive
NMIBC	Non-muscle invasive bladder cancer
NV UC	Non-variant urothelial bladder cancer
OR	Odds ratio
OS	Overall survival
PCMR	Proportionate cancer mortality ratio
PCV/PCV UC	Plasmacytoid variant
PFS	Progression-free survival

PSM	Positive surgical margins
PUC/UC	Plasmacytoid urothelial carcinoma
RC	Radical cystectomy
RR	Relative risk
SD	Standard deviation
SIR	Standardized incidence ratio
SmCC/SCC/SCCB	Small cell carcinoma
TCGA	The Cancer Genome Atlas
TUR	Transurethral resection
TURB/TURBT	Transurethral bladder tumour resection
UBC/UC	Urothelial bladder cancer
UM	Positive urethral margin
(UC)	Urothelial carcinoma

About the Authors

Sanchia S. Goonewardene, MBChB, BMedSc, MRCS, Dip.SSc, MPhil qualified from Birmingham Medical School with Honours in Clinical Science and a BMedSc Degree in Medical Genetics and Molecular Medicine. She has a specific interest in academia during her spare time, with over 627 publications to her name with 2 papers as a number 1 most cited in fields (Biomedical Library), and has significantly contributed to the Urological Academic World—she has since added a section to the European Association of Urology Congress on Prostate Cancer Survivorship and Supportive Care and is an associate member of an EAU guidelines panel on Chronic Pelvic Pain. She has been the UK lead in an EAU led study on Salvage Prostatectomy. She has also contributed to the BURST IDENTIFY study as a collaborator.

Her background with research entails an MPhil, the work from which went on to be drawn up as a document for PCUK then, NICE endorsed. She gained funding from the Wellcome Trust for her Research Elective. She is also an Alumni of the Urology Foundation, who sponsored a trip to USANZ trainee week. She also has four books published—Core Surgical Procedures for Urology Trainees (9828 downloads), Prostate Cancer Survivorship (6959 downloads), Basic Urological Management (11,945 downloads) and Management of Non-Muscle Invasive Bladder Cancer (11,313 downloads).

She has supervised her first thesis with Kings College London and Guys Hospital (BMedSci Degree gained first class, students' thesis score 95%). Recently she has gained her first Associate Editor position with the Journal of Robotic Surgery and is responsible as Urology Section Editor. She is an Editorial board member of the World Journal of Urology and was invited to be Guest Editor for a Special Issue on Salvage Therapy in Prostate Cancer. She is also a review board member for BMJ case reports. Additionally, she is on The International Continence Society Panel on Pelvic Floor Dysfunction, Good Urodynamic Practice Panel, is an ICS abstract reviewer and has been an EPoster Chair at ICS. More recently she has been an ICS Ambassador 2020 and is an ICS Mentor. She has also chaired semi live surgery at ERUS and presented her work as part of the Young Academic Urology Section at ERUS.

Karen Ventii, BSc, MSc, PhD is a Harvard-trained specialist in healthcare communications, with over 10 years of experience in oncology and urology. As a Visiting

Fellow at Harvard University, she conducted independent research on evolving trends in continuing medical education, with the aim of diminishing the gap between evidence and practice. Her research was conducted in collaboration with Dr. Aria F. Olumi (Janet & William DeWolf Professor of Surgery/Urology at Harvard Medical School, Chief of Urologic Surgery at Beth Israel Deaconess Medical Center, and Chair of Research for the American Urological Association).

Throughout her career, Dr. Ventii has worked on numerous medical education initiatives in the academic and pharmaceutical sectors, including the NIH Broadening Experience in Scientific Training (BEST) initiative to enhance training opportunities for early career scientists and prepare them for career options in the dynamic biomedical workforce landscape. Dr. Ventii has also authored many oncology- and urology-focused publications including a review article on Biomarkers in Prostate Cancer which was selected as one of the top Oncology reviews of 2014.

Dr. Ventii has worked with several global healthcare companies focused in oncology and has been responsible for content development, content editing, publications, and supporting strategic planning on several accounts.

Dr. Ventii holds a Doctorate in biochemistry from Emory University in Atlanta, GA, and a Bachelor of Science as well as a Master of Science degree in biology from Duquesne University in Pittsburgh, PA. Upon completing her Doctorate, Karen continued her research efforts at the Winship Cancer Institute investigating the biochemical properties of the breast cancer associated protein-1 (BAP1) tumor suppressor protein. Her research has been published in peer-reviewed journals such as Cancer Research, Biochemistry, and Oncology and she has presented her work in oral and poster formats at national conferences. Harvard University, Boston, MA, USA

Amit Bahl, MD, FRCP, FRCR, FFRRCSI is Consultant Clinical Oncologist at Bristol Cancer Institute, University Hospitals Bristol with a special interest in breast and urological cancers. He is the research lead for Uro-oncology at Bristol Haematology and Oncology Centre. He has led and developed the prostate brachytherapy service at Bristol. He has been an expert adviser to NICE for the technology appraisal on new drugs and an external service reviewer at oncology departments elsewhere in the country. Prior to his current roles, Professor Bahl became Member of the Royal College of Physicians (UK) and trained in Clinical Oncology, achieving the Fellowship of the Royal College of Radiologists qualification. He has been awarded the fellowship of the Royal College of Physicians. He is a current member of the National Cancer Research Institute Clinical Studies penile cancer subgroup. He has been college tutor of the Royal College of Radiologists for 10 years and has supervised several MD theses in breast and prostate cancer research. He has previously been in the NCRI Renal, Bladder and Prostate clinical studies group. He is an Executive Committee member of the British Uro-oncology group. Professor Bahl is actively involved in research into breast, prostate, bladder and penile cancers and has more than 100 publications in these research areas and has several presentations at national and international meetings. In 2012, Professor Bahl was awarded the Cochrane Shanks Jalil Professorship by the Royal College of Radiologists, London, and he is Visiting Professor to two international centres and at University of West of England. He is currently holding research grants in excess of £2 million and is Chief Investigator for several multicentre trials which are focussing on new modalities of treatment in breast and prostate cancer and also is leading the robotic brachytherapy project.   Bristol Cancer Institute, University Hospitals, Bristol, UK

Raj Persad, MB, BS, ChM, FRCS (Eng) appointed in 1996, is a Consultant Urological Surgeon and Andrologist in Bristol.

In his clinical role, he is one of the most experienced pelvic cancer surgeons in the UK and was one of the first in the UK to practice female neobladder reconstruction following cystectomy for invasive bladder cancer. He has subspecialised over many years in precise surgical techniques which improve both oncologic and functional outcomes. This includes techniques ranging from (1) the use of the Da Vinci Robot for performing Robot-Assisted Laparoscopic Radical Prostatectomy, (2) High Intensity Focused Ultrasound for minimally invasive non-surgical treatment of prostate cancer and (3) Rectal Spacer and Fiducial Marker precision placement for optimizing the outcomes of Image Guided Radiotherapy for prostate cancer.

In the field of Diagnostics he has been one of the National Leads in developing the prostate pre-biopsy MRI pathway for patients with elevated PSA. This has optimized the accuracy of cancer diagnosis minimized clinical risk and sepsis associated with transrectal biopsy. He has developed to a fine art both cognitive transperineal biopsies of the prostate as well as fusion biopsy of the prostate.

Professor Persad has been a National pioneer in minimally invasive techniques for the treatment of Symptomatic Benign Prostatic as an alternative to Transurethral Prostatectomy (TURP). These techniques include Urolift (prostatic urethral lift) procedure which he does under general or local anaesthetic depending on patient preference as well as REZUM, steam treatment of the prostate. He also treats BPH with Green Light Laser. All these techniques are offered by Professor Persad for BPH as well as traditional TURP if tablet therapy has failed or cannot be tolerated by the patient.

Professor Persad is also a National Authority in the treatment of Erectile Dysfunction. He practices optimum medical therapies for all male patients and has a large cohort of patients who are diabetic or who have had prostatectomy and in need of erectile function restoration. If conservative therapy fails with erectogenic pharmacotherapy or use of medical devices he can offer the insertion of state-of-the-art penile prosthetic devices. Professor Persad also treats deformity due to Peyronies across a range of severity, offering therapeutic injection in its early phases and various types of surgical correction if this fails according to patient needs.

Professor Persad has a 25-year experience in the restoration of fertility through microsurgical eversal of vasectomy and has some of the best results nationally. He also for more complex cases offers epididymo-vasovasostomy. In combination with the Bristol Centre for Reproductive Medicine, he will soon be offering male infertility procedures such as micro-TESE (testicular extraction of sperm) in order to optimize assisted conception techniques.

Academically, Prof Persad is involved in an extensive range of research with the Universities of Bristol, Pittsburgh, London and Oxford. These include the detection of early bladder and prostate cancer and novel imaging and treatment strategies for these diseases. He formerly led a team of researchers engaged in improving strategies for treatment of advanced prostate cancer in areas of hormonal treatment and immunotherapy (BPCRN). He has been Principal Investigator, Chief Investigator, and Collaborator in many National and International studies sponsored by the MRC, EORTC, CRUK, and NCRN. He has been a recipient of £4.5m research grants from UK bodies as well as the NIH USA, and has published over 300 scientific articles and 7 books in the field of Urology.

Together with Scientists and Clinicians in Bristol he is part of the productive BRC (Biomed Research Centre), which has a number of far-reaching clinical and scientific goals in the field of cancer and is Surgical Principle Investigator for the PreVent and Pre-Empt trials of lifestyle intervention in prostate cancer. He has an innovative research programme with Prof Chris Melhuish in Medical Robotics to enhance surgery and radiotherapy modalities with Robotic assistance.

In addition to his University and NHS Clinical commitments, he spends time visiting hospital units in the developing world (e.g. Tanzania), where he helps to train junior doctors and other healthcare professionals.

Hanif Motiwala, MB, BS, ChM, FRCS (Eng), FRCS (Urol) Mr Motiwala is well known to the community worldwide. He was Professor of Urology in India and has also served as an FRCS Urol Examiner. He has been training programme director for the London Deanery, Imperial Rotation, and was well liked by all of his trainees. He has also been a Lecturer for Institute of Urology and Oxford Trainees.

He has over 25 years' experience as a Consultant in urology and extensive exposure to senior leadership roles within healthcare provision and professional institutions including.

Chairman of the surgical division at Wexham Park Hospital. He also has a strong track record of achieving clinical targets within tightly controlled budgets, developing innovative strategies to improve patient care and optimise use of resources, for which he received a Bronze Award.

He is a dedicated and committed surgeon, utilising teaching, surgical and medical skills for the greater good through international voluntary work, building capability and skills in reconstructive surgery in India and Africa. He was conferred a position as Visiting Professor – University of Khartoum, Sudan, 2009 in recognition of voluntary work in Sudan, conducting final Urology Examinations to train qualified surgeons, providing training to surgeons in reconstruction and carrying out complex surgery.

David Albala, MD graduated with a geology degree from Lafayette College in Easton, Pennsylvania. He completed his medical school training at Michigan State University and went on to complete his surgical residency at the Dartmouth-Hitchcock Medical Center. Following this, Dr. Albala was an endourology fellow at

Washington University Medical Center under the direction of Ralph V. Clayman. He practiced at Loyola University Medical Center in Chicago and rose from the ranks of Instructor to full Professor in Urology and Radiology in 8 years. After 10 years, he became a tenured Professor at Duke University Medical Center in North Carolina. At Duke, he was Co-Director of the Endourology fellowship and Director for the Center of Minimally Invasive and Robotic Urological Surgery. He has over 180 publications in peer-reviewed journals and has authored 5 books in endourology and general urology. He is the Editor-in-Chief of the Journal of Robotic Surgery. He serves on the editorial board for Medical Reviews in Urology, Current Opinions in Urology and Urology Index and Reviews. He serves as a reviewer for eight surgical journals.

Presently he is Chief of Urology at Crouse Hospital in Syracuse, New York, and a physician at Associated Medical Professionals (a group of 29 urologists). He is considered a national and international authority in laparoscopic and robotic urological surgery and has been an active teacher in this area for over 20 years. His research and clinical interests have focused on robotic urological surgery. In addition, other clinical interests include minimally invasive treatment of benign prostatic hypertrophy (BPH) and the use of fibrin sealants in surgery. He has been a Visiting Professor at numerous institutions across the United States as well as overseas in countries such as India, China, Iceland, Germany, France, Japan, Brazil, Australia, and Singapore. In addition, he has done operative demonstrations in over 32 countries and 23 states. He has trained 16 fellows in endourology and advanced robotic surgery.

In addition, Dr. Albala is a past White House Fellow who acted as a special assistant to Federico Pena, Secretary of Transportation, on classified and unclassified public health related issues.

Part I
Introduction

Introduction to Muscle Invasive Bladder Cancer

Invasive bladder cancer is a common disease with a high mortality rate despite gold standard treatment [1]. The European Association of Urology (EAU) Muscle-invasive and Metastatic Bladder Cancer (MIBC) Guidelines provide information to optimise diagnosis, treatment, and follow-up of this aggressive disease [1]. There are a number of treatment strategies including radical therapy, bladder-sparing treatments and combinations of treatment modalities (different forms of surgery, radiation therapy, and chemotherapy) [1]. There are new organ-sparing approaches with minimally invasive surgery [1].

Organ preservation has been used more and more in the management of muscle-invasive bladder cancer [2]. Multiple bladder preservation options exist, although the approach of TURBT and chemoradiation is popular as trimodal therapy [2]. Phase III trials have shown superiority of chemoradiotherapy compared to radiotherapy alone [2]. Concurrent chemoradiotherapy gives local control outcomes comparable to those of radical surgery, but in comparison, better when considering quality of life [2].

Bladder-preserving techniques represent an alternative for patients who are unfit for cystectomy or decline major surgical intervention; however, need lifelong surveillance. It is important to emphasise to the patients opting for organ preservation the need for this, as risk of recurrence remains even years after radical chemoradiotherapy treatment [2].

Radical cystectomy and chemoradiation, are complimentary rather than competing treatments [2]. Meticulous patient selection is central to the success of recent trials within the field of bladder preservation [2]. However, close monitoring of patients who undergo bladder preservation are key to optimising outcomes [2].

S. S. Goonewardene et al., *Management of Muscle Invasive Bladder Cancer*, Management of Urology, https://doi.org/10.1007/978-3-030-57915-9_1

References

1. Alfred Witjes J, Lebret T, Compérat EM, Cowan NC, De Santis M, Bruins HM, Hernández V, Espinós EL, Dunn J, Rouanne M, Neuzillet Y, Veskimäe E, van der Heijden AG, Gakis G, Ribal MJ. Updated 2016 EAU guidelines on muscle-invasive and metastatic bladder cancer. Eur Urol. 2017;71(3):462–75.
2. El-Taji OM, Alam S, Hussain SA. Bladder sparing approaches for muscle-invasive bladder cancers. Curr Treat Options in Oncol. 2016;17(3):15.

Part II

Epidemiology and the Molecular Basis of Bladder Cancer

Epidemiology and Risk Factors in Muscle Invasive Bladder Cancer

2

2.1 Research Methods

A systematic review relating to bladder cancer epidemiology, risk factors and occupational hazards was conducted. This was to identify the bladder cancer epidemiology and risk factors in muscle invasive disease. The search strategy aimed to identify all references related to bladder cancer AND screening. Search terms used were as follows: (Bladder cancer) AND (Epidemiology) AND (Risk Factors). The following databases were screened from 1989 to June 2020:

- CINAHL
- MEDLINE (NHS Evidence)
- Cochrane
- AMed
- EMBASE
- PsychINFO
- SCOPUS
- Web of Science.

In addition, searches using Medical Subject Headings (MeSH) and keywords were conducted using Cochrane databases. Two UK-based experts in bladder cancer were consulted to identify any additional studies.

Studies were eligible for inclusion if they reported primary research focusing on bladder cancer and screening. Papers were included if published after 1984 and had to be in English. Studies that did not conform to this were excluded. Only primary research was included (Fig. 2.1). The overall aim was to identify bladder cancer risk factors and epidemiology in muscle invasive disease.

Abstracts were independently screened for eligibility by two reviewers and disagreements resolved through discussion or third-party opinion. Agreement

© The Editor(s) (if applicable) and The Author(s), under exclusive license to
Springer Nature Switzerland AG 2021
S. S. Goonewardene et al., *Management of Muscle Invasive Bladder Cancer*,
Management of Urology, https://doi.org/10.1007/978-3-030-57915-9_2

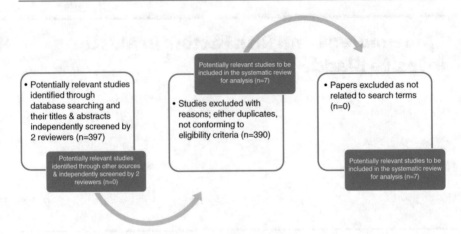

Fig. 2.1 Flow chart of studies identified through the systematic review. (Adapted from PRISMA)

level was calculated using Cohen's Kappa to test the intercoder reliability of this screening process. Cohens' Kappa allows comparison of inter-rater reliability between papers using relative observed agreement. This also takes account of the comparison occurring by chance. The first reviewer agreed all seven papers to be included, the second, agreed on seven. Cohens kappa was therefore 1.0.

Data extraction was piloted by the researcher and amended in consultation with the research team (author and two academic supervisors). Data collected included authors, year and country of publication, study aims, setting, intervention aims, number of participants, study design, intervention components and delivery methods, comparison groups and outcome measures, notes and follow-up questions for the authors. Studies were quality assessed using the PRISMA criteria for randomised controlled trials, Mays et al. [1, 2] for the action research and qualitative studies and the Critical Skills Appraisal programme for cohort studies. This was also applied to randomised controlled trials and qualitative studies.

The search identified 397 papers (Fig. 2.1). All seven mapped to the search terms and eligibility criteria. The current systematic reviews were examined to gain further knowledge about the subject. Three hundred and ninety papers were excluded due to not conforming to eligibility criteria or adding to the evidence. Of the seven papers left, relevant abstracts were identified, and the full papers obtained (all of which were in English), to quality assure against search criteria. There was considerable heterogeneity of design among the included studies therefore a narrative review of the evidence was undertaken. There was significant heterogeneity within studies, including clinical topic, numbers, outcomes, as a result a narrative review was thought to be best. There were seven cohort studies, with a moderate level of evidence. These were from a range of countries with minimal loss to follow-up. All participants were identified appropriately.

2.2   Flavonoids and Bladder Cancer Risk

Flavonoids have an antioxidant capacity and anti-carcinogenic effect in bladder cancer [3]. A number of studies have demonstrated inconsistent results [3]. Rossi analysed data from an Italian case-control study for acute, non-neoplastic, non-tobacco-related disease [3]. Rossi discovered inverse association between isoflavones (OR for the highest compared to the lowest quintile of intake = 0.56, 95% CI 0.37–0.84) and flavones (OR = 0.64, 95% CI 0.44–0.95) and bladder cancer [3]. A non-significant inverse association was found for flavan-3-ols (OR = 0.70), flavonols (OR = 0.85) and total flavonoids (OR = 0.76).

2.3   Metabolic Factors and Risk of Bladder Cancer

Teleka, assessed metabolic factors which may cause bladder cancer [4]. Among men, triglycerides and BP were positively associated with bladder cancer (BC) risk overall (hazard ratio [HR] per standard deviation [SD]: 1.17 [95% confidence interval (CI) 1.06–1.27] and 1.09 [1.02–1.17], respectively). Among women, BMI was inversely associated with risk (HR: 0.90 [0.82–0.99]) [4]. The associations for BMI and BP differed between men and women (p ≤ 0.005). Among men, BMI, cholesterol and triglycerides were positively associated with risk for NMIBC (HRs: 1.09 [95% CI 1.01–1.18], 1.14 [1.02–1.25], and 1.30 [1.12–1.48] respectively), and BP was positively associated with MIBC (HR: 1.23 [1.02–1.49]) [4]. Among women, glucose was positively associated with MIBC (HR: 1.99 [1.04–3.81]). This highlights the role of metabolic aberrations in BC risk [4].

2.4   Smoking Cessation and Bladder Cancer Risk

Soria assessed the impact of smoking cessation on oncological outcomes [5]. Smoking pattern, intensity, and duration result in an increased risk of developing bladder cancer (BCa). More aggressive tumour features at initial presentation were noted [5]. Tobacco consumption is associated with a higher risk of recurrence in NMIBC and impaired intravesical therapy outcomes [5]. Smoking cessation decreases the risk of BCa and improves treatment outcomes [5]. However, prospective series examining smoking cessation on outcomes are needed [5]. Brief counselling can significantly enhance smoking cessation rates. Adequate knowledge of association between tobacco and BCa, is central to better outcomes in clinical practice [5].

Ogihara investigated smoking cessation and preventative effects against bladder tumour recurrence [6]. Overall, 181 patients (28.5%) were classified as current smokers, 154 (24.3%) as former smokers, and 299 (47.2%) as non-smokers. Kaplan-Meier analysisdemonstrated recurrence rate was significantly lower in the non-smoking group than current- and former-smoker groups (p < 0.001 and p < 0.001, respectively) [6]. In the 154 former smokers, Kaplan-Meier analysishighlighted smoking intensity and duration was not associated with tumour recurrence rate [6]. Patients with a smoking cessation period of 15 years or more had a significantly lower tumor recurrence rate than their counterparts (p < 0.001) [6]. A multivariate analysis identified a smoking cessation period of <15 years (hazard ratio [HR] 2.20; p = 0.003) and T1 tumors (HR 1.99; p = 0.013) as independent risk factors for tumor recurrence in the former-smokers subgroup [6].

Rink investigated the association of pretreatment smoking status, cumulative exposure, and time since smoking cessation on outcomes of urothelial carcinoma of the bladder (UCB) treated with radical cystectomy (RC) [7]. Rink retrospectively collected clinicopathologic and smoking variables, including smoking status, number of cigarettes per day (CPD), duration in years, and time since smoking cessation, for 1506 patients treated with RC for UCB [7]. Lifetime cumulative smoking exposure was categorized as light short-term (≤20 CPD for ≤20 year), light long-term (≤20 CPD for >20 year), heavy short-term (>20 CPD for ≤20 year), and heavy long-term (>20 CPD for >20 year) [7]. There was no difference in clinicopathologic factors between patients who had never smoked (20%), former smokers (46%), and current smokers (34%). Smoking status was associated with cumulative incidence of disease recurrence (p = 0.004) and cancer-specific mortality (p = 0.016) in univariable analyses and disease recurrence in multivariable analysis (p = 0.02). Current smokers had the highest cumulative incidences of bladder cancer [7]. Among ever smokers, cumulative smoking exposure was associated with advanced tumor stages (p < 0.001), LN metastasis (p = 0.002), disease recurrence (p < 0.001), cancer-specific mortality (p = 0.001), and overall mortality (p = 0.037) [7]. In multivariable analyses that adjusted for standard characteristics; heavy long-term smokers had the worst outcomes, followed by light long-term, heavy short-term, and light short-term smokers [7]. Smoking cessation ≥10 year mitigated the risk of disease recurrence (hazard ratio [HR]: 0.44; p < 0.001), cancer-specific mortality (HR: 0.42; p < 0.001), and overall mortality (HR: 0.69; p = 0.012) in multivariable analyses. The study is limited by its retrospective nature [7].

2.5   Occupational Exposure in Muscle Invasive Bladder Cancer

Tobacco smoking and occupational exposures are the leading risk factors for developing urothelial bladder carcinoma (UBC), yet little is known about the contribution of these two factors to risk of UBC recurrence [8]. Wilcox evaluated whether smoking status and usual adult occupation are associated with time to UBC recurrence for 406 patients with muscle-invasive bladder cancer submitted to The Cancer Genome Atlas (TCGA) project [8]. Data on time to recurrence were available for 358 patients over a median follow-up time of 15 months. Of these, 133 (37.2%) experienced a recurrence [8]. Current smokers who smoked for more than 40 pack-years had an increased risk of recurrence compared to never smokers (HR 2.1, 95% CI 1.1, 4.1) [8]. Additionally, employment in a high-risk occupation was associated with a shorter time to recurrence (log-rank p = 0.005). There was an increased risk of recurrence for those employed in occupations with probable diesel exhaust exposure (HR 1.8, 95% CI 1.1, 3.0) and for those employed in production occupations (HR 2.0, 95% CI 1.1, 3.6) [8].

2.6 Androgen Suppression Therapy and Risk of Muscle Invasive Bladder Cancer

Shiota determined whether intravesical recurrence is affected by inhibition of androgen signaling in men with non-muscle invasive bladder cancer [9]. Shiota studied 228 men, including 32 with and 196 without androgen suppression therapy [9]. Intravesical recurrence developed in 4 (12.5%) and 59 men (30.1%) with and without androgen suppression therapy, respectively [9]. On multivariate analysis multiple tumours (HR 1.82, p = 0.027), a large tumour (HR 2.13, p = 0.043) and smoking history (HR 2.45, p = 0.020) and presence of androgen suppression therapy (HR 0.36, p = 0.024) were independent risk factors for intravesical recurrence [9]. Tumour progressed to muscle invasive bladder cancer in 6 men (3.1%) without androgen suppression therapy. No man with androgen suppression therapy progressed to muscle invasive bladder cancer [9].

2.7 Reviews Associated with Epidemiology and Risk Factors in Bladder Cancer

Westhoff systematically reviewed evidence on association between body mass index (BMI), diet, dietary supplements, and physical activity and bladder cancer prognosis [10]. In non-muscle invasive bladder cancer (NMIBC) patients, both overweight (three studies, pooled hazard ratio (HR) 1.29, 95% CI 1.05–1.58, $I^2 = 0\%$) as well as obesity (three studies, pooled HR 1.82, 95% CI 1.12–2.95, $I^2 = 79\%$) were associated with increased risk of recurrence when compared to normal weight [10]. No association with risk of progression was demonstrated. Results for BMI and prognosis in muscle-invasive or in all stages series were inconsistent [10]. Observational studies on diet and randomized controlled trials with dietary supplements gave variable outcomes. No studies on physical activity and prognosis have been published to date [10].

References

1. Moher D, Liberati A, Tetzlaff J, Altman DG. "Preferred Reporting Items for Systematic Reviews and Meta-Analyses: The Prisma Statement." [In English]. BMJ (Online) 339, no. 7716 (08 Aug 2009):332–36.
2. Mays N, Pope C, Popay J. "Systematically Reviewing Qualitative and Quantitative Evidence to Inform Management and Policy-Making in the Health Field." [In English]. Journal of Health Services Research and Policy 10, no. SUPPL. 1 (July 2005):6–20.

3. Rossi M, Strikoudi P, Spei ME, Parpinel M, Serraino D, Montella M, Libra M, La Vecchia C, Rosato V. Flavonoids and bladder cancer risk. Cancer Causes Control. 2019;30(5):527–35.
4. Teleka S, Häggström C, Nagel G, Bjørge T, Manjer J, Ulmer H, Liedberg F, Ghaderi S, Lang A, Jonsson H, Jahnson S, Orho-Melander M, Tretli S, Stattin P, Stocks T. Risk of bladder cancer by disease severity in relation to metabolic factors and smoking: a prospective pooled cohort study of 800,000 men and women. Int J Cancer. 2018;143(12):3071–82.
5. Soria F, Marra G, Čapoun O, Soukup V, Gontero P. Prevention of bladder cancer incidence and recurrence: tobacco use. Curr Opin Urol. 2018;28(1):80–7.
6. Ogihara K, Kikuchi E, Yuge K, Ito Y, Tanaka N, Matsumoto K, Miyajima A, Asakura H, Oya M. Refraining from smoking for 15 years or more reduced the risk of tumor recurrence in non-muscle invasive bladder cancer patients. Ann Surg Oncol. 2016;23(5):1752–9.
7. Rink M, Zabor EC, Furberg H, Xylinas E, Ehdaie B, Novara G, Babjuk M, Pycha A, Lotan Y, Trinh QD, Chun FK, Lee RK, Karakiewicz PI, Fisch M, Robinson BD, Scherr DS, Shariat SF. Impact of smoking and smoking cessation on outcomes in bladder cancer patients treated with radical cystectomy. Eur Urol. 2013;64(3):456–64.
8. Wilcox AN, Silverman DT, Friesen MC, Locke SJ, Russ DE, Hyun N, Colt JS, Figueroa JD, Rothman N, Moore LE, Koutros S. Smoking status, usual adult occupation, and risk of recurrent urothelial bladder carcinoma: data from The Cancer Genome Atlas (TCGA) Project. Cancer Causes Control. 2016;27(12):1429–35.
9. Shiota M, Kiyoshima K, Yokomizo A, Takeuchi A, Kashiwagi E, Dejima T, Takahashi R, Inokuchi J, Tatsugami K, Eto M. Suppressed recurrent bladder cancer after androgen suppression with androgen deprivation therapy or 5α-reductase inhibitor. J Urol. 2017;197(2):308–13.
10. Westhoff E, Witjes JA, Fleshner NE, Lerner SP, Shariat SF, Steineck G, Kampman E, Kiemeney LA, Vrieling A. Body mass index, diet-related factors, and bladder cancer prognosis: a systematic review and meta-analysis. Bladder Cancer. 2018;4(1):91–112.

Epidemiology, Risk Factors and Occupational Hazards

3

A systematic review relating to bladder cancer epidemiology, risk factors and occupational hazards was conducted. This was to identify the bladder cancer epidemiology, risk factors and occupational hazards. The search strategy aimed to identify all references related to bladder cancer AND screening. Search terms used were as follows: (Bladder cancer) AND (Epidemiology) AND (Risk Factors) AND (Occupational Hazards). The following databases were screened from 1989 to June 2020:

- CINAHL
- MEDLINE (NHS Evidence)
- Cochrane
- AMed
- EMBASE
- PsychINFO
- SCOPUS
- Web of Science.

In addition, searches using Medical Subject Headings (MeSH) and keywords were conducted using Cochrane databases. Two UK-based experts in bladder cancer were consulted to identify any additional studies.

Studies were eligible for inclusion if they reported primary research focusing on bladder cancer and screening. Papers were included if published after 1984 and had to be in English. Studies that did not conform to this were excluded. Only primary research was included (Fig. 3.1). The overall aim was to identify the role and components of bladder cancer screening.

Abstracts were independently screened for eligibility by two reviewers and disagreements resolved through discussion or third-party opinion. Agreement level

S. S. Goonewardene et al., *Management of Muscle Invasive Bladder Cancer*,
Management of Urology, https://doi.org/10.1007/978-3-030-57915-9_3

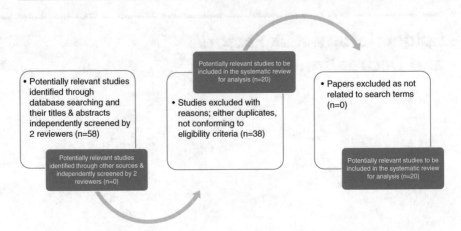

Fig. 3.1 Flow chart of studies identified through the systematic review. (Adapted from PRISMA)

was calculated using Cohen's Kappa to test the intercoder reliability of this screening process. Cohens' Kappa allows comparison of inter-rater reliability between papers using relative observed agreement. This also takes account of the comparison occurring by chance. The first reviewer agreed all 20 papers to be included, the second, agreed on 20.

Data extraction was piloted by the researcher and amended in consultation with the research team (author and two academic supervisors). Data collected included authors, year and country of publication, study aims, setting, intervention aims, number of participants, study design, intervention components and delivery methods, comparison groups and outcome measures, notes and follow-up questions for the authors. Studies were quality assessed using the PRISMA criteria for randomised controlled trials, Mays et al. [1, 2] for the action research and qualitative studies and the Critical Skills Appraisal programme for cohort studies. This was also applied to randomised controlled trials and qualitative studies.

The search identified 20 papers (Fig. 3.1). All 20 mapped to the search terms and eligibility criteria. The current systematic reviews were examined to gain further knowledge about the subject. Thirty-eight papers were excluded due to not conforming to eligibility criteria or adding to the evidence for bladder cancer screening. Of the 20 papers left, relevant abstracts were identified and the full papers obtained (all of which were in English), to quality assure against search criteria. There was considerable heterogeneity of design among the included studies therefore a narrative review of the evidence was undertaken. There was significant heterogeneity within studies, including clinical topic, numbers, outcomes, as a result a narrative review was thought to be best. There were 20 cohort studies, with a moderate level of evidence. These were from a range of countries with minimal loss to follow-up. All participants were identified appropriately.

3.1   Systematic Review Results on Bladder Cancer Epidemiology, Occupational Hazards and Risk Factors

3.1.1   Bladder Cancer Survival

The cause-specific mortality (1940–1993) of 2985 male workers employed in oil refineries was examined [3]. Separate analyses were undertaken by race, refinery, employment status (active and retired), and time since entry into employment [3]. Proportionate cancer mortality ratio (PCMR) analyses also were conducted. Significantly decreased mortality was observed for cancers of the bladder (PMR = 40) [3]. However, this may be explained by length of time in employment and exposure to carcinogens.

Darby et al. [4], studied the long term effects of atmospheric nuclear weapon tests and experimental programmes [4]. Greater than 10 years after initial participation the relative risk of death was raised for bladder cancer. However, the overall conclusion was participation in nuclear weapon tests had no detectable effect on expectation of life or on subsequent risk of developing cancer [4].

Exposure to occupational hazards among firefighters may lead to increased mortality from cancer [5]. Mortality from bladder cancer was increased and approached statistical significance (SMR = 1.79; 95% CI: 0.98–3.00). Firefighters certified between 1972 and 1976 had excess mortality from bladder cancer (SMR = 1.95; 95% CI: 1.04–3.33) [5]. This demonstrates the impact of exposure to occupational risk factors can have on mortality from cancer.

3.1.2   Carcinogenic Agents: Population Studies

Pukkala examined up to 45 years of cancer incidence data by occupational category [6]. Fifteen million people aged 30–64 years in the 1960, 1970, 1980/1981 and/or 1990 censuses in Denmark, Finland, Iceland, Norway and Sweden were included. High risk occupations were examined. The occupations with the highest risk factors included workers producing tobacco and chimney sweeps. Low risk factors were demonstrated in farmers, gardeners and teachers [6]. Waiters had the highest risk of bladder cancer in men and tobacco workers in women. This can be attributed to smoking [6]. Hairdressers also had a high-risk factor for bladder cancer—this may be due to exposure from hair dye. Chimney sweeps were exposed to polycyclic aromatic hydrocarbons from the chimney soot, and hairdressers' work environment is also rich in chemical agents [6].

3.1.3   Populations Studies with Women

The relation between occupation and bladder cancer in women was examined during the National Bladder Cancer Study [7]. This was a population-based, case-control study conducted in ten areas of the United States [7]. Increased risk of bladder cancer occurred in metal working and fabrication occupations (relative risk (RR) = 1.5; 95% confidence interval (CI) 0.9–2.6) [7]. Punch and stamping press operatives had a significant trend in risk with increasing duration of employment and an increased risk for women employed as chemical processing workers was also shown. The authors estimate that 11% of bladder cancer diagnosed among white women in the United States is attributable to occupational exposures [7].

The incidence of cancer of the urinary bladder is three- to fivefold lower in women than in men [8]. Kabat assessed the association of menstrual and reproductive factors and exogenous hormone use with the risk of incident transitional cell cancer of the urinary bladder in a cohort of 145,548 postmenopausal women (ages 50–79 years at baseline) enrolled in the Women's Health Initiative [8]. Relative to nulliparous women, parous women had a reduced risk of transitional cell cancer, however, there was no clear trend. Risk was significantly increased in women with a history of at least two miscarriages (HR 1.52, 95% CI 1.15–2.00) [8]. In conclusion Kabat found limited evidence for associations of reproductive factors or exogenous hormone use with the risk of bladder cancer [8].

3.1.4 Population Studies with Men

In nearly all populations studied, the risk of bladder cancer is two to four times as great in men as in women [9]. Hartge examined gender-specific incidence rates without known carcinogenic factors [9]. The data used were obtained from the National Bladder Cancer Study. Even in the absence of exposure to cigarettes, occupational hazards, or urinary tract infection, the gender-related risk persisted; the incidence of bladder cancer was 11.0 in men and 4.1 in women, yielding a ratio of 2.7 [9]. Possible explanations for the excessive risk in men include environmental and dietary exposures not yet identified and innate sexual characteristics such as anatomic differences, urination habits, or hormonal factors [9].

3.1.5 Arylamines

Cancer incidence was investigated in a cohort of 700 workers employed at a Connecticut chemical plant [10]. The plant produced a variety of chemicals, including arylamines such as dichlorobenzidine (DCB), o-dianisidine, o-tolidine, but not benzidine. The principal finding was a statistically significant increase in the standardized incidence ratio (SIR) for bladder cancer in men (SIR = 8.3; confidence interval, 3.3–17.0) [10]. The observed association between bladder cancer cases and exposure to arylamines increased with increasing exposure (SIRs = 0.0, 5.5, 16.4, for none, low, or moderate levels of exposure, respectively) [10]. Smoking probably contributed to the bladder cancer risk, as all case subjects were known to be current or former cigarette smokers [10].

Tomioka evaluate non-urological cancer risks associated with benzidine (BZ) and beta-naphthylamine (BNA), a historical cohort study was undertaken [11]. A total of 224 male workers exposed to BZ/BNA were followed from 1953 to 2011 [11]. Follow-up was successful for 216 (96.4%). Follow-up duration averaged 44.0 (SD 10.7) years. This study confirms the high risk of BC, suggesting that BZ/BNA have the potential to cause BC.

3.1.6   Anilene Dyes

Occupational exposure was examined in 258 industrial workers with bladder cancer versus 454 matched controls [12]. All participants were members of Tambov Province centers of chemical industry [12]. Statistical significance (relative risk-4.7) was established for exposure to aromatic amines [12]. For those contacting with aniline dyes the relative risk (RR) made up 2.4 [12]. The risk to develop bladder cancer in powder shops (RR 3.2) was attributed to the hazards of dyes and diphenyl-amine [12]. In leather-shoe and textile industry the exposure to dyes was not safe (RR 6.1), neither was it to chemicals, oil products, pesticides, overheating (RR 3.2, 1.6, 3.2 and 2.9, respectively) [12]. It is stated that in line with a significant risk to develop bladder cancer at exposure to aromatic amines there exist a number of occupational factors contributing to this risk.

3.1.7   Arsenic

Arsenic is a ubiquitous, naturally occurring metalloid that has significant risk of bladder cancer [13]. Individuals are exposed to naturally occurring levels of arsenic in grains, vegetables, meats and fish, as well as through food processed with water containing arsenic [13]. Oberoi et al. [13], examined the global burdens of disease for bladder cancers attributable to inorganic arsenic in food [13]. Oberoi used World Health Organization estimates of food consumption in 13 country clusters, in con-junction with reported measurements of total and inorganic arsenic in different foods. The conclusion was that each year 9129–119,176 additional cases of bladder cancer worldwide are attributable to inorganic arsenic in food.

3.1.8   Textile Industry

A case-control study on bladder cancer was carried out in Spain [14]. The study included 497 cases (438 males and 59 females), 583 hospital controls and 530 popu-lation controls. These patients were matched by sex, age and residence [14]. Among men, an increased risk of bladder cancer was discovered for textile workers (OR = 1.97, 95% CI 1.2–3.3), mechanics, maintenance workers (OR = 1.86, 95% CI 1.2–2.8), workers in the printing industry (OR = 2.06, 95% CI 1.0–4.3) and for managers (OR = 2.03, 95% CI 1.2–3.5) [14]. The risk was highest among those first employed <25 and prior to 1960. Among mechanics the risk was highest working >25 and after 1960 [14]. The OR for smokers who had also been employed in one of the high risk occupations was 7.82 (95% CI 4.4–14.0) which is compatible with a multiplicative effect of joint exposure to tobacco and occupational hazards [14].

In 1981–1982 a retrospective study was conducted in a polyamide-polyester factory in Lyon, France. This study evaluated the effect of exposure to phthalates, nickel catalysers, and other chemicals in the work environment [15]. An excess of cases of bladder cancer (based on seven cases) was noted among nylon workers [15]. The cohort is still young, however, and a continued follow up is required.

3.1.9 Metalworking Fluids Exposure

Occupations with mineral oil exposure have been associated with bladder cancer in population-based case-control studies [16]. Friesen et al. [16] examined bladder cancer incidence in relation to quantitative exposures to metalworking fluids (MWFs), based on 21,999 male automotive workers, Penalized splines were also fit to estimate the functional form of the exposure-response relation. Increased bladder cancer risk was associated with straight MWFs but not with any other exposure [16]. Calendar time windows relevant to polycyclic aromatic hydrocarbon exposure were examined but could not be distinguished from the lagged (10-, 20-year) metrics. The quantitative relation with straight MWFs strengthens the evidence for mineral oils as a bladder carcinogen [16].

3.1.10 Smoking and Bladder Cancer

Bladder cancer is associated with occupational hazards and smoking [17]. Sadetzki et al. [17] assessed risk factors for bladder cancer [17]. The study included 140 male patients and 280 matched controls [17]. This paper confirmed industrial employment as an occupational hazard (OR = 2.21; 95% Cl = 1. 21–4.02) and exposure to three or more metals (OR = 3.65; 95% Cl = 1.21–11.08) as risk factors. Smoking had infrequent association with higher rates in those smoking <18 years (OR = 2.64; 95% Cl = 1.4–4.99) and smoking >30 cigarettes per day (OR = 1.82; 95% Cl = 0.95–3.49) [17]. This paper suggests prevention of bladder cancer has a long way to go [17].

Occupation and bladder cancer in women was examined with the National Bladder Cancer Study, a population-based, case-control study [7]. Increased risk was apparent for women ever employed in metal working and fabrication occupations (relative risk (RR) = 1.5; 95% confidence interval (CI) 0.9–2.6) [7]. Stamping press operatives had a significant increase in risk with increasing duration of employment. There was also an increased risk for women employed as chemical processing workers. Eleven percent of bladder cancer diagnosed among women is attributable to occupational exposures [7].

Winters investigated the likelihood of smoking cessation after bladder cancer diagnosis in a population database [18]. The smoking cessation rate in patients with bladder cancer was 27% compared with 21% in noncancer controls [18]. There was no significant difference in the adjusted OR of quitting smoking in patients with bladder cancer (OR 1.3, 95% CI 0.7–2.5 vs. OR 1.2, 95% CI 0.4–3.6) [18]. Independent predictors of smoking cessation in patients with bladder cancer included age (p = 0.03), African American race (p = 0.03) and college education (p = 0.01) [18].

3.1.11   Impact of Occupational Risk Factors on Prognosis of Recurrent Bladder Cancer

The influence of occupational risk factors on bladder cancer is well known, studies on the influence on bladder cancer prognosis are rare. Primary relapses were examined in three case-control series [19]. Recurrent bladder tumour was noted in 416 cases (52%). Workers in the leather industry (n = 4), printing industry (n = 4), transportation (n = 43), and chemical industry (n = 40) and locksmiths/mechanics (n = 44) demonstrated shorter relapse-free times.

Mortality at two engine plants was analysed to review bladder cancer mortality among workers exposed to machining fluids [20]. Causes of death and work histories were available for 1870 decendents. Elevated mortality ratios for bladder cancer was not statistically significant in plantwide populations. Nitrosamines were probably present in camshaft and crankshaft grinding, which can also increase bladder cancer risk. Bladder cancer increased was also associated with duration among workers grinding in straight oil MF (OR = 3.0, 95% CI = 1.15, 7.8) and in machining/heat-treat operations (OR = 2.9, 95% CI = 1.14, 7.2).

3.1.12   Results from the Literature and Other Reviews on Bladder Cancer Epidemiology, Risk Factors, Occupational Exposure

Many epidemiological studies and reviews have been performed to identify the causes of bladder cancer [21]. Letastova reviewed the links between various environmental risk factors and cancer of the bladder. Risks identified include smoking, arsenic in drinking water at concentrations higher than 300 µg/l, exposure to aromatic amines (2-naphthylamine, 4-aminobiphenyl and benzidine) and 4,4′-methylenebis(2-chloroaniline). These are commonly found in chemical, dye and rubber industries as well as in hair dyes, paints, fungicides, cigarette smoke, plastics, metals and motor vehicle exhausts [21]. Other types of smoking besides cigarettes e.g. cigar, pipe, Egyptian waterpipe, smokeless tobacco and environmental tobacco smoking, can also have an effect. Other sources of arsenic exposure such as air, food, occupational hazards, and tobacco were also demonstrated as a risk [21]. This study highlighted it may be several years or decades between exposure and subsequent presentation of bladder cancer [21].

Each year, 430,000 people are diagnosed with bladder cancer [22]. This is a significant proportion of the population. Due to the aggressiveness of disease, prevention is paramount. Al-Zalabani et al. [22] reviewed all meta-analyses on modifiable risk factors of primary bladder cancer [22]. Statistically significant associations were found for current (RR 3.14) or former (RR 1.83) cigarette smoking, pipe (RR 1.9) or cigar (RR 2.3) smoking, antioxidant supplementation (RR 1.52), obesity (RR 1.10), higher physical activity levels (RR 0.86), higher body levels of selenium (RR 0.61) and vitamin D (RR 0.75), and higher intakes of: processed meat (RR 1.22), vitamin A (RR 0.82), vitamin E (RR 0.82), folate (RR 0.84), fruit (RR 0.77), vegetables (RR 0.83), citrus fruit (RR 0.85), and cruciferous vegetables (RR 0.84). Occupations with highest risk of exposure were tobacco workers (RR 1.72), dye workers (RR 1.58), and chimney sweeps (RR 1.53). Modification of lifestyle and occupational exposures can reduce this risk significantly. While smoking remains one of the key risk factors, also several diet-related and occupational factors are very relevant [22].

Workplace exposures account for 5–25% of all bladder cancer cases [23]. A critical review of the literature between 1938 and 2004 was performed, with a focus on occupational exposures [23]. Occupational exposure to bladder carcinogens, particularly to beta-naphthylamine occur in a number of industries, including aromatic amine manufacture, rubber and cable manufacture, and dyestuff manufacture and use [23] can have an impact on bladder cancer risk [23].

References

1. Moher D, Liberati A, Tetzlaff J, Altman DG. "Preferred Reporting Items for Systematic Reviews and Meta-Analyses: The Prisma Statement." [In English]. BMJ (Online) 339, no. 7716 (08 Aug 2009):332–36.
2. Mays N, Pope C, Popay J. "Systematically Reviewing Qualitative and Quantitative Evidence to Inform Management and Policy-Making in the Health Field." [In English]. Journal of Health Services Research and Policy 10, no. SUPPL. 1 (July 2005):6–20.
3. Dement JM, Hensley L, Kieding S, Lipscomb H. Proportionate mortality among union members employed at three Texas refineries. Am J Ind Med. 1998;33(4):327–40.
4. Darby SC, Kendall GM, Fell TP, Doll R, Goodill AA, Conquest AJ, Jackson DA, Haylock RG. Further follow up of mortality and incidence of cancer in men from the United Kingdom who participated in the United Kingdom's atmospheric nuclear weapon tests and experimental programmes. BMJ. 1993;307(6918):1530–5.
5. Ma F, Fleming LE, Lee DJ, Trapido E, Gerace TA, Lai H, Lai S. Mortality in Florida professional firefighters, 1972 to 1999. Am J Ind Med. 2005;47(6):50.
6. Pukkala E, Martinsen JI, Lynge E, Gunnarsdottir HK, Sparén P, Tryggvadottir L, Weiderpass E, Kjaerheim K. Occupation and cancer - follow-up of 15 million people in five Nordic countries. Acta Oncol. 2009;48(5):646–790.
7. Silverman DT, Levin LI, Hoover RN. Occupational risks of bladder cancer among white women in the United States. Am J Epidemiol. 1990;132(3):453–61.
8. Kabat GC, Kim MY, Luo J, Hou L, Cetnar J, Wactawski-Wende J, Rohan TE. Menstrual and reproductive factors and exogenous hormone use and risk of transitional cell bladder cancer in postmenopausal women. Eur J Cancer Prev. 2013;22(5):409–16.
9. Hartge P, Harvey EB, Linehan WM, Silverman DT, Sullivan JW, Hoover RN, Fraumeni JF Jr. Unexplained excess risk of bladder cancer in men. J Natl Cancer Inst. 1990;82(20):1636–40.
10. Ouellet-Hellstrom R, Rench JD. Bladder cancer incidence in arylamine workers. J Occup Environ Med. 1996;38(12):1239–47.

11. Tomioka K, Obayashi K, Saeki K, Okamoto N, Kurumatani N. Increased risk of lung cancer associated with occupational exposure to benzidine and/or beta-naphthylamine. Int Arch Occup Environ Health. 2015;88(4):455–65.
12. Nizamova RS. [Occupational hazards and bladder cancer]. Urol Nefrol (Mosk). 1991;(5):35–8.
13. Oberoi S, Barchowsky A, Wu F. The global burden of disease for skin, lung, and bladder cancer caused by arsenic in food. Cancer Epidemiol Biomark Prev. 2014;23(7):1187–94.
14. González CA, López-Abente G, Errezola M, Escolar A, Riboli E, Izarzugaza I, Nebot M. Occupation and bladder cancer in Spain: a multi-centre case-control study. Int J Epidemiol. 1989;18(3):569–77.
15. Hours M, Cardis E, Marciniak A, Quelin P, Fabry J. Mortality of a cohort in a polyamide-polyester factory in Lyon: a further follow up. Br J Ind Med. 1989;46(9):665–70.
16. Friesen MC, Costello S, Eisen EA. Quantitative exposure to metalworking fluids and bladder cancer incidence in a cohort of autoworkers. Am J Epidemiol. 2009;169(12):1471–8.
17. Sadetzki S, Bensal D, Blumstein T, Novikov I, Modan B. Selected risk factors for transitional cell bladder cancer. Med Oncol. 2000;17(3):179–82.
18. Winters BR, Wen L, Holt SK, et al. Does the diagnosis of bladder cancer lead to higher rates of smoking cessation? Findings from the Medicare Health Outcomes Survey. J Urol. 2019;202(2):241–6.
19. Selinski S, Bürger H, Blaszkewicz M, Otto T, Volkert F, Moormann O, Niedner H, Hengstler JG, Golka K. Occupational risk factors for relapse-free survival in bladder cancer patients. J Toxicol Environ Health A. 2016;79(22–23):1136–43.
20. Park RM, Mirer FE. A survey of mortality at two automotive engine manufacturing plants. Am J Ind Med. 1996;30(6):664–73.
21. Letašiová S, Medve'ová A, Šovčíková A, Dušinská M, Volkovová K, Mosoiu C, Bartonová A. Bladder cancer, a review of the environmental risk factors. Environ Health. 2012;11(Suppl 1):S11.
22. Al-Zalabani AH, Stewart KF, Wesselius A, Schols AM, Zeegers MP. Modifiable risk factors for the prevention of bladder cancer: a systematic review of meta-analyses. Eur J Epidemiol. 2016;31(9):811–51.
23. Olfert SM, Felknor SA, Delclos GL. An updated review of the literature: risk factors for bladder cancer with focus on occupational exposures. South Med J. 2006;99(11):1256–63.

The Molecular Basis of Muscle Invasive Bladder Cancer

4

4.1 Research Methods

A systematic review relating to muscle invasive bladder cancer and was conducted. This was to identify the molecular basis of muscle invasive disease. The search strategy aimed to identify all references related to bladder cancer AND muscle invasive disease AND molecular basis. Search terms used were as follows: (Bladder cancer) AND (muscle invasive disease) AND (Molecular Basis). The following databases were screened from 1989 to June 2020:

- CINAHL
- MEDLINE (NHS Evidence)
- Cochrane
- AMed
- EMBASE
- PsychINFO
- SCOPUS
- Web of Science.

In addition, searches using Medical Subject Headings (MeSH) and keywords were conducted using Cochrane databases. Two UK-based experts in bladder cancer were consulted to identify any additional studies.

Studies were eligible for inclusion if they reported primary research focusing on bladder cancer and the molecular basis. Papers were included if published after 1984 and had to be in English. Studies that did not conform to this were excluded. Only primary research was included (Fig. 4.1). The overall aim was to identify bladder cancer risk factors and epidemiology in muscle invasive disease.

© The Editor(s) (if applicable) and The Author(s), under exclusive license to Springer Nature Switzerland AG 2021
S. S. Goonewardene et al., *Management of Muscle Invasive Bladder Cancer*, Management of Urology, https://doi.org/10.1007/978-3-030-57915-9_4

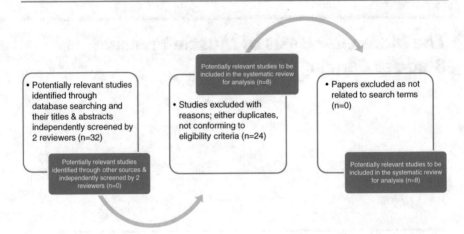

Fig. 4.1 Flow chart of studies identified through the systematic review. (Adapted from PRISMA)

Abstracts were independently screened for eligibility by two reviewers and disagreements resolved through discussion or third-party opinion. Agreement level was calculated using Cohen's Kappa to test the intercoder reliability of this screening process. Cohens' Kappa allows comparison of inter-rater reliability between papers using relative observed agreement. This also takes account of the comparison occurring by chance. The first reviewer agreed all eight papers to be included, the second, agreed on eight.

Data extraction was piloted by the researcher and amended in consultation with the research team (author and two academic supervisors). Data collected included authors, year and country of publication, study aims, setting, intervention aims, number of participants, study design, intervention components and delivery methods, comparison groups and outcome measures, notes and follow-up questions for the authors. Studies were quality assessed using the PRISMA criteria for randomised controlled trials, Mays et al. [1, 2] for the action research and qualitative studies and the Critical Skills Appraisal programme for cohort studies. This was also applied to randomised controlled trials and qualitative studies.

The search identified eight papers (Fig. 4.1). All eight mapped to the search terms and eligibility criteria. The current systematic reviews were examined to gain further knowledge about the subject. Twenty-four papers were excluded due to not conforming to eligibility criteria or adding to the evidence. Of the eight papers left, relevant abstracts were identified and the full papers obtained (all of which were in English), to quality assure against search criteria. There was considerable heterogeneity of design among the included studies therefore a narrative review of the evidence was undertaken. There was significant heterogeneity within studies, including clinical topic, numbers, outcomes, as a result a narrative review was thought to be best. There were eight cohort studies, with a moderate level of evidence. These were from a range of countries with minimal loss to follow-up. All participants were identified appropriately.

4.2   Systematic Review Results

4.2.1   The Molecular Basis of Bladder Cancer: Precision Diagnostics and Treatment

Bladder cancer (BC) can be classified into subtypes according to genetic background and clinical prognosis [3]. The gold standard in bladder cancer diagnostics is cystoscopy. One of the more challenging issues in bladder cancer is the high rate of recurrence [3]. Minimally invasive precision treatment technique, immunotherapy, chemotherapy, gene therapy, and targeted therapy of BC have been developed [3]. This results in an improved the prognosis and overall survival of BC patients [3].

Bladder cancers are biologically and clinically heterogeneous [4]. Recent large-scale transcriptomic profiling studies demonstrate molecularly distinct clusters explaining their heterogeneity [4]. Subtype-specific differential responses to cytotoxic chemotherapy and to therapies that inhibit a number of targets, including growth factors (EGFR, ERBB2, FGFR) and immune checkpoint (PD1, PDL1) inhibitors have been demonstrated [4]. Despite burgeoning evidence for important clinical implications, subtyping and precision diagnostics has yet to enter routine clinical practice [4].

4.2.2   PIK3CA Mutations in Muscle Invasive Bladder Cancer

Immune checkpoint inhibitors give better survival outcomes compared to chemotherapy. Borcoman discovered bladder cancer bearing *PIK3CA* gene mutations were significantly associated with lower expression of a defined immune gene sequence [5]. A reduced ten-gene immune gene sequence was identified that highlights muscle-invasive bladder cancer (MIBC) on a molecular basis, with immune infiltration and *PIK3CA* mutation [5]. Using qRT-PCR, increased chemokines and immune genes in *PIK3CA*-mutated tumors from mice, reflected an active immune infiltrate in comparison to untreated mice [5]. This highlights a rationale for combination strategies of PI3K inhibitors with immune checkpoint inhibitors as part of clinical strategy [5].

4.2.3   Epidermal Growth Factor in Muscle Invasive Bladder Cancer

Epidermal growth factor receptors (EGFr) have been measured on primary bladder cancer membranes by 125I-EGF ligand binding [6]. Muscle invasion had higher EGFr levels than superficial tumors or normal bladder mucosa ($p = 0.05$) [6]. When the two largest subgroups of superficial and invasive tumors were compared (15 pTa, 16 T3), the invasive tumours had significantly higher EGFr levels (p less than 0.05) [6]. EGFr may be involved in mechanisms of tumour progression [6]. EGFr can be a precision therapy with EGF-linked drugs in the appropriate subset of muscle invasive bladder cancers [6].

4.2.4   P53, pRB and RAS in Muscle Invasive Bladder Cancer

Advances have been made in molecular mechanisms of carcinogenesis in muscle invasive bladder cancer [7]. The subsets of urothelial carcinoma allow development of multifocal synchronous and metachronous tumours as a target [7]. Low-grade papillary carcinoma is associated with FGFR3 gene mutation or RAS gene mutation [7]. High-grade in situ/muscle-invasive carcinoma is associated with p53 and pRB. Loss of function results in loss of control of cell cycle and leads to an aggressive phenotype [7].

4.2.5   Transcriptome Profiling in Muscle Invasive Bladder Cancer

Zhang performed high-throughput transcriptome sequencing on a recurrent muscle-invasive cisplatin-resistant [8]. Zhang demonstrated five dysregulated genes, including CDH1, VEGFA, PTPRF, CLDN7, and MMP2 [8]. What was also demonstrated were 300 genes showed differential splicing patterns between normal and abnormal tissue [8]. Cancer splicing alternative genes were CD44, PDGFA, NUMB, and LPHN2 were also highlighted as being significant, in neoplastic disease [8].

4.2.6   Methylation Status in Bladder Cancer

The use of molecular markers may allow to predict for tumour aggressiveness [9]. Beukers highlighted methylation of GATA2, TBX2, TBX3, and ZIC4 genes could predict progression of superficial (Ta) tumours [9]. Beukers validated markers using DNA from tissue [9]. TBX2, TBX3, and ZIC4 were independent predictors of disease progression [9]. On the basis of this methylation state, three new molecular grade groups were formed [9]. Outcomes demonstrated 8% of patients in the low molecular grade group progressed within 5 years. Progression was 29% and 63% for the intermediate- and high-molecular grade groups [9]. This study demonstrated excellent markers for predicting progression to muscle-invasive bladder cancer in superficial cancer [9].

4.2.7   The Cancer Genome Project and the Molecular Basis of Bladder Cancer

Molecular subtypes in bladder cancer allows recognition of pathways driving different molecular groups and subsets [10]. The Cancer Genome Project (TCGA) project allows molecular analysis of 412 muscle-invasive bladder cancers [10]. This allows better insight into the molecular basis of this disease [10]. The DNA splices and alterations allow for precision diagnostic and therapeutic approaches [10]. Molecular subtypes of bladder cancer include distinct 'basal/squamous' and 'luminal' subtypes, papillary urothelial histology, immune checkpoint marker expression, and a 'neuronal' subtype [10]. The gene-level alterations and groups are relevant from translational science moving into clinical practice [10]. This highlights again, the role of basic science having an impact on diagnostics and therapeutics in muscle invasive bladder cancer.

References

1. Moher D, Liberati A, Tetzlaff J, Altman DG. "Preferred Reporting Items for Systematic Reviews and Meta-Analyses: The Prisma Statement." [In English]. BMJ (Online) 339, no. 7716 (08 Aug 2009):332–36.
2. Mays N, Pope C, Popay J. "Systematically Reviewing Qualitative and Quantitative Evidence to Inform Management and Policy-Making in the Health Field." [In English]. Journal of Health Services Research and Policy 10, no. SUPPL. 1 (July 2005):6–20.
3. Su H, Jiang H, Tao T, Kang X, Zhang X, Kang D, Li S, Li C, Wang H, Yang Z, Zhang J, Li C. Hope and challenge: precision medicine in bladder cancer. Cancer Med. 2019;8(4):1806–16.
4. Sjödahl G, Jackson CL, Bartlett JM, Siemens DR, Berman DM. Molecular profiling in muscle-invasive bladder cancer: more than the sum of its parts. J Pathol. 2019;247(5):563–73.
5. Borcoman E, De La Rochere P, Richer W, Vacher S, Chemlali W, Krucker C, Sirab N, Radvanyi F, Allory Y, Pignot G, Barry de Longchamps N, Damotte D, Meseure D, Sedlik C, Bieche I, Piaggio E. Inhibition of PI3K pathway increases immune infiltrate in muscle-invasive bladder cancer. Oncoimmunology. 2019;8(5):e1581556.
6. Smith K, Fennelly JA, Neal DE, Hall RR, Harris AL. Characterization and quantitation of the epidermal growth factor receptor in invasive and superficial bladder tumors. Cancer Res. 1989;49(21):5810–5.
7. Al Hussain TO, Akhtar M. Molecular basis of urinary bladder cancer. Adv Anat Pathol. 2013;20(1):53–60.
8. Zhang S, Liu Y, Liu Z, Zhang C, Cao H, Ye Y, Wang S, Zhang Y, Xiao S, Yang P, Li J, Bai Z. Transcriptome profiling of a multiple recurrent muscle-invasive urothelial carcinoma of the bladder by deep sequencing. PLoS One. 2014;9(3):e91466.
9. Beukers W, Kandimalla R, Masius RG, Vermeij M, Kranse R, van Leenders GJ, Zwarthoff EC. Stratification based on methylation of TBX2 and TBX3 into three molecular grades predicts progression in patients with pTa-bladder cancer. Mod Pathol. 2015;28(4):515–22.
10. Creighton CJ. The clinical applications of The Cancer Genome Atlas project for bladder cancer. Expert Rev Anticancer Ther. 2018;18(10):973–80.

Part III

Management of Histological Variants

Urothelial carcinoma (UC) with squamous differentiation (UC w/SD) is the most common variant [1]. Accurate identification is key although barriers exist; tumor heterogeneity, sampling limitation and pathologic interpretation of specimens [1]. Although many cases of UC w/SD present with muscle-invasive bladder cancer, those cancers that are confirmed to be truly non-muscle invasive can be managed with endoscopic resection, adjuvant intravesical therapies (i.e., Bacillus Calmette Guerin), and close surveillance [1]. Radical cystectomy series suggest that UC w/SD tends to present at a more advanced stage than pure UC does although survival outcomes are similar when controlling for standard clinicopathologic factors [1].

The true clinical significance of variant histology is challenging, especially with nonmuscle invasive disease [2]. This tends to identify a high-risk population with a worse prognosis and better suited for early aggressive intervention (i.e., radical cystectomy), then treatment recommendations should reflect this notion [2]. High-risk NMIBC or variant histology should be offered early cystectomy, especially if pure squamous, adenocarcinoma, sarcomatoid, plasmacytoid, or micropapillary disease [2]. For squamous differentiation, intravesical therapy is an option based on standard risk stratification in NMIBC [2]. With variant histology, there is a risk of understaging and also have close surveillance to not compromise the opportunity of cure [2]. The management of NMIBC and variant histology is difficult due to understaging and clinical controversies in management of high-risk NMIBC disease for standard urothelial cell carcinoma (early cystectomy vs. intravesical therapy) [2].

5.1   Risk Factors

Bladder cancer has the ninth highest incidence worldwide, but a small proportion (2–5%) are squamous cell carcinoma (SCC) [3]. The cohort of SCC were female (49% vs. 24%; p < 0.01) and African American (11% vs. 5%; p < 0.01) [3]. They presented at a higher stage than urothelial cancer. Muscle-invasive bladder cancer

S. S. Goonewardene et al., *Management of Muscle Invasive Bladder Cancer*,
Management of Urology, https://doi.org/10.1007/978-3-030-57915-9_5

(MIBC) was noted in 70% vs. 19% at diagnosis [3]. On multivariate analysis, SCC predicted poorer prognosis (hazard-ratio [HR] 1.79, p < 0.01) [3]. In contrast to urothelial disease, there was no benefit with neoadjuvant chemotherapy (NAC) over radical cystectomy alone (HR 0.93, p = 0.69). Muscle invasive SCC had a much worse prognosis and outcome when compared to urothelial histology.

5.2   Survival Outcomes

Vetterlein has examined outcomes from squamous carcinoma [4]. Overall, squamous cell (hazard ratio, 1.26; 95% confidence interval [CI], 1.07–1.49; p = 0.006) is associated with worse overall survival (OS) relative to urothelial bladder cancer [4]. Squamous cell carcinoma (odds ratio [OR], 1.58; 95% CI, 1.23–2.04; p < 0.001) was associated with greater risk of ≥pT3 disease [4]. In contrast, squamous cell variants were associated with decreased (OR, 0.66; 95% CI, 0.48–0.91; p = 0.012) odds of pN+ disease. Pure squamous cell and neuroendocrine carcinoma histologic types were associated with worse OS relative to urothelial bladder cancer.

Abdollah et al. [5] tested the effect of histological subtype (NBSCC vs. UC) on cancer-specific mortality (CSM), after adjusting for other-cause mortality (OCM) [5]. Abdollah identified 12,311 patients who were treated with radical cystectomy (RC) between 1988 and 2006, within 17 Surveillance, Epidemiology and End Results (SEER) registries [5]. Histological subtype was NBSCC in 614 (5%) patients vs. UC in 11,697 (95%) patients [5]. At RC, the rate of non-organ confined (NOC) disease was higher in NBSCC than UC (71.7% vs. 52.2%; p < 0.001). [5]. After adjustment for OCM, the 5-year cumulative CSM rates were 25.0% vs. 19.8% (p = 0.2) for patients with NBSCC vs. UC organ confined (OC) BCa, respectively [5]. The same rates were 46.3% vs. 49.3% in patients with NOC BCa (p = 0.1). At RC, the rate of NOC bladder cancer is higher in NBSCC patients than in their UC counterparts [5]. Despite a more advanced stage at surgery, NBSCC histological subtype is not associated with a less favourable CSM than UC histological subtype, after accounting for OCM and the extent of the disease (OC vs. NOC) [5].

5.3   Squamous Cell and Evidence of Metastatic Disease

Royce demonstrated squamous cell carcinoma (SCC, 2.4%) had a greater likelihood of presenting with metastatic disease at diagnosis, with impact on muscle invasive disease as a result [6] (11.5% for urothelial cancer (UC) vs. 31.3%, for SCC respectively, p < 0.001). Patients with non-urothelial bladder cancer were also more likely to have MIBC compared to UC (43% vs. 32.5%, respectively) [6]. The impact of this, is that UC were less likely to have radical surgery, chemotherapy, and radiation therapy (p < 0.001) [6]. Non urothelial bladder cancer as a result was associated with worse survival outcomes compared to UC (p < 0.001). This highlights just how different non urothelial bladder cancer disease is compared to UC. Most cases present with advanced disease, have more radical treatment, with inferior outcomes.

Minato et al. [7] identified the clinical significance of squamous differentiation in UC in radical cystectomy (RC) [7]. The 5-year OS rate of squamous differentiation and pure UC groups was 41.1% and 69.7% ($p = 0.002$) and the 5-year RFS rate was 51.8% and 59.5% ($p = 0.027$), respectively [7]. The Kaplan-Meier curves for squamous differentiation highlights rapid progression for squamous differentiation within the first 2 years than pure UC [7]. Multivariate analyses suggested that squamous differentiation in UC was significantly associated with poorer OS (hazard ratio [HR]: 4.22; 95% confidence interval [CI]: 1.20–14.8; $p = 0.024$) and close to significance for a lower recurrence free survival (HR: 2.13, 95% CI: 0.74–6.15, $p = 0.064$) [7].

References

1. Raman JD, Jafri SM. Surgical management of bladder urothelial carcinoma with squamous differentiation. Urol Oncol. 2015;33(10):429–33.
2. Porten SP, Willis D, Kamat AM. Variant histology: role in management and prognosis of non-muscle invasive bladder cancer. Curr Opin Urol. 2014;24(5):517–23.
3. Matulay JT, Woldu SL, Lim A, Narayan VM, Li G, Kamat AM, Anderson CB. The impact of squamous histology on survival in patients with muscle-invasive bladder cancer. Urol Oncol. 2019;37(6):353.
4. Vetterlein MW, Seisen T, Leow JJ, Preston MA, Sun M, Friedlander DF, Meyer CP, Chun FK, Lipsitz SR, Menon M, Kibel AS, Bellmunt J, Choueiri TK, Trinh QD. Effect of nonurothelial histologic variants on the outcomes of radical cystectomy for nonmetastatic muscle-invasive urinary bladder cancer. Clin Genitourin Cancer. 2017; https://doi.org/10.1016/j.clgc.2017.08.00.
5. Abdollah F, Sun M, Jeldres C, Schmitges J, Thuret R, Djahangirian O, Tian Z, Shariat SF, Perrotte P, Montorsi F, Karakiewicz PI. Survival after radical cystectomy of non-bilharzial squamous cell carcinoma vs urothelial carcinoma: a competing-risks analysis. BJU Int. 2012;109(4):564–9.
6. Royce TJ, Lin CC, Gray PJ, Shipley WU, Jemal A, Efstathiou JA. Clinical characteristics and outcomes of nonurothelial cell carcinoma of the bladder: results from the National Cancer Data Base. Urol Oncol. 2018;36(2):78.e1–78.e12.
7. Minato A, Noguchi H, Tomisaki I, Fukuda A, Kubo T, Nakayama T, Fujimoto N. Clinical significance of squamous differentiation in urothelial carcinoma of the bladder. Cancer Control. 2018;25(1):1073274818800269.

Histological Variants in Muscle Invasive Bladder Cancer: Adenocarcinoma

6

Bladder cancer (BC) has an incidence of 100,000 men and women each year in the European Union (EU) [1]. Variant histology account for up to 25%. There is evidence that additional variant histology results in impaired prognosis [1]. Aggressive behaviour and advanced stages at primary presentation are frequently observed in non-UC arguing for radical and sometimes different treatment strategies as compared to pure UC [1].

Mucinous adenocarcinoma represent 0.5–2% of all malignant epithelial bladder tumours [2]. Despite being rare, it has a poor prognosis due to presenting at diagnosis in advanced stages [2]. There is no consensus on the treatment of adenocarcinoma of bladder. Surgery would be the only curative treatment. Due to the aggressiveness of the conditions, it is curative in just a small number of cases [2].

6.1 Survival Outcomes in Bladder Adenocarcinoma: Radical Surgery vs. Resection

Martínez-Piñeiro examined 11 cases of primary adenocarcinoma of the bladder [3]. Nine cases were muscle invasive at diagnosis. Two patients were submitted to radical cystectomy, lymphadenectomy and Wallace II cutaneous uretero-ileostomy. One patient underwent partial cystectomy and lymphadenectomy. Six were submitted to transurethral resection [3]. Excision of the urachal tumor was by en bloc partial cystectomy. The 5-year survival of patients with infiltrating tumors, excluding the urachal tumor, was 33%, 67% died within the first year of follow-up [3]. The only case of superficial adenocarcinoma is alive and tumor-free at 94 months [3]. Primary adenocarcinoma of the bladder is an aggressive tumour. Although it may be superficial at the time of diagnosis, it soon develops into an infiltrating tumour if untreated [3]. Treatment and survival depend on tumor stage, although as this is very aggressive, most present with muscle invasive disease [3].

S. S. Goonewardene et al., *Management of Muscle Invasive Bladder Cancer*,
Management of Urology, https://doi.org/10.1007/978-3-030-57915-9_6

Jue investigated perioperative factors on overall survival treated with radical cystectomy with adenocarcinoma of the bladder [4]. The National Cancer Data Base was utilized to identify patients diagnosed with muscle-invasive bladder cancer (cT2–4, N0, M0) from 2004 to 2013. Variant histology bladder cancers (adenocarcinoma) were compared to urothelial carcinoma regarding overall survival. Significant predictors of worse overall survival included: African-American ancestry (aHR = 1.24, 95% CI: 1.03–1.48, p = 0.021), age (1.03, 1.02–1.03, p < 0.001), comorbidity (1.30, 1.20–1.40, p < 0.001), cT3 stage (1.41, 1.26–1.57, p < 0.001), and cT4 stage (1.59, 1.38–1.84, p < 0.001). Non-mucinous adenocarcinoma (1.15–2.20, p = 0.005) was a significant predictor of worse overall survival compared to urothelial carcinoma [4]. This re-enforces the prior studies above.

Palmero Marti report six cases with mucinous adenocarcinoma of the bladder [2]. One case had a radical cystectomy, the other had TURBT (superficial disease). Only one survived, who did not have muscle invasive disease [2]. These findings show the discouraging results of this entity closely intertwined with the pathologic stage.

Primary Bladder Adenocarcinoma is a rare malignancy that has been observed in a heterogeneous patient population [5]. Uhlig presents muscle invasive adenocarcinoma at diagnosis [5]. After transurethral resection and cystectomy with an orthotopic neobladder and adjuvant radiochemotherapy was conducted [5]. Twenty-four months later, a symptomatic fistula between neobladder and ileoileal anastomosis was excised, resulting in urinary incontinence [5]. This patient had no recurrence but had issues with small bladder capacity. This highlights a good outcome from muscle invasive adenocarcinoma, although this is rare [5].

6.2   CEA and CA 19-9 in Diagnostics in Muscle Invasive Adenocarcinoma of the Bladder

Iwaki report a case of primary adenocarcinoma of the bladder producing carcinoembryonic antigen (CEA) and carbohydrate antigen 19-9 (CA19-9) [6]. The initial presentation was with gross hematuria. CT demonstrated a mass on the urinary bladder and locally invasive disease. CEA and CA19-9 levels were increased to 8.9 ng/ml (normal <2.5) and 870 U/ml (normal <37), respectively [6]. Radical cystectomy and bilateral cutaneous ureterostomy were performed. Pathology demonstrated a well-differentiated adenocarcinoma with invasion through the entire muscle layer [6]. Postoperatively, the serum CEA and CA19-9 levels decreased to 5.4 ng/ml and 53 U/ml, respectively, and both CEA and CA19-9 were detected by immunohistochemical examination of the tumor [6]. This highlights a potential role for CEA and CA 19-9 in diagnostics of histological variants.

6.3   Muscle Invasive Adenocarcinoma of the Bladder Mimicking a Ureterocoele

Yenilmez reported a case of adenocarcinoma of the urinary bladder. This presented like a simple ureterocele with irritative bladder symptoms [7]. An IVU demonstrated a dilated left distal ureter resembling a cobra-head appearance [7]. Cystoscopy revealed abnormal mucosa in that distal portion [7]. Transurethral biopsy revealed a muscle-invasive adenocarcinoma [7]. There were no metastatic lesions on computed tomography. The patient underwent radical cystectomy and urinary diversion successfully [7].

6.4   Partial Cystectomy and Radiotherapy in Adenocarcinoma of the Bladder

Nocks reviewed 17 patients with adenocarcinoma of the urinary bladder [8]. Five patients had urachal adenocarcinoma; 8 pure adenocarcinoma; 4 mixed adenocarcinoma and transitional cell carcinoma [8]. Twelve of 17 patients (71%) had muscle invasion (T2–T3). There were no cases with regional or distant metastases at initial presentation. Treatment used included: transurethral resection in 3 patients; radical cystectomy in 4; simple cystectomy in 2; salvage radical cystectomy in 1; and partial cystectomy in 7 (3 of whom also received radiotherapy) [8]. Three and 5-year survival rates were 60% and 27%, respectively [8]. Five of 8 patients who died had evidence of metastatic disease. Only 1 patient with muscle invasive disease was alive more than 5 years [8]. However, 2 of 3 patients with invasive urachal adenocarcinoma who had preoperative radiotherapy plus partial cystectomy are free of disease at 38 and 60 months [8].

6.5   Neoadjuvant Chemotherapy in Bladder Adenocarcinoma

Neoadjuvant chemotherapy is of unknown benefit in adenocarcinoma of the bladder [9]. Vetterlein assessed neoadjuvant chemotherapy on non-organ-confined disease and overall survival after radical cystectomy (RC) in adenocarcinoma of the bladder [9]. Patients with adenocarcinoma (OR, 0.24; 95% CI, 0.06–0.91 [p = 0.035]) were more likely to have organ confined disease at the time of RC when treated with neoadjuvant chemotherapy [9]. However, a statistically significant overall survival benefit was not demonstrated due to aggressive tumour behaviour [9].

6.6   Adjuvant Therapy in Adenocarcinoma of the Bladder

Regarding variant histology, it is unknown whether adjuvant therapy (AC) works post radical cystectomy (RC) [10]. Berg assessed the effect of AC on overall survival (OS) [10]. The objective of this study was pure urothelial carcinoma, urothelial carcinoma with concomitant variant histology, or another pure variant histology [10]. Within the National Cancer Data Base, 15,397 patients who underwent RC for nonmetastatic, localized carcinoma with positive lymph nodes (T2N+) or locally advanced stage (≥T3N0/N+) were identified, excluding prior neoadjuvant chemotherapy [10]. In multivariable landmark analyses, AC compared with initial observation was associated with an OS benefit for pure urothelial carcinoma (hazard ratio, 0.87; 95% confidence interval, 0.82–0.91). There was no significant difference for those with variant histology [10].

6.7   Novel Chemotherapeutic Agents for Metastatic Adenocarcinoma of the Bladder

Teo et al. highlighted initial presentation of adenocarcinoma of the bladder with intermittent macroscopic haematuria, chronic left-sided hydronephrosis and intestinal metaplasia of the bladder [11]. Cystoscopy revealed a mass at the dome, which was resected [11]. Pathology confirmed muscle-invasive adenocarcinoma [11]. Radical cystectomy was initially planned, but subsequent CT confirmed metastatic disease. Due to histologic similarity between this patient's tumor and colorectal cancer, palliative FOLFOX6 (folinic acid, 5-fluorouracil and oxaliplatin) chemotherapy plus bevacizumab was administered [11]. After 3 months of treatment a good response was attained, which was sustained for more than 10 months after initial diagnosis [11].

6.8   Systematic Reviews Related: Lymphadenectomy in Adenocarcinoma of the Bladder

Crozier explored the impact of lymphadenectomy in non-urothelial bladder cancer [12]. Practice of lymphadenectomy in combination with partial or radical cystectomy when treating variant histology is common [12]. Pelvic recurrence following radical or partial cystectomy was more commonly reported in non-lymphadenectomy cohorts. The exception to this observation was the adenocarcinoma cohort [12]. Current evidence supporting lymphadenectomy in the surgical management of bladder cancer is largely based on studies limited to urothelial cancer [12]. Despite this, the practice of lymphadenectomy in non-urothelial cancer is common. However, due to the aggressiveness of adenocarcinoma, lymphadenectomy is often conducted as standard practice.

References

1. Klaile Y, Schlack K, Boegemann M, Steinestel J, Schrader AJ, Krabbe LM. Variant histology in bladder cancer: how it should change the management in non-muscle invasive and muscle invasive disease? Transl Androl Urol. 2016;5(5):692–701.
2. Palmero Martí JL, Queipo Zaragozá JA, Bonillo García MA, Budía Alba A, Vera Sempere FJ, Jiménez Cruz JF. Mucinous adenocarcinoma of the bladder. Actas Urol Esp. 2003;27(4):274–80.
3. Martínez-Piñeiro L, González-Peramato P, Hidalgo L, de la Peña J, Cisneros J, Cozar JM, Martínez-Piñeiro JA. Primary bladder adenocarcinoma: retrospective study of 11 cases and general review. Arch Esp Urol. 1991;44(2):131–8.
4. Jue JS, Koru-Sengul T, Moore KJ, Miao F, Alameddine M, Nahar B, Punnen S, Parekh DJ, Ritch CR, Gonzalgo ML. Sociodemographic and survival disparities for histologic variants of bladder cancer. Can J Urol. 2018;25(1):9179–85.
5. Uhlig A, Behnes CL, Strauss A, Trojan L, Uhlig J, Leitsmann C. Primary bladder adenocarcinoma: case report with long-term follow-up. Urol Case Rep. 2018;18:64–6.
6. Iwaki H, Omatsu S, Konishi T, Moritani S. Adenocarcinoma of the bladder producing carcinoembryonic antigen and carbohydrate antigen 19-9: report of a case. Hinyokika Kiyo. 1997;43(5):355–8.
7. Yenilmez A, Donmez T, Acikalin MF, Kale M. Adenonocarcinoma of the urinary bladder mimicking simple ureterocele: a case report. Int Urol Nephrol. 2007;39(2):465–6.
8. Nocks BN, Heney NM, Daly JJ. Primary adenocarcinoma of urinary bladder. Urology. 1983;21(1):26–9.
9. Vetterlein MW, Wankowicz SAM, Seisen T, Lander R, Löppenberg B, Chun FK, Menon M, Sun M, Barletta JA, Choueiri TK, Bellmunt J, Trinh QD, Preston MA. Neoadjuvant chemotherapy prior to radical cystectomy for muscle-invasive bladder cancer with variant histology. Cancer. 2017;123(22):4346–55.
10. Berg S, D'Andrea D, Vetterlein MW, Cole AP, Fletcher SA, Krimphove MJ, Marchese M, Lipsitz SR, Sonpavde G, Noldus J, Shariat SF, Kibel AS, Trinh QD, Mossanen M. Impact of adjuvant chemotherapy in patients with adverse features and variant histology at radical cystectomy for muscle-invasive carcinoma of the bladder: does histologic subtype matter? Cancer. 2019;125(9):1449–58.
11. Teo M, Swan NC, McDermott RS. Sustained response of adenocarcinoma of the urinary bladder to FOLFOX plus bevacizumab. Nat Rev Urol. 2011;8(5):282–5.
12. Crozier J, Demkiw S, Lawrentschuk N. Utility of lymphadenectomy following cystectomy for non-urothelial bladder cancer: a systematic review. Minerva Urol Nefrol. 2016;68(2):185–91.

Histological Variants in Muscle Invasive Bladder Cancer: Sarcomatoid Cancer

7

Invasive urothelial carcinoma, can have for divergent differentiation [1]. Several 'variant' types are classified in the 2004 World Health Organization Classification [1]. These histological variants have a significant diagnostic and therapeutic impact. Insight into how aggressive these can be of are central to understanding pathology of disease. This enhances prognosis prediction. Often, specific therapies used in urothelial carcinoma are used in this group, but with worse outcomes [1]. Especially therapeutic protocols and outcomes are completely different with Sarcomatoid bladder cancer.

7.1 Causes of Sarcomatoid Bladder Cancer

Sarcomatoid urothelial bladder cancer (SARC) often presents with distant metastasis and is associated with short survival [2]. Guo conducted a genomic analysis of 28 cases of SARC and 84 cases of standard urothelial carcinoma (UC) [2]. SARCs demonstrated precise genome mapping, with enrichment of TP53, RB1, and PIK3CA mutations [2]. They are related to the basal molecular subtype of conventional UCs. They are divided into epithelial-basal and more aggressive mesenchymal subsets based on TP63 expression [2]. SARCs are driven by downregulation of homotypic adherence genes and dysregulation of the EMT network [2]. This is demonstrated within an infiltrated phenotype. This has significant impact for therapeutic targets.

Sanfrancesco et al. [3] examined immunohistochemical markers in sarcomatoid UCa, including epithelial-to-mesenchymal transition in 28 cases [3]. The histopathology demonstrated spindled, myxoid, pseudoangiosarcomatous, and malignant fibrous histiocytoma-like undifferentiated features [3]. The sarcomatoid component was immunoreactive for pancytokeratin (22 of 26; 85%), p63 (20 of 26; 77%), cytokeratin 903 (17 of 26; 65%), cytokeratin 7 (16 of 26; 62%), GATA3 (16 of 26; 62%),

S. S. Goonewardene et al., *Management of Muscle Invasive Bladder Cancer*, Management of Urology, https://doi.org/10.1007/978-3-030-57915-9_7

and cytokeratin 5/6 (16 of 26; 62%). Smooth muscle actin demonstrated focal immunoreactivity (22 of 26; 85%) [3]. Epithelial-to-mesenchymal transition markers were frequently expressed, including vimentin (26 of 26; 100%), FoxC2 (26 of 26; 100%), SNAIL (23 of 26; 88.5%), and ZEB1 (18 of 26; 69.2%) [3]. Sixteen of 28 patients (57%) died of disease (overall mean survival, 9.1 months). The presence of myxoid or chordoid features was associated with worse outcomes and decreased survival (p < 0.05) [3].

7.2   Diagnostics in Sarcomatoid Bladder Cancer

Sarcomatoid carcinoma is an extremely rare aggressive tumor variant comprising about 0.3% of all primary tumours of the urinary bladder and carries an overall dismal prognosis [4]. Immunohistochemistry plays an important role in establishing diagnosis. Daga demonstrated patients can present with obstructive voiding symptoms, intermittent haematuria and a bladder mass [4]. MRI was used in diagnosis [4]. Patients were treated with transurethral resection. Histopathology demonstrated pT1 high-grade malignant spindle cell tumour [4]. A radical cystoprostatectomy with bilateral extended pelvic lymphadenectomy with ileal conduit was conducted [4]. After cystectomy, histopathology revealed high-grade muscle invasive spindle cell tumor [4].

Wang reported an unusual case of high-grade bladder cancer in a paediatric case who complained of painless haematuria and urinary frequency [5]. The tumour displayed sarcomatoid differentiation with aggressive behaviour, requiring adjuvant chemotherapy [5]. However, the disease advanced, resulting in survival only 6 months after surgery [5]. Paediatric bladder cancers are normally low-grade and presenting early. In contrast sarcomatoid differentiation with a high-grade urothelial carcinoma leads to a poor prognosis [5]. Frank haematuria in pediatric cases, must be thoroughly investigated [5]. Urothelial neoplasia management in young patients should be based on grade and stage as opposed to age of the patient [5].

7.3   Clinicopathological and Immunohistochemical Diagnosis of Sarcomatoid Bladder Cancer

Terada examined the histopathology and immunohistochemical diagnosis of sarcomatoid bladder cancer [6]. Histologically, the tumor was composed of malignant round cells with hyperchromatic nuclei [6]. Many intracytoplasmic vacuoles were present [6]. Immunohistochemically, the tumor cells were positive for cytokeratin (CK) 18, vimentin, p53 and Ki-67 (labeling 80%) [6]. Because the CK18 was diffusely expressed, the pathological diagnosis was sarcomatoid carcinoma [6].

Jones reviewed 25 sarcomatoid carcinomas of the urinary bladder [7]. On cystoscopy, the appearance can vary from a large polypoid mas, an intramural mass with bladder wall thickening with necrosis and ulceration. Microscopy demonstrated a tapering spindle cells and cohesive non-spindled cells [7]. Twenty-two cases had an invasive overtly epithelial carcinomatous component. In situ transitional carcinoma was present in 12 cases. Myxoid change, ranging from extensive to focal, separating the spindle cells was present [7]. The spindle cells were immunoreactive for cytokeratin (12 of 19), vimentin (16 of 17), carcinoembryonic antigen (3 of 15) and muscle-specific actin (4 of 16) [7]. The epithelioid carcinomatous areas were highlighted by the cytokeratin immunostain. These features distinguish this tumour from reactive of neoplastic mesenchymal lesions [7].

Daga has previously examined immunohistochemistry in a single case report [4]. The diagnosis was uncertain and two differential diagnosis were kept, sarcomatoid carcinoma and pleomorphic sarcoma [4]. Sarcomatoid carcinoma as it was positive for cytokeratin, CK-8/18, GATA 3. All lymph nodes were negative for metastasis (pT2, N0, Mx) [4]. Early recognition, with immunohistochemistry is key to early diagnosis and management in histochemical analysis.

7.4 Survival Outcomes with Radical Cystectomy and Sarcomatoid Carcinoma

A patient was diagnosed with muscle invasive sarcomatous and carcinomatous elements [8]. Immunohistochemical examination showed that the sarcomatous component did not stain for S-100 protein or for smooth muscle actin but it stained for epithelial markers [8]. Under the diagnosis of sarcomatoid carcinoma, we performed a total cystectomy and ileal conduit without chemotherapy or radiation. A follow-up CT taken at 4 months postoperatively showed no evidence of recurrence [8].

7.5 Adjuvant Chemotherapy in Sarcomatoid Bladder Cancer

The use of adjuvant chemotherapy (AC) in pure urothelial carcinoma of the bladder is established. Regarding variant histology, standard guidelines concerning the optimal treatment after radical cystectomy (RC) are unknown [9]. Berg examined the role of adjuvant therapy in sarcomatoid differentiation [9]. AC compared with initial observation was associated with an OS benefit in pure urothelial carcinoma (hazard ratio, 0.87; 95% confidence interval, 0.82–0.91). No differences in variant histology [9]. Multivariable Cox regression landmark analysis revealed a survival benefit from AC in pure urothelial carcinoma. However, a survival benefit of AC for variant histology or other pure variant histology was not demonstrated [9]. This demonstrates how therapies for urothelial cancer, may not necessarily give good outcomes in variant histology.

Tanuma reported a sarcomatoid tumour with an osteosarcoma element [10]. Abdominal computed tomography (CT) and magnetic resonance imaging revealed a 3 cm non-papillary bladder tumor with muscle invasion without calcification [10]. On TURBT and re-TURBT histologically, the non-papillary part was composed of sarcomatous elements including osteosarcoma, chondrosarcoma, and spindle cell sarcoma [10]. The papillary part was composed of high-grade urothelial carcinoma and spindle cell sarcoma. Muscularis propria was not present in the specimen [10]. Staging CT was negative and total cystectomy with an ileal conduit was performed [10]. The pathological findings were identical to those of the re-TURBT specimens, pTxN0 sarcomatoid urothelial carcinoma [10]. The patient received adjuvant chemotherapy with two courses of gemcitabine and cisplatin [10]. There was neither recurrence nor metastases during the 20-month follow-up [10].

References

1. Amin MB. Histological variants of urothelial carcinoma: diagnostic, therapeutic and prognostic implications. Mod Pathol. 2009;22(Suppl 2):S96–S118.
2. Guo CC, Majewski T, Zhang L, Yao H, Bondaruk J, Wang Y, Zhang S, Wang Z, Lee JG, Lee S, Cogdell D, Zhang M, Wei P, Grossman HB, Kamat A, Duplisea JJ, Ferguson JE III, Huang H, Dadhania V, Gao J, Dinney C, Weinstein JN, Baggerly K, McConkey D, Czerniak B. Dysregulation of EMT drives the progression to clinically aggressive sarcomatoid bladder cancer. Cell Rep. 2019;27(6):1781–1793.e4.
3. Sanfrancesco J, McKenney JK, Leivo MZ, Gupta S, Elson P, Hansel DE. Sarcomatoid urothelial carcinoma of the bladder: analysis of 28 cases with emphasis on clinicopathologic features and markers of epithelial-to-mesenchymal transition. Arch Pathol Lab Med. 2016;140(6):543–51.
4. Daga G, Kerkar P. Sarcomatoid carcinoma of urinary bladder: a case report. Indian J Surg Oncol. 2018;9(4):644–6.
5. Wang Z, Xiong W, Pan C, Zhu L, Wang X, Huang Z, Zhao X, Zhong Z. Aggressive muscle-invasive bladder cancer with sarcomatoid differentiation in a 10-year-old girl: a case report. Exp Ther Med. 2016;11(3):985–7.
6. Terada T. Sarcomatoid carcinoma in the pelvic cavity. Int J Clin Exp Pathol. 2013;6(4):795–7.
7. Jones EC, Young RH. Myxoid and sclerosing sarcomatoid transitional cell carcinoma of the urinary bladder: a clinicopathologic and immunohistochemical study of 25 cases. Mod Pathol. 1997;10(9):908–16.
8. Oka D, Noda Y, Takada S, Fujimoto N, Koide T, Yamazaki M, Kobayashi Y. Sarcomatoid carcinoma of the urinary bladder: a case report. Hinyokika Kiyo. 2002;48(6):375–7.
9. Berg S, D'Andrea D, Vetterlein MW, Cole AP, Fletcher SA, Krimphove MJ, Marchese M, Lipsitz SR, Sonpavde G, Noldus J, Shariat SF, Kibel AS, Trinh QD, Mossanen M. Impact of adjuvant chemotherapy in patients with adverse features and variant histology at radical cystectomy for muscle-invasive carcinoma of the bladder: does histologic subtype matter? Cancer. 2019;125(9):1449–58.
10. Tanuma K, Kawai K, Tsuchiya H, Matsumoto Y, Kandori S, Kojima T, Kimura T, Joraku A, Miyazaki J, Nishiyama H, Sakata A. Sarcomatoid urothelial carcinoma of the bladder including an osteosarcoma element. Hinyokika Kiyo. 2017;63(11):487–92.

Carcinosarcoma of the urinary bladder is <0.05% of urothelial tumours and is a biphasic malignant neoplasm [1]. Histologically, it demonstrates epithelial and mesenchymal differentiation with the presence or absence of heterologous elements [1]. It is present in adults after 60 years, and has a poor prognosis [1]. It is a tumour found more frequently in men than women, with an age range of 33–83 [2]. The prognosis is poor [2]. Seventy percent death rate within 2 years, but it seems to be improved by radical cystectomy and adjuvant therapy [2].

8.1 The Genetic Basis of Carcinosarcoma

Sarcomatoid urothelial carcinoma is a rare neoplasm. It has a biphasic morphology exhibiting both epithelial and sarcomatoid elements [3]. Pathology is uncertain, whether it arises from a single cancer stem cell with subsequent differentiation or two separate cancer stem cells is debatable [3]. To clarify its' clonal origin, the TP53 mutation status of a series of 17 sarcomatoid urothelial carcinomas was analysed using single-strand conformation polymorphism, DNA sequencing and p53 immunohistochemistry [3]. Five out of the 17 sarcomatoid urothelial carcinomas contained TP53 point mutations in exons 5 and 8 [3]. In all 5 cases, the TP53 point mutations were identical in both the epithelial and sarcomatoid components [3]. The sarcomatoid and epithelial tumour components in all 17 cases showed concordant p53 expression patterns [3]. This highlights, despite divergence at the phenotypic level, the sarcomatoid and carcinomatoid elements of this uncommon tumour share a common clonal origin [3].

Carcinosarcomas of the urinary bladder are malignant biphasic tumours with an epithelial and a spindle cell component [4]. The immunohistology revealed a poorly differentiated urothelial carcinoma (GIII) and a co-existing pleomorphic, spindle cell leiomyosarcoma (GIII) [4]. The two components were analysed for gains and

S. S. Goonewardene et al., *Management of Muscle Invasive Bladder Cancer*,
Management of Urology, https://doi.org/10.1007/978-3-030-57915-9_8

losses of chromosomal material using comparative genomic hybridization [4]. The tumour components revealed as overlapping core aberrations losses on the short arm of chromosome 9 and on the long arm of chromosome 11 [4]. However, both components showed additional aberrations exclusively detected in one of the components [4]. The occurrence of overlapping aberrations strongly argues for a monoclonal origin of this tumour with a common ancestor [4]. The additional aberrations of the components point to an independent and divergent course of tumour progression in both components [4].

8.2   Histopathology of Carcinosarcoma

Carcinosarcoma of the urinary bladder is rare with a poor prognosis [5]. The majority are not diagnosed until advanced [5]. Superficial carcinosarcoma has always invaded the lamina propria [5]. In addition to the carcinomatous degeneration of the mucosa, sarcomatous degeneration of the underlying submucosal stroma is also present [5]. Any local surgical treatment, such as TUR or partial cystectomy, involves the risk of incomplete tumour removal, because the sarcomatous elements typically invade the submucosa while the overlying mucosa remains intact [5]. Therefore, radical cystectomy appears to be the treatment of choice for both superficial and invasive carcinosarcoma of the urinary bladder [5].

Non-urothelial BC and variants of UC account for up to 25% of all BCs [6]. Further discrimination can be made into epithelial and non-epithelial non-UC [6]. Most of the non-UCs are of epithelial origin (approximately 90%) including squamous-cell carcinoma, adenocarcinoma and small-cell carcinoma [6]. Non-epithelial tumours are rare and include variants as sarcoma, carcinosarcoma, paraganglioma, melanoma and lymphoma [6]. Accordingly, aggressive behaviour and often advanced stages at primary presentation are frequently observed in non-UC arguing for radical and sometimes different treatment strategies as compared to pure UC [6].

The clinicopathologic, immunohistochemical, and ultrastructural features of eight cases were analysed [7]. Microscopically, the tumours consisted mostly of a varied mixture of high-grade transitional cell carcinoma with chondrosarcoma, osteosarcoma, rhabdomyosarcoma, and undifferentiated spindle cell (leiomyosarcoma-like) components with occasional transitional features between one component and another [7]. All tumours but one invaded the muscularis propria or the perivesical fatty tissue [7]. Immunohistochemically, keratin expression was observed focally in the sarcoma component as well as the carcinoma component [7]. Reactivity for vimentin, desmin, muscle specific actin, and S-100 protein were observed in poorly differentiated areas.

Haj Salah reviewed three male patients age 76–86 years were found to have polypoid masses in the urinary bladder [1]. In all cases, microscopic examination revealed biphasic neoplasms with distinct mesenchymal and epithelial components [1]. The two first cases were remarkable respectively by the presence of chondrosarcomatous and osteosarcomatous components [1].

A case of synchronically coexistent carcinosarcoma and transitional cell carcinoma was presented by González-Carreró et al. [8]. Carcinosarcoma was formed by an epithelial component represented by a high-level transitional cell carcinoma and a mesenchymal component characterized by an unspecific fusocellular sarcoma with chondrosarcomatous differentiation [8]. An immunohistochemical analysis was performed, confirming the dual nature of the carcinosarcoma [8].

By immunohistochemical examination, the carcinoma element and the sarcomatous element demonstrated positive immunoreaction for cytokeratin (CK), epithelial membrane antigen (EMA) and carcinoembryonic antigen [9]. Some sarcomatous elements expressed smooth muscle actin and muscle specific actin (MSA) and occasional epithelioid are as demonstrated a positive immunoreaction for desmin, MSA and myoglobin, indicating leiomyosarcomatous and rhabdomyosarcomatous differentiation, respectively [9]. Unexpectedly, tumour cells in the chondrosarcomatous element revealed a simultaneous positivity of CK and EMA as well as S-100 protein [9]. Both epithelial and sarcomatous elements showed an intensive positive immunoreaction for p53 and heat shock protein (HSP) 70 [9]. However, HSP27 and HSP60 were detected in most epithelial elements and only in a small number of tumour cells in the sarcomatous area [9]. These findings indicate that sarcomatous elements, including heterologous elements, may derive from epithelial elements with partial or complete loss of epithelial features, and different factors other than p53 and HSP70 may associate with the morphological alteration of carcinoma [9].

Histologic and immunohistochemical examinations were performed on bladder tumours from four patients [10]. Four patients (three men, one woman) age 54–77 years were found to have polypoid masses in the urinary bladder [10]. In all cases, histologic examination showed biphasic neoplasms with distinct mesenchymal and epithelial components [10]. One of the cases was remarkable for the presence of liposarcoma, malignant peripheral nerve sheath tumour, and micropapillary urothelial carcinoma [10]. Two of the patients died 2 years after diagnosis, which is consistent with the previously reported aggressive nature of urinary bladder carcinosarcomas [10]. Because of the aggressive biologic behaviour of these tumours, they should be identified promptly and treated appropriately [10].

A case of carcinosarcoma of the urinary bladder in a 2-year-old girl is reported [11]. The tumour, measuring $34 \times 20 \times 18$ mm, was located in the peri-trigone area of the urinary bladder with polypoid features [11]. Histologic examination revealed transitional cell carcinoma at the tumour surface with downward invasion [11]. Concurrently, a sarcomatous area was found beneath the carcinoma, with these two different malignant components sharing on apparent transition without distinct boundaries [11]. Sarcomatous components included immature round cells focally showing rhabdoid features [11]. No rhabdomyomatous component was observed. Immunohistochemistry disclosed vimentin and cytokeratin-double positive cells at the transposition between carcinoma and sarcomatous components [11]. In addition, ultrastructural analysis revealed that the epithelial cells had a distinct junctional complex, and the sarcomatous cells occasionally had a meshwork of cytoplasmic intermediate filaments, indicating bidirectional cytodifferentiation to epithelial and mesenchymal elements [11]. The extremely young age at which this case of carcinosarcoma occurred suggests that the tumour may be of mesodermal stem cell origin [11].

8.3   Clinical Presentation of Carcinosarcoma

A 74 year-old woman presented with a polypoid tumour of the bladder with haematuria [2]. On histology, this was carcinosarcoma with a weak epithelial composition. It was confirmed by immunolabelling with keratin demonstrating chondrosarcomatous material [2]. Six months later, the patient developed metastases in the kidney, in the paravertebral muscles, and in the right para-ureteral lymph nodes [2].

Li described carcinosarcoma of the urinary bladder with a large cell neuroendocrine epithelial component [12]. A 61-year-old man presented with gross haematuria and underwent resection of a biphasic bladder tumour [12]. The malignant epithelial component demonstrated large cell neuroendocrine differentiation with immunohistochemical reactivity for neurone specific enolase, synaptophysin, and chromogranin [12]. The malignant mesenchymal component did not demonstrated differentiation by histology or immunohistochemistry [12].

Urinary bladder sarcomatoid carcinoma (carcinosarcoma) is rare [13]. A total of 221 histology confirmed cases were identified between 1973 and 2004, this accounted for approximately 0.11% of all primary bladder tumours during the study period. Median age of the patients was 75 years (range 41–96) [13]. Of the patients with a known tumour stage (N = 204), 72.5% had a regional or distant stage; 98.4% of patients with known histology grade (N = 127), had poorly or undifferentiated histology [13]. Multiple primary tumours were identified in about 40% of study subjects.

8.4   Survival Outcomes

Carcinosarcoma (CS) of the bladder is a rare malignancy, highly aggressive with unfavourable prognosis [14]. There is little evidence on recurrence after definitive surgical therapy [14]. Urethral recurrence of CS after radical cystoprostatectomy can occur despite radical therapy [14].

Sarcomatoid carcinoma and carcinosarcoma of the bladder are rare tumours that contain epithelial and mesenchymal elements. These have a worse prognosis than conventional urothelial carcinoma [15]. Wright investigated the survival of patients with the two tumour subtypes compared to survival in those with urothelial carcinoma [15]. Overall unadjusted survival rates for urothelial carcinoma, sarcomatoid carcinoma and carcinosarcoma were 77%, 54% and 48% at 1 year, and 47%, 37% and 17% at 5 years, respectively [15]. Sarcomatoid carcinoma and carcinosarcoma presented at a similar age but with a higher T stage and with more frequent regional and distant metastases compared to urothelial carcinoma [15]. On multivariate analysis sarcomatoid carcinoma (HR 1.18, 95% CI 0.91–1.52) and carcinosarcoma (HR 2.00, 95% CI 1.65–2.41) were at higher risk for death compared to those with urothelial carcinoma [15]. Overall mortality was worse with carcinosarcoma than with sarcomatoid carcinoma (HR 1.70, 95% CI 1.23–2.34) [15].

8.5 Surgical Treatment for Carcinosarcoma

Sanchez Bernal presented a new case of carcinosarcoma of the bladder [16]. This tumour is generally considered to be a rare one, has an uncertain aetiology and very poor prognosis, composed by mesenchymal and epithelial elements [16]. It is an aggressive tumour with a short clinical course [16]. At present radical cystectomy is the treatment of choice [16].

Hara reported a case of carcinosarcoma arising from a bladder diverticulum [17]. A 71-year-old male was referred to our hospital for macroscopic haematuria [17]. Two diverticula were identified in the left wall of the urinary bladder, one of which showed a broad-based tumour [17]. The bladder tumour was resected using a transurethral approach and the tumour was histologically diagnosed as leiomyosarcoma [17]. The patient underwent partial resection of the bladder including the two diverticula and the tumour [17]. Pathological examination revealed that the resected specimen was composed of three elements, transitional cell carcinoma (G3), squamous cell carcinoma, and leiomyosarcoma [17]. He died 5 months after surgery to remove the panperitonitis carcinomatosa [17]. This suggests partial resection may not be an option in this group of patients.

This was again confirmed by Nuwahid et al. [18]. A 47-year-old man presented with hematuria and dysuria [18]. He was found to have a carcinosarcoma originating from a bladder diverticulum. He underwent a partial cystectomy and received postoperative chemotherapy [18]. One year later, he presented with a large local recurrence and died shortly afterward [18].

8.6 Adjuvant Therapy in Carcinosarcoma

Carcinosarcoma of the bladder is a rare neoplasm characterized by carcinoma and malignant soft tissue neoplasm [19]. Treatment included cystectomy in 11 patients with (4) and without (7) radiation therapy, and transurethral resection in 4 with (1) and without (3) radiation therapy [19]. A total of 11 patients died of cancer at 1–48 months (mean 17.2) and 2 survived for 8–131 months [19]. Other treatment included transurethral resection in 17 patients with (7) and without (10) radiation therapy, including 1 who also received chemotherapy, and only cystectomy in 5, including 2 who also underwent radiation therapy and 1 who also received chemotherapy [19]. Mean follow-up available in 21 cases was 49 months (range 1–420). A total of 17 patients died of cancer at 1–73 months (mean 9.8), 1 was alive at 140 months and 3 died of unrelated causes.

Wang et al. reviewed the impact of adjuvant radiotherapy in combination with surgery [13]. The majority of patients (95.9%) received cancer directed surgery, 35.8% had radical or partial cystectomy, 15.8% of patients received radiation therapy combination with surgery [13]. The median overall survival was 14 months (95% CI 7–21 months). 1-, 5-, and 10-year cancer specific survival rate were 53.9%, 28.4% and 25.8% [13]. In a multivariate analysis, only tumour stage was found to be a significant prognostic factor for disease-specific survival [13]. Urinary bladder carcinosarcoma commonly presented as high grade, advanced stage and aggressive behaviour with a poor prognosis [13]. Emphasis on early detection, including identification of risk factors is needed to improve the outcome for patients with this malignancy [13].

Damiano presented a 73-year-old man with a history of transitional cell carcinoma of the bladder, an ulcerated mass on the left hemitrigone and left hydronephrosis who underwent radical cystoprostatectomy and urinary diversion followed by cisplatin-gemcitabine chemotherapy [20]. At 24 months of follow-up the patient is alive and free from recurrent disease, with good quality of life and preserved renal function [20]. Among all the studied prognostic factors, pathological stage is the main predictor of survival [20]. The outcome of our patient suggests that the relatively well tolerated gemcitabine-cisplatin regimen after surgical treatment of invasive carcinosarcoma of the bladder might improve the currently dismal prognosis of selected elderly patients [20].

Bladder carcinosarcoma commonly presents as high-grade, advanced stage, and aggressive behaviour with a poor prognosis [21]. An 83-year-old male presented with painless gross haematuria [21]. Cystoscopy revealed massive non-papillary bladder tumour on the right wall [21]. The 91 g tumour could be completely removed with transurethral resection [21]. Histology of the tumour was diagnosed as carcinosarcoma with no submucosal invasion composed of biphasic malignant epithelial and mesenchymal cells [21]. Epithelial malignancy was urothelial cancer and mesenchymal one was chondrosarcoma and leiomyosarcoma [21]. The specimens taken at the second-look TURBT revealed that carcinoma in situ (urothelial cancer) but not sarcoma existed at the mucosa surrounding the previous tumor site [21]. Eighty milligram of BCG instillation intravesically every week for 6 weeks was successfully administered to the patient [21]. There was no tumour recurrence for 6 months after treatments.

8.7   Neoadjuvant Chemotherapy in Carcinosarcoma

Patient with carcinosarcoma usually present with a high stage malignancy [22]. Cystectomy or transurethral resection is the preferred treatment, often followed by radiation therapy, although prognosis is very bad [22]. Hoshi, reported a case of carcinosarcoma of bladder obtained pathologically complete response by neoadjuvant chemoradiotherapy [22]. There was no evidence of disease 30 months after the operation [22].

References

1. Haj Salah MB, Mekni A, Nouira Y, Haha-Bellil SB, Bellil K, Kchir N, Haouet S, Horchani A, Zitouna M. Carcinosarcoma of the urinary bladder. Report of three cases. Tunis Med. 2007;85(11):982–4.
2. Jlidi R, Remadi S, Gloor J, Chatelanat F. Carcinosarcoma of the urinary bladder and renal metastasis. Ann Pathol. 1991;11(1):42–6.
3. Armstrong AB, Wang M, Eble JN, MacLennan GT, Montironi R, Tan PH, Lopez-Beltran A, Zhang S, Baldridge LA, Spartz H, Cheng L. TP53 mutational analysis supports monoclonal origin of biphasic sarcomatoid urothelial carcinoma (carcinosarcoma) of the urinary bladder. Mod Pathol. 2009;22(1):113–8.
4. Gronau S, Menz CK, Melzner I, Hautmann R, Möller P, Barth TF. Immunohistomorphologic and molecular cytogenetic analysis of a carcinosarcoma of the urinary bladder. Virchows Arch. 2002;440(4):436–40.
5. Kuntz RM, Geyer V, Savvas V, Grosse G. Carcinosarcoma of the urinary bladder. Urologe A. 1993;32(1):59–63.
6. Klaile Y, Schlack K, Boegemann M, Steinestel J, Schrader AJ, Krabbe LM. Variant histology in bladder cancer: how it should change the management in non-muscle invasive and muscle invasive disease? Transl Androl Urol. 2016;5(5):692–701.
7. Perret L, Chaubert P, Hessler D, Guillou L. Primary heterologous carcinosarcoma (metaplastic carcinoma) of the urinary bladder: a clinicopathologic, immunohistochemical, and ultrastructural analysis of eight cases and a review of the literature. Cancer. 1998;82(8):1535–49.
8. González-Carreró J, Nogueira March JL, Ojea A, Figueiredo L, Jamardo D, Guate JL, Cunqueiro R. Carcinosarcoma and papillary transitional cell carcinoma coexisting in the same bladder. Actas Urol Esp. 1990;14(4):286–8.
9. Kamishima T, Fukuda T, Usuda H, Takato H, Iwamoto H, Kaneko H. Carcinosarcoma of the urinary bladder: expression of epithelial markers and different expression of heat shock proteins between epithelial and sarcomatous elements. Pathol Int. 1997;47(2–3):166–73.
10. Baschinsky DY, Chen JH, Vadmal MS, Lucas JG, Bahnson RR, Niemann TH. Carcinosarcoma of the urinary bladder—an aggressive tumor with diverse histogenesis. A clinicopathologic study of 4 cases and review of the literature. Arch Pathol Lab Med. 2000;124(8):1172–8.
11. Inagaki T, Nagata M, Kaneko M, Amagai T, Iwakawa M, Watanabe T. Carcinosarcoma with rhabdoid features of the urinary bladder in a 2-year-old girl: possible histogenesis of stem cell origin. Pathol Int. 2000;50(12):973–8.
12. Li Y, Outman JE, Mathur SC. Carcinosarcoma with a large cell neuroendocrine epithelial component: first report of an unusual biphasic tumour of the urinary bladder. J Clin Pathol. 2004;57(3):318–20.
13. Wang J, Wang FW, Lagrange CA, Hemstreet GP III, Kessinger A. Clinical features of sarcomatoid carcinoma (carcinosarcoma) of the urinary bladder: analysis of 221 cases. Sarcoma. 2010;2010:454792.
14. Bivalacqua TJ, Bagga HS, Patil K, Magheli A, Taube JM, Guzzo TJ, Gonzalgo ML. Urethral carcinosarcoma from bladder carcinosarcomatous lesions: analysis of clinicopathological features. Can J Urol. 2009;16(1):4512–5.
15. Wright JL, Black PC, Brown GA, Porter MP, Kamat AM, Dinney CP, Lin DW. Differences in survival among patients with sarcomatoid carcinoma, carcinosarcoma and urothelial carcinoma of the bladder. J Urol. 2007;178(6):2302–6.
16. Sánchez Bernal C, Báez Perea JM, Bachiller Burgos J, Soto Delgado M, Juárez Soto A, Beltrán Aguilar V. Bladder carcinosarcoma: case report with immunohistologic study. Actas Urol Esp. 1998;22(7):557–60.
17. Hara S, Miyazaki S, Yamazaki T, Hara I, Fujisawa M, Gohji K, Okada H, Arakawa S, Kamidono S, Hanioka K. A case of true carcinosarcoma in bladder diverticulum. Hinyokika Kiyo. 1999;45(4):265–8.

18. Nuwahid F, German K, Campbell F, Stephenson T. Carcinosarcoma in a bladder diverticulum. Urology. 1994;44(5):775–8.
19. Lopez-Beltran A, Pacelli A, Rothenberg HJ, Wollan PC, Zincke H, Blute ML, Bostwick DG. Carcinosarcoma and sarcomatoid carcinoma of the bladder: clinicopathological study of 41 cases. J Urol. 1998;159(5):1497–503.
20. Damiano R, D'Armiento M, Cantiello F, Amorosi A, Tagliaferri P, Sacco R, Venuta S. Gemcitabine and cisplatin following surgical treatment of urinary bladder carcinosarcoma. Tumori. 2004;90(5):458–60.
21. Zaitsu M, Yamanoi M, Mikami K, Tonooka A, Uekusa T, Takeuchi T. A case of giant bladder carcinosarcoma without submucosal invasion. Case Rep Med. 2011;2011:349518.
22. Hoshi S, Sasaki M, Muto A, Suzuki K, Kobayashi T, Tukigi M, Ono K, Sugano O, Saso S. Case of carcinosarcoma of urinary bladder obtained a pathologically complete response by neoadjuvant chemoradiotherapy. Int J Urol. 2007;14(1):79–81.

Muscle Invasive Bladder Cancer: Small Cell

9

9.1   Neuroendocrine Markers in Small Cell Bladder Cancer

Most SmCCs expressed neuroendocrine markers synaptophysin (41/56), chromogranin (26/55), and CD56 (39/41) [1]. Some SmCCs showed focal expression of CK5/6 (9/25), a marker for the basal molecular subtype [1]. Expression of the retinoblastoma 1 (RB1) gene protein was lost in most bladder SmCCs (2/23) [1]. The patients' survival was significantly associated with cancer stage, but with no significant difference between mixed and pure SmCCs [1]. In this study SmCC had a worse prognosis, when compared with conventional UC but only with metastatic disease [1]. A fraction of SmCCs show a basal molecular subtype, which highlights its good response to chemotherapy [1]. Inactivation of the RB1 gene may be implicated in the oncogenesis of bladder SmCC [1].

9.2   Cytological and Immunological Analyses in Small Cell Bladder Carcinoma

The incidence of primary small cell carcinoma (SCC) is extremely rare [2]. Sharma analysed cytological and immunophenotypic features of SCC in urine [2]. On cytologic and histopathologic examination, typical SCC morphology was present [2]. On immunohistochemistry, synaptophysin and CD56 were positive, while chromogranin was positive in only 50% [2]. The Ki-67 labelling index ranged from 30% to 100% [2]. SCC should be kept in the differential diagnosis, when high-grade urothelial carcinoma is suspected in a urine cytology specimen, as this distinction has important therapeutic and prognostic implications [2].

Van Hoeven reviewed urinary cytology specimens with histologically proven tumours [3]. In four tumours, small cell carcinoma was the sole malignant cellular

© The Editor(s) (if applicable) and The Author(s), under exclusive license to Springer Nature Switzerland AG 2021
S. S. Goonewardene et al., *Management of Muscle Invasive Bladder Cancer*, Management of Urology, https://doi.org/10.1007/978-3-030-57915-9_9

component: all 11 urinary specimens harboured cells with features of an undifferentiated small cell carcinoma [3]. In the remaining nine tumours, small cell carcinoma appeared with transitional, squamous cell or adenocarcinoma, but in four, small cell carcinoma was the sole invasive component [3]. Almost one third of urinary specimens in this group lacked a small cell component. Neuroendocrine differentiation was confirmed by immunopathology in 11 cases (neuron specific enolase positive in 11 of 12, synaptophysin in 2/11, chromogranin in 2/13, Leu 7 in 2/7), and by ultrastructural analysis in 2 [3]. Small cell carcinoma is a cytologically recognizable variant of bladder cancer, but admixture with other malignant components may mask its appearance in urinary specimens [3].

9.3   Survival Outcomes

Small cell carcinomas of the bladder (SCCB) account for fewer than 1% of all urinary bladder tumours. There is no consensus regarding the optimal treatment for SCCB [4]. The study included 107 patients (mean [±standard deviation, SD] age, 69.6 [±10.6] years; mean follow-up time, 4.4 years) with primary bladder SCC, with 66% of these patients having pure SCC [4]. Seventy-two percent and 12% of the patients presented with T2-4N0M0 and T2-4N1-3M0 stages, respectively, and 16% presented with synchronous metastases [4]. The most frequent curative treatments were radical surgery and chemotherapy, sequential chemotherapy and radiation therapy, and radical surgery alone [4]. The median (interquartile range, IQR) OS and DFS times were 12.9 months (IQR, 7–32 months) and 9 months (IQR, 5–23 months), respectively. The metastatic, T2-4N0M0, and T2-4N1-3M0 groups differed significantly ($p = 0.001$) in terms of median OS and DFS [4]. In a multivariate analysis, impaired creatinine clearance (OS and DFS), clinical stage (OS and DFS), a Karnofsky performance status <80 (OS), and pure SCC histology (OS) were independent and significant adverse prognostic factors [4]. In the patients with nonmetastatic disease, the type of treatment (i.e. radical surgery with or without adjuvant chemotherapy vs. conservative treatment) did not significantly influence OS or DFS ($p = 0.7$) [4].

9.4   Prognostic Factors in Diagnosis of Small Cell Bladder Cancer

No prognostic factor has been established in small cell bladder cancer [5]. Naito reviewed 31 patients with primary SCCB [5]. The association of various clinicopathological, such as the serum NSE value, with cancer-specific survival (CSS) were assessed [5]. Nineteen (61.3%) died of SCCB during the follow-up, with a median survival time of 12.7 months [5]. Univariate analysis demonstrated that stage (extensive disease) and serum NSE ≥25 ng/ml were significantly associated with worse CSS [5]. Multivariate analysis identified increased serum NSE value as a sole independent predictor of CSS (hazard ratio 18.52, p = 0.0022) [5].

GATA3 is a sensitive marker for urothelial carcinoma [6]. Nuclear GATA3 expression was encountered in 7 bladder (7/22, 32%) and 2 lung (2/15, 13%) small cell carcinomas [6]. Among bladder tumours, strong and diffuse (>75%) GATA3 labelling was seen in 3 cases (3/22, 14%); focal positivity was observed in the 4 remaining cases (4/22, 18%) [6]. The novel finding of GATA3 positivity in one-third of bladder small cell carcinoma is of potential value in differentiating small cell carcinomas of prostate origin from those of bladder origin [6].

The predictive factors of prognosis and treatment for small-cell carcinoma (SCC) are controversial [7]. Chang collected data of patients who were diagnosed with genitourinary SCC (GSCC) [7]. Primary tumour resection was attempted in 13 of 18 patients (72.2%). Radical surgery was performed in 6 of 14 (42.9%) limited disease patients [7]. Most of the patients (13, 72.2%) received cisplatin-based chemotherapy. Patients who had normal lactic dehydrogenase (LDH) levels showed a significantly higher median PFS and overall survival (OS) compared with patients with high LDH levels (p = 0.030, p = 0.010) [7]. Patients with limited disease treated with a radical operation experienced a non-significant (p = 0.211) longer PFS compared with patients who were not treated, but this reached statistical significance after analyzing OS (p = 0.211, p = 0.039) [7]. Serum LDH levels beyond the normal range indicate a poor prognosis [7]. For GSCC patients who are diagnosed with limited disease, radical surgery is strongly recommended along with cisplatin-based chemotherapy [7].

9.5   Clinical Presentation of Small Cell Bladder Cancer

Li presents a case of an 87-year-old man who presented with haematuria and was found to have an ill-defined mass in the urinary bladder on computed tomography and cystoscopic examination [8]. On pathological examination following tumour biopsy, the mucosa of the bladder wall was found to be extensively infiltrated by neuroendocrine carcinoma, positive for CD56 and synaptophysin and negative for epithelial membrane antigen, consistent with SCNEC of the urinary bladder [8]. The patient refused further surgical treatment and succumbed to the disease 2 months after the diagnosis [8].

Small cell carcinoma (SmCC) of the bladder is a rare disease. Wang studied a large series of bladder SmCC from a single institution [1]. The patients included 69 men and 12 women with a mean age of 68 years [1]. Most bladder SmCCs were presented at advanced stage, with tumours invading the muscularis propria and beyond (n = 77) [1]. SmCC was pure in 27 cases and mixed with other histologic types in 54 cases, including urothelial carcinoma (UC) (n = 32), UC in situ (n = 26), glandular (n = 14), micropapillary (n = 4), sarcomatoid (n = 4), squamous (n = 3), and plasmacytoid (n = 1) features [1].

9.6   Surgical Outcomes

Small cell carcinoma of the bladder has a low incidence and poor survival. Due to the paucity of evidence, algorithms based on randomized trials are unavailable [9]. Pesquera-Ortega, conducted an observational retrospective study of ten patients diagnosed with small cell carcinoma [9]. Four cases presented high-grade papillary urothelial carcinoma with small cell carcinoma [9]. Radical cystectomy was performed in 40% patients, in combination with chemotherapy, radiotherapy or both [9]. Median survival was 330 days (IC 95%: 40.757–619.243). One patient showed complete response [9]. Even though small cell carcinoma has a low incidence tumour, the prognosis is worse than urothelial carcinoma [9]. Survival at local stages is optimized by neoadjuvant chemotherapy, followed by radical resection [9].

In patients with small cell carcinoma, 65% had a history of cigarette smoking, and 88% presented with haematuria [10]. All but one had muscle-invasive disease at presentation [10]. Thirty-eight patients (59%) underwent cystectomy [10]. Sixty-six percent had lymph node metastasis at radical cystectomy [10]. Twenty patients (32%) had pure small cell carcinoma, and 44 patients (68%) had small cell carcinoma with other histologic types (35 patients had urothelial carcinoma, 4 patients had adenocarcinoma, 2 patients had sarcomatoid urothelial carcinoma, and 3 patients had both adenocarcinoma and urothelial carcinoma) [10]. With a mean follow-up of 21 months, 68% died of bladder carcinoma. No significant survival difference was demonstrated between patients who did and did not undergo cystectomy (p = 0.65) [10]. Organ-confined disease had marginally better survival than non-organ confined disease (p = 0.06) [10]. The overall, 1-year, 18-month, 3-year, and 5-year disease-specific survival rates were 56%, 41%, 23%, and 16%, respectively [10]. The prognosis for small cell carcinoma remains poor, even though the overall survival for bladder carcinoma has improved significantly over the last decade [10].

Small cell carcinoma of the bladder (SCCB) is a rare and lethal disease [11]. Van de Kamp reported on a bladder sparing strategy with platinum-etoposide-based chemotherapy followed by radiotherapy of the bladder [11]. Of the 110 patients with SCCB (82% male), 89 patients (81%) had SCCB [11]. Of these, 65 were treated with chemotherapy and radiotherapy, with a median overall recurrence free survival of 22 months (CI: 14–30). Of 65 patients, 23 (35%) progressed to distant metastasis without intravesical recurrence (CI: 8–11), whereas 14 patients (22%) developed isolated intravesical recurrence at a median of 24 months (CI: 14–34) [11]. Local recurrence contained SCCB, urothelial carcinoma, and carcinoma in situ and was treated with various local salvage treatments including TURB, cystectomy, neoadjuvant chemotherapy, and BCG [11]. Following salvage treatment a complete response was seen in 64%. Median overall survival for intravesical vs. systemic recurrence was different, with 28 (CI: 9–47) and 8 (CI: 5–11) months, respectively (p < 0.001) [11]. This demonstrates a bladder sparing approach can be a reasonable alternative to major surgery [11]. However, in those surviving long enough isolated intravesical recurrence occurs even after many years [11].

Small cell carcinoma of the bladder is an uncommon but clinically aggressive disease [12]. Eswara examined long term outcomes in bladder preservation [12]. The median follow-up for survivors was 34 months [12]. Presentation most commonly was with muscle-invasive disease (T2–4—89%). Twenty-one percent had lymph node/distant metastases at presentation. Tobacco use and chemical exposure were noted in 64% and 4% of patients, respectively. T1-2N0M0 disease had a median survival of 22 months, compared to 8 months with more advanced disease (p = 0.03). Patients with T3–4 or nodal/metastatic disease who were given chemotherapy had an improved survival compared to those with T3–4 or nodal/metastatic disease who did not undergo chemotherapy (13 vs. 4 months, p = 0.005). The median time to recurrence of the entire cohort was 8 months, overall and cancer-specific survival was 14 months, and 5-year survival was 11%.

9.7 Neoadjuvant Chemotherapy in Small Cell Bladder Cancer

Small-cell carcinoma is a poorly differentiated neoplasm that is aggressive [13]. Thirty-eight patients were treated for small-cell carcinoma of the bladder [13]. Median survival was 11.8 months. The overall survival rates after 1, 3, and 5 years were 46.6%, 26.2%, and 14%, respectively [13]. Survival analysis showed that no single treatment strategy was significantly superior (95% confidence interval [CI], 0.26–3.03; p = 0.860 for surgery; 95% CI, 0.31–2.87; p = 0.928 for neoadjuvant chemotherapy; 95% CI, 0.65–5.49; p = 0.238 for radiation) [13]. Among the 20 patients who received neoadjuvant chemotherapy, downstaging occurred in 9 (45%) [13]. Neoadjuvant chemotherapy might halt the progression of the disease until cystectomy and lead to downstaging [13]. However, it is important to note, that this is an incredibly aggressive form of cancer, that very often presents as locally advanced. Whilst neoadjuvant chemotherapy is important, it is also important for this cohort of patients to receive radical therapy such as radical cystectomy.

Patel identified patients with localized/locally advanced (cTis-cT4, cN0 or cM0) bladder small cell carcinoma diagnosed between 1998 and 2010 from the National Cancer Database (NCDB) [14]. A total of 625 patients met study inclusion criteria. Median age at diagnosis was 73 years (range 36–90) and 65% of patients presented with cT2 disease [14]. Patients were treated with bladder preservation therapy (174 or 27.8%), bladder preservation therapy plus multimodal treatment (333 or 53.3%), radical cystectomy alone (46 or 7.4%) and radical cystectomy plus multimodal treatment (72 or 11.5%). The 3-year overall survival rate was 23% (95% CI 15–32), 35% (95% CI 30–45), 38% (95% CI 17–60) and 30.1% (95% CI 16–47), respectively [14]. Overall survival was most favourable for radical cystectomy alone plus neoadjuvant chemotherapy with a 3-year rate of 53% (95% CI 19–79) [14].

9.8   Radiotherapy in Small Cell Cancer of the Bladder

Small cell carcinoma of the urinary bladder (SCCB) is rare [15]. Mattes reported using definitive external beam radiation therapy (EBRT) as part of multimodality management of SCCB [15]. Median follow-up was 26 months [15]. Three patients had in-bladder recurrence (2-year local recurrence, 25%), two being non-invasive and successfully managed with transurethral resection. The third case was invasive but managed with chemotherapy alone, due to simultaneous distant metastases [15]. No patient underwent salvage cystectomy. Six patients had recurrence distantly (2-year distant recurrence, 40%), predominantly bone metastases (n = 3). No patients developed brain metastases [15]. Two-year disease-free and overall survival were 51% and 78%, respectively. The 2-year distant metastasis-free survival for node-negative and node-positive patients was 76% and 26%, respectively (p = 0.04) [15]. The 2-year incidence of distant metastases for ≥ 4 cycles of doublet chemotherapy was 27%, compared with 75% with less chemotherapy (p = 0.01) [15]. The incidence of grade ≥ 2 acute and late genitourinary or gastrointestinal toxicity was 69% and 7%, respectively [15].

9.9   Adjuvant Therapy in Small Cell Cancer of the Bladder

Small-cell carcinoma of the urinary bladder (SCCUB) accounts for less than 1% of all cancers arising in the urinary bladder [16]. Many patients with SCCUB undergo local resection. Platinum-etoposide combination chemotherapy is employed as the main systemic treatment option for SCCUB [16]. Chemotherapy is usually combined with other therapeutic modalities, especially in patients whose disease is limited to the locoregional area [16]. Owing to the rarity of this malignancy, no prospective study has been performed that establishes the efficacy and duration of chemotherapy or the relative efficacy of platinum-etoposide versus other chemotherapeutic regimens [16].

Kaushik reviewed radical cystectomy for small cell carcinoma of the bladder, to compare outcomes with a cohort of patients with urothelial carcinoma, and to determine the effect of adjuvant chemotherapy [17]. Among the 68 small cell carcinoma of the bladder patients, 37 (54%) were found to have small cell carcinoma of the bladder only after pathology re-review. Patients with small cell carcinoma of the bladder had a higher rate of advanced (pT3/4) tumour stage (84% vs. 46%; p < 0.0001) and pN+ disease (37% vs. 20%; p = 0.001) compared with patients with urothelial carcinoma [17]. When matched for stage and lymph node status, no significant difference in 5-year cancer-specific survival was observed between the two groups (27% vs. 29%; p = 0.64) [17]. Among small cell carcinoma of the bladder patients, those receiving adjuvant chemotherapy had improved 5-year overall survival compared with patients who did not receive adjuvant chemotherapy (43% vs. 20%; p = 0.03), and a trend toward superior cancer-specific survival (40% vs. 23%; p = 0.07) [17].

Schreiber utilized the Surveillance, Epidemiology, and End Results Database to examine small cell carcinoma in a large population-based sample [18]. A total of 663 patients were identified. Most patients had either stage II (38.8%) or stage IV (35.4%) disease [18]. The median OS for was 12 months [95% confidence interval (CI), 10.9–13.1] [18]. After excluding distant metastatic disease at presentation or unknown treatment, there were no significant differences in survival between cystectomy (median survival, 21 months; 95% CI, 14.3–27.7) and external beam radiation (median survival, 17 months; 95% CI, 13.4–20.6) [18]. On multivariate analysis, both cystectomy (hazard ratio, 0.53; 95% CI, 0.4–0.71; p < 0.001) and radiation (hazard ratio, 0.66; 95% CI, 0.5–0.88; p = 0.005) were associated with improved survival [18].

Undifferentiated small cell carcinoma of the bladder is a rare tumour with pathologic features similar to those of oat cell carcinoma of the lung [19]. This neuroendocrine neoplasm of the bladder has a highly malignant biological behaviour. Presentation is with either locally advanced or distant metastatic disease [19]. Two patients with advanced small cell carcinoma of the bladder who were treated successfully with radical cystoprostatectomy and adjuvant methotrexate, vinblastine, doxorubicin, and cisplatin chemotherapy (M-VAC) [19]. Both had regional lymph node involvement and are disease free at follow-up of 1 year and 2.5 years, respectively [19]. This demonstrates radical cystectomy and M-VAC chemotherapy in the treatment of undifferentiated small cell carcinoma of the bladder [19].

9.10   Chemotherapy and Radiotherapy in Metastatic Small Cell Carcinoma of the Bladder

Naito reported a 59-year-old male patient with metastatic small cell carcinoma of the bladder treated with systemic chemotherapy including an amrubicin. The patient initially presented with visible haematuria [20]. A cytoscopy revealed a non-papillary, broad-based tumour extending from the right to the posterior wall of the bladder [20]. A computed tomography showed bilateral hydronephrosis caused by the bladder tumour and multiple metastases to the para-aortic and common iliac lymph nodes [20]. The histopathological findings following a transurethral resection of the bladder tumour revealed a T2N3M1, LYM, stage IV small cell carcinoma [20].

Ismaili reviewed recurrent and metastatic disease in small cell cancer [21]. The median age as 63 years, with stage IV disease [21]. Nine patients were treated by chemotherapy. Four were treated by local radiotherapy (three with radiotherapy without previous surgery and one with surgery followed by radiotherapy) and chemotherapy [21]. One patient was treated by whole brain radiotherapy [21]. One patient died before treatment. After 52.4 months median follow up, 12 patients died. Median overall survival was 7.6 months [21]. Survival probability at 1 year was 33%. Median overall survival was 9.9 months in the mixed small cell carcinoma group, and was only 4.6 months in the pure small cell carcinoma group [21].

Survival probability at 1 year in the mixed small cell carcinoma group was 44% as compared to 17% in the pure small cell carcinoma group (Log-rank test: p = 0.228) [21].

Meijer assessed the long-term outcome and the risk of recurrence in small cell carcinoma of the bladder (SCCB) treated with neoadjuvant chemotherapy followed by external beam radiotherapy (sequential chemoradiation) [22]. Median time to recurrence was 20 months, median overall survival 26 months, 5-year overall survival 22.2%, median cancer-specific survival 47 months and 5-year cancer-specific survival 39.6% [22]. For complete responders after neoadjuvant chemotherapy (n = 19), median cancer-specific survival was 52 months with a 5-year cancer-specific survival 45.9% versus a median cancer-specific survival of 22 months and 5-year cancer-specific survival 0.0% for incomplete responders (n = 8; p = 0.034) [22]. Eight patients (29.6%) underwent transurethral resections (TUR-BT) for local recurrences in the bladder [22]. At the end of follow up, four patients had undergone cystectomy for recurrence of disease resulting in a bladder-preservation rate of 85.2% [22].

References

1. Wang G, Xiao L, Zhang M, Kamat AM, Siefker-Radtke A, Dinney CP, Czerniak B, Guo CC. Small cell carcinoma of the urinary bladder: a clinicopathological and immunohistochemical analysis of 81 cases. Hum Pathol. 2018;79:57–65.
2. Sharma A, Sharma S, Patnaik N, Pradhan D, Satapathy K, Pradhan MR, Mohanty SK. Cytomorphologic and immunophenotypic profile of a cohort of small cell carcinoma of the urinary bladder. Acta Cytol. 2016;60(5):475–80.
3. van Hoeven KH, Artymyshyn RL. Cytology of small cell carcinoma of the urinary bladder. Diagn Cytopathol. 1996;14(4):292–7.
4. Pasquier D, Barney B, Sundar S, Poortmans P, Villa S, Nasrallah H, Boujelbene N, Ghadjar P, Lassen-Ramshad Y, Senkus E, Oar A, Roelandts M, Amichetti M, Vees H, Zilli T, Ozsahin M. Small cell carcinoma of the urinary bladder: a retrospective, multicenter rare cancer network study of 107 patients. Int J Radiat Oncol Biol Phys. 2015;92(4):904–10.
5. Naito A, Taguchi S, Nakagawa T, Matsumoto A, Nagase Y, Tabata M, Miyakawa J, Suzuki M, Nishimatsu H, Enomoto Y, Takahashi S, Okaneya T, Yamada D, Tachikawa T, Minowada S, Fujimura T, Fukuhara H, Kume H, Homma Y. Prognostic significance of serum neuron-specific enolase in small cell carcinoma of the urinary bladder. World J Urol. 2017;35(1):97–103.
6. Bezerra SM, Lotan TL, Faraj SF, Karram S, Sharma R, Schoenberg M, Bivalacqua TJ, Netto GJ. GATA3 expression in small cell carcinoma of bladder and prostate and its potential role in determining primary tumor origin. Hum Pathol. 2014;45(8):1682–7.
7. Chang K, Dai B, Kong YY, Qu YY, Gan HL, Gu WJ, Ye DW, Zhang HL, Zhu Y, Shi GH. Genitourinary small-cell carcinoma: 11-year treatment experience. Asian J Androl. 2014;16(5):705–9.
8. Li Z, Lin C, Wang D, Xie J, Zhou C, Chen P, Yang Y, Sun S, Peng J, Yang S, Lai Y. Primary small-cell neuroendocrine carcinoma of the urinary bladder: a rare case and a review of the literature. Mol Clin Oncol. 2018;9(3):335–8.
9. Pesquera-Ortega L, Calleja-Escudero J, Pascual-Fernández Á, Calvo-González R, Muñoz-Moreno M, Cortiñas-González JR. [Small cell carcinoma of the bladder: our experience]. Arch Esp Urol. 2015;68(7):602–8.

10. Cheng L, Pan CX, Yang XJ, Lopez-Beltran A, MacLennan GT, Lin H, Kuzel TM, Papavero V, Tretiakova M, Nigro K, Koch MO, Eble JN. Small cell carcinoma of the urinary bladder: a clinicopathologic analysis of 64 patients. Cancer. 2004;101(5):957–62.

11. van de Kamp M, Meijer R, Pos F, Kerst M, van Werkhoven E, van Rhijn B, Horenblas S, Bex A. Intravesical recurrence after bladder sparing treatment of small cell carcinoma of the bladder: characteristics, treatment, and outcome. Urol Oncol. 2018;36(6):307.e1–8.

12. Eswara JR, Heney NM, Wu CL, McDougal WS. Long-term outcomes of organ preservation in patients with small cell carcinoma of the bladder. Urol Int. 2015;94(4):401–5.

13. Jung K, Ghatalia P, Litwin S, Horwitz EM, Uzzo RG, Greenberg RE, Viterbo R, Geynisman DM, Kutikov A, Plimack ER, Smaldone MC, Wong YN, Bilusic M. Small-cell carcinoma of the bladder: 20-year single-institution retrospective review. Clin Genitourin Cancer. 2017;15(3):e337–43.

14. Patel SG, Stimson CJ, Zaid HB, Resnick MJ, Cookson MS, Barocas DA, Chang SS. Locoregional small cell carcinoma of the bladder: clinical characteristics and treatment patterns. J Urol. 2014;191(2):329–34.

15. Mattes MD, Kan CC, Dalbagni G, Zelefsky MJ, Kollmeier MA. External beam radiation therapy for small cell carcinoma of the urinary bladder. Pract Radiat Oncol. 2015;5(1):e17–22.

16. Pan CX, Zhang H, Lara PN Jr, Cheng L. Small-cell carcinoma of the urinary bladder: diagnosis and management. Expert Rev Anticancer Ther. 2006;6(12):1707–13.

17. Kaushik D, Frank I, Boorjian SA, Cheville JC, Eisenberg MS, Thapa P, Tarrell RF, Thompson RH. Long-term results of radical cystectomy and role of adjuvant chemotherapy for small cell carcinoma of the bladder. Int J Urol. 2015;22(6):549–54.

18. Schreiber D, Rineer J, Weiss J, Leaf A, Karanikolas N, Rotman M, Schwartz D. Characterization and outcomes of small cell carcinoma of the bladder using the surveillance, epidemiology, and end results database. Am J Clin Oncol. 2013;6(2):126–31.

19. Oesterling JE, Brendler CB, Burgers JK, Marshall FF, Epstein JI. Advanced small cell carcinoma of the bladder. Successful treatment with combined radical cystoprostatectomy and adjuvant methotrexate, vinblastine, doxorubicin, and cisplatin chemotherapy. Cancer. 1990;65(9):1928–36.

20. Naito A, Matsumoto A, Odani K, Sato Y, Azuma T, Ishizawa M, Nagase Y, Oshi M, Homma Y. Metastatic small cell carcinoma of the urinary bladder treated with systematic chemotherapy including amrubicin: a case report. Nihon Hinyokika Gakkai Zasshi. 2016;107(1):34–8.

21. Ismaili N, Heudel PE, Elkarak F, Kaikani W, Bajard A, Ismaili M, Errihani H, Droz JP, Flechon A. Outcome of recurrent and metastatic small cell carcinoma of the bladder. BMC Urol. 2009;9:4.

22. Meijer RP, Meinhardt W, van der Poel HG, et al. Local control rate and prognosis after sequential chemoradiation for small cell carcinoma of the bladder. Int J Urol. 2013;20(8):778–84.

MIBC Plasmacytoid Bladder Cancer

10

10.1 Clinical Presentation of Plasmacytoid Bladder Cancer

Plasmacytoid bladder cancer can present with direct intraperitoneal metastases complicated with massive ascites [1]. A case report and literature review [1]. Shao presented a 74-year-old male patient with massive ascites and bilateral lower leg oedema [1]. Colonoscopy showed a 3-cm lesion in the sigmoid colon and an oedematous nonpapillary tumour was found by cystoscopy [1]. Histopathology demonstrated adenocarcinoma of colon and Plasmacytoid Urothelial Cancer (PUC) of bladder. The diagnosis of PUC with peritoneal carcinomatosis was then confirmed by immunohistochemical stain [1].

10.2 Immunohistochemical Diagnosis in Plasmacytoid Cancer

Plasmacytoid urothelial carcinoma (UC) is a rare variant of UC that can histologically mimic metastatic cancer involving the urinary bladder [2]. Forty-five cases of plasmacytoid UC reviewed histologically [2]. GCPDFP-15, PR, CDX2 and p-CEA showed positive staining in 11 (24.4%), 6 (13.3%), 8 (17.7%), and 22 (48.8%) cases, respectively. GCPDFP-15 was expressed in 4/8 female cases, 1 concurrently focally (+2) expressing PR [2]. GATA 3 and uroplakin II was positive in 37/45 cases (82.2%) and 15/45 (33.3%) cases, respectively [2].

A plasmacytoid bladder cancer is recognised in the World Health Organization classification system [3]. It is characterised by discohesive growth of plasmacytoid cells. In addition there are eccentric nuclei. This can extend into the bladder wall and perivesical adipose tissue [3]. Tumour cells had identified cytokeratins, epithelial membrane antigen, GATA-3 (endothelial transcription factor 3), CD15, p53, and p16 [3]. Malignant cells strongly stained with CD138 [3]. Electron microscopy demonstrated divergent squamous and glandular differentiation [3]. Unlike

S. S. Goonewardene et al., *Management of Muscle Invasive Bladder Cancer*, Management of Urology, https://doi.org/10.1007/978-3-030-57915-9_10

urothelial carcinoma, the analysis of exons 4–9 of TP53 had no alterations. Plasmacytoid carcinoma has specific immunohistochemical markers, including positivity for GATA-3 [3].

Immunohistochemical study also demonstrated tumour cells were strongly positive for AE1/AE3, epithelial membrane antigen, CK7 and CK18. CK20 and uroplakin III were also expressed [4]. CEA, p53, CD138, p63 and E-cadherin were positive in 12, 13, 15, 11 and 10 cases, respectively [4]. The Ki-67 index ranged from 5% to 70% (mean = 30%). Three patients died of distant metastasis at 3, 27- and 60-months post-surgery respectively [4]. Ten patients were alive and disease free at 7–120 months [4]. This demonstrates the aggressive nature of this disease.

Makise reported diverse histology of squamous, glandular, and plasmacytoid components of bladder cancer in one tumour [5]. This presented with gross haematuria [5]. Due to the locally invasive extent, a radical cystectomy was performed [5]. The plasmacytoid UC component was composed of discohesive cancer cells with eccentric nuclei and eosinophilic cytoplasm, that diffusely entered the bladder wall [5]. Immunohistochemically, the loss of membranous E-cadherin expression was highlighted in the plasmacytoid UC component. The patient developed local recurrences 2 months postoperatively and died of the disease 6 months postoperatively [5].

10.3   Survival Outcomes

Cockerill evaluated oncological outcomes after radical cystectomy (RC) in plasmacytoid urothelial carcinoma (UC) versus pure UC of the bladder [6]. Patients with plasmacytoid UC were more likely to have extravesical disease ($\geq$pT3) (83% vs. 43%, $p < 0.0001$) and positive margins (31% vs. 2.1%, $p < 0.0001$) than pure UC [6]. Plasmacytoid UC was associated with decreased overall survival (27% vs. 45% at 5 years, relative risk [RR] 1.4, $p = 0.04$), cancer-specific survival (36% vs. 57% at 5 years, RR 1.7, $p = 0.01$), and local recurrence-free survival (63% vs. 81% at 5 years, RR 2, $p = 0.01$) [6]. When plasmacytoid UC were matched to pure UC, there were no significant differences in 5-year overall, cancer-specific, and local or distant recurrence-free survival [6].

Keck reviewed 205 tumour samples from locally advanced bladder cancer treated via the randomized AUO-AB05/95 trial [7]. This included radical cystectomy and adjuvant cisplatin-based chemotherapy for histologic subtypes [7]. One hundred and seventy-eight UC, 18 plasmacytoid (PUC) and 9 micropapillary (MPC) carcinomas [7]. PUC have the worst clinical outcome and overall survival compared to conventional UC or MPC—these have the best clinical outcome (27.4 months, 62.6 months, and 64.2 months, respectively; $p = 0.013$ by Kaplan Meier analysis) [7]. Backward multivariate Cox's proportional hazards regression analysis (adjusted to relevant clinicopathological parameters) showed a hazard ratio of 3.2 ($p = 0.045$) for PUC in contrast to patients suffering from MPC [7].

Monn evaluated pathologic and survival outcomes among patients with variant histology (VH) urothelial carcinoma of the bladder [8]. In total, 624 patients were identified. Overall, 26% (n = 162) had VH, with the most common being squamous differentiation (n = 68), micropapillary variant (MPV, n = 28), plasmacytoid variant (PCV, n = 25), and sarcomatoid variant (n = 15); 64% of MPV and 72% of PCV had positive lymph nodes [8]. PCV were independently associated with twice the risk of all-cause mortality compared with nonvariant, when adjusting for demographics, American Society of Anesthesiologists class, transurethral resection of bladder tumour stage, cystectomy stage, positive lymph nodes, and reception of chemotherapy (odds ratio = 2.20, 95% CI: 1.28–3.78; p = 0.004; odds ratio = 2.42, 95% CI: 1.33–4.42; p = 0.004, respectively) [8]. PCV are associated with increased risk of mortality. Improved recognition of VH will enable larger cohorts of study and better prognostic understanding of the significance of specific VH involvement [8].

The true clinical significance of variant histology is controversial, and diagnosis is challenging, especially in the setting of non-muscle invasive (NMI) disease [9]. Patients with high-risk NMI tumours and variant histology should be offered early cystectomy, especially if harbouring pure squamous, adenocarcinoma, sarcomatoid, plasmacytoid, or micropapillary disease [9]. Diligence is needed in the presence of variant histology to minimize the risk of understaging as well as close surveillance to not compromise the opportunity of cure [9]. The management of non-muscle invasive bladder cancer with variant histology is challenging, largely in part to the high risk of understaging and the background of already existing controversy regarding the management of high-risk NMI disease for standard urothelial cell carcinoma (early cystectomy vs. intravesical therapy) [9].

10.4   Surgical Outcomes in Plasmacytoid Bladder Cancer

Kaimakliotis identified prognostic factors in tumour behaviour to improve outcomes in PCV UC [10]. PCV UC is often diagnosed at a higher stage at cystectomy (73% pT3–4 vs. 40%, p = 0.001), were more likely to have lymph node involvement (70% vs. 25%, p < 0.001). Positive surgical margins were found in 40% of patients with PCV UC vs. 10% of patients with normal urothelial carcinoma (UC) (p < 0.001) [10]. Median overall survival and disease-specific survival were 19 and 22 months for PCV, respectively [10]. Median overall survival and disease-specific survival had not been reached for NV at 68 months (p < 0.001) [10]. Presence of PCV UC on transurethral resection of bladder tumour was associated with non-organ-confined disease (odds ratio = 4.02; 95% CI: 1.06–15.22; p = 0.040), and PCV at cystectomy was associated with increased adjusted risk of mortality (hazard ratio = 2.1; 95% CI: 1.2–3.8; p = 0.016) [10].

Bladder plasmacytoid carcinoma is an invasive urothelial carcinoma subtype that is emphasized for its morphological overlap with plasma cells and metastatic carcinoma [11]. Ricardo-Gonzalez reviewed outcomes post cystectomy. One tumour was pT2, 11 pT3 and 3 pT4. Six of 15 patients (40%) presented with lymph node metastasis and 5 (33%) had intraperitoneal metastasis at cystectomy [11]. These initial sites of metastatic spread included the pre-rectal space, ovary and vagina, ovary and fallopian tube, bowel serosa, and omentum and bowel serosa in 1 case each [11].

Three patients had subsequent metastasis involving the pre-rectal space, pleural fluid and small bowel serosa, and bowel serosa in 1 each [11]. Eight patients had follow-up information available, including 3 who died of disease, 3 with disease and 2 with no evidence of disease [11].

10.5 Patterns of Metastases: Plasmacytoid Bladder carcinoma

Kaimakliotis examined differences in disease progression and nature of tumour invasion to see if prediction of tumour behaviour and improved management options for plasmacytoid variant cancer (PCV) was possible [12]. Of 510 patients, 30 had a positive urethral margin (+UM) on final pathology [12]. The incidence of +UM in N patients was 17 of 457 (3.7%), in MPV 5 of 28 (17.9%), and in PCV 8 of 25 (32.0%) (p < 0.001) [12]. Carcinoma in situ on the luminal margin was noted for all cases, except in 5 of the 8 PCV patients with +UM. In these retrograde longitudinal invasion along the subserosal and adventitia was highlighted [12]. Positive surgical margins (+PSM) and positive lymph nodes (+LN) were significantly higher for both PCV (28.0%, 72.0%) and Micropapillary Variants (MPV) (10.7%, 64.3%) than normal urothelial cancer (2.6%, 18.6%, p < 0.001, each) [12].

PCV exhibits a unique pattern of spread along the ureter [12]. This highlights a new potential route of invasion along the fascial sheath [12]. The incidence of +PSM and +LN liken PCV to the known aggressive MPV, and in conjunction with the increased incidence of +UM, may lead to a paradigm shift, with surgeons and pathologists being more vigilant with surgical margins [12].

Pereira highlighted, the range of presentation, with 81-year-old man who presented with pelvic pain and evolving urinary retention over 3 months [13]. The patient was found to have a tense glans and penile shaft with surrounding induration consistent with malignant priapism [13]. The extent of the induration included the suprapubic region, scrotum, left iliac region and left flank [13]. A CT scan demonstrated an enhancing, pedunculated lesion arising from the anterior bladder wall measuring $30 \times 31 \times 20$ mm [13]. There were multiple enlarged left inguinal lymph nodes [13]. Core biopsies of the subcutaneous tissue on the anterior abdominal wall demonstrated plasmacytoid urothelial carcinoma [13]. The majority of patients with plasmacytoid variant of transitional cell carcinoma will present with >stage 3 bladder disease [13].

10.6 Neoadjuvant Chemotherapy in Plasmacytoid Bladder Cancer

Pokuri presents a 41-year-old Asian man, referred with macroscopic haematuria [14]. Cystoscopy detected a non-papillary tumour. Transurethral resection revealed a pT1N0M0 bladder cancer [14]. A pathological examination demonstrated a high-grade invasive urothelial carcinoma and a component of signet ring cell carcinoma

[14]. A follow-up of the transurethral resection with radical cystectomy demonstrated infiltrating urothelial carcinoma, with partial features of the plasmacytoid variant [14]. Neoadjuvant chemotherapy treatment with gemcitabine and cisplatin was administered for two cycles [14]. There has been no recurrence for 2 years. This highlights a role for neoadjuvant chemotherapy in muscle invasive plasmacytoid bladder cancer.

10.7   Recurrence in Plasmacytoid Bladder Cancer

Plasmacytoid urothelial carcinoma is a rare variant histology with poorly defined clinical behaviour [15]. Dayyani identified 31 patients with a median age of 63.5 years, of whom 83.3% were male [15]. TNM stage was cT1N0 in 4 patients, cT2N0 in 7, cT3b-4aN0 in 5 and cT4b, N+ or M+ in 15 [15]. Median overall survival was 17.7 months (stage I–III vs. IV 45.8 vs. 13.3) [15]. Five of the 16 patients with potentially surgically resectable plasmacytoid urothelial carcinoma (pT4aN0M0 or less) received neoadjuvant chemotherapy, 10 underwent initial surgery and 1 was treated only with transurethral resection of bladder tumour [15]. Despite pathological down staging in 80% of the patients who received neoadjuvant chemotherapy, relapses were common [15]. There was no survival difference between patients treated with neoadjuvant chemotherapy or initial surgery, although 7 received adjuvant chemotherapy [15]. Surgical up staging with positive margins was also common for surgery alone. The most common site of recurrence was in the peritoneum (19 of 23 patients) with relapses even in those with a pathological complete response at surgery [15]. In patients who presented with metastatic disease and were treated with chemotherapy median survival was 12.6 months.

The clinical significance of the plasmacytoid variant (PCV) in urothelial carcinoma (UC) is currently lacking [16]. Patients with PCV UC were more likely to have advanced tumour stage (p = 0.001), positive lymph nodes (p = 0.038), and receive neoadjuvant chemotherapy than those with pure UC (46% vs. 22%, p < 0.0001) [16]. The rate of positive soft tissue surgical margins was over five times greater in the PCV UC group compared with the pure UC group (21% vs. 4.1%, respectively, p < 0.0001) [16]. Median OS for the pure UC versus the PCV patients were 8 year and 3.8 year, respectively [16]. On univariable analysis, PCV was associated with an increased risk of overall mortality (hazard ratio = 1.34, 95% confidence interval: 1.02–1.78, p = 0.039) [16]. However, on multivariable analysis adjusted for age, sex, neoadjuvant chemotherapy received, lymph node status, pathologic stage, and soft margin status, the association between PCV and OS was no longer significant (hazard ratio = 1.06, 95% confidence interval: 0.78, 1.43, p = 0.7) [16].

Data regarding PUC shows that this neoplasia presents a distinctive clinical outcome represented by aggressive behaviour and poor survival rate [17]. Da Fonseca reported a case of a 57-year-old male patient with a 3-month history of haematuria and pelvic pain [17]. Radical cystectomy with lymphadenectomy was performed and pathological examination showed a pT3pN0 PUC of the bladder [17]. The patient remained free of recurrence for 8 months, but the disease recurred involving the abdominal wall and subcutaneous tissue [17]. Chemotherapy provided a positive clinical response and relief of symptoms [17]. This highlights the aggressiveness of this rare variant of bladder cancer and recommend radical surgery and multidisciplinary management of this neoplasm [17].

References

1. Shao YH, Kao CC, Tang SH, Cha TL, Tsao CW, Meng E, Yu DS, Sun GH, Wu ST. Unusual presentation of direct intraperitoneal metastases complicated with massive ascites from plasmacytoid variant of bladder cancer and adenocarcinoma of colon: a case report and literature review. Medicine (Baltimore). 2017;96(7):e5816.
2. Borhan WM, Cimino-Mathews AM, Montgomery EA, Epstein JI. Immunohistochemical differentiation of plasmacytoid urothelial carcinoma from secondary carcinoma involvement of the bladder. Am J Surg Pathol. 2017;41(11):1570–5.
3. Raspollini MR, Sardi I, Giunti L, Di Lollo S, Baroni G, Stomaci N, Menghetti I, Franchi A. Plasmacytoid urothelial carcinoma of the urinary bladder: clinicopathologic, immunohistochemical, ultrastructural, and molecular analysis of a case series. Hum Pathol. 2011;F42(8):1149–58.
4. Zhang W, Jiang YX, Liu Y, Yu WJ, Zhao H, Li YJ. Plasmacytoid urothelial carcinoma of the urinary bladder: a clinicopathologic study of 16 cases. Zhonghua Bing Li Xue Za Zhi. 2013;42(7):433–7.
5. Makise N, Morikawa T, Takeshima Y, Homma Y, Fukayama M. A case of urinary bladder urothelial carcinoma with squamous, glandular, and plasmacytoid differentiation. Case Rep Oncol. 2014;7(2):362–8.
6. Cockerill PA, Cheville JC, Boorjian SA, Blackburne A, Thapa P, Tarrell RF, Frank I. Outcomes following radical cystectomy for plasmacytoid urothelial carcinoma: defining the need for improved local cancer control. Urology. 2017;102:143–7.
7. Keck B, Wach S, Stoehr R, Kunath F, Bertz S, Lehmann J, Stöckle M, Taubert H, Wullich B, Hartmann A. Plasmacytoid variant of bladder cancer defines patients with poor prognosis if treated with cystectomy and adjuvant cisplatin-based chemotherapy. BMC Cancer. 2013;13:71.
8. Monn MF, Kaimakliotis HZ, Pedrosa JA, Cary KC, Bihrle R, Cheng L, Koch MO. Contemporary bladder cancer: variant histology may be a significant driver of disease. Urol Oncol. 2015;33(1):18.e15–18.e2.
9. Porten SP, Willis D, Kamat AM. Variant histology: role in management and prognosis of non-muscle invasive bladder cancer. Curr Opin Urol. 2014;24(5):517–23.
10. Kaimakliotis HZ, Monn MF, Cary KC, Pedrosa JA, Rice K, Masterson TA, Gardner TA, Hahn NM, Foster RS, Bihrle R, Cheng L, Koch MO. Plasmacytoid variant urothelial bladder cancer: is it time to update the treatment paradigm? Urol Oncol. 2014a;32(6):833–8.
11. Ricardo-Gonzalez RR, Nguyen M, Gokden N, Sangoi AR, Presti JC Jr, McKenney JK. Plasmacytoid carcinoma of the bladder: a urothelial carcinoma variant with a predilection for intraperitoneal spread. J Urol. 2012;187(3):852–5.
12. Kaimakliotis HZ, Monn MF, Cheng L, Masterson TA, Cary KC, Pedrosa JA, Foster RS, Koch MO, Bihrle R. Plasmacytoid bladder cancer: variant histology with aggressive behavior and a new mode of invasion along fascial planes. Urology. 2014b;83(5):1112–6.
13. Pereira R, Perera M, Rhee H. Metastatic plasmacytoid bladder cancer causing malignant priapism. BMJ Case Rep. 2019;12(7):e228088.
14. Pokuri VK, Syed JR, Yang Z, Field EP, Cyriac S, Pili R, Levine EG, Azabdaftari G, Trump DL, Guru K, George S. Predictors of complete pathologic response (pT0) to neoadjuvant chemotherapy in muscle-invasive bladder carcinoma. Clin Genitourin Cancer. 2016;14(1):e59.

15. Dayyani F, Czerniak BA, Sircar K, Munsell MF, Millikan RE, Dinney CP, Siefker-Radtke AO. Plasmacytoid urothelial carcinoma, a chemosensitive cancer with poor prognosis, and peritoneal carcinomatosis. J Urol. 2013;189(5):1656–61.
16. Li Q, Assel M, Benfante NE, Pietzak EJ, Herr HW, Donat M, Cha EK, Donahue TF, Bochner BH, Dalbagni G. The impact of plasmacytoid variant histology on the survival of patients with urothelial carcinoma of bladder after radical cystectomy. Eur Urol Focus. 2019;5(1):104–8.
17. da Fonseca LG, Souza CE, Mattedi RL, Girardi DM, Sarkis ÁS, Hoff PMG. Plasmacytoid urothelial carcinoma: a case of histological variant of urinary bladder cancer with aggressive behaviour. Autops Case Rep. 2014;4(4):57–61.

11.1 Histopathology of Micropapillary Bladder Carcinoma

The micropapillary variant of urothelial carcinoma (MPUC) is a rare but well-recognized tumour [1]. It is more aggressive compared to conventional urothelial carcinoma. They demonstrate variable keratin 7, keratin 20 and human epidermal growth factor receptor 2 (Her 2)neu expression [1]. The tumour presents with haematuria [1]. The micropapillary pattern was seen in 20–95% [1]. All showed extensive lymphatic emboli with detrusor muscle invasion [1]. Lymph node metastasis was present in all except one. They all underwent cystoprostatectomy [1]. Keratin 7 and abluminal pattern of EMA positivity were seen in 100%. Keratin 20 was positive in five cases (71%). Her 2neu positivity was seen in four cases [1]. Three patients died 2, 3, and 6 months after initial diagnosis—two were Her 2 positive, one was Her 2 negative [1]. There was no clear prognostic significance of Her 2 positivity.

Micropapillary carcinoma (MPC) is so aggressive and needs early recognition and treatment [2]. González-Peramato et al. [2] determined whether this can be recognized with cytology. On histology, 14 cases were infiltrative, while 6 were exclusively superficial [2]. Cytology was characterized by numerous small, cohesive groups and single neoplastic cells [2]. Pseudopapillae were present in 17 cases and in 9 they were a relevant finding. Morules were present in 15 cases. Isolated microacini were seen in 14 cases. Infiltrative tumours showed more neoplastic groups [2]. Cellular atypia was prominent in 17 cases. In 15 cases, a cytologic diagnosis of urothelial carcinoma was made. One case was diagnosed as adenocarcinoma. The remaining 4 cases were considered suspicious of malignancy [2].

Immunohistochemical staining demonstrated that both micropapillary and associated conventional urothelial carcinomas were positive for MUC1 and 2, cytokeratin 7, PTEN, p53, and Ki-67. Her2Neu, uroplakin, cytokeratin 20, 34betaE12, CA125, and p16 were positive in 4, 10, 8, 7, 3, and 3 cases, respectively [3].

S. S. Goonewardene et al., *Management of Muscle Invasive Bladder Cancer*,
Management of Urology, https://doi.org/10.1007/978-3-030-57915-9_11

MUC5A, MUC6, and CDX2 were negative in all micropapillary cases [3]. Follow-up information was available in all cases (range, 2–21 months; mean, 10 months) [3]. Eleven of patients died of disease from 2 to 14 months, and 2 patients were alive with disease at 14 and 21 months. Univariate statistical analysis showed survival differences between invasive micropapillary and conventional urothelial carcinomas (p < 0.0001) [3].

11.2   Clinical Presentation of Micropapillary Bladder Cancer

Kumari reported the case of a 58-year-old man who presented with macroscopic haematuria [4]. The diagnosis was high-grade urothelial carcinoma and with recurrence after 16 months [4]. Histopathology after transurethral biopsy revealed a non-muscle invasive high-grade bladder tumour at first presentation [4]. The histopathology demonstrated a recurrent high-grade, muscle invasive, micropapillary variant of urothelial carcinoma with focal adenomatous morphology. Immunohistochemical expression of CK7/CK20, negativity for PSA, AMACR, and CDX2 aided in identifying the primary tumour. Radical cystectomy was performed. The patient had no distant metastases on follow-up.

Sanjo reported a case of metastatic micropapillary variant of the bladder. This progressed from low grade non-muscle invasive bladder carcinoma, highlighting how aggressive the disease process can be [5]. Lung, para-aortic and pelvic lymph nodes metastatic lesions were found in a 62-year-old woman, after non-muscle invasive bladder carcinoma [5]. The bladder wall was thickened on computerized tomography (CT). Transurethral resection of bladder tumour (TURBT) was conducted 12 months apart, followed by intravesical therarubicin and bacille Calmette-Guérin therapy, respectively [5]. Both TURBT specimens showed low grade, non-muscle invasive urothelial carcinoma. The thickened bladder wall was resected transurethrally and the pathological examination revealed that the recurrent tumour was entirely composed of micropapillary variant component [5]. There must have been tiny lesions of a micro papillary variant component after the second TURBT. Several reports suggest that intravesical BCG therapy was ineffective for micropapillary variant. So the UC component was substituted for micropapillary component [5].

A 69-year-old man was admitted with lymphatic oedema of left arm [6] and a past history of TURBT 5 years ago, a urothelial carcinoma with micropapillary variant, G3 = G2, pT1 [6]. CT scan revealed bladder tumour with invasion of the rectum, and multiple lymph nodes swelling in the axilla, retroperitoneum and pelvis (cT4bN3M1) [6]. Biopsies were taken of the bladder wall and the left axillary lymph nodes. Histology revealed micropapillary carcinoma [6]. Five courses of gemcitabine plus cisplatin (GC therapy) were administered. The bladder tumour and lymph node metastases reduced remarkably, with serum CA19-9 level decreasing from 172,000 to 106 U/ml [6]. Unfortunately, the patient died from recurrence 23 months after the start of GC therapy [6].

11.3   Clinical Risk Stratification in Micropapillary Bladder Cancer

Fernandez analysed survival in clinically localised, surgically resectable micropapillary bladder cancer (MPBC) [7]. This was in radical cystectomy (RC) with and without neoadjuvant chemotherapy (NAC) and then they looked to develop risk stratification based on outcome data [7]. For the entire cohort, estimated 5-year overall survival and disease-specific survival (DSS) rates were 52% and 58%, respectively [7]. CART analysis identified three risk subgroups: low-risk: cT1, no hydronephrosis; high-risk: ≥cT2, no hydronephrosis; and highest-risk: cTany with tumour-associated hydronephrosis [7]. The 5-year DSS for the low-, high-, and highest-risk groups were 92%, 51%, and 17%, respectively (p < 0.001) [7]. Patients down-staged at RC <pT1 regardless of the use of NAC had the best survival (5-year DSS of 96% vs. 45% for those not down-staged; p < 0.001). Those who were not down-staged despite NAC had 5-year DSS of only 17% [7].

11.4   Survival Outcomes in Micropapillary Bladder Cancer

Vourganti elucidated the oncologic behaviour of micropapillary urothelial bladder carcinoma (MPBC) [8]. MPBC presented with more high grade (86.1% vs. 38.7%, p < 0.0001) and more high stage disease (40.8% NMI vs. 90.4% NMI, p < 0.0001) than UC [8]. Low grade (LG) NMI MPBC had worse OS and CSS compared to LG UC (p = 0.0037, p < 0.0001 respectively), and did no better than high grade (HG) NMI MPBC [8]. No difference was detected between HG NMI MPBC and HG NMI UC pts. A CPH model controlling for stage, grade, treatment, age, race, and sex detected no significant survival difference in MPBC vs. UC (HR 1.04, p = 0.7966) [8]. For NMI MPBC (n = 49), only 4 patients underwent definitive therapy, of whom none died of disease. However, in those not receiving definitive therapy (n = 45), 7 cancer specific deaths occurred (15.6%) [8].

Wang examined the epidemiology, natural history, and prognostic factors of MPBC using a population-based registry [9]. MPBC accounted for approximately 0.01% of primary bladder tumours [9]. 56.1% had muscle invasive disease. 75.5% had poor or undifferentiated histology. 30.6% had a radical or partial cystectomy [9]. The 1-, 3-, and 5-year overall survival rates for the SEER cohort were estimated at 84.5%, 57.3%, and 42.3%, respectively [9]. On multivariate analysis, tumour stage and marital status were the most significant predictors for cancer-specific survival [9]. When comparing published single-institution studies to the SEER cohort, significant differences existed in demographic characteristics including age at diagnosis, male-to-female ratio, tumour stage, cystectomy treatment, and survival outcomes, likely reflecting differences in practice patterns [9]. This is the first population-based study to analyse MPBC's epidemiology, tumour characteristics, and survival rates. Emphases on early detection, cystectomy, and multimodality in treatment are needed [9].

Micropapillary carcinoma (MPC) is an aggressive variant of urothelial carcinoma (UC) [10]. In the TURBT, 12 had pTa, 33 pT1 and 27 pT2 tumours with 23% also displaying urothelial carcinoma in situ (CIS) [10]. On cystectomy, the MPC component was upstaged in 79% [10]. Twenty-five (35%) had metastases at presentation or nodal metastases at cystectomy and 27 patients (38%) died of disease [10]. Mean survival was 17.8 months. Of 12 pTa MPC cases, 8 were treated with cystectomy, all displaying invasive carcinoma including 5 (62%) with pT2–pT4 disease [10]. Three (25%) of these patients died of disease. Seven patients had a MPC component of <10% all had cystectomy [10]. Six of these had invasive carcinoma including 2 (33%) with pT2–pT4 disease. One (15%) of these patients died of disease.

11.5   Neoadjuvant Chemotherapy in Micropapillary Bladder Cancer

Meeks describe the pathological outcomes of muscle-invasive micropapillary bladder cancer with neoadjuvant chemotherapy [11]. A total of 82 patients with muscle-invasive micropapillary bladder cancer were treated [11]. Neoadjuvant chemotherapy was initiated in 29 (66%) patients and all patients underwent RC (93%) or partial cystectomy (7%) [11]. Micropapillary histology was diagnosed at resection in 37 (84%) patients [11]. Final RC pathology revealed pT0 in 15 (34%) patients and positive lymph nodes in 13 (31%) patients [11]. Down-staging to pT0 occurred in 13 (45%) with neoadjuvant chemotherapy compared with 2 (13%) who had none (p = 0.049) [11]. pT0 disease with micropapillary histology had higher overall survival rates (25% vs. 92%) and lower rates of recurrence (21% vs. 79%) [11].

11.6   Trimodal Therapy in Micropapillary Bladder Cancer

Sui sought to use a population-level cancer database to assess survival outcomes in patients treated with surgery, radiation therapy and/or chemotherapy [12]. Overall 869 patients with MPBC and 389,603 patients with UC met the inclusion criteria [12]. Median age of the MPBC cohort was 69.9 years (58.9–80.9) with the majority of the cohort presenting with high-grade (89.3%) and muscle invasive or locally advanced disease (47.6%) [12]. For cT1 MPBC, outcomes of RC and BPS were not statistically different. For ≥cT2 disease, NAC showed a survival benefit compared with RC alone for UC but not for MPBC [12]. On multivariable analysis, MPBC histology independently predicted worse increased risk of death. On subanalysis of the MBC RC patients, NAC did not improve survival outcomes compared with RC alone [12].

11.7   Surgical Outcomes in Micropapillary Bladder Cancer

Li investigated the clinico-pathological characteristics, treatment, and prognosis of MPBC to improve the understanding of this invasive disease. 81.8% had cT1 above or with lymph node and distant metastasis (cT2N0 in 18.2%, cT3-4N0 in 13.6%, cTanyN+ in 43.2%, and cTanyM+ in 6.8%) [13]. There was a high grade in 70.5% of patients. Lymphovascular invasion (LVI) was present in 61.4%and LVI in cT2 was more common than in cT1 (71.4% vs. 22.2%). 52.3% had radical cystectomy (RC) [13]. At 16 months, 77.3% developed distant metastases, and 47.7% died of the disease [13]. The mean overall survival (OS) was 28.9 months and the median OS was 20 months, and the amount of micropapillary (MPP) is correlated inversely with prognosis [13].

Jackson reviewed the outcomes of micropapillary urothelial carcinoma (MPUC) [14]. Sixteen of 40 patients died after a median follow-up of 37 months [14]. Tumour stage was strongly predictive of OS (p < 0.0001). LVI was associated with increased mortality (hazard ratio 12.4, 95% CI: 3.5–44.5, p = 0.0001), higher pathological stage (p = 0.001), lymph node involvement (p = 0.001) and iMP differentiation (p = 0.006) [14]. In NMI cases not undergoing cystectomy (n = 17), NMI-sMP compared with NMI-iMP differentiation was associated with an improved OS when compared with iMP (63 vs. 47 months, p = 0.05) [14].

Willis reported on cT1 micropapillary bladder cancer [15]. In this cohort of 72 patients, 40 received primary intravesical bacillus Calmette-Guérin and 26 underwent up-front radical cystectomy [15]. Of patients who received bacillus Calmette-Guérin 75%, 45% and 35% experienced disease recurrence, progression and lymph node metastasis, respectively [15]. Up-front cystectomy had improved survival compared to treatment with primary bacillus Calmette-Guérin (5-year disease specific survival 100% vs. 60% p = 0.006). Delayed cystectomy after recurrence had a 5-year disease specific survival 62% (p = 0.015) [15]. Prognosis was especially poor in cases who waited for progression before undergoing radical cystectomy. The estimated 5-year disease specific survival was 24% with a median survival of 35 months [15]. Up-front cystectomy had pathological up-staging in 27%, including 20% with lymph node metastasis [15].

Kamat reviewed the records of 100 consecutive patients with micropapillary bladder cancer [16]. The TNM stage of disease at the time of presentation was Ta in 5 patients, carcinoma in situ (CIS) in 4 patients, T1 in 35 patients, T2 in 26 patients, T3 in 7 patients, T4 in 6 patients; N+ in 9 patients, and M+ in 8 patients [16]. Kaplan-Meier estimates of 5-year and 10-year overall survival (OS) rates were 51% and 24%, respectively [16]. Bladder-sparing therapy with intravesical bacillus Calmette-Guerin therapy was attempted in 27 of 44 patients with nonmuscle-invasive disease. Sixty-seven percent (18 patients) developed disease progression (≥cT2), including 22% who developed metastatic disease [16]. Of 55 patients undergoing radical cystectomy for surgically resectable disease (≤cT4a), 23 received neoadjuvant chemotherapy and 32 were treated with initial cystectomy, with no significant difference noted in stage distribution between the two groups [16]. For the 23 patients treated with neoadjuvant chemotherapy, the median OS was 43.2 months with 32% of patients still alive at 5 years [16]. For the 32 patients treated with initial cystectomy, the median survival had not been reached at the time of last follow-up, with 71% still alive at 5 years [16].

11.8   Adjuvant Therapy in Micropapillary Bladder Cancer

Micropapillary bladder cancer is a rare and aggressive variant of urothelial carcinoma [17]. A retrospective review of our experience in management of patients with muscle-invasive or metastatic micropapillary bladder cancer was performed to better define the behavior of this disease [17]. Mean patients age was 60 years. The majority of patients (72%) were diagnosed after 2004 [17]. After a median follow-up of 31.7 months, median overall survival was 19 months. Two patients presented with stage II, one with stage III and eight with stage IV disease. All five patients who had node positive metastases and treated with radical surgery and adjuvant chemotherapy relapsed and had a disease free survival of 9.6 months [17].

Masson-Lecomte assessed the oncological outcomes of radical cystectomy (RC) and adjuvant chemotherapy to treat muscle-invasive bladder cancer (MIBC) with a micropapillary component (MPC), and to compare outcomes with those from pure urothelial carcinoma (PUC) [18]. Median survival was 29 months in the MPC versus 31 months in the PUC group [18]. The median number of treatment cycles administered was 6 (3–8) in the PUC versus 5 (3–8) in the MPC group (p = 0.45) [18]. Five-year disease-free recurrence and cancer-specific survival (CSS) rates were 15% and 24%, respectively, in the MPC versus 42% and 47%, respectively, in the PUC group (p = 0.007 and 0.058) [18]. In multivariate analyses, ASA score, soft tissue surgical margins, and MPC were associated with disease recurrence (p = 0.022, 0.001, and 0.015, respectively) [18].

References

1. Chatterjee D, Das A, Radotra BD. Invasive micropapillary carcinoma of urinary bladder: a clinicopathological study. Indian J Pathol Microbiol. 2015;58(1):2–6.
2. González-Peramato P, Jiménez-Heffernan JA, Vicandi B, López-Ferrer P, Bárcena C, Alvarez-Rodríguez F, Picazo ML, Viguer JM. Micropapillary carcinoma of the urinary tract: a cytologic study of urine and fine-needle aspirate samples. Acta Cytol. 2014;58(3):269–74.
3. Lopez-Beltran A, Montironi R, Blanca A, Cheng L. Invasive micropapillary urothelial carcinoma of the bladder. Hum Pathol. 2010;41(8):1159–64.
4. Kumari N, Jha A, Vasudeva P, Agrawal U. High-grade urothelial carcinoma of bladder transforming to micropapillary variant on follow-up. Iran J Med Sci. 2017;42(3):318–21.
5. Sanjo H, Ito Y, Osaka K, Komiya A, Kobayashi K, Sakai N, Noguchi S, Kishi H. Metastatic micropapillary variant of the urinary bladder: progression from low grade non-muscle invasive bladder carcinoma. Hinyokika Kiyo. 2012;58(8):447–51.
6. Ishii T, Matsubara T, Taira H, Hiratsuka Y. Metastatic micropapillary variant of urothelial carcinoma of the urinary bladder responding to gemcitabine and cisplatin chemotherapy. Nihon Hinyokika Gakkai Zasshi. 2013;104(3):540–4.
7. Fernández MI, Williams SB, Willis DL, Slack RS, Dickstein RJ, Parikh S, Chiong E, Siefker-Radtke AO, Guo CC, Czerniak BA, McConkey DJ, Shah JB, Pisters LL, Grossman HB, Dinney CP, Kamat AM. Clinical risk stratification in patients with surgically resectable micropapillary bladder cancer. BJU Int. 2017;119(5):684–91.
8. Vourganti S, Harbin A, Singer EA, Shuch B, Metwalli AR, Agarwal PK. Low grade micropapillary urothelial carcinoma, does it exist? - analysis of management and outcomes from the surveillance, epidemiology and end results (SEER) database. J Cancer. 2013;4(4):336–42.

9. Wang J, Wang FW. The natural history, treatment pattern, and outcomes of patients with micropapillary bladder carcinoma. Am J Clin Oncol. 2015;38(5):472–8.
10. Compérat E, Roupret M, Yaxley J, Reynolds J, Varinot J, Ouzaïd I, Cussenot O, Samaratunga H. Micropapillary urothelial carcinoma of the urinary bladder: a clinicopathological analysis of 72 cases. Pathology. 2010;42(7):650–4.
11. Meeks JJ, Taylor JM, Matsushita K, Herr HW, Donat SM, Bochner BH, Dalbagni G. Pathological response to neoadjuvant chemotherapy for muscle-invasive micropapillary bladder cancer. BJU Int. 2013;111(8):E325–30.
12. Sui W, Matulay JT, James MB, Onyeji IC, Theofanides MC, RoyChoudhury A, DeCastro GJ, Wenske S. Micropapillary bladder cancer: insights from the National Cancer Database. Bladder Cancer. 2016;2(4):415–23.
13. Li Z, Liao H, Tan Z, Mao D, Wu Y, Xiao YM, Yang SK, Zhong L. Micropapillary bladder cancer: a clinico-pathological characterization and treatment analysis. Clin Transl Oncol. 2017;19(10):1217–24.
14. Jackson BL, Mohammed A, Mayer N, Dormer J, Griffiths TR. Is immediate radical cystectomy necessary for all patients with non-muscle-invasive micropapillary bladder cancer? Urol Int. 2016;96(1):32–8.
15. Willis DL, Fernandez MI, Dickstein RJ, Parikh S, Shah JB, Pisters LL, Guo CC, Henderson S, Czerniak BA, Grossman HB, Dinney CP, Kamat AM. Clinical outcomes of cT1 micropapillary bladder cancer. J Urol. 2015;193(4):1129–34.
16. Kamat AM, Dinney CP, Gee JR, Grossman HB, Siefker-Radtke AO, Tamboli P, Detry MA, Robinson TL, Pisters LL. Micropapillary bladder cancer: a review of the University of Texas M. D. Anderson Cancer Center experience with 100 consecutive patients. Cancer. 2007;110(1):62–7.
17. Heudel P, El Karak F, Ismaili N, Droz JP, Flechon A. Micropapillary bladder cancer: a review of Léon Bérard Cancer Center experience. BMC Urol. 2009;9:5.
18. Masson-Lecomte A, Xylinas E, Bouquot M, Sibony M, Allory Y, Comperat E, Zerbib M, de la Taille A, Rouprêt M. Oncological outcomes of advanced muscle-invasive bladder cancer with a micropapillary variant after radical cystectomy and adjuvant platinum-based chemotherapy. World J Urol. 2015;33(8):1087–93.

Part IV
Assessment and Diagnosis in MIBC

MIBC Bladder Cancer Assessment and Diagnosis

Bladder cancer is the fourth most common cancer with an estimated 15,580 deaths in 2014 [1]. Initial presentation is usually with clinically localized disease [1]. Once bladder cancer invades beyond the muscularis propria, the likelihood of development of metastatic disease increases substantially [1]. In the case of histological variants, presentation is very often muscle invasive.

12.1 Clinical Presentation of Bladder Cancer

Haematuria has a prevalence of 0.1–2.6% [2]. Twenty percent of patients with haematuria have a urological tumour. Twenty percent will have significant underlying pathology [2]. Haematuria is the 'classic' presentation, 70–80% will have painless, visible haematuria [2]. Ramirez determined whether the severity of haematuria (microscopic or gross) impacted disease stage [3]. Presentation was with visible haematuria (GH; 1083, 78.3%), microscopic haematuria (MH; 189, 13.7%) or without haematuria (112, 8.1%) [3]. High-grade disease was found in 64% and 57.1%, respectively. Severity of haematuria was not associated with higher grade disease [3]. Stage of disease for MH was Ta/carcinoma in situ (CIS) in 68.8%, T1 in 19.6%, and $\geq$T2 in 11.6% [3]. Stage of disease at diagnosis for GH was Ta/CIS in 55.9%, T1 in 19.6%, and $\geq$T2 in 17.9% [3]. On multivariate analyses, GH was associated with $\geq$T2 disease (odds ratio 1.69, 95% confidence interval 1.05–2.71, p = 0.03) [3]. Earlier detection of disease, could influence survival [3].

Cha hypothesized that in asymptomatic haematuria, the risk of bladder cancer can be predicted with high accuracy [4]. Of the 1182 subjects who presented with asymptomatic haematuria, 245 (20.7%) had bladder cancer. Increasing age (OR = 1.03, p < 0.0001), smoking history (OR = 3.72, p < 0.0001), gross haematuria (OR = 1.71, p = 0.002), and positive cytology (OR = 14.71, p < 0.0001) were independent predictors of bladder cancer [4]. The multivariable model achieved 83.1% accuracy for predicting the presence of bladder cancer [4].

© The Editor(s) (if applicable) and The Author(s), under exclusive license to
Springer Nature Switzerland AG 2021
S. S. Goonewardene et al., *Management of Muscle Invasive Bladder Cancer*,
Management of Urology, https://doi.org/10.1007/978-3-030-57915-9_12

Ordell Sundelin investigated asymptomatic microscopic haematuria, and if this was predictive of urinary tract cancer [5]. In total, 1305 patients (492 males and 813 females) were included [5]. Eleven patients (0.8%) were diagnosed with cancer, including non-invasive Ta bladder cancer (n = 6), invasive bladder cancer (n = 2) and carcinoma in situ (n = 1) [5]. None of the patients had renal cancer or upper urinary tract tumours as the final diagnosis [5].

Diagnosis is dependent on investigation of symptoms, most commonly visible haematuria [6].

Non-visible haematuria was associated with bladder cancer: odds ratio (OR) 20 (95% confidence interval [CI] = 12–33) [6]. The PPV of non-visible haematuria was 1.6% (95% CI = 1.2–2.1) in those aged ≥60 years and 0.8% (95% CI = 0.1–5.6) in 40–59-year-olds [6]. The PPV of visible haematuria was 2.8% (95% CI = 2.5–3.1) and 1.2% (95% CI = 0.6–2.3) for the same age groups respectively [6]. Both non-visible and visible haematuria are associated with bladder cancer. Visible haematuria confers nearly twice the risk of cancer compared with the non-visible form [6].

Bladder cancer can also present as perineal pain and priapism [7]. This has been treated with radiotherapy to the whole penis. This gives rapid clinical benefit and persistent control of the disease [7]. Penile metastases are very rare. No consensus exists on treatment, but radiotherapy is a promising treatment to palliate pain and control the disease [7].

Bladder cancer can present as LUTS, but this was thought to be low [8]. Dobbs evaluated the prevalence and clinical characteristics and LUTS in the absence of gross or microscopic haematuria in bladder cancer diagnostics [8]. 4.1% (14/340) presented solely with LUTS [8]. Of the 14 patients presenting with LUTS, 9 (64.3%), 4 (28.6%), and 1 (7.1%) presented with clinical stage Ta, carcinoma in Situ (CIS), and T2 disease [8]. Recurrence occurred in 7 (50.0%), with progression occurring in 1 (7.1%). Eleven (78.6%) are alive and currently disease free, and 3 (21.4%) had died, with only 1 (7.1%) death attributable to bladder cancer [8].

12.2   Diagnosis and Assessment in Bladder Cancer

Bladder cancer most commonly presents with asymptomatic haematuria, leading to diagnostics-cystoscopy, renal function testing, and upper urinary tract imaging. This should occur in adults 45 years and older and in those with irritative voiding symptoms, risk factors for bladder cancer, or gross haematuria [9]. Transurethral resection of the bladder tumour allows for definitive diagnosis, staging, and primary treatment [9]. Non-muscle-invasive disease is treated with transurethral resection. This can be followed by intravesical bacille Calmette-Guérin or intravesical chemotherapy [9]. Bladder cancer with muscle invasion is treated with radical cystectomy and neoadjuvant chemotherapy due to higher rates of progression and recurrence [9].

Five percent of asymptomatic microscopic haematuria will have tumour present [10]. Persistent microscopic haematuria with urinary tract infection requires investigation [10]. The upper urinary tract is best evaluated with multiphasic computed tomography urography, to identify renal and ureteral lesions [10]. The lower urinary tract is assessed cystoscopy for urethral stricture disease, benign prostatic hyperplasia, and bladder cancer [10]. Voided urine cytology is no longer recommended as part of the routine evaluation of asymptomatic microscopic haematuria, unless there are risk factors for malignancy [10].

Viswanath assessed routine urine cytology in primary evaluation at a one-stop haematuria clinic [11]. Overall, 986 samples of urine were sent for cytology [11]. In 126 patients, the report was abnormal; of these 71 were found to have bladder transitional cell carcinoma by flexible cystoscopy and 3 had upper tract transitional cell carcinoma diagnosed radiologically [11]. The remaining 52 patients with abnormal cytology were not found to have cancer on further investigations.

12.3   The Role of Haematuria Clinics in Bladder Cancer

Elmussareh reviewed haematuria referrals to evaluate the pattern of referrals and the cancer detection rates [12]. The study included 1577 patients [12]. Of these, 56.4% had visible haematuria (VH) and 43.6% had non-visible haematuria (NVH). In total, 228 malignancies were detected (14.5% cancer detection rate) [12]. Overall, 11.2% had bladder cancer, 1.8% renal cancer and 0.4% upper tract transitional cell carcinoma [12]. In the VH group, 205 malignancies were detected (23% cancer detection rate) [12]. The detection rate was higher for asymptomatic VH (24.6%) than for those with symptomatic VH (15.4%) [12]. The cancer detection rate for symptomatic NVH was 9.1% [12]. For asymptomatic NVH, the cancer detection rate was only 1.5% [12]. The overall cancer detection rate of 14.5%, and 23% for VH is an important validation of previous studies [12]. A cancer detection rate of greater than 30% was present in VH over 70 years old [12].

McCombie examined delays in diagnosis and initial treatment of patients with bladder cancer [13]. Of 1365 attendances, 151 were diagnosed with a bladder tumour [13]. For visible haematuria the median (range) waiting time from initial bleeding to surgery was 69.5 (9–1165) days [13]. Reasons for prolonged waiting times included poor public awareness, patient fear and anxiety, delayed and non-referral from primary care, administrative delays, and resource limitations [13]. Many patients experience significant delays in the diagnosis and treatment of their bladder cancer [13].

Sapre, report the outcomes of the first 3 years of a dedicated haematuria clinic [14]. A total of 643 patients were seen with non-visible (170, 26%) and visible haematuria (463, 72%) [14]. Sixty-five (10%) were diagnosed with urothelial carcinoma. Sixty-three percent had lower tract disease [14]. Forty-eight percent of the bladder urothelial carcinomas were invasive or high-grade [14]. Moving towards a 'one-stop' approach are helping to further decrease the number of patients requiring a second clinic visit [14].

Nilbert assessed a national healthcare intervention to reduce the time between diagnosis and treatment of urinary tract malignancy [15]. Bladder cancer was the most common malignant diagnosis (83%) [15]. Cancers were diagnosed in 23% of males and 13% of females and showed a strong correlation with age: cancer diagnosis in 2% aged <50 years and in 44% aged ≥90 years [15]. Results were affected by bacteriuria but not by anticoagulant medication, with 12%/22% and 19%/19% cancer detection, respectively [15]. The standardized care pathway shortened the diagnostic delay to a median of 25 days compared to 35 days for regular referral (p = 0.01) [15].

12.4   Bladder Cancer Screening

No major organization recommends screening asymptomatic adults for bladder cancer, and the U.S. Preventive Services Task Force concluded that current evidence is insufficient to assess the balance of benefits and harms of screening. No major organization recommends screening asymptomatic adults for bladder cancer [9].

12.5   Biomarkers in Bladder Cancer Diagnostics

Precision medicine can improve management by guiding therapy based on molecular characteristics [16]. In bladder cancer, application of biomarkers appears especially promising [16]. The high heterogeneity and recurrence rates, suggest precise intervention, continuous monitoring, and the development of alternative treatment could be accomplished by proteomics-guided personalized approaches [16]. This notion is backed by studies presenting biomarkers that are of value in patient stratification and prognosis, and by recent studies demonstrating the identification of promising therapeutic targets [16].

With a lack of disease-specific symptoms, diagnosis and follow-up of bladder cancer has remained a challenge [17]. Numerous molecular assays for diagnostics have been developed and assessed regarding clinical use [17]. These assays have superior sensitivity compared to urine cytology, yet none are included in clinical guidelines [17]. The reason for this is lack of incorporation into clinical decision-making so far [17]. Current data suggest that some markers may have a role in screening and surveillance [17].

O'Sullivan investigated whether the RNA assay uRNA® and its derivative Cxbladder® has greater sensitivity for the detection of bladder cancer than cytology, NMP22™ BladderChek™ and NMP22™ ELISA, and the role in risk stratification [18]. uRNA detected 41 of 66 urothelial carcinoma cases (62.1% sensitivity, 95% CI 49.3–73.8) compared with NMP22 ELISA (50.0%, 95% CI 37.4–62.6), BladderChek (37.9%, 95% CI 26.2–50.7) and cytology (56.1%, 95% CI 43.8–68.3) [18]. Cxbladder, which was developed on the study data, detected 82%, including 97% of the high-grade tumours and 100% of tumours stage 1 or greater [18]. The cutoffs for uRNA and Cxbladder were prespecified to give a specificity of 85% [18]. The specificity of cytology was 94.5% (95% CI 91.9–96.5), NMP22 ELISA 88.0%, (95% CI 84.6–91.0) and BladderChek 96.4% (95% CI 94.2–98.0) [18]. Cxbladder distinguished between low grade Ta tumours and other detected urothelial carcinoma with a sensitivity of 91% and a specificity of 90% [18].

12.6   Guidelines and Diagnostics in Bladder Cancer

Karl determined the adherence to guideline recommendations, performing a large retrospective database analysis [19]. There was a significant trend over the years to a higher use of cytologic analysis, standard urinalysis, and CT/MRI [19]. A significant trend toward a lower rate of IVP and a stable use of RPG was observed [19]. Despite published recommendations on the initial investigations, less than half received all the factors required for an initial diagnosis of bladder cancer [19]. Greater adherence to recommendations may ensure best treatment and outcomes [19]. Appropriate treatment is critical to patient outcomes, because evidence-based therapeutic management can be practiced only if an accurate assessment of the disease takes place at the time of initial diagnosis [19].

In 2007 the World Cancer Research Fund (WCRF) and the American Institute of Cancer Research (AICR) issued 8 recommendations (plus 2 special recommendations) on diet, physical activity, and weight management for cancer prevention on the basis of the most comprehensive collection of available evidence [20]. Concordance with WCRF/AICR recommendations demonstrated the score was significantly associated with decreased risk of cancer [20]. Adherence to the WCRF/AICR recommendations for cancer prevention may lower the risk of developing most types of cancer.

12.7   Diagnostic Imaging in Bladder Cancer

Trinh determine test characteristics of CT urography for detecting bladder cancer in patients with haematuria and those undergoing surveillance, and to analyze reasons for false-positive and false-negative results [21]. Ninety-five bladder cancers were detected. CT urography accuracy: was 91.5% (650/710), sensitivity 86.3% (82/95), specificity 92.4% (568/615), positive predictive value 63.6% (82/129), and negative predictive value was 97.8% (568/581) [21]. Of 43 false positives, the majority of interpretation errors were due to benign prostatic hyperplasia (n = 12), trabeculated bladder (n = 9), and treatment changes (n = 8) [21]. CT urography is an accurate test for diagnosing bladder cancer; however, in protocols relying predominantly on excretory phase images, overall sensitivity remains insufficient to obviate cystoscopy [21]. Awareness of bladder cancer mimics may reduce false-positive results [21].

Gandrup compared split-bolus computed tomography urography (CTU), magnetic resonance urography (MRU) and flexible cystoscopy in patients with macroscopic haematuria regarding the diagnosis of bladder tumours [22]. At flexible cystoscopy, MRU and CTU, 32, 19 and 15 bladder lesions were identified, respectively [22]. Histopathology showed that 13 of the 29 biopsied lesions were transitional cell carcinomas [22]. Compared with the histopathology, the sensitivity and specificity for detection of tumours by CTU and MRU were 61.5% and 94.9%, and 79.9% and 93.4%, respectively [22]. False-positive detection of bladder tumours, compared with histopathology, was reported in seven CTUs and nine MRUs, whereas the number of false-negative findings was five for CTUs and three for MRUs [22].

Blick evaluated the diagnostic accuracy of CT urography in patients with visible haematuria aged >40 years and to determine if CT urography has a role for diagnosing bladder cancer [23].

The prevalence of bladder cancer in the clinical cohort was 20% (156/778). For the diagnostic strategy using CT urography sensitivity was 1.0 (95% confidence interval [CI] 0.98–1.00), specificity was 0.94 (95% CI 0.91–0.95), the positive predictive value (PPV) was 0.80 (95% CI 0.73–0.85) and the negative predictive value (NPV) was 1.0 (95% CI 0.99–1.00) [23]. For the diagnostic strategy using CT urography as a replacement test for flexible cystoscopy sensitivity was 0.95 (95% CI 0.90–0.97), specificity was 0.83 (95% CI 0.80–0.86), the PPV was 0.58 (95% CI 0.52–0.64), and the NPV was 0.98 (95% CI 0.97–0.99) [23]. Similarly using flexible cystoscopy for diagnosing bladder cancer sensitivity was 0.98 (95% CI 0.94–0.99), specificity was 0.94 (95% CI 0.92–0.96), the PPV was 0.80 (95% CI 0.73–0.85) and the NPV was 0.99 (95% CI 0.99–1.0) [23]. There is a clear advantage for the diagnostic strategy using CT urography and flexible cystoscopy as a triage test for rigid cystoscopy and follow-up.

Gross and microscopic haematuria both are a common cause of referral for primary diagnosis of bladder cancer [24]. Ahmed conducted a study to assess and compare the findings and diagnostic competency of transabdominal ultrasonography (US) versus cystourethroscopy for haematuria of lower urinary tract origin [24]. One hundred and nine patients were studied [24]. Fifty-four patients (49.5%) presented with macroscopic haematuria, while 55 patients presented with microscopic haematuria [24]. The sensitivity and specificity of US in detecting prostate enlargement, vesical stones, bladder wall tumour, cystitis and schistosomiasis were [(84, 80%); (82.6, 97.7%); (64.7, 92.1%); (15.3, 96.8%); and (15.3, 98.9%)], respectively, as compared to cystoscopic diagnosis as the gold standard [24].

12.8   Novel Methods for Diagnosis of Bladder Cancer

Although haematuria (blood in urine) is the most common symptom of bladder cancer, 70–98% of haematuria cases are benign [25]. These haematuria patients unnecessarily undergo costly, invasive, and expensive evaluation for bladder cancer [25]. Therefore, there remains a need for non-invasive office-based tests that can rapidly and reliably rule out bladder cancer in patients undergoing haematuria evaluation [25]. Herein, a clinical assay for matrix metalloproteinases ("Ammps") is presented, which generates a visual signal based on the collagenase activity (in urine of patients) on the Ammps substrates [25]. Ammps substrates are generated by crosslinking gelatin with Fe(II) chelated alginate nanoparticles, which precipitate in urine samples [25]. The cleavage of gelatin-conjugated alginate (Fe(II)) nanoparticles by collagenases generates free-floating alginate (Fe(II)) nanoparticles that participate in Fenton's reaction to generate a visual signal [25]. In a pilot study of 88 patients, Ammps had 100% sensitivity, 85% specificity, and a negative predictive value (NPV) of 100% for diagnosing bladder cancer [25]. This high NPV can be useful in ruling out bladder cancer in patients referred for haematuria evaluation [25].

Wang determined the clinical bladder cancer-specific antigen-1 (BLCA-1) in the diagnosis of bladder cancer (BC) [26]. Urine BLCA-1 levels in BC patients were significantly higher than that found in healthy controls (p < 0.01) [26]. BLCA-1 levels in the urine of patients without mucus membrane invasion (Ta) were significantly different from urine levels found in patients with mucus membrane invasion (T1–T4; p = 0.022). BLCA-1 levels in the serum of patients without muscular coat invasion (Ta–T1) were significantly different than serum levels of patients with muscular coat invasion (T2–T4; p = 0.042) [26]. Clinical detection of serum and urine BLCA-1 protein levels showed a high level of sensitivity and specificity in diagnosing BC [26].

12.9   Gender Discrepancies in Bladder Cancer Diagnostics

The incidence of bladder cancer is three to four times greater in men than in women [27]. However, women are diagnosed with more advanced disease at presentation and have less favourable outcomes after treatment [27]. It has been shown that the gender difference in bladder cancer incidence is independent of differences in exposure risk, including smoking status [27]. Importantly, gender differences exist in the timeliness and completeness of haematuria evaluation, with women experiencing a significantly greater delay in urologic referral and undergoing guideline-concordant imaging less frequently [27]. Correspondingly, women have more advanced tumours at the time of bladder cancer diagnosis. Interestingly, higher cancer-specific mortality has been noted among women even after adjusting for tumour stage and treatment modality [27].

Men are diagnosed with bladder cancer at three times the rate of women [28]. However, women present with advanced disease and have poorer survival, suggesting delays in bladder cancer diagnosis [28]. Haematuria is the presenting symptom in most cases. Garg assessed gender differences in haematuria evaluation in older adults with bladder cancer [28]. Of 35,646 patients with a haematuria claim in the year preceding bladder cancer diagnosis 97% had a urology visit claim [28]. Mean time to urology visit was 27 days (range 0–377). Time to urology visit was longer for women than for men (adjusted HR 0.9, 95% CI 0.87–0.92) [28]. Women were more likely to undergo delayed (after greater than 30 days) haematuria evaluation (adjusted OR 1.13, 95% CI 1.07–1.21) [28]. These findings may explain stage differences in bladder cancer diagnosis and inform efforts to decrease gender disparities in bladder cancer stage and outcomes [28].

Han assessed geographic variation in cystoscopy rates among women vs. men with suspected bladder cancer, lending insight into gender-specific differences in cystoscopic evaluation [29].

Overall, 173,551 women (n = 14.8 million) and 286,090 men (n = 11.5 million) underwent cystoscopy in 2014. While women received less cystoscopies compared to men (mean 11.0 vs. 23.5 per 1000, p < 0.001), there was greater variation in cystoscopy rates among women (coefficient of variation 27.5 vs. 23.5, p = 0.010) [29]. When restricting to ICD-9 codes for haematuria only, women continued to demonstrate greater variation in cystoscopy rates (coefficient of variation 27.8 vs. 24.2, p = 0.022) [29].

References

1. Tsao CK, Liaw BC, Oh WK, Galsky MD. Muscle invasive bladder cancer: closing the gap between practice and evidence. Minerva Urol Nefrol. 2015;67(1):65–73.
2. King K, Steggall M. Haematuria: from identification to treatment. Br J Nurs. 2014;23(9):S28–32.
3. Ramirez D, Gupta A, Canter D, Harrow B, Dobbs RW, Kucherov V, Mueller E, Streeper N, Uhlman MA, Svatek RS, Messing EM, Lotan Y. Microscopic haematuria at time of diagnosis is associated with lower disease stage in patients with newly diagnosed bladder cancer. BJU Int. 2016;117(5):783–6.
4. Cha EK, Tirsar LA, Schwentner C, Hennenlotter J, Christos PJ, Stenzl A, Mian C, Martini T, Pycha A, Shariat SF, Schmitz-Dräger BJ. Accurate risk assessment of patients with asymptomatic hematuria for the presence of bladder cancer. World J Urol. 2012;30(6):847–52.
5. Ordell Sundelin M, Jensen JB. Asymptomatic microscopic hematuria as a predictor of neoplasia in the urinary tract. Scand J Urol. 2017;51(5):373–5.
6. Price SJ, Shephard EA, Stapley SA, Barraclough K, Hamilton WT. Non-visible versus visible haematuria and bladder cancer risk: a study of electronic records in primary care. Br J Gen Pract. 2014;64(626):e584–9.
7. Galot R, Christian N, Bitar M, Seront E. Unusual presentation of bladder cancer resurgence and efficacy of radiotherapy. BMJ Case Rep. 2016;2016:bcr2015213538.
8. Dobbs RW, Hugar LA, Revenig LM, Al-Qassab S, Petros JA, Ritenour CW, Issa MM, Canter DJ. Incidence and clinical characteristics of lower urinary tract symptoms as a presenting symptom for patients with newly diagnosed bladder cancer. Int Braz J Urol. 2014;40(2):198–203.
9. DeGeorge KC, Holt HR, Hodges SC. Bladder cancer: diagnosis and treatment. Am Fam Physician. 2017;96(8):507–14.
10. Sharp VJ, Barnes KT, Erickson BA. Assessment of asymptomatic microscopic hematuria in adults. Am Fam Physician. 2013;88(11):747–54.
11. Viswanath S, Zelhof B, Ho E, Sethia K, Mills R. Is routine urine cytology useful in the haematuria clinic? Ann R Coll Surg Engl. 2008;90(2):153–5.
12. Elmussareh M, Young M, Ordell Sundelin M, Bak-Ipsen CB, Graumann O, Jensen JB. Outcomes of haematuria referrals: two-year data from a single large university hospital in Denmark. Scand J Urol. 2017;51(4):282–9.
13. McCombie SP, Bangash HK, Kuan M, Thyer I, Lee F, Hayne D. Delays in the diagnosis and initial treatment of bladder cancer in Western Australia. BJU Int. 2017;120(Suppl 3):28–34.
14. Sapre N, Hayes E, Bugeja P, Corcoran NM, Costello AJ, Anderson PD. Streamlining the assessment of haematuria: 3-year outcomes of a dedicated haematuria clinic. ANZ J Surg. 2015;85(5):334–8.
15. Nilbert M, Bläckberg M, Ceberg J, Hagberg O, Stenhoff R, Liedberg F. Diagnostic pathway efficacy for urinary tract cancer: population-based outcome of standardized evaluation for macroscopic haematuria. Scand J Urol. 2018;52(4):237–43.
16. Latosinska A, Frantzi M, Vlahou A, Merseburger AS, Mischak H. Clinical proteomics for precision medicine: the bladder cancer case. Proteomics Clin Appl. 2018;12(2).
17. Schmitz-Dräger BJ, Droller M, Lokeshwar VB, Lotan Y, Hudson MA, van Rhijn BW, Marberger MJ, Fradet Y, Hemstreet GP, Malmstrom PU, Ogawa O, Karakiewicz PI, Shariat SF. Molecular markers for bladder cancer screening, early diagnosis, and surveillance: the WHO/ICUD consensus. Urol Int. 2015;94(1):1–24.

18. O'Sullivan P, Sharples K, Dalphin M, Davidson P, Gilling P, Cambridge L, Harvey J, Toro T, Giles N, Luxmanan C, Alves CF, Yoon HS, Hinder V, Masters J, Kennedy-Smith A, Beaven T, Guilford PJ. A multigene urine test for the detection and stratification of bladder cancer in patients presenting with hematuria. J Urol. 2012;188(3):741–7.

19. Karl A, Adejoro O, Saigal C, Konety B, Urologic Diseases in America Project. General adherence to guideline recommendations on initial diagnosis of bladder cancer in the United States and influencing factors. Clin Genitourin Cancer. 2014;12(4):270–7.

20. Romaguera D, Vergnaud AC, Peeters PH, van Gils CH, Chan DS, Ferrari P, Romieu I, Jenab M, Slimani N, Clavel-Chapelon F, Fagherazzi G, Perquier F, Kaaks R, Teucher B, Boeing H, von Rüsten A, Tjønneland A, Olsen A, Dahm CC, Overvad K, Quirós JR, Gonzalez CA, Sánchez MJ, Navarro C, Barricarte A, Dorronsoro M, Khaw KT, Wareham NJ, Crowe FL, Key TJ, Trichopoulou A, Lagiou P, Bamia C, Masala G, Vineis P, Tumino R, Sieri S, Panico S, May AM, Bueno-de-Mesquita HB, Büchner FL, Wirfält E, Manjer J, Johansson I, Hallmans G, Skeie G, Benjaminsen Borch K, Parr CL, Riboli E, Norat T. Is concordance with World Cancer Research Fund/American Institute for Cancer Research guidelines for cancer prevention related to subsequent risk of cancer? Results from the EPIC study. Am J Clin Nutr. 2012;96(1):150–63.

21. Trinh TW, Glazer DI, Sadow CA, Sahni VA, Geller NL, Silverman SG. Bladder cancer diagnosis with CT urography: test characteristics and reasons for false-positive and false-negative results. Abdom Radiol (NY). 2018;43(3):663–71.

22. Gandrup KL, Løgager VB, Bretlau T, Nordling J, Thomsen HS. Diagnosis of bladder tumours in patients with macroscopic haematuria: a prospective comparison of split-bolus computed tomography urography, magnetic resonance urography and flexible cystoscopy. Scand J Urol. 2015;49(3):224–9.

23. Blick CG, Nazir SA, Mallett S, Turney BW, Onwu NN, Roberts IS, Crew JP, Cowan NC. Evaluation of diagnostic strategies for bladder cancer using computed tomography (CT) urography, flexible cystoscopy and voided urine cytology: results for 778 patients from a hospital haematuria clinic. BJU Int. 2012;110(1):84–94.

24. Ahmed FO, Hamdan HZ, Abdelgalil HB, Sharfi AA. A comparison between transabdominal ultrasonographic and cystourethroscopy findings in adult Sudanese patients presenting with haematuria. Int Urol Nephrol. 2015;47(2):223–8.

25. Acharya AP, Theisen KM, Correa A, Meyyappan T, Apfel A, Sun T, Tarin TV, Little SR. An inexpensive, point-of-care urine test for bladder cancer in patients undergoing hematuria evaluation. Adv Healthc Mater. 2017;6(22).

26. Wang Z, Li H, Chi Q, Qiu Y, Li X, Xin L. Clinical significance of serological and urological levels of bladder cancer-specific antigen-1 (BLCA-1) in bladder cancer. Med Sci Monit. 2018;24:3882–7.

27. Dobruch J, Daneshmand S, Fisch M, Lotan Y, Noon AP, Resnick MJ, Shariat SF, Zlotta AR, Boorjian SA. Gender and bladder cancer: a collaborative review of etiology, biology, and outcomes. Eur Urol. 2016;69(2):300–10.

28. Garg T, Pinheiro LC, Atoria CL, Donat SM, Weissman JS, Herr HW, Elkin EB. Gender disparities in hematuria evaluation and bladder cancer diagnosis: a population-based analysis. J Urol. 2014;192(4):1072–7.

29. Han DS, Zhou W, Seigne JD, Lynch KE, Schroeck FR. Geographic variation in cystoscopy rates for suspected bladder cancer between female and male Medicare beneficiaries. Urology. 2018;122:83–8.

Bladder Cancer Screening

13

A systematic review relating to bladder cancer screening was conducted. The search strategy aimed to identify all references related to bladder cancer AND screening. Search terms used were as follows: (Bladder cancer) AND (Screening). The following databases were screened from 1989 to June 2020:

- CINAHL
- MEDLINE (NHS Evidence)
- Cochrane
- AMed
- EMBASE
- PsychINFO
- SCOPUS
- Web of Science.

In addition, searches using Medical Subject Headings (MeSH) and keywords were conducted using Cochrane databases. Two UK-based experts in bladder cancer were consulted to identify any additional studies.

Studies were eligible for inclusion if they reported primary research focusing on bladder cancer and screening. Papers were included if published after 1984 and had to be in English. Studies that did not conform to this were excluded. Only primary research was included (Fig. 13.1). The overall aim was to identify bladder cancer risk factors and epidemiology in muscle invasive disease.

Abstracts were independently screened for eligibility by two reviewers and disagreements resolved through discussion or third party opinion. Agreement level was calculated using Cohen's Kappa to test the intercoder reliability of this screening process . Cohens' Kappa allows comparison of inter-rater reliability between papers using relative observed agreement. This also takes account of the comparison occurring by chance. The first reviewer agreed all 40 papers to be included, the second, agreed on 40. Cohens kappa was therefore 1.0.

© The Editor(s) (if applicable) and The Author(s), under exclusive license to
Springer Nature Switzerland AG 2021
S. S. Goonewardene et al., *Management of Muscle Invasive Bladder Cancer*,
Management of Urology, https://doi.org/10.1007/978-3-030-57915-9_13

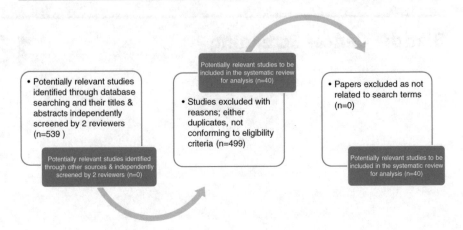

Fig. 13.1 Flow chart of studies identified through the systematic review. (Adapted from PRISMA)

Data extraction was piloted by the researcher and amended in consultation with the research team (author and two academic supervisors). Data collected included authors, year and country of publication, study aims, setting, intervention aims, number of participants, study design, intervention components and delivery methods, comparison groups and outcome measures, notes and follow-up questions for the authors. Studies were quality assessed using the PRISMA criteria for randomised controlled trials, Mays et al. [1, 2] for the action research and qualitative studies and the Critical Skills Appraisal programme for cohort studies. This was also applied to randomised controlled trials and qualitative studies.

The search identified 539 papers (Fig. 13.1). All 40 mapped to the search terms and eligibility criteria. The current systematic reviews were examined to gain further knowledge about the subject. Three hundred and ninety papers were excluded due to not conforming to eligibility criteria or adding to the evidence. Of the 40 papers left, relevant abstracts were identified and the full papers obtained (all of which were in English), to quality assure against search criteria. There was considerable heterogeneity of design among the included studies therefore a narrative review of the evidence was undertaken. There was significant heterogeneity within studies, including clinical topic, numbers, outcomes, as a result a narrative review was thought to be best. There were 34 cohort studies, with a moderate level of evidence, and 6 trials with a good level of evidence. These were from a range of countries with minimal loss to follow-up. All participants were identified appropriately.

13.1   Systematic Review Results

13.1.1 Urinary Metabolomes in Bladder Cancer Screening

Loras examined changes in the urinary metabolome of bladder cancer before and after TURBT and during surveillance [3]. Analysis of metabolic profiles, displayed negative predictive values for low, low-intermediate, high-intermediate and high risk groups of 96.5%, 94.0%, 92.9% and 76.1% respectively [3]. Detailed analysis revealed several candidate metabolites—phenylalanine, arginine, proline and tryptophan metabolisms emerged as potential biomarkers [3]. These results give strong support for the clinical use of metabolomic profiling in assessing bladder cancer recurrence [3].

13.1.2 CellDetect in Bladder Cancer Screening

Davis validated the performance of this assay in a controlled, blinded, multicenter study [4]. Two hundred and seventeen voided urine specimens were included [4]. Ninety-six (44%) were positive by histology and 121 (56%) were negative by either cystoscopy or histology [4]. The overall sensitivity of CellDetect was 84% [4]. The sensitivity for low-grade nonmuscle-invasive bladder cancer tumors was greater than this of BTA stat (78% vs. 54%), more than twofold higher compared with standard cytology (33%, $p \leq 0.05$) [4]. The specificity was 84% in routine surveillance by cystoscopy [4]. At 9 months, 21% were positive CellDetect and negative reference standard developed UCC, which was significantly higher compared with the 5% of the true negative cases [4].

13.1.3 Blue Light Flexible Cystoscopy

Daneshmand compared blue and white light flexible cystoscopy for the detection of bladder cancer during surveillance [5]. Following surveillance 103 of the 304 patients were referred, 63 with confirmed malignancy, 26 with carcinoma in situ [5]. In 13 patients (20.6%, 95% CI 11.5–32.7) recurrence was seen only with blue light flexible cystoscopy ($p < 0.0001$) [5]. Five were confirmed as carcinoma in situ [5]. Operating room assessment confirmed carcinoma in situ in 26 of 63 patients (41%), which was detected only with blue light cystoscopy in 9 of the 26 (34.6%, 95% CI 17.2–55.7, $p < 0.0001$) [5]. Blue light cystoscopy identified additional malignant lesions in 29 of the 63 patients (46%) [5]. The false-positive rate was 9.1% for white and blue light cystoscopy [5].

Nakai confirmed effectiveness in photodynamic diagnosis of bladder cancer using 5-aminolevulinic acid as part of a prospective multicenter non-randomized phase III trial [6]. The sensitivity of the fluorescent light source (79.6%) was significantly higher ($p < 0.001$) than white light source (54.1%) [6]. In total, 25.4% (46/181) of specimens were diagnosed as positive with only the fluorescent light source [6]. In 9 (15%) of 60 patients, the risk classification and treatment after TURBT were changed depending on the additional types of tumour diagnosed by the fluorescent light source [6]. The specificity of the fluorescent light versus white light source was 80.6% versus 95.5%. No grade 4 or 5 adverse events were noted [6]. Hypotension and urticaria were severe adverse events whose relationship to oral 5-aminolevulinic acid could not be excluded [6].

Smith evaluated blue-light flexible cystoscopy (BLFC) in surveillance for bladder cancer with a high risk of recurrence [7]. A total of 304 patients were enrolled, 103 were referred for investigation [7]. Sixty-three were found to have histologically confirmed malignancy [7]. Pain levels were low, anxiety levels decreased after BLFC ($\Delta = -2.6$), with a greater decrease in negative pathology results (p = 0.051) [7]. No differences in anxiety were noted or test performance (true-positive/false-positive) [7]. Most patients found BLFC 'worthwhile' (94%), would 'do it again' (94%) and 'would recommend it to others' (91%), with no differences based on BLFC results or test performance [7].

Inoue examined the utility and safety of photodynamic diagnosis (PDD) after oral administration of 5-aminolevulinic acid (5-ALA) (ALA-PDD) in bladder cancer [8]. Regarding safety, the adverse drug reactions were observed as grade 1 pruritus in 1 patient (0.6%) [8]. Efficacy, specificity and positive predictability were lower than a WL-source, sensitivity was higher with FL-source than WL-source [8]. The proportion of tumours detected only by FL-cystoscopy was greater than the proportion of patients with tumours detected only by conventional WL-cystoscopy [8]. Moreover, not only sensitivity, but also the proportion of patients with tumours detected only by FL-cystoscopy, was highest among patients who received 5-ALA at $\geq$20 mg/kg/body [8].

Daniltchenko conducted a prospective randomized trial comparing bladder tumour resection (TUR) under standard white light versus ALA induced fluorescence were evaluated [9]. Median time to recurrence was 5 months in the standard and 12 months in the ALA group. Recurrence-free survival was 25% in the standard group versus, 41% in the ALA group. The recurrence rate at 2, 12, 36 and 60 months after initial TUR was 41%, 61%, 73% and 75%, and 16%, 43%, 59% and 59% in the white light and ALA groups, respectively. The total number of recurrences were 82 in the standard and 61 in the ALA group. Tumour progression occurred in 9 patients in the standard and 4 in the ALA group. Cost analysis suggests a considerable economical advantage of ALA fluorescence assisted TUR compared to the standard procedure.

Lapini evaluated hexaminolevulinate hydrochloride (Hexvix(®)) PDD cystoscopy compared with standard white light cystoscopy (WLC) [10]. Overall, 234 suspicious lesions were detected; 108 (46.2%) were histologically confirmed to be bladder tumours/carcinoma in situ (CIS) [10]. The sensitivity of BLC biopsies was significantly higher than for WLC technique (99.1% vs. 76.8%; p < 0.00001) [10]. The relative sensitivity of BLC versus WLC was 1.289, showing superiority of BLC of 28.9%. [10]. The specificity of BLC biopsies was not significantly different compared with WLC (36.5% vs. 30.2%) [10]. Positive predictive value for BLC- and WLC-guided biopsies was 54.9% and 50.9%, respectively [10]. Negative predictive value per biopsy for BLC- and WLC-guided biopsies was 97.4% and 64.8%, respectively. BLC and WLC had true positive rates of 97.9% and 88.5% respectively [10]. This difference was statistically significant (p = 0.0265) [10].

Grossman compared hexaminolevulinate fluorescence cystoscopy with white light cystoscopy for detecting Ta and T1 papillary lesions in patients with bladder cancer [11]. Non-invasive pTa tumours were found in 108 of 196 evaluable patients

(55.1%). In 31 patients (29%) at least 1 more tumour was detected by HAL than by white light cystoscopy (p < 0.05) [11]. Six had no lesions detected by white light, 12 had 1 lesion detected by white light and more than 1 by HAL, and 13 had multiple Ta lesions detected by the 2 methods [11]. At least 1 more tumour was detected by white light cystoscopy than by HAL cystoscopy in 10 patients (9%, 95% CI 5–16) [11]. Tumours invading the lamina propria (T1) were found in 20 patients (10.2%) [11]. At least 1 additional T1 tumour was detected by HAL but not by white light cystoscopy in 3 (15%). At least 1 more T1 tumour was detected by white light cystoscopy than by HAL cystoscopy in 1 patient (5%, 95% CI 0–25) [11]. Detection rates for Ta tumours were 95% for HAL cystoscopy and 83% for white light cystoscopy (p = 0.0001) [11]. Detection rates were 95% and 86%, respectively, for T1 tumours (p = 0.3) [11].

Palou assessed the sensitivity and specificity of blue-light cystoscopy (BLC) with hexaminolevulinate as an adjunct to white-light cystoscopy (WLC) vs. WLC alone [12]. In all, 1569 lesions were identified from 283 patients: 621 were tumour lesions according to histology and 948 were false-positives. Of the 621 tumour lesions, 475 were detected by WLC (sensitivity 76.5%, 95% confidence interval [CI] 73.2–79.8) and 579 were detected by BLC (sensitivity 93.2%, 95% CI 91.0–95.1; p < 0.001) [12]. There was a significant improvement in the sensitivity in the detection of all types of NMIBC lesions with BLC compared with WLC. Of 219 patients with tumours, 188 had NMIBC [highest grade: carcinoma in situ (CIS), n = 36; Ta, n = 87; T1, n = 65). CIS lesions were identified more with BLC (n = 27) than with WLC [n = 19; sensitivity: BLC 75.0% (95% CI 57.8–87.9) vs. WLC 52.8% (95% CI 35.5–69.6); p = 0.021]. Results varied across centres [12].

Photodynamic diagnosis (PDD) of non-muscle-invasive bladder cancer (NMIBC) following transurethral administration of a hexalated form of 5-aminolevulinic acid (5-ALA), 5-ALA hexyl ester, is widely performed in Western countries [13]. In this study, effectiveness and safety of the oral administration of 5-ALA is assessed in a phase II/III study of PDD for NMIBC in comparison to those of conventional white-light endoscopic diagnosis [13]. All 62 enrolled patients completed the clinical trial [13]. The sensitivities of PDD were higher (84.4% and 75.8% in the 10 and 20 mg/kg-groups, respectively) than those of conventional endoscopic diagnosis (67.5% and 47.6%, respectively) (p = 0.014 and p < 0.001, respectively) [13]. Five episodes of serious adverse events developed in four patients; whereas a causal relationship with the investigational agent was ruled out in all episodes [13].

Geavlete evaluate the impact of hexaminolevulinate blue-light cystoscopy and transurethral resection of bladder tumors (TURBT) upon the short-term recurrence rate in high-risk nonmuscle-invasive bladder cancer (NMIBC) compared with conventional cystoscopy and resection [14]. The proportions of CIS, pTaG3, and pT1 cases in the initial series were 13.1%, 5.7%, and 22.2% in the blue light series and 11.3%, 5.7%, and 23.3% in the white light series [14]. In total, 72 and 64 high-risk cases, respectively, were diagnosed in the blue- and white-light series [14]. The overall short-term recurrence rate at Re-TURBT was 11.1% for the blue-light group and 31.2% for the white-light group [14]. The recurrence rates were 4.3% versus 27.8% for CIS, 10% versus 22.2% for pTaG3, and 15.4% versus 35.1% for pT1 cases, in favor of the blue-light arm [14]. The recurrence rate in patients presenting with high-grade tumors was 17.2% in the blue-light group and 37% in the white-light group [14].

Denzinger performed a prospective, randomized trial to investigate whether the long-term tumor recurrence and residual tumor rates can be decreased using 5-ALA fluorescence diagnosis (FD) [15]. Of the 301 patients, 191 were available for the efficacy analysis [15]. The residual tumor rate was 25.2% in the WL arm versus 4.5% in the FD arm (p < 0.0001) [15]. The RFS rate after 2, 4, 6, and 8 years was 73%, 64%, 54%, and 45% in the WL group and 88%, 84%, 79%, and 71% in the FD group, respectively, revealing a statistically significant difference in favor of fluores-cent TUR (p = 0.0003) [15].

Jichlinski examined the sensitivity and specificity of Hexvix (PhotoCure ASA, Oslo, Norway) hexyl aminolevulinate (HAL) fluorescence cystoscopy in patients with superficial bladder cancer [16]. A total of 422 biopsies obtained in fluorescing (165) and nonfluorescing (257) areas, including 5 random biopsies per patient, were analyzed to provide the best reference for the calculation of sensitivity and specific-ity [16]. There were a total of 143 histologically verified tumors in 45 patients, including carcinoma in situ (CIS), Ta or T1 lesions [16]. A total of 43 patients were diagnosed by fluorescence cystoscopy compared with 33 diagnosed by white light for 96% and 73% per-patient sensitivity, respectively [16]. HAL cystoscopy was found particularly useful for finding CIS tumors. Of 13 patients with CIS tumors all except 1 were diagnosed or confirmed by HAL cystoscopy [16]. HAL cystoscopy was well tolerated with no definite drug related adverse events reported, including effects on standard blood parameters [16].

Witjes evaluated whether the technique of fluorescence cystoscopy with HAL was also feasible with a specially designed flexible fluorescence cystoscope (FFC) [17]. In these 20 patients (mean age 71 years (49–89), 3 females) mean HAL instil-lation time was 81 min [17]. Overall 27 histologically confirmed lesions were found in 19 patients [17]. Detection rates in these 19 patients were 14 with FFC, 17 with RFC and 15 with RWLC [17]. Of the 27 lesions 19 were detected with FFC, 23 with RFC and 20 with RWLC [17]. Overall fluorescence intensity using the flexible sys-tem was 76% (30–147%) as compared to RFC using a visual analogue score. No side effects were noted which were attributable to HAL [17].

Cheng determined whether fluorescence cystoscopy after intravesical adminis-tration of 5-aminolevulinic acid (5-ALA) is more sensitive in detection of dysplasia and bladder cancer when compared with conventional cystoscopy and determined the safety of using 5-ALA [18]. Among the 175 biopsies obtained, the sensitivity of the fluorescence cystoscopy was greater than that of conventional cystoscopy (89.1% vs. 65.6%, p < 0.05) [18]. Specificity was at 64.8% and 83.8% respectively with p < 0.05 [18]. Duration of ALA instillation did not seem to affect the sensitivity and specificity of photodynamic diagnosis [18]. The procedures were well tolerated by all patients with no additional complication.

Zaak investigated 5-aminolevulinic acid (5-ALA) induced fluorescence endos-copy (AFE) have promised a procedure with an outstanding sensitivity for the detection of early stage bladder cancer [19]. Two thousand four hundred seventy-five specimens were obtained (2.4 biopsies per AFE) [19]. In 552 AFEs (54.5%), neoplastic urothelial lesions were detected, in 34.2% only because of their positive fluorescence; 38.7% of these additionally detected neoplastic foci had poorly differentiated histologic features [19].

Filbeck performed a prospective, single institution, randomized trial to investigate whether the residual tumour rate and long-term tumour recurrence can be decreased by fluorescence diagnosis [20]. A total of 191 patients with superficial bladder carcinoma were available for efficacy analysis [20]. The residual tumor rate was 25.2% in the white light arm versus 4.5% in the fluorescence diagnosis arm (p < 0.0001) [20]. Median follow-up in the white light arm in 103 cases was 21.2 months (range 4–40) compared with 20.5 (range 3–40) in the 88 in the fluorescence diagnosis arm [20]. Recurrence-free survival in the fluorescence diagnosis group was 89.6% after 12 and 24 months compared with 73.8% and 65.9%, respectively, in the white light group (p = 0.004) [20]. This superiority proved to be independent of risk group [20]. The adjusted hazard ratio of fluorescence diagnosis versus white light transurethral resection was 0.33 (95% confidence interval 0.16–0.67) [20].

13.1.4   Bladder Epicheck in Bladder Cancer Screening

Witjes assessed the performance of Bladder Epicheck for bladder cancer recurrence [21]. This was a blinded, single-arm, prospective multicenter study [21]. Out of 440 patients recruited, 353 were eligible for analysis [21]. Overall sensitivity, specificity, NPV, and positive predictive value were 68.2%, 88.0%, 95.1%, and 44.8%, respectively [21]. Excluding low-grade (LG) Ta recurrences, the sensitivity was 91.7% and NPV was 99.3% [21]. The area under receiver operating characteristic (ROC) curves with and without LG Ta lesions was 0.82 and 0.94, respectively [21].

13.1.5   Urinary miRNA-96 in Bladder Cancer Diagnosis

Eissa explored the efficacy of urinary miRNA-96 as molecular marker in bladder cancer diagnosis and its relation to bilharziasis [22]. Urine cytology, serologic assessment of schistosomiasis and estimation of miRNA-96 by real-time PCR were carried out for 94 bladder cancer patients, 30 benign bladder lesions and 60 healthy individuals [22]. Expression of miRNA-96 showed a significant difference among the three tested groups and also between benign and malignant bilharzial cases [22]. Urinary miRNA-96 is a good noninvasive diagnostic biomarker for bladder cancer [22].

13.1.6   Urinary Cytology in Bladder Cancer Screening

Tan determined the diagnostic accuracy of urinary cytology to diagnose bladder cancer in haematuria [23]. Of the 3556 patients recruited, urine cytology was performed in 567 (15.9%) patients [23]. Bladder cancer was diagnosed in 39 (6.9%)

patients and UTUC in 8 (1.4%) patients [23]. The accuracy of urinary cytology was sensitivity 43.5%, specificity 95.7%, positive predictive value (PPV) 47.6% and negative predictive value (NPV) 94.9% [23]. A total of 21 bladder cancers and 5 UTUC were missed. Bladder cancers missed were: 4 (19%) were ≥pT2, 2 (9.5%) were G3 pT1, 10 (47.6%) were G3/2 pTa and 5 (23.8%) were G1 pTa [23]. High-risk cancer was confirmed in 8 (38%) patients. There was a small increase in sensitivity (57.7%) for high-risk cancers [23]. When urine cytology was combined with imaging, the diagnostic performance improved with CTU (sensitivity 90.2%, specificity 94.9%) superior to RBUS (sensitivity 66.7%, specificity 96.7%) [23]. False positive cytology results were confirmed in 22–12 (54.5%) had further invasive tests and 5 (22.7%) had a repeat cytology [23]. No cancer was identified in these.

13.1.7 Porphyrins as Urinary Biomarkers

Inoue et al. [24] evaluated the use of urine samples from bladder cancer patients as tumour biomarkers [24]. Almost all of the urinary porphyrin concentrations from bladder cancer were higher than patients with no pathology [24]. Moreover, 8 h after ALA administration, urinary UPI and CPI showed high sensitivity (100 for UPI and CPI) and specificity (96.4 for UPI and 91.4 for CPI) [24].

13.1.8 Quantitative mRNA Determination in Bladder Cancer Screening

March-Villalba studied the relationship between quantitative mRNA determination (hTERT) in bladder tumour, history of bladder tumour, and in patients with no history [25]. Differences were observed in mean $hTERT_N$ levels in each of the groups: tumour presence 21.33 ± 40.66, tumour history 2.16 ± 2.67, controls 0.9 ± 1, 75 (p < 0.001) [25]. In patients with tumour, there was no difference in mean $hTERT_N$ levels between the different grades and stages, although there was a tendency: low grade tumour 9.04 ± 16.95, high grade 28.95 ± 48.36 (p = .069), stage Ta 10.33 ± 19.39, T1 17.88 ± 27.14, T2 54.8 ± 74.05 (p = .056) [25]. In addition, the sensitivity of $hTERT_N$ was superior to that of other test (76%), although specificity and positive and negative predictive values were better for cytology (94%, 88.4% and 72.3% respectively) and NMP22 (88%, 80.6% and 73.3% respectively) [25].

13.1.9 Biomarkers in Bladder Cancer Screening

Bell analysed whether baseline C, ImmunoCyt (I), BTA Stat (B), haemoglobin dipstick (H), and NMP22 BladderChek (N) can predict recurrence and progression [26].On univariate analysis, C (HR 1.36; p = 0.26), I (HR 0.89; p = 0.66), B (HR 0.80; p = 0.42), H (HR 0.75; p = 0.30), and N (HR 0.82; p = 0.48) were not associated with recurrence-free survival (RFS). With regard to progression-free survival

(PFS), C was significantly prognostic (HR 2.67; p = 0.017), whereas I, B, H, and N were not [26]. On multivariable analysis, NMP22 was the only marker to be independently associated with RFS (HR 0.41, p < 0.01) and PFS (HR 0.32, p = 0.02) [26].

13.1.10 Cytokeratin 20 and IGF2 in Bladder Cancer Screening

Salomo assessed Cytokeratin 20 (CK20) and insulin-like growth factor 2 (IGF2) were assessed against voided urine cytology (VUC) [27]. Relative transcript levels were significantly elevated 3.4/11-fold for CK20 and 188/64-fold for IGF2 (p < 0.001) in urine sediments of bladder cancer patients compared to controls in the TC and VC, respectively [27]. In a combined analysis, the resulting sensitivity (SN) (SN_{TC}: 77.9%; SN_{VC}: 90.3%) and specificity (SP) (SP_{TC}: 88.0%; SP_{VC}: 84.0%) were similar to that of VUC [27]. The sensitivity of VUC in combination with CK20 and IGF2 was considerably increased (SN_{TC}: 94.6%; SN_{VC}: 93.2%) while specificity was reduced (SP_{TC}: 72.0%; SP_{VC}: 82.0%) compared to VUC alone in the test and validation cohort [27].

13.1.11 Angiogenin and Clusterin in Urinary Cytology in Bladder Cancer Screening

Shabayek evaluated angiogenin and clusterin in comparison and combination with voided urine cytology in bladder cancer screening [28]. This study includes malignant (bladder cancer patients, n = 50), benign (n = 20) and healthy (n = 20) groups [28]. All groups had cystoscopic examination, detection of bilharzial antibodies, urine cytology, and estimation of urinary angiogenin and clusterin by ELISA [28]. The overall sensitivity and specificity were 66% and 75% for angiogenin, 70% and 82.5% for clusterin and 46% and 80% for voided urine cytology [28]. Combined sensitivity of voided urine cytology with the two studied biomarkers was 88% which is higher than the combined sensitivity of both markers alone (82%) and that of the cytology with each marker (76% and 80%) for angiogenin and clusterin respectively [28].

13.1.12 Methylation and Line 1 in Bladder Cancer Screening

Andreotti examined the association between LINE1 total percent 5-methylcytosine and bladder cancer risk using pre-diagnostic blood DNA from Prostate, Lung, Colorectal, Ovarian Cancer Screening Trial (PLCO) (299 cases/676 controls), and the Alpha-Tocopherol, Beta-Carotene Cancer Prevention (ATBC) cohort of Finnish male smokers (391 cases/778 controls) [29]. In PLCO, higher, although non-significant, bladder cancer risks were observed in the highest three quartiles (Q2–Q4) compared with the lowest quartile (Q1) (OR = 1.36, 95% CI: 0.96–1.92) [29]. The association was stronger in males (Q2–Q4 vs. Q1 OR = 1.48, 95% CI:

1.00–2.20) and statistically significant among male smokers (Q2–Q4 vs. Q1 OR = 1.83, 95% CI: 1.14–2.95) [29]. No association was found among females or female smokers. Findings for male smokers were validated in ATBC (Q2–Q4 vs. Q1: OR = 2.31, 95% CI: 1.62–3.30) and a highly trend was observed (p = 8.7 × 10⁻⁷) [29]. These findings suggest that higher global methylation levels prior to diagnosis may increase bladder cancer risk, particularly among male smokers [29].

13.1.13   Metabolomic Urinary Profiles in Bladder Cancer Screening

Jin used high-performance liquid chromatography-quadrupole time-of-flight mass spectrometry (HPLC-QTOFMS) to profile urine metabolites of 138 with bladder cancer and 121 control subjects (69 healthy people and 52 patients with haematuria due to non-malignant diseases) [30]. Multivariate statistical analysis demonstrated bladder cancer could be clearly distinguished from the control groups on the basis of their metabolomic profiles [30]. Muscle invasive disease could be distinguished using metabolomic profiles [30]. Twelve differential metabolites were identified distinguishing between BC and control groups, and many were involved in glycolysis and betaoxidation [30]. This association was confirmed by microarray results showing that carnitine transferase and pyruvate dehydrogenase complex expressions are significantly altered in bladder cancer [30]. In terms of clinical applicability, the differentiation model diagnosed BC with a sensitivity and specificity of 91.3% and 92.5%, respectively. Comparable results were obtained by receiver operating characteristic analysis (AUC = 0.937) [30]. Multivariate regression also suggested that the metabolomic profile correlates with cancer-specific survival time [30].

13.1.14   Mitochondrial DNA in Bladder Cancer Screening

Guney investigated the Mitochondrial DNA (mtDNA) alterations in bladder cancer cases. Mitochondrial genes ATPase6, CytB, ND1, and D310 region were amplified by polymerase chain reaction and then sequenced. This study indicated that G8697A, G14905A, C15452A, and A15607G mutations are frequent in bladder cancers (p < 0.05). In addition, the incidence of A3480G, T4216C, T14798C, and G9055A mutations were higher in patients with bladder tumours [31].

13.1.15   Tyr-Phosphorylated Proteins in Bladder Cancer Screening

Khadjavi demonstrated that the levels of Tyr-phosphorylated proteins (TPPs) are highly increased in bladder cancer tissues and that soluble TPPs can also be detected in urine samples, then assessed levels in urine [32]. Due to their low abundance Tyr evidenced that both phosphoprotein enrichment step and very sensitive detection methods are required to detect TPPs in urine samples [32].

13.1.16   GC-Globulin in Bladder Cancer Screening

Li identified 16 proteins including Gc-globulin (GC) in urine from bladder cancer and normal controls by two-dimensional fluorescent differential gel electrophoresis (2D-DIGE) and matrix-assisted laser desorption time-of-flight mass spectrometry (MALDI-TOF/TOF MS) [33]. Bioinformatics analyses indicated GC played important roles in the regulation of growth, apoptosis, death and epidermal growth factor receptor activity [33]. ELISA quantification by correcting for creatinine expression showed GC-Cr was significantly increased in bladder cancer than in benign bladder damage cases and normal controls (1013.70 ± 851.25 versus 99.34 ± 55.87, 105.32 ± 47.81 ng/mg, respectively) [33]. Receiver operating characteristic (ROC) analysis suggested that at 161.086 ng/mg urinary GC, bladder cancer could be detected with 92.31% sensitivity and 83.02% specificity, and at 1407.481 ng/mg urinary GC with 82.61% sensitivity and 88.24% specificity [33]. Taken together, GC was identified as a potential novel urinary biomarker for the early detection and surveillance of bladder cancer.

13.1.17   Methylation Status with p16 and p14 in Bladder Cancer Screening

Kawamoto examined whether the methylation status of p16(INK4a) and p14(ARF), genes located upstream of the RB and p53 pathway, is a useful biomarker in bladder cancer [34]. Using methylation-specific PCR (MSP), Kawamoto examined the methylation status of p16(INK4a) and p14(ARF) in 64 samples from 45 bladder cancer patients (34 males, 11 females) [34]. The methylation rate for p16(INK4a) and p14(ARF) was 17.8% and 31.1%, respectively, in the 45 patients [34]. The incidence of p16(INKa) and p14(ARF) methylation was significantly higher in invasive ($\geq$pT2) than superficial bladder cancer (pT1) (p = 0.006 and p = 0.001, respectively) [34]. No MSP bands for p16(INK4a) and p14(ARF) were detected in superficial, non-recurrent tumours [34]. In 19 patients with tumour recurrence, the p16(INK4a) and p14(ARF) methylation status of the primary and recurrent tumours was similar [34]. Of the 22 patients who had undergone cystectomy, 8 (36.4%) manifested p16(INKa) methylation; p16(INK4a) was not methylated in 23 patients without cystectomy (p = 0.002) [34]. Kaplan-Meier analysis revealed that patients with p14(ARF) methylation had a significantly poorer prognosis than those without (p = 0.029) [34].

13.1.18   Urine Tumour Associated Trypsin Inhibitor

Gkialas assessed the value of urine tumour-associated trypsin inhibitor (TATI), CYFRA 21-1, which measures cytokeratin 19 fragment, and urinary bladder carcinoma antigen (UBC) in detection of high-grade bladder carcinoma [35]. The TATI measurements were significant greater in group 1 compared with groups 2 and 3. The overall sensitivity was 85.7% for TATI, 61.9% for CYFRA 21-1, 50% for UBC, and 42.8% for cytology. TATI was significantly more sensitive in Stage Ta (80%) than CYFRA 21-1 (32%), UBC (12%), and cytology (20%). TATI was also more sensitive compared with other tumour markers for Stage T1 but not for Stage T2 or T3 [35].

13.1.19   mRNA in Bladder Cancer Screening

Forty-four mRNA transcripts were monitored blindly in urine samples from 196 subjects with bladder cancer (89 with active BCa) using quantitative real-time PCR (RT-PCR) [36]. Statistical analyses defined associations of individual biomarkers with clinical data and the performance of predictive multivariate models was assessed using ROC curves [36]. The majority of the candidate mRNA targets were associated with BCa over other clinical variables [36]. Multivariate models identified an optimal 18-gene diagnostic signature that predicted BCa with a sensitivity of 85% and a specificity of 88% (AUC 0.935) [36]. Analysis of urinary mRNA signatures can provide valuable information on investigation for BCa [36]. Additional refinement and validation will allow development of accurate assays for the non-invasive detection and monitoring of BCa [36].

13.1.20   Urinary Basic Fetoprotein and BTA Test in Urinary Cytology

Imamura compared the results of urinary basic fetoprotein (BFP) and the BTA test with urinary cytology in bladder cancer [37]. The sensitivity of urinary BFP for Ta, 1 bladder cancer was significantly higher than urinary cytology ($p < 0.05$) [37]. The urinary cytology positive rate for Ta, T1 bladder cancer improved when combined with urinary BFP and the BTA test [37]. The urinary BFP positive rate for benign diseases was significantly higher in patients with pyuria than in patients without pyuria ($p < 0.05$) [37]. The BTA test positive rate for benign diseases was higher in pyuria without [37]. The urinary BFP and the BTA test positive rates for postoperative bladder cancer with no evidence of recurrence was significantly higher in urinary diversion than without (BFP: $p < 0.01$, BTA: $p < 0.05$) [37].

13.1.21   BTA Stat Test vs. NMP 22 vs. Urine Cytology

Gutiérrez Baños compared the sensitivity and specificity of the BTA stat test, NMP-22 and voided urine cytology in the diagnosis of bladder cancer [38]. Two patients were excluded from the study. The overall sensitivity was 76.47% for cytology, 78.43% for the BTA stat test and 84.31% for NMP-22 ($p = $ n.s.) [38]. The specificity was 91.49%, 87.23% and 87.23% respectively ($p = $ n.s.) [38]. By grade and stage, NMP-22 showed the best results followed by the BTA stat test and lastly cytology, although the differences were not significant [38]. The ideal cut-off for NMP-22 in our series was 6 U/ml and not the generally recognized 10 U/ml [38].

Raitanen evaluate the role of a positive BTA stat Test result in patients with negative cystoscopic findings [39]. Of 501 patients, 133 (26.5%) had bladder cancer recurrence at cystoscopy, of which the BTA stat Test detected 71 (53.4%); only 21 of the cases (17.9%) were detected by cytologic examination [39]. Of the remaining 368 patients with no visible tumour at cystoscopy, 96 (26.1%) had a positive BTA stat Test result. Fifty-five of those (57.3%) underwent intravenous urography or renal ultrasound and random biopsies, and an additional 9 recurrences (16.4%) were detected [39]. Of those 46 patients who had a true false-positive BTA stat Test, 3 (3 of 43, 7.0%) had recurrence at the next follow-up cystoscopy, 4 (8.7%) had a urine infection, and 8 (17.4%) had ongoing intravesical instillations; the latter 2% were significantly higher than among those with true-negative BTA stat Test results (0% and 6.8%, respectively) [39].

13.1.22 NMP 22 as a Screening Test in Bladder Cancer

Miyoshi evaluated the usefulness of urinary nuclear matrix protein 22 (NMP22) compared to urinary cytology in the detection of urothelial transitional cell carcinoma (TCC) [40]. Twenty-four patients (10.6%) had urothelial TCC [40]. The urinary NMP22 level was significantly higher in urinary TCC compared to without [40]. The sensitivity and specificity of the results obtained with urinary NMP22 were 58.3% and 84.2%, respectively, and those obtained by urinary cytology were 45.8% and 98.0%, respectively [40]. False-positive results were obtained with urinary NMP22 can occur in urinary diversion using intestine, bladder invasion from other cancers, urinary tract infection, and urolithiasis [40]. The urinary NMP22 level was significantly associated with tumour stage, suggesting its usefulness for detection of urothelial TCC [40]. However, although urinary NMP22 showed equal sensitivity for the detection of TCC, it was not superior to urinary cytology [40].

13.1.23 Urinary Fibrin as a Screening Test for Bladder Cancer

Oeda assessed utility of urine fibrin/fibrinogen degradation products (FDP) in screening for bladder cancer [41]. Histologically confirmed bladder cancer was found in 14 cases [41]. Overall sensitivity of urinary FDP, NMP22, BTA and cytology were 79%, 64%, 36% and 36%, respectively [41]. While the sensitivity of FDP was significantly higher than that of BTA and cytology, no significant difference was found between FDP and NMP22 [41]. Overall specificity of these four methods were 69%, 78%, 92% and 90%, respectively [41]. The specificity of FDP and NMP22 were significantly lower than that of BTA and Cytology, but satisfactory as a screening test [41]. The sensitivity of the four methods for low-grade and non-invasive tumours were 70%, 50%, 30% and 10% (G1 or G2, n = 10), and 75%, 58%, 33% and 25% (Ta or T1, n = 12), respectively [41]. FDP might have a high sensitivity for even low-grade and non-invasive tumours [41].

13.1.24 DNA Image Cytometry in Bladder Cancer Screening

Planz assessed the potential of DNA image cytometry in screening for bladder cancer, compare it with conventional urinary cytology, and evaluate its possible use in routine urinary evaluation [42]. Urinary cytology yielded an overall sensitivity of 47.5% [42]. Conventional analysis of DNA histograms measuring the presence of DNA stemline aneuploidy (1.8c > stemline ploidy [STP] > 2.2c) revealed a sensitivity of 62.5% [42]. The specificity of both methods was 100%. DNA image cytometry demonstrated a high sensitivity in grade 1 tumours (70.4%) compared with cytology (26%) [42].

13.1.25 Matrix Metalloproteinases in Bladder Cancer Screening

Monier examined matrix metalloproteinases in bladder cancer screening [43]. Three metalloproteinases with gelatinolytic activity were isolated from urine in untreated high-grade bladder cancer or with functioning renal grafts (control) [43]. Urinary proteins were by continuous-elution SDS-polyacrylamide gel electrophoresis [43]. This isolated the gelatinase species from crude urine samples: (1) a 72 kDa progelatinase A (MMP-2) and its activated 68 kDa form; (2) a 92 kDa progelatinase B (MMP-9); (3) a higher molecular weight (HMW) complex (115 kDa) which was identified as progelatinase B associated with lipocalin, NGAL [43]. A similar marker profile was observed in bladder cancer tissues. The current study demonstrated the efficiency of continuous elution electrophoresis [43]. It offered two main advantages: (1) the separation of latent from active gelatinase isoforms with no interference from the TIMPs and (2) the identification and isolation in a single step of large amounts of urine gelatinase species with both high recovery and significant specific activities [43]. Continuous-elution electrophoresis can be used for correlation with clinical events of bladder cancer diagnosis and prognosis [43].

13.1.26 Microsatellite Markers in Bladder Cancer Screening

Molina Burgos evaluate the use of microsatellite markers and the utility of loss of heterozigosity (LOH) and microsatellite instability (MSI) in exfoliated cells from urine sediment [44]. In 111 samples LOH/MSI (sensitivity 74%) was demonstrated [44]. The cytology was positive only in 60 patients (sensitivity 40%) [44]. We found a bigger number of microsatellite alterations (AM) in superficial tumours (sensibility 77.3% vs. 28.8% for the cytology) and these were significant when comparing tumours GI-II vs. GIII (MSI p < 0.001—LOH p < 0.004). The marker with more sensibility was D4S243 with 40%. One patient with prostate carcinoma and another one with chronic cystitis gave false positive results.

13.1.27 Conclusion

The overall conclusion from this systematic review are that there are a number of new ways forward in bladder cancer screening including molecular techniques. However, as yet, no clinical guidelines has included any of the molecular markers within their content.

References

1. Moher D, Liberati A, Tetzlaff J, Altman DG. "Preferred Reporting Items for Systematic Reviews and Meta-Analyses: The Prisma Statement." [In English]. BMJ (Online) 339, no. 7716 (08 Aug 2009):332–36.
2. Mays N, Pope C, Popay J. "Systematically Reviewing Qualitative and Quantitative Evidence to Inform Management and Policy-Making in the Health Field." [In English]. Journal of Health Services Research and Policy 10, no. SUPPL. 1 (July 2005):6–20.
3. Loras A, Trassierra M, Sanjuan-Herráez D, et al. Bladder cancer recurrence surveillance by urine metabolomics analysis. Sci Rep. 2018;8(1):9172.
4. Davis N, Shtabsky A, Lew S, et al. A novel urine-based assay for bladder cancer diagnosis: multi-institutional validation study. Eur Urol Focus. 2018;4(3):388–94.
5. Daneshmand S, Patel S, Lotan Y, et al. Efficacy and safety of blue light flexible cystoscopy with hexaminolevulinate in the surveillance of bladder cancer: a phase III, comparative, multicenter study. J Urol. 2018;199(5):1158–65. [Published correction appears in J Urol. 2019;201(5):1017].
6. Nakai Y, Inoue K, Tsuzuki T, et al. Oral 5-aminolevulinic acid-mediated photodynamic diagnosis using fluorescence cystoscopy for non-muscle-invasive bladder cancer: a multicenter phase III study. Int J Urol. 2018;25(8):723–9.
7. Smith AB, Daneshmand S, Patel S, et al. Patient-reported outcomes of blue-light flexible cystoscopy with hexaminolevulinate in the surveillance of bladder cancer: results from a prospective multicentre study. BJU Int. 2019;123(1):35–41.
8. Inoue K, Matsuyama H, Fujimoto K, et al. The clinical trial on the safety and effectiveness of the photodynamic diagnosis of non-muscle-invasive bladder cancer using fluorescent light-guided cystoscopy after oral administration of 5-aminolevulinic acid (5-ALA). Photodiagn Photodyn Ther. 2016;13:91–6.
9. Daniltchenko DI, Riedl CR, Sachs MD, et al. Long-term benefit of 5-aminolevulinic acid fluorescence assisted transurethral resection of superficial bladder cancer: 5-year results of a prospective randomized study. J Urol. 2005;174(6):2129–33.
10. Lapini A, Minervini A, Masala A, et al. A comparison of hexaminolevulinate (Hexvix(®)) fluorescence cystoscopy and white-light cystoscopy for detection of bladder cancer: results of the HeRo observational study. Surg Endosc. 2012;26(12):3634–41.
11. Grossman HB, Gomella L, Fradet Y, et al. A phase III, multicenter comparison of hexaminolevulinate fluorescence cystoscopy and white light cystoscopy for the detection of superficial papillary lesions in patients with bladder cancer. J Urol. 2007;178(1):62–7.
12. Palou J, Hernández C, Solsona E, et al. Effectiveness of hexaminolevulinate fluorescence cystoscopy for the diagnosis of non-muscle-invasive bladder cancer in daily clinical practice: a Spanish multicentre observational study. BJU Int. 2015;116(1):37–43.
13. Inoue K, Anai S, Fujimoto K, et al. Oral 5-aminolevulinic acid mediated photodynamic diagnosis using fluorescence cystoscopy for non-muscle-invasive bladder cancer: a randomized, double-blind, multicentre phase II/III study. Photodiagn Photodyn Ther. 2015;12(2):193–200.

14. Geavlete B, Jecu M, Multescu R, Georgescu D, Geavlete P. HAL blue-light cystoscopy in high-risk nonmuscle-invasive bladder cancer—re-TURBT recurrence rates in a prospective, randomized study. Urology. 2010;76(3):664–9.
15. Denzinger S, Burger M, Walter B, et al. Clinically relevant reduction in risk of recurrence of superficial bladder cancer using 5-aminolevulinic acid-induced fluorescence diagnosis: 8-year results of prospective randomized study. Urology. 2007;69(4):675–9.
16. Jichlinski P, Guillou L, Karlsen SJ, et al. Hexyl aminolevulinate fluorescence cystoscopy: new diagnostic tool for photodiagnosis of superficial bladder cancer—a multicenter study. J Urol. 2003;170(1):226–9.
17. Witjes JA, Moonen PM, van der Heijden AG. Comparison of hexaminolevulinate based flexible and rigid fluorescence cystoscopy with rigid white light cystoscopy in bladder cancer: results of a prospective phase II study. Eur Urol. 2005;47(3):319–22.
18. Cheng CW, Lau WK, Tan PH, Olivo M. Cystoscopic diagnosis of bladder cancer by intravesical instillation of 5-aminolevulinic acid induced porphyrin fluorescence—the Singapore experience. Ann Acad Med Singap. 2000;29(2):153–8.
19. Zaak D, Kriegmair M, Stepp H, et al. Endoscopic detection of transitional cell carcinoma with 5-aminolevulinic acid: results of 1012 fluorescence endoscopies. Urology. 2001;57(4):690–4.
20. Filbeck T, Pichlmeier U, Knuechel R, Wieland WF, Roessler W. Clinically relevant improvement of recurrence-free survival with 5-aminolevulinic acid induced fluorescence diagnosis in patients with superficial bladder tumors. J Urol. 2002;168(1):67–71.
21. Witjes JA, Morote J, Cornel EB, et al. Performance of the bladder EpiCheck™ methylation test for patients under surveillance for non-muscle-invasive bladder cancer: results of a multicenter, prospective, blinded clinical trial. Eur Urol Oncol. 2018;1(4):307–13.
22. Eissa S, Habib H, Ali E, Kotb Y. Evaluation of urinary miRNA-96 as a potential biomarker for bladder cancer diagnosis. Med Oncol. 2015;32(1):413.
23. Tan WS, Sarpong R, Khetrapal P, et al. Does urinary cytology have a role in haematuria investigations? BJU Int. 2019;123(1):74–81.
24. Inoue K, Ota U, Ishizuka M, et al. Porphyrins as urinary biomarkers for bladder cancer after 5-aminolevulinic acid (ALA) administration: the potential of photodynamic screening for tumors. Photodiagn Photodyn Ther. 2013;10(4):484–9.
25. March-Villalba JA, Panach-Navarrete J, Herrero-Cervera MJ, Aliño-Pellicer S, Martínez-Jabaloyas JM. hTERT mRNA expression in urine as a useful diagnostic tool in bladder cancer. Comparison with cytology and NMP22 BladderCheck Test®. Expresión de ARNm de hTERT en orina como herramienta diagnóstica útil en cáncer de vejiga. Comparación con citología y NMP22 BladderCheck Test®. Actas Urol Esp. 2018;42(8):524–30.
26. Bell MD, Yafi FA, Brimo F, et al. Prognostic value of urinary cytology and other biomarkers for recurrence and progression in bladder cancer: a prospective study. World J Urol. 2016;34(10):1405–9.
27. Salomo K, Huebner D, Boehme MU, et al. Urinary transcript quantitation of CK20 and IGF2 for the non-invasive bladder cancer detection. J Cancer Res Clin Oncol. 2017;143(9):1757–69.
28. Shabayek MI, Sayed OM, Attaia HA, Awida HA, Abozeed H. Diagnostic evaluation of urinary angiogenin (ANG) and clusterin (CLU) as biomarker for bladder cancer. Pathol Oncol Res. 2014;20(4):859–66.
29. Andreotti G, Karami S, Pfeiffer RM, et al. LINE1 methylation levels associated with increased bladder cancer risk in pre-diagnostic blood DNA among US (PLCO) and European (ATBC) cohort study participants. Epigenetics. 2014;9(3):404–15.
30. Jin X, Yun SJ, Jeong P, Kim IY, Kim WJ, Park S. Diagnosis of bladder cancer and prediction of survival by urinary metabolomics. Oncotarget. 2014;5(6):1635–45.
31. Guney AI, Ergec DS, Tavukcu HH, et al. Detection of mitochondrial DNA mutations in non-muscle invasive bladder cancer. Genet Test Mol Biomarkers. 2012;16(7):672–8.
32. Khadjavi A, Notarpietro A, Mannu F, et al. A high-throughput assay for the detection of Tyr-phosphorylated proteins in urine of bladder cancer patients. Biochim Biophys Acta. 2013;1830(6):3664–9.

33. Li F, Chen DN, He CW, et al. Identification of urinary Gc-globulin as a novel biomarker for bladder cancer by two-dimensional fluorescent differential gel electrophoresis (2D-DIGE). J Proteomics. 2012;77:225–36.
34. Kawamoto K, Enokida H, Gotanda T, et al. p16INK4a and p14ARF methylation as a potential biomarker for human bladder cancer. Biochem Biophys Res Commun. 2006;339(3):790–6.
35. Gkialas I, Papadopoulos G, Iordanidou L, et al. Evaluation of urine tumor-associated trypsin inhibitor, CYFRA 21-1, and urinary bladder cancer antigen for detection of high-grade bladder carcinoma. Urology. 2008;72(5):1159–63.
36. Urquidi V, Netherton M, Gomes-Giacoia E, et al. Urinary mRNA biomarker panel for the detection of urothelial carcinoma. Oncotarget. 2016;7(25):38731–40.
37. Imamura M, Inoue K, Megumi Y, Nishimura M, Ohmori K, Nishimura K. Clinical evaluation of urinary basic fetoprotein and the BTA test for detection of bladder cancer. Hinyokika Kiyo. 2000;46(10):705–9.
38. Gutiérrez Baños JL, Rebollo Rodrigo MH, Antolín Juarez F, et al. Estudio comparativo entre el BTA stat test, NMP-22 y citología en el diagnóstico del cáncer vesical [Comparative study of BTA stat test, NMP-22, and cytology in the diagnosis of bladder cancer]. Arch Esp Urol. 2000;53(1):21–7.
39. Raitanen MP, Kaasinen E, Lukkarinen O, et al. Analysis of false-positive BTA STAT test results in patients followed up for bladder cancer. Urology. 2001;57(4):680–4.
40. Miyoshi Y, Matsuzaki J, Miura T. Evaluation of usefulness of urinary nuclear matrix protein 22 (NMP22) in the detection of urothelial transitional cell carcinoma. Hinyokika Kiyo. 2001;47(6):379–83.
41. Oeda T, Manabe D. The usefulness of urinary FDP in the diagnosis of bladder cancer: comparison with NMP22, BTA and cytology. Nihon Hinyokika Gakkai Zasshi. 2001;92(1):1–5.
42. Planz B, Synek C, Robben J, Böcking A, Marberger M. Diagnostic accuracy of DNA image cytometry and urinary cytology with cells from voided urine in the detection of bladder cancer. Urology. 2000;56(5):782–6.
43. Monier F, Surla A, Guillot M, Morel F. Gelatinase isoforms in urine from bladder cancer patients. Clin Chim Acta. 2000;299(1–2):11–23.
44. Molina Burgos R, Millán Salvador JM, Oltra Soler JS, Jiménez Cruz JF. Análisis de microsatélites en células exfoliadas del sedimento urinario. Su utilidad para la detección del cáncer vesical. Estudio comparativo con citología urinaria [Microsatellite analysis in exfoliated cells from urinary sediment. Its utility for the detection of bladder cancer. Comparison with urinary cytology]. Actas Urol Esp. 2003;27(8):618–28.

A Systematic Review on Blue Light Cystoscopy in Bladder Cancer Diagnostics

14

14.1 Systematic Review Methods

A systematic review relating to blue light cystoscopy and bladder cancer was conducted. The search strategy aimed to identify all references related to Blue Light Cystoscopy and Bladder Cancer. Search terms used were as follows: (Bladder cancer) AND (Blue light cystoscopy). The following databases were screened from 1989 to June 2020:

- CINAHL
- MEDLINE (NHS Evidence)
- Cochrane
- AMed
- EMBASE
- PsychINFO
- SCOPUS
- Web of Science.

In addition, searches using Medical Subject Headings (MeSH) and keywords were conducted using Cochrane databases. Two UK-based experts in bladder cancer were consulted to identify any additional studies.

Studies were eligible for inclusion if they reported primary research focusing on bladder cancer and screening. Papers were included if published after 1984 and had to be in English. Studies that did not conform to this were excluded. Only primary research was included.

Abstracts were independently screened for eligibility by two reviewers and disagreements resolved through discussion or third party opinion (Fig. 14.1). Agreement level was calculated using Cohen's Kappa to test the intercoder reliability of this screening process. Cohens' Kappa allows comparison of inter-rater reliability between papers using relative observed agreement. This also takes account

S. S. Goonewardene et al., *Management of Muscle Invasive Bladder Cancer*,
Management of Urology, https://doi.org/10.1007/978-3-030-57915-9_14

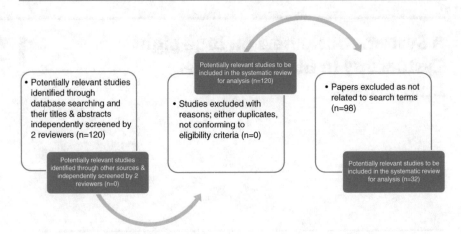

Fig. 14.1 Flow chart of studies identified through the systematic review. (Adapted from PRISMA)

of the comparison occurring by chance. The first reviewer agreed all 32 papers to be included, the second, agreed on 32. Cohens' Kappa was 1.0.

Data extraction was piloted by the researcher and amended in consultation with the research team (author and two academic supervisors). Data collected included authors, year and country of publication, study aims, setting, intervention aims, number of participants, study design, intervention components and delivery methods, comparison groups and outcome measures, notes and follow-up questions for the authors. Studies were quality assessed using the PRISMA criteria for randomised controlled trials, Mays et al. [1, 2] for the action research and qualitative studies and the Critical Skills Appraisal programme for cohort studies. This was also applied to randomised controlled trials and qualitative studies. There were 32 cohort studies.

14.2   Systematic Review Results

Photodynamic diagnostic technique with blue light cystoscopy (BLC) uses preferential uptake and accumulation of protoporphyrins in neoplastic tissue which emit a red fluorescence when illuminated with blue light (360–450 nm wavelengths) [3]. This allows enhanced visualization of small papillary tumours and flat carcinoma in situ lesions that might have been missed on white light cystoscopy (WLC) [3].

14.2.1   Blue Light vs. White Light Cystoscopy

In a multicentre study, Schmidbauer compared hexaminolevulinate (HAL) fluorescence cystoscopy and standard white light cystoscopy in carcinoma in situ (CIS) detection [4]. Of 211, 83 (39%) had CIS, of whom 18 (22%) were detected by HAL cystoscopy only, 62 (75%) were detected by standard and HAL cystoscopy, 2 (2%) were detected by standard cystoscopy only and 1 (1%) was detected by nonguided biopsy [4]. Therefore, HAL cystoscopy identified 28% more patients with CIS than standard cystoscopy. The side effects were negligible, and no unexpected events were reported [4]. HAL fluorescence cystoscopy improves the detection of bladder CIS significantly, improving prognosis [4]. The procedure is easily implemented as an adjunct to standard cystoscopy and it adds no significant risk of complications [4].

Lapini, evaluated hexylaminolevulinate hydrochloride (Hexvix($^{®}$)) PDD cystoscopy compared with standard WLC [5]. Overall, 234 suspicious lesions were detected; 108 (46.2%) were bladder tumours/carcinoma in situ (CIS) [5]. The sensitivity of BLC biopsies was significantly higher than for WLC technique (99.1% vs. 76.8%; p < 0.00001) [5]. The relative sensitivity of BLC versus WLC was 1.289, showing superiority of BLC of 28.9% [5]. The specificity of BLC biopsies was not significantly different compared with WLC (36.5% vs. 30.2%) [5]. Positive predictive value for BLC- and WLC-guided biopsies was 54.9% and 50.9%, respectively [5]. Negative predictive value per biopsy for BLC- and WLC-guided biopsies was 97.4% and 64.8%, respectively. BLC and WLC reached the correct diagnosis in 97.9% and 88.5% of patients, respectively [5].

Geavlete et al. [6] assessed Hexvix blue light cystoscopy (BLC) and compared it to standard white light cystoscopy (WLC). WLC identified 40 suspicious lesions (37 pathologically confirmed), while BLC detected 58 apparent tumours (52 pathologically confirmed). WLC correctly diagnosed 68.5%, with a rate of 7.5% false-positive results, while BLC diagnosed 96.3%, presenting a 10.3% rate of false-positive results. Twenty-two cases of the study group diagnosed with SBT were followed. The tumour recurrence rate after 18 weeks was 4.5% for the study group and 22.7% for the control group. Hexvix fluorescence cystoscopy is a valuable diagnostic method, with considerably better results by comparison to WLC. The improved diagnostic accuracy may have a significant impact upon the recurrence rate.

Burgués reviewed the benefit of PDD vs. conventional white light cystoscopy (WL) [7]. A total of 1659 lesions were biopsied: 522 were identified with PDD and WL, 237 only with PDD, 19 only with WL and 881 random biopsies [7]. Of the 600 tumours, PDD detected 563, WL 441 and random biopsies 29 (20 CIS) [7]. The mean over detection rate for PDD over WL was 31.9% for all bladder tumours, but it was 209% for carcinoma in situ (CIS) [7]. Sensitivity was 93.8% for PDD and 78.2% for WL [7]. Specificity was 81.5% for PDD and 90.5% for WL. In 23% PDD detected at least one additional lesion compared to WL [7].

14.2.2   Efficacy and Safety of Blue Light vs. White Light in Bladder Cancer Diagnostics

Lee evaluated the efficacy and safety of hexaminolevulinate fluorescence cystoscopy in the diagnosis of bladder cancer [8]. From 30 patients 134 specimens were extracted

[8]. One hundred and one specimens showed positive results by blue light cystoscopy (BLC) [8]. The sensitivity of BLC and white light cystoscopy (WLC) was 92.3% and 80.8%, respectively (p = 0.021) [8]. The specificity of BLC and WLC was 48% and 49.1%, respectively (p > 0.05) [8]. The positive and negative predictive values of BLC were 71.2% and 81.8%, respectively, those of WLC were 72.0% and 68.6%, respectively [8]. With WLC, 48 specimens showed negative findings, but of that group, 15 specimens (31.2%) were revealed to be malignant with BLC [8].

Inoue report on intravesical 5-aminolevulinic acid (5-ALA) in diagnostics [9]. From 76 cases, 36 were from a polypoid lesion and 40 from a non-polypoid lesion (including 19 carcinoma in situ). Twenty-one patients with dysplasia were detected pathologically, with a sensitivity of 89.5% and specificity of 58.5%. The predictive accuracy was 77.0% [9]. The AUC in blue light endoscopy was more than that in white light endoscopy in not only all cases (p = 0.010) but also in cases with non-polypoid lesion (p = 0.007) and recurrent cases (p = 0.002) [9]. Duration of 5-ALA instillation with a median time of 80 (range 30–150) min did not seem to affect the accuracy of photodynamic diagnosis [9]. Procedures were well tolerated by all patients with mild bladder irritability but no systemic side effects [9].

Lane examined the tolerability of the repeat use of white light cystoscopy with blue light cystoscopy [10]. Eighty-nine adverse events out of 269 procedures (33%), of which 66 (74%) occurred after the first white light cystoscopy with blue light cystoscopy; 14 (16%) after the second time and 9 (10%) after the third time or more [10]. There was no statistically significant difference in adverse events undergoing 1 vs. 2 or more white light cystoscopy with blue light cystoscopy procedures (p = 0.134) [10]. Lane observed 1 grade 3 adverse event and no grade 4 or 5 adverse events [10]. None of the adverse events were classified as related to hexaminolevulinate hydrochloride [10].

Grossman compared hexaminolevulinate fluorescence cystoscopy with white light cystoscopy for detecting Ta and T1 papillary lesions in patients with bladder cancer [11]. At least 1 additional T1 tumour was detected by HAL but not by white light cystoscopy in 3 of these patients (15%), while at least 1 more T1 tumour was detected by white light cystoscopy than by HAL cystoscopy in 1 patient (5%, 95% CI 0–25) [11]. Detection rates for Ta tumours were 95% for HAL cystoscopy and 83% for white light cystoscopy (p = 0.0001) [11]. Detection rates were 95% and 86%, respectively, for T1 tumours (p = 0.3). HAL instillation was well tolerated with few local or systemic side effects [11].

14.2.3   Blue Light Cystoscopy and Early Detection of Bladder Cancer

5-Aminolevulinic acid-induced fluorescence endoscopy (AFE) has increased the effectiveness of bladder cancer detection [12]. Application of 5-aminolevulinic acid (5-ALA) endogenous protoporphyrin IX (PP IX) accumulates in tumour tissue [12]. When such tissue is then irradiated with blue light, the neoplastic areas can be identified by red fluorescence and, in the case of the bladder, can be removed by transurethral resection (TUR) or laser coagulation in the same endoscopic session [12]. The great advantage of this highly sensitive technique (95%) is to be seen in particular in the detection of flat urothelial neoplastic lesions—until recently a deficit in conventional white-light endoscopy [12]. Initial investigations show that improved early detection and the reduction in the residual tumor rate lead to longer recurrence-free intervals [12].

14.2.4 Blue Light Cystoscopy and Malignant vs. Benign Lesions

5-Aminolevulinic acid induced fluorescence endoscopy has outstanding sensitivity for detecting early stage bladder cancer [13]. Nevertheless, a third of the lesions that show specific fluorescence are histologically benign [13]. Zaak decreased the false-positive rate of 5-aminolevulinic acid induced fluorescence endoscopy by incorporating protoporphyrin IX fluorescence quantification into the standard cystoscopy procedure [13]. Malignant fluorescence positive lesions showed significantly stronger fluorescence intensity than fluorescing lesions with benign histology [13]. A threshold was established that decreased the false-positive rate by 30% without affecting sensitivity [13]. Fluorescence image quantification is a new endoscopic method for objectively selecting multicolor fluorescence bladder lesion images for biopsy [13]. It has the potential of eliminating human error by different surgeons with variable experience in fluorescence endoscopy [13].

Ferre conducted a prospective evaluation of bladder tumour targeting by Hexvix(®) fluorescence [14]. From the 107 patients, 67 have been identified with bladder cancer and 328 samples have shown positive fluorescence in blue light [14]. Compared to white light, 13 additional tumours have been diagnosed by Hexvix(®) for 11 patients: Cis (n = 6), LMP (n = 3), pTa low grade (n = 3), pT1 low grade (n = 1) (p = 0.003) [14]. The false positive rate for Hexvix(®) was 53.4% versus 52% for white light [14]. Previous TCC history, multifocality and EORTC score for recurrence and progression have been associated with better bladder cancer targeting by Hexvix(®) (p = 0.007; p = 0.01; p = 0.03; p = 0.04) [14].

Koenig reported the results of a clinical study investigating the diagnosis of malignant and dysplastic bladder lesions by protoporphyrin IX (PPIX) fluorescence and to compare them with those from earlier studies [15]. There were 63 benign and 67 malignant/dysplastic areas biopsied; 10 malignant/dysplastic lesions (4 transitional cell carcinoma, 2 carcinoma in situ, 4 dysplasia) were not detected during routine white-light cystoscopy but were identified under blue light [15]. Fluorescence cystoscopy improved the overall diagnosis of malignant/dysplastic bladder lesions by 18% over standard white-light cystoscopy [15]. The improvement was greater for dysplastic lesions and carcinoma in situ (50%) [15].

Ehsan evaluated the efficiency of endoscopic fluorescence diagnosis of superficial malignant bladder tumours following intravesical instillation of delta-aminolevulinic acid [16]. A clear strong red fluorescence colour was observed emitting from all malignant vesical lesions [16]. A diagnostic sensitivity of 98% and specificity of 65% has been determined for this novel diagnostic modality [16].

14.2.5   Role of Blue Light Cystoscopy in Detection of CIS

Fradet, compared hexaminolevulinate (Hexvix) fluorescence cystoscopy with white light cystoscopy for carcinoma in situ [17]. Of 196 evaluable patients 29.6% had carcinoma in situ, including 18 with carcinoma in situ alone,35 with carcinoma in situ and concomitant papillary disease, which was detected on random biopsy in 5 [17]. Of the 18 patients with no concomitant papillary disease carcinoma in situ was detected only by hexaminolevulinate fluorescence in 4 and only by white light in 4 [17]. In the group with concomitant papillary disease carcinoma in situ was found only by hexaminolevulinate fluorescence in 5 patients and only by white light in 3 [17]. The proportion of patients in whom 1 or more carcinoma in situ lesions were found only by hexaminolevulinate cystoscopy was greater than the hypothesized 5% (p = 0.0022) [17]. Overall more carcinoma in situ lesions were found by hexaminolevulinate than by white light cystoscopy in 22 of 58 patients (41.5%), while the converse occurred in 8 of 58 (15.1%) [17].

14.2.6   Blue Light Cystoscopy in Atypical Bladder Cancer Diagnosis

Pederzoli retrospectively reviewed transurethral biopsies of bladder tumors in which both WLC and BLC evaluations were performed including in atypical bladder carcinomas [18]. Review of BLC(+)/atypical cases showed a mean agreement of 79%, and none of the cases showed staining pattern consistent with CIS [18]. All patients with BLC(+)/atypical lesions had history of intravesical BCG and/or mitomycin [18]. Using final pathology as the reference, sensitivity, specificity and negative predictive value (NPV) of BLC were 93% (CI 80.1–98.5%), 46% (CI 35.4–56.3%) and 94% (CI 82.5–97.8%), respectively [18].

14.2.7   Role of Blue Light Cystoscopy in Positive Cytology

Ray investigated the value of photodynamic diagnosis (PDD) using hexylaminolaevulinate (Hexvix) in positive urine cytology with negative standard primary investigations [19]. Twenty-five PDD-assisted cystoscopies were carried out on 23 patients [19]. Of the 23 patients, 17 (74%) were previously untreated for transitional cell carcinoma (TCC), 6 were under surveillance for previous TCC [19]. Nineteen (83%) cytology specimens were confirmed as suspicious or positive [19]. TCC of the bladder or preneoplastic lesions were diagnosed in 6 patients, i.e. 6 (26%) of those investigated and 6 of 19 (32%) with confirmed positive cytology [19]. Additional pathology was detected in 5 of the 6 patients, including 2 carcinoma in situ (CIS), 1 CIS + G3pT1 tumour, and 2 dysplasia [19].

14.2.8   Blue Light Cystoscopy and Role in Bladder Cancer Surveillance

Loidl assessed flexible cystoscopy assisted by hexaminolevulinate (HAL) fluorescence [20]. In the 45 patients studied 41 (91%) patients had exophytic tumours, of which 39 (95.1%) were detected by HAL flexible cystoscopy and 40 (97.5%) by HAL rigid cystoscopy [20]. Seventeen (37.8%) patients had concomitant or carcinoma in situ only, which was identified by HAL flexible cystoscopy in 14 (82.3%), by HAL rigid cystoscopy in 15 (88.2%), by flexible standard in 11 (64.7%) and by standard white light rigid cystoscopy in 13 (76.7%) patients [20]. HAL fluorescence flexible cystoscopy compared to HAL rigid cystoscopy showed almost equivalent results in detecting papillary and flat lesions in bladder cancer patients [20]. Both procedures were superior to standard white light flexible cystoscopy [20].

14.2.9   Blue Light Cystoscopy in Detection of Recurrence

Stenzl assessed the impact that improved detection with hexaminolevulinate fluorescence cystoscopy may have on early recurrence rates [21]. Detection was performed as a within patient comparison in the fluorescence group [21]. In this group 286 patients had at least 1 Ta or T1 tumour (intent to treat) [21]. In 47 patients (16%) at least 1 of the tumours was seen only with fluorescence (p = 0.001) [21]. During the 9-month follow up (intent to treat) there was tumour recurrence in 128 of 271 patients (47%) in the fluorescence group and 157 of 280 (56%) in the white light group (p = 0.026) [21]. The relative reduction in recurrence rate was 16% [21].

Fanari reviewed cases of WLC and FC in a single moment with HAL in the diagnosis and follow-up of bladder cancer [22]. 26.1% of the lesions were found only by the PDD method [22]. The false positivity due to the method adopted was 21.2% [22]. The gain in terms of recurrence-free survival (compared with historical reference group treated only with WL) was 22.3% at 12 months and 24.4% at 20 months [22].

Daneshmand compared blue light flexible cystoscopy with white light flexible cystoscopy for the detection of bladder cancer during surveillance [23]. Following surveillance 103 of the 304 patients were referred, 63 with confirmed malignancy, 26 of the 63 had carcinoma in situ. In 13 of the 63 patients (20.6%, 95% CI 11.5–32.7) recurrence was seen only with blue light flexible cystoscopy (p < 0.0001) [23]. Five of these cases were confirmed as carcinoma in situ. Operating room examination confirmed carcinoma in situ in 26 of 63 patients (41%), which was detected only with blue light cystoscopy in 9 of the 26 (34.6%, 95% CI 17.2–55.7, p < 0.0001) [23]. Blue light cystoscopy identified additional malignant lesions in 29 of the 63 patients (46%) [23]. The false-positive rate was 9.1% for white and blue light cystoscopy. None of the 12 adverse events during surveillance were serious [23].

Burger assessed blue light (BL) HAL cystoscopy for detection of Ta/T1 and carcinoma in situ (CIS) tumours, and recurrence [24]. BL cystoscopy detected significantly more Ta tumours (14.7%; p < 0.001; odds ratio [OR]: 4.898; 95% CI, 1.937–12.390) and CIS lesions (40.8%; p < 0.001; OR: 12.372; 95% CI, 6.343–24.133) than WL [24]. There were 24.9% with at least one additional Ta/T1 tumour seen with BL (p < 0.001), significant also in patients with primary (20.7%; p < 0.001) and recurrent cancer (27.7%; p < 0.001), and in high risk (27.0%; p < 0.001) and intermediate risk cases (35.7%; p = 0.004) [24]. In 26.7% of patients, CIS was detected only by BL (p < 0.001) and was significant in primary (28.0%; p < 0.001) and recurrent cancer (25.0%; p < 0.001) [24]. Recurrence rates up to 12 months were significantly lower overall with BL, 34.5% versus 45.4% (p = 0.006; RR: 0.761 [0.627–0.924]), and lower in patients with T1 or CIS (p = 0.052; RR: 0.696 [0.482–1.003]) [24], Ta (p = 0.040; RR: 0.804 [0.653–0.991]), and in high-risk (p = 0.050) and low-risk (p = 0.029) subgroups.

14.2.10   Blue Light Cystoscopy in High Risk Patients

Blanco evaluated fluorescence cystoscopy with hexaminolevulinate (HAL) in the early detection of dysplasia (DYS) and carcinoma in situ (CIS) in select high risk patients [25]. The overall incidence was 43.3% dysplasia, 23.3% CIS, and 13.3% superficial transitional cell cancer [25]. In 21 patients, HAL cystoscopy was positive with one or more fluorescent flat lesions. Of the positive cases, there were 4 CIS, 10 DYS, 2 association of CIS and DYS, 4 well-differentiated non-infiltrating bladder cancers, and 1 chronic cystitis [25]. In 9 patients with negative HAL results, random biopsies showed 1 CIS and 1 DYS. HAL cystoscopy showed 90.1% sensitivity and 87.5% specificity with 95.2% positive predictive value and 77.8% negative predictive value [25].

14.2.11   Blue Light Cystoscopy in Progression of Bladder Cancer

Kamat reviewed whether blue light cystoscopy with hexaminolevulinate (HAL) impacts the rate of progression and time to progression using the revised definition [26]. In the original analysis, after 4.5 years (median), 8 HAL and 16 WL patients were deemed to have progressed (transition from NMIBC to muscle invasive bladder cancer, (T2–4)) [26]. According to the new definition, additional patients in both groups were found to have progressed: 31 (12.2%) HAL vs. 46 (17.6%) WL (p = 0.085) with 4 (1.6%) HAL and 11 (4.2%) WL patients progressing from Ta to CIS. Time to progression was longer in the HAL group (p = 0.05) [26].

14.2.12   Accuracy of Blue vs. White Light Cystoscopy

Pagliarulo compared the accuracy of white light cystoscopy (WLC) and blue light cystoscopy (BLC) in previously resected urothelial bladder cancer [27]. Sixty-four patients underwent WLC and BLC prior to cystectomy [27]. Residual disease was found in 31/64 (48.4%) patients, including 27 (42.1%) cases of carcinoma in situ (CIS) [27]. The accuracy of BLC was much higher than WLC, both in the diagnosis of residual disease (87.1% vs. 32.3%, and 87.9% vs. 51.5%, for sensitivity and specificity, respectively), as of CIS only (92.6% vs. 29.6% and 83.8% vs. 51.4%) [27]. Detection rates were much better for BLC vs. WLC, both overall (86.2% vs. 31%, and 98.3% vs. 93.3%, for sensitivity and specificity, respectively), and when CIS only was considered (89.6% vs. 31.2% and 96.9% vs. 92.8%) [27].

Geavlete evaluated the impact of hexaminolevulinate blue-light cystoscopy (HAL-BLC) on the diagnostic accuracy compared with standard white-light cystoscopy (WLC) [28]. In the 142 patients tumour detection rates significantly improved for carcinoma in situ, pTa and overall cases [28]. In 35.2% of the cases, additional malignant lesions were found by HAL-BLC and consequently, the recurrence- and progression-risk categories of patients and subsequent treatment improved in 19% of the cases due to fluorescence cystoscopy [28]. The recurrence rate at 3 months was lower in the HAL-BLC series (7.2% vs. 15.8%) due to fewer 'other site' recurrences when compared with the WLC series (0.8% vs. 6.1%) [28]. The 1 and 2 year recurrence rates were significantly decreased in the HAL-BLC group compared with the WLC group (21.6% vs. 32.5% and 31.2% vs. 45.6%, respectively) [28].

Jichlinski examined the sensitivity and specificity of hexyl aminolevulinate (HAL) fluorescence cystoscopy in bladder cancer [29]. A total of 422 biopsies obtained in fluorescing (165) and non-fluorescing (257) areas, including 5 random biopsies per patient, were analyzed for sensitivity and specificity [29]. There were 143 histologically verified tumours in 45 patients, including carcinoma in situ (CIS), Ta or T1 lesions [29]. Forty-three patients were diagnosed by fluorescence cystoscopy compared with 33 diagnosed by white light for 96% and 73% sensitivities, respectively [29]. HAL cystoscopy was useful for detection of CIS [29]. Of 13 with CIS tumours all except 1 were diagnosed or confirmed by HAL cystoscopy [29]. HAL cystoscopy was well tolerated with no definite drug related adverse events reported, including effects on standard blood parameters [29].

Jocham determined if improved tumour detection using hexaminolevulinate (HAL) fluorescence cystoscopy could lead to improved treatment in patients with bladder cancer [30]. HAL imaging improved overall tumour detection [30]. Of all tumours 96% were detected with HAL imaging compared with 77% using standard cystoscopy [30]. This difference was particularly noticeable for dysplasia (93% vs. 48%), carcinoma in situ (95% vs. 68%) and superficial papillary tumours (96% vs. 85%) [30]. As a result of improved detection, additional postoperative procedures were recommended in 15 patients (10%) and more extensive treatment was done intraoperatively in a further 10 [30]. Overall 17% of patients received more appropriate treatment at the time of the study following blue light fluorescence cystoscopy, that is 22% or 1 of 5 if patients without tumors were excluded [30].

Palou assess the sensitivity and specificity of blue-light cystoscopy (BLC) with hexaminolevulinate as an adjunct to white-light cystoscopy (WLC) vs. WLC alone [31]. In all, 1569 lesions were identified from 283 patients: 621 were tumour lesions according to histology and 948 were false-positives [31]. Of the 621 tumour lesions, 475 were detected by WLC (sensitivity 76.5%, 95% confidence interval [CI] 73.2–79.8) and 579 were detected by BLC (sensitivity 93.2%, 95% CI 91.0–95.1; $p < 0.001$) [31]. There was a significant improvement in the sensitivity in the detection of all types of NMIBC lesions with BLC compared with WLC. Of 219 patients with tumours, 188 had NMIBC [highest grade: carcinoma in situ (CIS), n = 36; Ta, n = 87; T1, n = 65] [31]. CIS lesions were identified more with BLC (n = 27) than with WLC [n = 19; sensitivity: BLC 75.0% (95% CI 57.8–87.9) vs. WLC 52.8% (95% CI 35.5–69.6); p = 0.021] [31].

14.2.13   Reviews Related to Systematic Review

Malmstrom reports the outcomes of the discussion at the Nordic expert panel meeting, concluding that, in line with European guidance, HAL-FC has an important role in the initial detection of NMIBC and for follow-up of patients to assess tumour recurrence after WLC [32]. It provides practical advice, with an algorithm on the use of this diagnostic procedure for urologists managing NMIBC [32].

14.2.14   Grey Literature Related to Systematic Review

A European expert panel was convened to review the evidence for hexaminolevulinate-guided fluorescence cystoscopy in the diagnosis and management of NMIBC (identified through a PubMed MESH search) and available guidelines from across Europe [33]. On the basis of this information and drawing on the extensive clinical experience of the panel, specific indications for the technique were then identified through discussion [33]. The panel recommends that hexaminolevulinate-guided fluorescence cystoscopy be used to aid diagnosis at initial transurethral resection following suspicion of bladder cancer and in patients with positive urine cytology but negative white-light cystoscopy for the assessment of tumour recurrences in patients not previously assessed with hexaminolevulinate, in the initial follow-up of patients with carcinoma in situ (CIS) or multifocal tumours, and as a teaching tool [33]. The panel does not currently recommend the use of hexaminolevulinate-guided fluorescence cystoscopy in patients for whom cystectomy is indicated or for use in the outpatient setting with flexible cystoscopy [33].

14.2.15   Conclusions

This review demonstrates a role for HAL in the diagnosis and detection of bladder tumours and CIS, which surpass white light cystoscopy.

References

1. Moher D, Liberati A, Tetzlaff J, Altman DG. "Preferred Reporting Items for Systematic Reviews and Meta-Analyses: The Prisma Statement." [In English]. BMJ (Online) 339, no. 7716 (08 Aug 2009):332–36.
2. Mays N, Pope C, Popay J. "Systematically Reviewing Qualitative and Quantitative Evidence to Inform Management and Policy-Making in the Health Field." [In English]. Journal of Health Services Research and Policy 10, no. SUPPL. 1 (July 2005):6–20.

3. Pietzak EJ. The impact of Blue Light Cystoscopy on the diagnosis and treatment of bladder cancer. Curr Urol Rep. 2017;18(5):39.

4. Schmidbauer J, Witjes F, Schmeller N, Donat R, Susani M, Marberger M, Hexvix PCB301/01 Study Group. Improved detection of urothelial carcinoma in situ with hexaminolevulinate fluorescence cystoscopy. J Urol. 2004;171(1):135–8.

5. Lapini A, Minervini A, Masala A, Schips L, Pycha A, Cindolo L, Giannella R, Martini T, Vittori G, Zani D, Bellomo F, Cosciani Cunico S. A comparison of hexaminolevulinate (Hexvix(®)) fluorescence cystoscopy and white-light cystoscopy for detection of bladder cancer: results of the HeRo observational study. Surg Endosc. 2012;26(12):3634–41.

6. Geavlete B, Mulţescu R, Georgescu D, Geavlete P. Hexvix induced fluorescence blue light cystoscopy—a new perspective in superficial bladder tumors diagnosis. Chirurgia (Bucur). 2008;103(5):559–64.

7. Burgués JP, Conde G, Oliva J, Abascal JM, Iborra I, Puertas M, Ordoño F, Grupo BLUE (Blue Light Urologic Endoscopy). Hexaminolevulinate photodynamic diagnosis in non-muscle invasive bladder cancer: experience of the BLUE group. Actas Urol Esp. 2011;35(8):439–45.

8. Lee JS, Lee SY, Kim WJ, Seo SI, Jeon SS, Lee HM, Choi HY, Jeong BC. Efficacy and safety of hexaminolevulinate fluorescence cystoscopy in the diagnosis of bladder cancer. Korean J Urol. 2012;53(12):821–5.

9. Inoue K, Karashima T, Kamada M, Kurabayashi A, Ohtsuki Y, Shuin T. Clinical experience with intravesical instillations of 5-aminolevulinic acid (5-ALA) for the photodynamic diagnosis using fluorescence cystoscopy for bladder cancer. Nihon Hinyokika Gakkai Zasshi. 2006;97(5):719–29.

10. Lane GI, Downs TM, Soubra A, Rao A, Hemsley L, Laylan C, Shi F, Konety B. Tolerability of repeat use of Blue Light Cystoscopy with hexaminolevulinate for patients with urothelial cell carcinoma. J Urol. 2017;197(3 Pt 1):596–601.

11. Grossman HB, Gomella L, Fradet Y, Morales A, Presti J, Ritenour C, Nseyo U, Droller MJ, PC B302/01 Study Group. A phase III, multicenter comparison of hexaminolevulinate fluorescence cystoscopy and white light cystoscopy for the detection of superficial papillary lesions in patients with bladder. J Urol. 2007;178(1):62–7.

12. Zaak D. Fluorescent endoscopy superior to white light endoscopy. Detecting cancers of the urinary bladder earlier. MMW Fortschr Med. 2002;144(13):24–6.

13. Zaak D, Frimberger D, Stepp H, Wagner S, Baumgartner R, Schneede P, Siebels M, Knüchel R, Kriegmair M, Hofstetter A. Quantification of 5-aminolevulinic acid induced fluorescence improves the specificity of bladder cancer detection. J Urol. 2001;166(5):1665–8.

14. Ferré A, Cordonnier C, Demailly M, Hakami F, Sevestre H, Saint F. Bladder tumor targeting by Hexvix(®) fluorescence: 4 years results after prospective monocentric evaluation. Prog Urol. 2013;23(3):195–202.

15. Koenig F, McGovern FJ, Larne R, Enquist H, Schomacker KT, Deutsch TF. Diagnosis of bladder carcinoma using protoporphyrin IX fluorescence induced by 5-aminolaevulinic acid. BJU Int. 1999;83(1):129–35.

16. Ehsan A, Sommer F, Haupt G, Engelmann U. Significance of fluorescence cystoscopy for diagnosis of superficial bladder cancer after intravesical instillation of delta aminolevulinic acid. Urol Int. 2001;67(4):298–304.

17. Fradet Y, Grossman HB, Gomella L, Lerner S, Cookson M, Albala D, Droller MJ, PC B302/01 Study Group. A comparison of hexaminolevulinate fluorescence cystoscopy and white light cystoscopy for the detection of carcinoma in situ in patients with bladder cancer: a phase III, multicenter study. J Urol. 2007;178(1):68–73.

18. Pederzoli F, Amador BM, Samarska I, Lombardo KA, Kates M, Bivalacqua TJ, Matoso A. Diagnosis of urothelial carcinoma in situ using blue light cystoscopy and the utility of immunohistochemistry in blue light-positive lesions diagnosed as atypical. Hum Pathol. 2019;90:1–7.

19. Ray ER, Chatterton K, Khan MS, Thomas K, Chandra A, O'Brien TS. Hexylaminolaevulinate 'blue light' fluorescence cystoscopy in the investigation of clinically unconfirmed positive urine cytology. BJU Int. 2009;103(10):1363–7.

20. Loidl W, Schmidbauer J, Susani M, Marberger M. Flexible cystoscopy assisted by hexaminolevulinate induced fluorescence: a new approach for bladder cancer detection and surveillance? Eur Urol. 2005;47(3):323–6.
21. Stenzl A, Burger M, Fradet Y, Mynderse LA, Soloway MS, Witjes JA, Kriegmair M, Karl A, Shen Y, Grossman HB. Hexaminolevulinate guided fluorescence cystoscopy reduces recurrence in patients with nonmuscle invasive bladder cancer. J Urol. 2010;184(5):1907–13.
22. Fanari M, Serra S, Corona A, De Lisa A. Fluorescence cystoscopy with hexaminolevulinate: our preliminary experience of 184 procedures. Urologia. 2011;78(3):187–9.
23. Daneshmand S, Patel S, Lotan Y, Pohar K, Trabulsi E, Woods M, Downs T, Huang W, Jones J, O'Donnell M, Bivalacqua T, DeCastro J, Steinberg G, Kamat A, Resnick M, Konety B, Schoenberg M, Jones JS, Flexible Blue Light Study Group Collaborators. Efficacy and safety of Blue Light flexible cystoscopy with hexaminolevulinate in the surveillance of bladder cancer: a phase III, comparative, multicenter study. J Urol. 2018;199(5):1158–65.
24. Burger M, Grossman HB, Droller M, Schmidbauer J, Hermann G, Drăgoescu O, Ray E, Fradet Y, Karl A, Burgués JP, Witjes JA, Stenzl A, Jichlinski P, Jocham D. Photodynamic diagnosis of non-muscle-invasive bladder cancer with hexaminolevulinate cystoscopy: a meta-analysis of detection and recurrence based on raw data. Eur Urol. 2013;64(5):846–54.
25. Blanco S, Raber M, Leone BE, Nespoli L, Grasso M. Early detection of urothelial premalignant lesions using hexaminolevulinate fluorescence cystoscopy in high risk patients. J Transl Med. 2010;8:122.
26. Kamat AM, Cookson M, Witjes JA, Stenzl A, Grossman HB. The impact of Blue Light Cystoscopy with hexaminolevulinate (HAL) on progression of bladder cancer - a new analysis. Bladder Cancer. 2016;2(2):273–8.
27. Pagliarulo V, Alba S, Gallone MF, Di Stasi S, Cormio L, Petitti T, Buscarini M, Minafra P, Carrieri G. Diagnostic accuracy of hexaminolevulinate in a cohort of patients undergoing radical cystectomy. J Endourol. 2017;31(4):405–11.
28. Geavlete B, Multescu R, Georgescu D, Jecu M, Stanescu F, Geavlete P. Treatment changes and long-term recurrence rates after hexaminolevulinate (HAL) fluorescence cystoscopy: does it really make a difference in patients with non-muscle-invasive bladder cancer (NMIBC)? BJU Int. 2012;109(4):549–56.
29. Jichlinski P, Guillou L, Karlsen SJ, Malmström PU, Jocham D, Brennhovd B, Johansson E, Gärtner T, Lange N, van den Bergh H, Leisinger HJ. Hexyl aminolevulinate fluorescence cystoscopy: new diagnostic tool for photodiagnosis of superficial bladder cancer—a multicenter study. J Urol. 2003;170(1):226–9.
30. Jocham D, Witjes F, Wagner S, Zeylemaker B, van Moorselaar J, Grimm MO, Muschter R, Popken G, König F, Knüchel R, Kurth KH. Improved detection and treatment of bladder cancer using hexaminolevulinate imaging: a prospective, phase III multicenter study. J Urol. 2005;174(3):862–6; discussion 866.
31. Palou J, Hernández C, Solsona E, Abascal R, Burgués JP, Rioja C, Cabrera JA, Gutiérrez C, Rodríguez O, Iborra I, Herranz F, Abascal JM, Conde G, Oliva J. Effectiveness of hexaminolevulinate fluorescence cystoscopy for the diagnosis of non-muscle-invasive bladder cancer in daily clinical practice: a Spanish multicentre observational study. BJU Int. 2015;116(1):37–43.
32. Malmström PU, Grabe M, Haug ES, Hellström P, Hermann GG, Mogensen K, Raitanen M, Wahlqvist R. Role of hexaminolevulinate-guided fluorescence cystoscopy in bladder cancer: critical analysis of the latest data and European guidance. Scand J Urol Nephrol. 2012;46(2):108–16.
33. Witjes JA, Redorta JP, Jacqmin D, Sofras F, Malmström PU, Riedl C, Jocham D, Conti G, Montorsi F, Arentsen HC, Zaak D, Mostafid AH, Babjuk M. Hexaminolevulinate-guided fluorescence cystoscopy in the diagnosis and follow-up of patients with non-muscle-invasive bladder cancer: review of the evidence and recommendations. Eur Urol. 2010;57(4):607–14.

Muscle Invasive Bladder Cancer and the Staging Conundrum: Which Imaging Modality Is Best?

15

Urinary bladder cancer is a heterogeneous disease with a variety of pathologic features, cytogenetic [1]. Early detection is important, since up to 47% of bladder cancer-related deaths may have been avoided [1]. The role of newer MR imaging sequences (e.g., diffusion-weighted imaging) in the diagnosis and local staging of bladder cancer is still evolving [1]. Substantial advances in MR imaging technology have made multiparametric MR imaging a feasible and reasonably accurate technique for the local staging of bladder cancer to optimize treatment [1].

15.1 MRI in Bladder Cancer

Yamada assessed diffusion-weighted magnetic resonance imaging (DW-MRI) to conventional MRI for T staging and the correlation between apparent diffusion coefficient (ADC) values and clinicopathological parameters for patients with bladder cancer [2]. Yamada, retrospectively reviewed the records of 160 patients with bladder cancer who underwent MRI [2]. In 160 patients, 127 (79.4%) tumours were detectable by MRI. For T staging, the accuracy for distinguishing muscle invasion (T $\leq$ 1 vs. T $\geq$ 2) with DW-MRI (83.0%) was superior to that without DW-MRI (66.7%). The accuracy for distinguishing perivesical fat invasion (T $\leq$ 2 vs. T $\geq$ 3) with DW-MRI (98.0%) was also superior to that without DW-MRI (92.6%).

Ohgiya evaluated the ability of diffusion-weighted imaging (DWI) at 3 T for diagnosing T stage and detecting stalks in bladder cancer [3]. Thirty-nine consecutive patients with bladder tumours underwent magnetic resonance (MR) imaging that included T2-weighted imaging (T2WI) and DWI using a 3 T MR scanner [3]. Specificity and accuracy in differentiating T1 tumours from T2 to T4 tumours were significantly better with T2WI plus DWI (83% [20/24] and 85% [33/39]) than T2WI (50% [12/24] and 67% [26/39]; p = 0.02), and accuracy for diagnosing tumour stage was significantly better with T2WI plus DWI (82% [32/39]) than T2WI alone (59% [23/39]; p = 0.03) [3]. The observers identified stalks in 11 tumours by T2WI (48%

S. S. Goonewardene et al., *Management of Muscle Invasive Bladder Cancer*, Management of Urology, https://doi.org/10.1007/978-3-030-57915-9_15

[11/23]) and 17 by DWI (74% [17/23]) (p < 0.03) [3]. DWI at 3 T was superior to T2WI for evaluating the T stage of bladder cancer, particularly in differentiating T1 tumours from those T2 or higher, and in detecting stalks of papillary bladder tumours [3].

Daneshmand evaluated the accuracy of dynamic gadolinium-enhanced magnetic resonance imaging (DGE-MRI) to detect extravesical bladder cancer (BC) and lymph node-positive disease in invasive BC [4]. Pathologic examination revealed invasive BC in 80/122 (65.5%), including stage pT4 in 15/122 (12.3%), pT3 in 27/122 (22.1%), and pT2 in 38/122 (31.1%), and 27 patients (22.1%) had node-positive disease. The sensitivity, specificity, and accuracy of DGE-MRI in differentiating lymph node-negative organ-confined from nonorgan-confined BC was 87.5%, 47.6%, and 74% and for the detection of positive nodal disease was 40.7%, 91.5%, and 80.3%, respectively. Although DGE-MRI improved T and N staging of invasive BC, it is still not the ideal modality and needs a standardized protocol for interpretation of the imaging findings.

Nguyen, assessed T2-weighted magnetic resonance imaging (T2W-MRI) and the additional diagnostic value of dynamic contrast-enhanced MRI (DCE-MRI) using multitransmit 3 T in the localization of bladder cancer [5]. The sensitivity, specificity, and accuracy of the localization with T2W-MRI alone were 81% (29/36), 63% (5/8), and 77% (34/44) for observer 1 and 72% (26/36), 63% (5/8), and 70% (31/44) for observer 2 [5]. With additional DCE-MRI available, these values were 92% (33/36), 75% (6/8), and 89% (39/44) for observer 1 and 92% (33/36), 63% (5/8), and 86% (38/44) for observer 2 [5]. Of 11 malignant tumours within the bladder wall thickening, 6 (55%) were found on T2W images and 10 (91%) were found on DCE maps [5]. Compared with conventional T2W-MRI alone, the addition of DCE-MRI improved interobserver agreement as well as the localization of small malignant tumours and those within bladder wall thickening [5].

Bashir determine the diagnostic accuracy of high-resolution MR imaging done at 1.5 T in distinguishing bladder-restricted tumour from non-bladder-restricted tumour and compare the mean short axis dimension of metastatic pelvic lymph nodes with benign pelvic lymph nodes [6]. The accuracy of MRI in differentiating distinguishing bladder-restricted tumour from non-bladder-restricted tumour was 67.72%. The mean short axis diameter of metastatic lymph nodes was greater than that of non-metastatic lymph nodes, i.e., 7.4 mm and 5.4 mm respectively.

Diffusion weighted magnetic resonance imaging (DWI) and dynamic contrast-enhanced (DCE) MRI have been considered useful for pathological staging and histological grading in bladder cancer [7]. A total of 59 patients with 69 pathologically confirmed tumour lesions were included in this study. All patients underwent MR examination at 3.0 T basing on DWI and DCE imaging [7]. Aggressiveness of bladder cancer is negatively correlated with ADC value (r = −0.705, p < 0.0001) and wash-out rate (r = −0.719, p < 0.0001) [7]. The tumour ADC value is positively correlated with wash-out rate (r = 0.555, p < 0.0001). The diagnostic specificity and accuracy using tumour ADC value and wash-out for the tumour with size <24 mm were better than that tumours with size ≥24 mm [7]. The sensitivity, specificity and accuracy of ADC and wash-out rate in combination in diagnosis of bladder cancer aggressiveness were 96.7%, 94.9% and 95.7%, respectively [7]. ROC curve revealed the diagnostic performance of aggressiveness of bladder cancer using ADC value and wash-out rate were 0.928 (cut-off value: 0.905×10^{-3} mm²/s) and 0.891 (cut-off value: 0.685 min⁻¹), respectively [7]. ADC and wash-out rate derived from DWI and DCE-MRI at 3.0 T have good potential to assess the aggressiveness of bladder cancer and the accuracy was greater for ADC than for semi-quantitative parameters.

The correlation between clinical tumour stage and pathological tumour stage in radical cystectomy specimens in locally advanced bladder cancer is suboptimal [8]. MRI overestimated tumour stage in 23 out of 47 patients (49%), whereas 6 patients (13%) were understaged [8]. In the three groups of patients (those with the same stage group at MRI as in the cystectomy specimen, overestimated tumour stage and understaged patients), the time interval between transurethral resection of the bladder (TURB) and MRI did not differ significantly. Preoperative MRI overestimated tumour stage in almost half of the patients investigated in this study. Postoperative changes could have contributed to such overstaging with MRI.

15.2   PET Imaging in Bladder Cancer

Since the introduction of combined radiologic-nuclear imaging procedures like PET/CT and PET/MRI, new and promising diagnostic tools in bladder and prostate cancer imaging are available to physicians [9]. Although PET-based hybrid imaging in bladder cancer is currently utilized only in selected cases, an increase in PET imaging can be observed in prostate cancer due to the development of cancer-specific PET tracers [9]. Especially novel ligands of prostate-specific membrane antigen (PSMA) exhibit great potential to effectively influence future staging of prostate cancer [9]. However, before recommendations for implication in routine staging can be given, evaluation in the context of prospective multicenter clinical trials are mandatory.

The treatment and prognosis of bladder cancer are based on the depth of primary tumour invasion. Bashir determine the diagnostic accuracy of high-resolution MR imaging done at 1.5 T in distinguishing bladder-restricted tumor from non-bladder-restricted tumor and compare the mean short axis dimension of metastatic pelvic lymph nodes with benign pelvic lymph nodes [6].

The accuracy of MRI in differentiating distinguishing bladder-restricted tumor from non-bladder-restricted tumor was 67.72%. The mean short axis diameter of metastatic lymph nodes was greater than that of non-metastatic lymph nodes, i.e., 7.4 mm and 5.4 mm respectively.

A highly accurate preoperative tumour, node, metastasis (TNM) staging is critical to proper patient management and treatment [10]. This study retrospectively investigated the value of ¹⁸F-fluorodeoxyglucose (FDG) positron emission tomography/computed axial tomography (¹⁸F-FDG PET/CT) and magnetic resonance imaging (MRI) for preoperative N staging of bladder cancer [10]. ¹⁸F-FDG PET/CT and MRI were performed in 18 patients [10]. The specificities for detection of lymph-node metastases for MRI and ¹⁸F-FDG PET/CT were 80% (n = 15) and 93.33%

(n = 15), respectively [10]. The negative predictive values were 80% (n = 15) and 87.5% (n = 16) for MRI and ^{18}F-FDG PET/CT, respectively [10].

In patients with bladder cancer (BCa) preoperative staging with (11)C-choline positron emission tomography-computed tomography (PET/CT) could be used to derive prognostic information and hence stratify patients preoperatively with respect to disease management [11]. There was no statistically significant difference in OS and CSD between the patient groups when stratified for organ-confined versus non-organ-confined disease or lymph node involvement defined by either (11)C-choline PET/CT (OS: p = 0.262, hazard ratio [HR] = 1.60; p = 0.527, HR = 0.76; CSD: p = 0.144, HR = 2.25; p = 0.976, HR = 0.98) or CT (OS: p = 0.518, HR = 1.34; p = 0.228, HR = 1.67; CSD: p = 0.323, HR = 1.90; p = 0.136, HR = 2.38). The limitation of this study is the small number of included patients [11]. In this prospective trial neither CT nor (11)C-choline PET/CT were able to sufficiently predict OS or CSD in BCa patients treated with radical cystectomy albeit trends and moderately increased HRs could be demonstrated without significant differences between CT or (11)C-choline PET/CT [11].

Mertens investigated the association between extravesical (18) F-fluorodeoxyglucose (FDG) avid lesions on FDG-positron emission tomography/ computed tomography (PET/CT) and mortality in patients with muscle-invasive bladder cancer [12]. Of the 211 patients, 98 (46.4%) had 1 or more extravesical lesions on PET/CT, 113 (53.5%) had a negative PET/CT. Conventional CT revealed extravesical lesions in 51 patients (24.4%) [12]. Patients with a positive PET/CT had a significantly shorter OS and DSS (median OS: 14 vs. 50 months, p = 0.001; DSS: 16 vs. 50 months, p < 0.001). On the basis of our results, the presence of extravesical FDG-avid lesions on PET/CT might be considered an independent indicator of mortality.

Positron emission tomography/computed tomography (PET/CT) with (18) F-fluorodeoxyglucose (FDG) has been used with limited success in the past in primary diagnosis and locoregional staging of urinary bladder cancer, mainly because of the pharmacokinetics of renal excretion of (18)F-FDG [13]. Nayak evaluated the potential application of diuretic (18)F-FDG PET/CT in improving detection and locoregional staging of urinary bladder tumours [13]. Of the 25 patients, CECT detected a primary tumour in 23 (sensitivity 92%), while (18)F-FDG PET/CT was positive in 24 patients (sensitivity 96%). Mean size and maximum standardized uptake value of the bladder tumours were 3.33 cm (range 1.6–6.2) and 5.3 (range 1.3–11.7), respectively [13]. Of the 25 patients, only 10 patients underwent radical cystectomy based on disease status on TURBT [13]. Among those 10 patients, 9 had locoregional metastases. Among the 9 patients who had positive lymph nodes for metastasis on histopathology, CECT and PET/CT scan had a sensitivity of 44% and 78%, respectively [13]. (18)F-FDG PET/CT was found to be superior to CECT in the detection of the primary tumour and locoregional staging (p < 0.05) [13]. Diuretic (18)F-FDG PET/CT is highly sensitive and specific and plays an important role in improving detection of the primary tumour and locoregional staging of urinary bladder tumours. Diuretic (18)F-FDG PET/CT demonstrated a higher diagnostic value when compared with CECT in these patients.

Kollberg evaluated the clinical use of [(18)F]fluorodeoxyglucose-positron emission tomography/computed tomography (FDG-PET/CT) in addition to conventional preoperative radiological investigations in a defined group of patients with high-risk muscle-invasive bladder cancer [14]. Compared to CT alone, FDG-PET/CT provided more supplemental findings suggesting malignant manifestations in 48 (47%) of the 103 patients [14]. The additional FDG-PET/CT findings led to an altered provisional treatment plan in 28 out of 103 patients (27%), detection of disseminated bladder cancer and subsequent cancellation of the initially intended cystectomy in 16 patients, and identification of disseminated disease and treatment with induction chemotherapy before radical cystectomy in 12 patients [14]. Preoperative FDG-PET/CT changed the treatment plan for a considerable proportion (27%) of the present patients [14]. Accordingly, such examination can potentially improve the preoperative staging of cystectomy patients with high-risk features, and may also reduce the number of futile operations in patients with advanced disease who are beyond cure [14].

References

1. Verma S, Rajesh A, Prasad SR, Gaitonde K, Lall CG, Mouraviev V, Aeron G, Bracken RB, Sandrasegaran K. Urinary bladder cancer: role of MR imaging. Radiographics. 2012;32(2):371–87.
2. Yamada Y, Kobayashi S, Isoshima S, Arima K, Sakuma H, Sugimura Y. The usefulness of diffusion-weighted magnetic resonance imaging in bladder cancer staging and functional analysis. J Cancer Res Ther. 2014;10(4):878–82.
3. Ohgiya Y, Suyama J, Sai S, Kawahara M, Takeyama N, Ohike N, Sasamori H, Munechika J, Saiki M, Onoda Y, Hirose M, Gokan T. Preoperative T staging of urinary bladder cancer: efficacy of stalk detection and diagnostic performance of diffusion-weighted imaging at 3T. Magn Reson Med Sci. 2014;13(3):175–81.
4. Daneshmand S, Ahmadi H, Huynh LN, Dobos N. Preoperative staging of invasive bladder cancer with dynamic gadolinium-enhanced magnetic resonance imaging: results from a prospective study. Urology. 2012;80(6):1313–8.
5. Nguyen HT, Pohar KS, Jia G, Shah ZK, Mortazavi A, Zynger DL, Wei L, Clark D, Yang X, Knopp MV. Improving bladder cancer imaging using 3-T functional dynamic contrast-enhanced magnetic resonance imaging. Investig Radiol. 2014;49(6):390–5.
6. Bashir U, Ahmed I, Bashir O, Azam M, Faruqui ZS, Uddin N. Diagnostic accuracy of high resolution MR imaging in local staging of bladder tumors. J Coll Physicians Surg Pak. 2014;24(5):314–7.
7. Zhou G, Chen X, Zhang J, Zhu J, Zong G, Wang Z. Contrast-enhanced dynamic and diffusion-weighted MR imaging at 3.0T to assess aggressiveness of bladder cancer. Eur J Radiol. 2014;83(11):2013–8.
8. Liedberg F, Bendahl PO, Davidsson T, Gudjonsson S, Holmer M, Månsson W, Wallengren NO. Preoperative staging of locally advanced bladder cancer before radical cystectomy using 3 tesla magnetic resonance imaging with a standardized protocol. Scand J Urol. 2013;47(2):108–12.
9. Maurer T, Eiber M, Krause BJ. [Molecular multimodal hybrid imaging in prostate and bladder cancer]. Urologe A. 2014a;53(4):469–83.
10. Jensen TK, Holt P, Gerke O, Riehmann M, Svolgaard B, Marcussen N, Bouchelouche K. Preoperative lymph-node staging of invasive urothelial bladder cancer with 18F-fluorodeoxyglucose positron emission tomography/computed axial tomography and

magnetic resonance imaging: correlation with histopathology. Scand J Urol Nephrol. 2011;45(2):122–8.

11. Maurer T, Horn T, Souvatzoglou M, Eiber M, Beer AJ, Heck MM, Haller B, Gschwend JE, Schwaiger M, Treiber U, Krause BJ. Prognostic value of 11C-choline PET/CT and CT for predicting survival of bladder cancer patients treated with radical cystectomy. Urol Int. 2014b;93(2):207–13.

12. Mertens LS, Mir MC, Scott AM, Lee ST, Fioole-Bruining A, Vegt E, Vogel WV, Manecksha R, Bolton D, Davis ID, Horenblas S, van Rhijn BW, Lawrentschuk N. 18F-Fluorodeoxyglucose—positron emission tomography/computed tomography aids staging and predicts mortality in patients with muscle-invasive bladder cancer. Urology. 2014;83(2):393–8.

13. Nayak B, Dogra PN, Naswa N, Kumar R. Diuretic 18F-FDG PET/CT imaging for detection and locoregional staging of urinary bladder cancer: prospective evaluation of a novel technique. Eur J Nucl Med Mol Imaging. 2013;40(3):386–93.

14. Kollberg P, Almquist H, Bläckberg M, Cronberg C, Garpered S, Gudjonsson S, Kleist J, Lyttkens K, Patschan O, Liedberg F. [(18)F]Fluorodeoxyglucose - positron emission tomography/computed tomography improves staging in patients with high-risk muscle-invasive bladder cancer scheduled for radical cystectomy. Scand J Urol. 2015;49(4):296–301.

A Systematic Review on the Staging Conundrum in Bladder Cancer

16

A systematic review relating to staging, imaging and bladder cancer was conducted. The search strategy aimed to identify all references related to the Staging conundrum and Bladder Cancer. Search terms used were as follows: (Bladder cancer) AND (Staging) AND (Imaging). The following databases were screened from 1989 to June 2020:

- CINAHL
- MEDLINE (NHS Evidence)
- Cochrane
- AMed
- EMBASE
- PsychINFO
- SCOPUS
- Web of Science.

In addition, searches using Medical Subject Headings (MeSH) and keywords were conducted using Cochrane databases. Two UK-based experts in bladder cancer were consulted to identify any additional studies.

Studies were eligible for inclusion if they reported primary research focusing on bladder cancer and screening. Papers were included if published after 1984 and had to be in English. Studies that did not conform to this were excluded. Only primary research was included.

Abstracts were independently screened for eligibility by two reviewers and disagreements resolved through discussion or third party opinion (Fig. 16.1). Agreement level was calculated using Cohen's Kappa to test the intercoder reliability of this screening process. Cohens' Kappa allows comparison of inter-rater reliability between papers using relative observed agreement. This also takes account of the comparison occurring by chance. The first reviewer agreed all 14 papers to be included, the second, agreed on 14. Cohens' Kappa was 1.0.

© The Editor(s) (if applicable) and The Author(s), under exclusive license to
Springer Nature Switzerland AG 2021
S. S. Goonewardene et al., *Management of Muscle Invasive Bladder Cancer*,
Management of Urology, https://doi.org/10.1007/978-3-030-57915-9_16

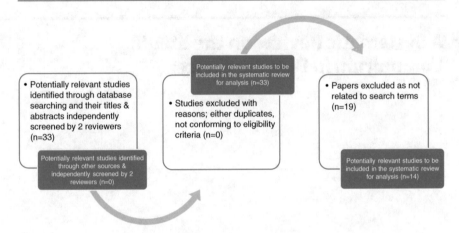

Fig. 16.1 Flow chart of studies identified through the systematic review. (Adapted from PRISMA)

Data extraction was piloted by the researcher and amended in consultation with the research team (author and two academic supervisors). Data collected included authors, year and country of publication, study aims, setting, intervention aims, number of participants, study design, intervention components and delivery methods, comparison groups and outcome measures, notes and follow-up questions for the authors. Studies were quality assessed using the PRISMA criteria for randomised controlled trials, Mays et al. [1, 2] for the action research and qualitative studies and the Critical Skills Appraisal programme for cohort studies. This was also applied to randomised controlled trials and qualitative studies. There were 14 cohort studies.

16.1   Systematic Review Results

16.1.1 Variation in Imaging for Bladder Cancer Staging

McInnes tested the hypotheses that use of preoperative imaging for muscle-invasive bladder cancer (MIBC) conforms to practice guidelines and preoperative imaging with accurate staging is related to improved outcomes [3]. Two thousand eight hundred and two patients with MIBC underwent cystectomy during 1994–2008 [3]. Over the three 5-year study periods there was an increase in preoperative chest X-ray (55%, 64%, 63%, p < 0.001), chest computed tomography (CT) (10%, 10%, 21%, p < 0.001), bone scan (30%, 34%, 36%; p = 0.04) and CT/magnetic resonance imaging/ultrasonography abdomen/pelvis (80%, 87%, 90%, p ≤ 0.001) [3]. Use of chest imaging was associated with age (odds ratio [OR] 1.24–1.59 compared with the youngest age group), N-stage (OR 0.79 for the NX group compared with the N+ group), surgeon volume (OR 0.47–0.53 compared with the highest volume quartile) and geographic region (OR 0.47–2.19 compared with the largest region) [3]. Use of bone scan was associated with

N-stage (OR 0.57 for the NX group compared with the N+ group) and geographic region (OR 0.71–1.34 compared with the largest region) [3].

16.1.2 MRI in Detection of NMIBC vs. MIBC

Panebianco determined multi-parametric magnetic resonance imaging (mpMRI) to differentiate muscle invasive bladder cancer (MIBC) from non-muscle invasive bladder cancer (NMIBC) [4]. Ninety-six percent of T1-labeled tumours by the T2W + DWI + PWI image set were confirmed to be NMIBC at histopathology [4]. Overall accuracy of the complete mpMRI protocol was 94% in differentiating NMIBC from MIBC [4]. PWI, DWI and DTI quantitative parameters were shown to be significantly different in cancerous versus non-cancerous areas within the bladder wall in T2-labelled lesions [4].

Preoperative discrimination between nonmuscle-invasive bladder carcinomas (NMIBC) and the muscle-invasive ones (MIBC) is very crucial in the management of patients with bladder cancer (BC) [5]. An optimal subset involving 19 features was selected from T_2 W and DW sequences, which outperformed the other subsets selected from T_2 W or DW sequence in muscle invasion discrimination [5]. The best performance for the differentiation task was achieved by the SVM-RFE + SMOTE classifier, with averaged sensitivity, specificity, accuracy, and area under the curve of receiver operating characteristic of 92.60%, 100%, 96.30%, and 0.9857, respectively, which outperformed the diagnostic accuracy by experts [5].

Pre-operative differentiation is vital for NMIBC or MIBC. Wang investigate whether intravoxel incoherent motion (IVIM) diffusion-weighted imaging (DWI) can differentiate NMIBC from MIBC [6]. Comparisons were made between the MIBC and NMIBC group, and differences were analyzed by comparing the areas under the curve (AUCs) [6]. The ADC and D value were significantly lower in patients with MIBC compared to those with NMIBC ($p < 0.01$) [6]. The AUC of D value (0.894) was significantly ($p < 0.05$) larger than the ADC value (0.786), with sensitivities and specificities of 95% and 87.5% (D) and 80% and 68.7% (ADC), respectively [6]. The D value obtained from IVIM exhibited better performance than conventional DWI for distinguishing NMIBC from MIBC and may serve as a potential imaging biomarker for bladder cancer invasion [6].

16.1.3 MRI in Low Grade vs. High Grade Bladder Cancer

The diagnostic performance of diffusion-weighted magnetic resonance imaging (DW-MRI) in bladder cancer was investigated by Kobayashi et al. [7]. In detecting bladder cancer, DW-MRI exhibited high sensitivity equivalent to that of T2W-MRI (>90%) [7]. Interobserver agreement was good for DW-MRI (κ score, 0.88), though moderate for T2W-MRI (0.67) [7]. ADC values were significantly lower in high-grade (vs. low-grade, $p < 0.0001$) and high-stage (T2 vs. T1 vs. Ta, $p < 0.0001$) tumours [7]. At a cut-off ADC value determined by partition analysis, clinically aggressive phenotypes including muscle-invasive bladder cancer (MIBC) and high-grade T1 disease were differentiated from less aggressive phenotypes with a sensitivity of 88%, a specificity of 85% and an accuracy of 87% [7].

16.1.4   Sensitivity and Specificity of MRI vs. CT Urogram

Extension through the deep muscle of the bladder wall was present in 20 of the 40 patients and was diagnosed with a sensitivity of 95% and a specificity of 95% [8]. Extension to perivesical fat was present in 18 of 40 patients, with a sensitivity of 66% and a specificity of 100% [8]. Invasion of the adjacent organs was present in 9 of 40 patients, with a sensitivity of 44% and a specificity of 96% [8]. On the basis of the MR findings, the tumour was correctly staged. In 24 of 40 (60%) patients, tumour extension was overestimated in 3 of 40 (7.5%) patients, and tumour extension was underestimated in 13 of 40 (32.5%) patients [8]. MR imaging has been shown to be accurate in identification of macroscopic lymph node involvement and deep muscle involvement [8]. It appears to be at least as useful as computed tomography (CT) in the evaluation of perivesical fat involvement and to be superior to CT in the detection of invasion of adjacent organs [8]. One limitation of MR imaging is in the evaluation of tumour extension into the periurethral glands [8].

16.1.5   The Role of High Resolution Ultrasound in Bladder Cancer Staging

Magnetic resonance imaging (MRI) has been proposed as a staging tool for bladder cancer (BC), but its use has been limited by its high costs and limited availability [9]. Saita tested the feasibility of high-resolution mUS in BC and ability to differentiate between non-muscle-invasive BC (NMIBC) and muscle-invasive BC (MIBC) [9]. Micro-US was accurate in differentiating the three layers of the bladder wall [9]. Bladder cancers were identified as heterogeneous structures protruding from the normal bladder wall. In 14 cases the lesions appeared confined to the lamina propria, and in all cases NMIBC was confirmed by the final pathological report. In other cases, the lesions extended into the muscular layer, but MIBC was confirmed in five out of seven cases (71.4%) [9].

16.1.6   Staging and VIRADS

Ueno evaluated the interobserver agreement and diagnostic performance of VI-RADS [10]. Data was assessed for 74 bladder cancers who had undergone mp-MRI before transurethral resection [10]. Five readers assessed the probability of MIBC using VI-RADS scores [10]. Interobserver agreement was excellent (ICC 0.85, 95% confidence interval 0.80–0.89) and the diagnostic performance of VI-RADS was represented as a pooled AUC of 0.90 (95% confidence interval

0.87–0.93) [10]. VI-RADS is suitable as a comprehensive tool for appropriate treatment planning for patients with bladder cancer [10].

Barchetti evaluated accuracy with Vesical Imaging-Reporting and Data System (VI-RADS) for differentiation of non-muscle invasive bladder cancer (NMIBC) and muscle-invasive bladder cancer (MIBC) [11]. Sensitivity and specificity were 91% and 89% for reader 1 and 82% and 85% for reader 2 respectively when the cutoff VI-RADS >2 was used to define MIBC [11]. At the same cutoff, PPV and NPV were 77% and 96% for reader 1 and 69% and 92% for reader 2 [11]. When the cutoff VI-RADS >3 was used, sensitivity and specificity were 82% and 94% for reader 1 and 77% and 89% for reader 2. Corresponding PPV and NPV were 86% and 93% for reader 1 and 74% and 91% for reader 2 [11]. Area under curve was 0.926 and 0.873 for reader 1 and 2 respectively. Inter-reader agreement was good for the overall score ($K = 0.731$) [11].

16.1.7   The Role of FDG PET in Bladder Cancer Staging

Goodfellow determine whether to use (18) F-fluorodeoxyglucose positron emission tomography (FDG PET) scans in the preoperative staging of bladder cancer (BC) [12]. The PET scan was able to detect metastatic disease outside of the pelvis with a sensitivity of 54% compared with 41% for the staging CT (N = 207) [12]. Both scans had similar specificities of 97% and 98% [12]. There were 13 PET avid lesions not visualised on the corresponding staging CT scans [12]. These proved to be metastatic BC (6 patients), a synchronous primary colonic cancer (1), colonic adenomas (1), basal cell tumour of the parotid gland (1) and inflammatory lesions (4) [12]. The sensitivity and specificity of the CT scans for pelvic LN involvement was 45% and 98%, respectively (N = 93) [12]. Using a combination of the PET and CT scan, the sensitivity for detecting metastatic disease in LNs increased to 69% with a 3% reduction in specificity to 95% [12].

16.1.8   Reviews Related to Systematic Review

Magnetic resonance imaging (MRI) has shown potential for local tumour detection and staging, but the accuracy for LNM detection remains disappointingly low [13]. The LN staging accuracy is improved with ultra-small super-paramagnetic particles of iron oxide (USPIO) [13]. This, however, is not commercially available at the moment [13]. Positron emission tomography (PET), a functional imaging technique most commonly accompanied with computed tomography (PET/CT), may also have a role in the detection of bladder cancer LNM in the future [13]. According to the currently available scientific evidence, recommendations include, use of pelvic MRI for primary tumour evaluation and local LNM detection acknowledging limited nodal imaging accuracy, pelvic/abdominal/chest CT for evaluation of distant metastasis [13]. The scientific evidence does not support the routine use of PET/CT (18F-FDG, 18F/11C-choline, 11C-acetate) in bladder cancer staging or in LNM detection [13].

Malayeri, reviewed papers related to cross-sectional imaging to assess local, nodal, and distant metastases in MIBC [14]. CT with contrast is a practical approach, but potential for understaging of small lymph nodes or foci of metastasis is present [14]. Multiparametric MRI is emerging as the imaging modality of choice in tumour staging, with a reported accuracy of more than 90% [14]. Locoregional lymph node metastasis can also be accurately evaluated using functional MRI [14]. PET/CT with conventional radiotracers is a common imaging modality for staging distant metastases [14].

Early and accurate diagnosis of Bladder cancer (BCa) will contribute extensively to the management of the disease [15]. A total of 81 published papers were reviewed [15]. For patients with haematuria and suspected of BCa, cystoscopy and CT are most commonly recommended [15]. Ultrasonography, MRI, PET/CT using ^{18}F-FDG or ^{11}C-choline and recently PET/MRI using ^{18}F-FDG also play a prominent role in detection of BCa [15].

16.1.9   Grey Literature Related to Systematic Review

Muscle-invasive bladder cancer (MIBC) has a tendency toward urothelial multifocality and is at risk for local and distant spread, most commonly to the lymph nodes, bone, lung, liver, and peritoneum [16]. Pretreatment staging of MIBC should include imaging of the urothelial upper tract for synchronous lesions; imaging of the chest, abdomen, and pelvis for metastases; and MRI pelvis for local staging. CT abdomen and pelvis without and with contrast (CT urogram) is recommended to assess the urothelium and abdominopelvic organs [16]. Pelvic MRI can improve local bladder staging accuracy [16]. Chest imaging is also recommended with chest radiograph usually being adequate [16]. FDG-PET/CT may be appropriate to identify nodal and metastatic disease [16].

16.1.10   Systematic Review Conclusion

CT is used in two modes, CT and computed tomographic urography (CTU), both for diagnosis and staging of BCa [15]. However, they cannot differentiate T1 and T2 BCa [15]. MRI is performed to diagnose invasive BCa and can differentiate muscle invasive bladder carcinoma (MIBC) from non-muscle invasive bladder carcinoma (NMIBC) [15]. However, CT and MRI have low sensitivity for nodal staging [15]. For nodal staging PET/CT is preferred [15]. PET/MRI provides better differentiation of normal and pathologic structures as compared with PET/CT [15].

References

1. Moher D, Liberati A, Tetzlaff J, Altman DG. "Preferred Reporting Items for Systematic Reviews and Meta-Analyses: The Prisma Statement." [In English]. BMJ (Online) 339, no. 7716 (08 Aug 2009):332–36.
2. Mays N, Pope C, Popay J. "Systematically Reviewing Qualitative and Quantitative Evidence to Inform Management and Policy-Making in the Health Field." [In English]. Journal of Health Services Research and Policy 10, no. SUPPL. 1 (July 2005):6–20.

3. McInnes MD, Siemens DR, Mackillop WJ, Peng Y, Wei S, Schieda N, Booth CM. Utilisation of preoperative imaging for muscle-invasive bladder cancer: a population-based study. BJU Int. 2016;117(3):430–8.
4. Panebianco V, De Berardinis E, Barchetti G, Simone G, Leonardo C, Grompone MD, Del Monte M, Carano D, Gallucci M, Catto J, Catalano C. An evaluation of morphological and functional multi-parametric MRI sequences in classifying non-muscle and muscle invasive bladder cancer. Eur Radiol. 2017;27(9):3759–66.
5. Xu X, Zhang X, Tian Q, Wang H, Cui LB, Li S, Tang X, Li B, Dolz J, Ayed IB, Liang Z, Yuan J, Du P, Lu H, Liu Y. Quantitative identification of nonmuscle-invasive and muscle-invasive bladder carcinomas: a multiparametric MRI radiomics analysis. J Magn Reson Imaging. 2019;49(5):1489–98.
6. Wang F, Wu LM, Hua XL, Zhao ZZ, Chen XX, Xu JR. Intravoxel incoherent motion diffusion-weighted imaging in assessing bladder cancer invasiveness and cell proliferation. J Magn Reson Imaging. 2018;47(4):1054–60.
7. Kobayashi S, Koga F, Yoshida S, Masuda H, Ishii C, Tanaka H, Komai Y, Yokoyama M, Saito K, Fujii Y, Kawakami S, Kihara K. Diagnostic performance of diffusion-weighted magnetic resonance imaging in bladder cancer: potential utility of apparent diffusion coefficient values as a biomarker to predict clinical aggressiveness. Eur Radiol. 2011;21(10):2178–86.
8. Buy JN, Moss AA, Guinet C, Ghossain MA, Malbec L, Arrive L, Vadrot D. MR staging of bladder carcinoma: correlation with pathologic findings. Radiology. 1988;169(3):695–700.
9. Saita A, Lughezzani G, Buffi NM, Hurle R, Nava L, Colombo P, Diana P, Fasulo V, Paciotti M, Elefante GM, Lazzeri M, Guazzoni G, Casale P. Assessing the feasibility and accuracy of high-resolution microultrasound imaging for bladder cancer detection and staging. Eur Urol. 2019;18:e2230.
10. Ueno Y, Takeuchi M, Tamada T, Sofue K, Takahashi S, Kamishima Y, Hinata N, Harada K, Fujisawa M, Murakami T. Diagnostic accuracy and interobserver agreement for the vesical imaging-reporting and data system for muscle-invasive bladder cancer: a multireader validation study. Eur Urol. 2019;76(1):54–6.
11. Barchetti G, Simone G, Ceravolo I, Salvo V, Campa R, Del Giudice F, De Berardinis E, Buccilli D, Catalano C, Gallucci M, Catto JWF, Panebianco V. Multiparametric MRI of the bladder: inter-observer agreement and accuracy with the Vesical Imaging-Reporting and Data System (VI-RADS) at a single reference center. Eur Radiol. 2019;29:5498–506.
12. Goodfellow H, Viney Z, Hughes P, Rankin S, Rottenberg G, Hughes S, Evison F, Dasgupta P, O'Brien T, Khan MS. Role of fluorodeoxyglucose positron emission tomography (FDG PET)-computed tomography (CT) in the staging of bladder cancer. BJU Int. 2014;114(3):389–95.
13. Salminen AP, Jambor I, Syvänen KT, Boström PJ. Lymph node imaging in bladder cancer. Minerva Urol Nefrol. 2015.
14. Malayeri AA, Pattanayak P, Apolo AB. Imaging muscle-invasive and metastatic urothelial carcinoma. Curr Opin Urol. 2015;25(5):441–8.
15. Salmanoglu E, Halpern E, Trabulsi EJ, Kim S, Thakur ML. A glance at imaging bladder cancer. Clin Transl Imaging. 2018;6(4):257–69.
16. Expert Panel on Urologic Imaging, van der Pol CB, Sahni VA, Eberhardt SC, Oto A, Akin O, Alexander LF, Allen BC, Coakley FV, Froemming AT, Fulgham PF, Hosseinzadeh K, Maranchie JK, Mody RN, Schieda N, Schuster DM, Venkatesan AM, Wang CL, Lockhart ME. ACR appropriateness criteria® pretreatment staging of muscle-invasive bladder cancer. J Am Coll Radiol. 2018;15(5S):S150–9.

Current State of Investigations and Limitations in Muscle Invasive Bladder Cancer

17

17.1 MIBC: Is Upper Tract Imaging Required?

Al-Mula Abed conducted a single-center prospective study to examine the usefulness of investigating the upper tract in visible haematuria [1]. In total, 57 patients (aged 23–95 years) with initial or terminal VH were identified [1]. Of these, 56 had FC and 9 patients were subsequently diagnosed with a LUT malignancy [1]. With regards to upper urinary tract (UUT), 35 patients (61.4%) had an USS, 46 (80.7%) underwent a CTU, and 25 (43.9%) patients had both [1]. In this group, no UUT malignancy was identified on upper tract imaging [1]. FC is recommended, but a non-invasive USS can be a safe initial investigation for the UUT, with a CTU subsequently considered in those with abnormalities on USS and those with ongoing bleeding [1].

17.2 MIBC: Is There a Role for Urine Cytology in Haematuria Investigations?

Urine cytology has been a long-standing first line investigation for haematuria and is recommended in current major guidelines [2]. Mishriki determined the contribution of urine cytology in haematuria investigations. Patients with positive urine cytology as the only finding underwent further cystoscopy, retrograde studies or ureteroscopy with biopsy under general anaesthesia [2]. Of the patients 124 (4.5%) had malignant cells and 260 (9.4%) had atypical/suspicious results [2]. For urothelial cancer cytology demonstrated 45.5% sensitivity and 89.5% specificity [2]. Two patients with urine cytology as the only positive finding had urothelial malignancy on further investigation [2].

S. S. Goonewardene et al., *Management of Muscle Invasive Bladder Cancer*, Management of Urology, https://doi.org/10.1007/978-3-030-57915-9_17

17.3   Is Cystoscopy Required for Investigation of Microscopic Haematuria?

The non-invasive bladder cancer urine test system (CXbladder) for asymptomatic microscopic haematuria (AMH), may suggest cystoscopy and invasive tests are not required [3]. Physicians reduced invasive procedures for individuals identified as having a low probability of UC with Cxbladder [3]. The intensity of investigation was targeted and increased, including use of total procedures and cystoscopy, for patients identified by Cxbladder tests as having a high probability of UC [3]. The outcome resulted in patients with a high risk of UC receiving appropriate guideline-recommended invasive diagnostic tests [3]. Patients who tested negative were offered fewer and significantly less invasive procedures [3].

Rodgers determine the most effective diagnostic strategy for investigating haematuria in adults [4]. Eighteen out of 19 identified studies evaluated dipstick tests, suggesting moderate usefulness in establishing the presence of haematuria [4]. Twenty-eight studies included data on the accuracy of laboratory tests (tumour markers, cytology) for the diagnosis of bladder cancer [4]. The majority of tumour marker studies evaluated nuclear matrix protein 22 or bladder tumour antigen. The sensitivity and specificity ranges suggested that neither are useful either for diagnosing bladder cancer or for ruling out further investigation (cystoscopy) [4]. Fifteen studies evaluating urine cytology, with high specificity, suggesting some possible utility in confirming malignancy [4].

Regine investigates the sensitivity of virtual CT in assessing lesion of the bladder wall to compare it with that of conventional endoscopy, and outlines the indications, advantages and disadvantages of virtual CT-pneumocystography [5]. Thirty lesions (24 pedunculated, 6 sessile) were detected at conventional cystoscopy in 16 patients (multiple polyposis in 3 cases) [5]. Virtual cystoscopy identified 23 lesions (19 pedunculated and 4 sessile) [5]. The undetected lesions were pedunculated <5 mm (5 cases) and sessile (2 cases). One correctly identified pedunculated lesion was associated with a bladder stone [5].

17.4   Role of Biomarkers as a Replacement for Haematuria Investigations

Urinary markers simplify surveillance schedules and improve early detection of tumours, especially in NMIBC [6]. Several biomarkers show a higher sensitivity than urinary cytology [6]. Molecular biomarkers in this field are strongly desired [6]. Molecular profiling using is more feasible with recent developments in sequencing technologies [6]. Currently, molecular profiling is are being used for early detection, prediction of prognosis, and drug sensitivity [6]. Furthermore, several groups used transcriptome profiling to classify MIBC into various distinct subtypes, showing distinct clinical behaviours and responses to chemotherapy and immune checkpoint inhibitors [6]. However, guidelines have yet to take this into account.

References

1. Al-Mula Abed OWS, Srirangam SJ, Wemyss-Holden GD. Upper tract imaging in patients with initial or terminal hematuria suggestive of bleeding from the lower urinary tract: how often is the upper urinary tract responsible for the hematuria? Oman Med J. 2018;33(5):374–9.
2. Mishriki SF, Aboumarzouk O, Vint R, Grimsley SJ, Lam T, Somani B. Routine urine cytology has no role in hematuria investigations. J Urol. 2013;189(4):1255–8.
3. Lough T, Luo Q, Luxmanan C, Anderson A, Suttie J, O'Sullivan P, Darling D. Clinical utility of a non-invasive urine test for risk assessing patients with no obvious benign cause of hematuria: a physician-patient real world data analysis. BMC Urol. 2018;18(1):18.
4. Rodgers M, Nixon J, Hempel S, Aho T, Kelly J, Neal D, Duffy S, Ritchie G, Kleijnen J, Westwood M. Diagnostic tests and algorithms used in the investigation of haematuria: systematic reviews and economic evaluation. Health Technol Assess. 2006;10(18):iii–iv, xi–259.
5. Regine G, Atzori M, Buffa V, Miele V, Ialongo P, Adami L. Virtual CT-pneumocystoscopy: indications, advantages and limitations. Our experience. Radiol Med. 2003;106(3):154–9.
6. Kojima T, Kawai K, Miyazaki J, Nishiyama H. Biomarkers for precision medicine in bladder cancer. Int J Clin Oncol. 2017;22(2):207–13.

Bladder Cancer Surveillance

18

18.1 Research Methods

A systematic review relating to bladder cancer surveillance was conducted. This was to identify the bladder cancer epidemiology and risk factors in muscle invasive disease. The search strategy aimed to identify all references related to bladder cancer AND surveillance. Search terms used were as follows: (Bladder cancer) AND (Surveillance). The following databases were screened from 1989 to June 2020:

- CINAHL
- MEDLINE (NHS Evidence)
- Cochrane
- AMed
- EMBASE
- PsychINFO
- SCOPUS
- Web of Science.

In addition, searches using Medical Subject Headings (MeSH) and keywords were conducted using Cochrane databases. Two UK-based experts in bladder cancer were consulted to identify any additional studies.

Studies were eligible for inclusion if they reported primary research focusing on bladder cancer and screening. Papers were included if published after 1984 and had to be in English. Studies that did not conform to this were excluded. Only primary research was included (Fig. 18.1). The overall aim was to identify bladder cancer risk factors and epidemiology in muscle invasive disease.

Abstracts were independently screened for eligibility by two reviewers and disagreements resolved through discussion or third party opinion. Agreement level was calculated using Cohen's Kappa to test the intercoder reliability of this screening process. Cohens' Kappa allows comparison of inter-rater reliability between papers

© The Editor(s) (if applicable) and The Author(s), under exclusive license to
Springer Nature Switzerland AG 2021
S. S. Goonewardene et al., *Management of Muscle Invasive Bladder Cancer*,
Management of Urology, https://doi.org/10.1007/978-3-030-57915-9_18

using relative observed agreement. This also takes account of the comparison occurring by chance. The first reviewer agreed all 14 papers to be included, the second, agreed on 14. Cohens kappa was therefore 1.0.

Data extraction was piloted by the researcher and amended in consultation with the research team (author and two academic supervisors). Data collected included authors, year and country of publication, study aims, setting, intervention aims, number of participants, study design, intervention components and delivery methods, comparison groups and outcome measures, notes and follow-up questions for the authors. Studies were quality assessed using the PRISMA criteria for randomised controlled trials, Mays et al. [1, 2] for the action research and qualitative studies and the Critical Skills Appraisal programme for cohort studies. This was also applied to randomised controlled trials and qualitative studies.

The search identified 708 papers (Fig. 18.1). All 14 out of 708 mapped to the search terms and eligibility criteria. The current systematic reviews were examined to gain further knowledge about the subject. Three hundred and ninety papers were excluded due to not conforming to eligibility criteria or adding to the evidence. Of the 14 papers left, relevant abstracts were identified and the full papers obtained (all of which were in English), to quality assure against search criteria. There was considerable heterogeneity of design among the included studies therefore a narrative review of the evidence was undertaken. There was significant heterogeneity within studies, including clinical topic, numbers, outcomes, as a result a narrative review was thought to be best. There were 12 cohort studies, with a moderate level of evidence and two trials, with a good level of evidence. These were from a range of countries with minimal loss to follow-up. All participants were identified appropriately.

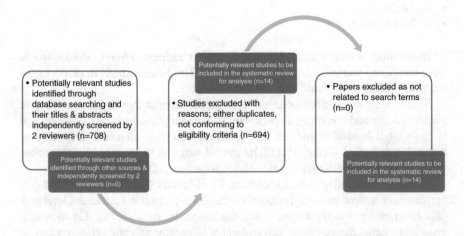

Fig. 18.1   Flow chart of studies identified through the systematic review. (Adapted from PRISMA)

18.2   Systematic Review Results

18.2.1 Urinary Metabolites in Bladder Cancer Surveillance

Loras examined changes in the urinary metabolome of NMBIC patients before and after TURBT, as well during the subsequent surveillance period [3]. Adjusting by prior probability of recurrence per risk, discriminant analysis of UPLC-MS metabolic profiles, displayed negative predictive values for low, low-intermediate, high-intermediate and high risk patient groups of 96.5%, 94.0%, 92.9% and 76.1% respectively [3]. Detailed analysis revealed several candidate metabolites and perturbed phenylalanine, arginine, proline and tryptophan metabolisms as potential biomarkers [3]. A pilot retrospective analysis of longitudinal trajectories of a BC metabolic biomarkers during post TURBT surveillance was carried out and the results give strong support for the clinical use of metabolomic profiling in assessing NMIBC recurrence [3].

Jin used high-performance mass spectrometry (HPLC-QTOFMS) to profile urine metabolites of 138 patients with BC and 121 control subjects [4]. Multivariate statistical analysis revealed that the cancer group could be clearly distinguished from the control groups on the basis of their metabolomic profiles [4]. Patients with muscle-invasive BC could also be distinguished from patients with non-muscle-invasive BC on the basis of their metabolomic profiles [4]. Successive analyses identified 12 differential metabolites distinguishing between the BC and control groups, and many of them turned out to be involved in glycolysis and betaoxidation [4]. The association of these metabolites with cancer was corroborated by microarray results. This demonstrated carnitine transferase and pyruvate dehydrogenase complex expressions are significantly altered in cancer groups [4]. In terms of clinical applicability, the differentiation model diagnosed BC with a sensitivity and specificity of 91.3% and 92.5%, respectively, and comparable results were obtained by receiver operating characteristic analysis (AUC = 0.937) [4]. Multivariate regression also suggested that the metabolomic profile correlates with cancer-specific survival time [4].

18.2.2 CellDetect in Bladder Cancer Surveillance

CellDetect is a unique histochemical stain enabling colour and morphological discrimination between malignant and benign cells based on differences in metabolic signature [5]. The overall sensitivity of CellDetect was 84% [5]. Sensitivity for detecting low-grade nonmuscle-invasive bladder cancer was greater than BTA stat (78% vs. 54%) and more than twofold higher compared with standard cytology (33%, p ≤ 0.05) [5]. The specificity was 84% in routine surveillance by cystoscopy. At a median follow-up of 9 months, 21% with positive CellDetect and negative reference standard developed UCC, which was significantly higher compared with the 5% of the true negative cases [5]. Limitations include the lack of instrumental urine samples and the lack of patients with nongenitourinary cancers in the study population [5].

18.2.3 NMP 22 in Bladder Cancer Surveillance

Akaza determined the clinical usefulness of NMP22 (Nuclear Matrix Protein 22) as a urinary marker in bladder cancer surveillance compared with urine cytology [6]. Urinary NMP22 values were determined for 144 patients with histologically diagnosed bladder cancer, 65 patients with other urological cancers, and 171 healthy volunteers by use of a UNMP22 Test kit (an enzyme-linked immunosorbent assay) [6]. The sensitivities of urinary NMP22 and voided urine cytology were 61.1% (88/144) and 33.8% (48/144), respectively, a significant difference (p < 0.00001) [6]. Multivariate analysis revealed that tumour size affected the urinary NMP22 values [6]. The positive rate by tumour size was 42.3%, 59.1%, and 85.0% for tumours of <10 mm, 10–30 mm, and >30 mm, respectively [6]. Urinary NMP22 values decreased postoperatively in 82.9% of the patients [6]. The median NMP22 values for prostate cancer and renal cancer were 4.4 U/ml (95% CI: 2.2–6.7) and 6.2 U/ml (95% CI: 3.6–12.5) [6]. The positive rates were 24.2% and 31.3%, respectively, both of which were significantly lower than for bladder cancer [6].

18.2.4 5-Aminolevulinic Acid-Induced Fluorescence Endoscopy in Bladder Cancer Surveillance

Kriegmair determined whether neoplastic disease, missed under white light can be detected during transurethral resection with 5-aminolevulinic acid-induced porphyrin fluorescence [7]. In 82 (25%) cases additional neoplastic lesions were found due to red porphyrin fluorescence which was induced by 5-aminolevulinic acid. Thirty-one percent of these neoplastic foci which were found in normal and nonspecific inflamed mucosa had a poorly differentiated histology [7].

Loidl assessed flexible cystoscopy assisted by hexaminolevulinate (HAL) fluorescence [8]. In the 45 patients studied 41 (91%) had exophytic tumours, of which 39 (95.1%) were detected by HAL flexible cystoscopy and 40 (97.5%) by HAL rigid cystoscopy [8]. Seventeen (37.8%) had concomitant or carcinoma in situ only, which was identified by HAL flexible cystoscopy in 14 (82.3%), by HAL rigid cystoscopy in 15 (88.2%), by flexible standard in 11 (64.7%) and by standard white light rigid cystoscopy in 13 (76.7%) patients [8].

Daneshmand compared blue light flexible cystoscopy with white light flexible cystoscopy in surveillance [9]. Following surveillance 103 of the 304 patients were referred, including 63 with confirmed malignancy, 26 had carcinoma in situ [9]. In 13 of the 63 (20.6%, 95% CI 11.5–32.7) recurrence was seen only with blue light flexible cystoscopy (p < 0.0001) [9]. Five of these cases were confirmed as carcinoma in situ [9]. Operating room examination confirmed carcinoma in situ in 26 of 63 (41%), which was detected only with blue light cystoscopy in 9 of the 26 (34.6%, 95% CI 17.2–55.7, p < 0.0001) [9]. Blue light cystoscopy identified additional malignant lesions in 29 of the 63 patients (46%) [9]. The false-positive rate was

9.1% for white and blue light cystoscopy. None of the 12 adverse events during surveillance were serious [9].

Drejer examined whether photodynamic diagnosis (PDD) in addition to flexible cystoscopy reduces risk of tumour recurrence in prior non-muscle invasive bladder cancer [10]. PDD is an optical technique that enhances the visibility of pathologic tissue and helps guidance tumour resection [10]. A total of 351 patients were allocated to the intervention group (flexible PDD), and 348 to the control group (flexible white light) [10]. After randomization, only 117 patients in the intervention group had at least 1 tumour recurrence compared to 143 patients in the control group (p = 0.049) [10]. Odds ratio of 0.67 (p = 0.02, 95% CI: 0.48–0.95) correlates with a tumour reduction of 33% in favour of the intervention group [10].

18.2.5 The BTA Stat Test in Bladder Cancer Surveillance

Pode assessed the sensitivity and specificity of the non-invasive BTA stat urine test for detection of primary and recurrent bladder cancer with special reference to the size, grade and stage of the tumours, and examine the effect of intravesical bacillus Calmette-Guerin treatment on the results [11]. No tumour was found in 122 patients, primary transitional cell carcinoma was found in 71 and cystoscopy revealed recurrent tumours in 57 [11]. Overall sensitivity of the BTA stat test was 82.8% and specificity was 68.9% [11]. Sensitivity of urine cytology was 39.8% and specificity was 95.1% [11]. The BTA stat test detected 90.1% of the primary and 73.7% of the recurrent tumours [11]. All patients with carcinoma in situ, high grade tumors, muscle invasive cancer and tumors larger than 2 cm were diagnosed by the BTA stat test [11].

18.2.6 Bladder EpiCheck in Bladder Cancer Surveillance

Witjes assessed Bladder EpiCheck (BE) is a novel urine assay that uses 15 proprietary DNA methylation biomarkers to assess the presence of bladder cancer [12]. Out of 440 patients recruited, 353 were eligible for the performance analysis [12]. Overall sensitivity, specificity, NPV, and positive predictive value were 68.2%, 88.0%, 95.1%, and 44.8%, respectively [12]. Excluding low-grade (LG) Ta recurrences, the sensitivity was 91.7% and NPV was 99.3% [12]. The area under receiver operating characteristic (ROC) curves with and without LG Ta lesions was 0.82 and 0.94, respectively [12].

18.2.7 Microsatellite Analysis in Bladder Cancer Surveillance

de Bekker-Grob determined how good microsatellite analysis (MA) markers in voided urine samples should be to make a surveillance procedure cost-effective in which cystoscopy is partly replaced by MA for patients with non-muscle-invasive urothelial carcinoma (NMI-UC) [13]. The probability of being without recurrence after 2 years of surveillance was similar (86.6% conventional arm vs. 86.3% test arm) with currently available MA markers (sensitivity of 58% and specificity of 73%) [13].

van der Aa compared, in non-muscle-invasive low-grade (pTa/pT1, G1/G2) urothelial cell carcinoma of the urinary bladder, flexible cystoscopy or surveillance by microsatellite analysis (MA) in voided urine, in patients under regular cystoscopic surveillance (CUS) [14]. The introduction of the cystoscope was reported to cause discomfort in 39% and pain in 35% of the responses to the questionnaires; the waiting time for the results of MA was reported as burdensome in 19% [14]. Painful micturition was significantly more frequent in the week after CUS than after MA (30% and 12%, respectively) [14]. The frequency of fever (1% and 2%) and haematuria (7% and 6%) was similar in both groups [14]. Older patients reported significantly less pain and discomfort from cystoscopy, and this was not related to having more previous cystoscopies [14].

18.2.8 Urinary Cytology, BTA Trak and Cytokeratin's 8 and 18

Babjuk compared results of urinary cytology, quantitative detection of human complement factor H-related protein (BTA TRAK), and urinary fragments of cytokeratins 8 and 18 (UBC IRMA) with the recurrence status in pTapT1 bladder cancer to look for a role in a surveillance protocol [15]. The sensitivity and specificity of cytology, BTA, and UBC were 19.8% and 99%, 53.8% and 83.9%, and 12.1% and 97.2%, respectively [15]. The sensitivity of pTis detection was 66.6%, 0%, and 100%, respectively [15]. With cutoffs set to a sensitivity of 90%, the specificity of BTA and UBC dropped to 24.8% and 20.4%, respectively [15].

18.2.9 Urotel in Bladder Cancer Surveillance

The urine postal cytology kit Urotel was assessed against standard cytological method; 184 patients attending for routine surveillance cystourethroscopy provided free flow urine specimens [16]. The urine cytology was reported blind. Comparison of the two tests showed similar specificity but significantly higher sensitivity with the Urotel kit [16]. These kits may have a place in the surveillance of patients at high risk of recurrent tumour or those with carcinoma in situ [16].

References

1. Moher D, Liberati A, Tetzlaff J, Altman DG. "Preferred Reporting Items for Systematic Reviews and Meta-Analyses: The Prisma Statement." [In English]. BMJ (Online) 339, no. 7716 (08 Aug 2009):332–36.

2. Mays N, Pope C, Popay J. "Systematically Reviewing Qualitative and Quantitative Evidence to Inform Management and Policy-Making in the Health Field." [In English]. Journal of Health Services Research and Policy 10, no. SUPPL. 1 (July 2005):6–20.
3. Loras A, Trassierra M, Sanjuan-Herráez D, et al. Bladder cancer recurrence surveillance by urine metabolomics analysis. Sci Rep. 2018;8(1):9172.
4. Jin X, Yun SJ, Jeong P, Kim IY, Kim WJ, Park S. Diagnosis of bladder cancer and prediction of survival by urinary metabolomics. Oncotarget. 2014;5(6):1635–45.
5. Davis N, Shtabsky A, Lew S, et al. A novel urine-based assay for bladder cancer diagnosis: multi-institutional validation study. Eur Urol Focus. 2018;4(3):388–94.
6. Akaza H, Miyanaga N, Tsukamoto T, Ishikawa S, Noguchi R, Ohtani M, Kawabe K, Kubota Y, Fujita K, Obata K, Hirao Y, Kotake T, Ohmori H, Kumazawa J, Koiso K. [Evaluation of urinary NMP22 (nuclear matrix protein 22) as a diagnostic marker for urothelial cancer–NMP22 as a urinary marker for surveillance of bladder cancer. NMP22 Study Group]. Gan To Kagaku Ryoho. 1997 May;24(7):829–36.
7. Kriegmair M, Zaak D, Stepp H, et al. Transurethral resection and surveillance of bladder cancer supported by 5-aminolevulinic acid-induced fluorescence endoscopy. Eur Urol. 1999;36(5):386–92.
8. Loidl W, Schmidbauer J, Susani M, Marberger M. Flexible cystoscopy assisted by hexaminolevulinate induced fluorescence: a new approach for bladder cancer detection and surveillance? Eur Urol. 2005;47(3):323–6.
9. Daneshmand S, Patel S, Lotan Y, et al. Efficacy and safety of blue light flexible cystoscopy with hexaminolevulinate in the surveillance of bladder cancer: a phase III, comparative, multicenter study. J Urol. 2018;199(5):1158–65. [Published correction appears in J Urol. 2019;201(5):1017].
10. Drejer D, Moltke AL, Nielsen AM, Lam GW, Jensen JB. DaBlaCa-11: photodynamic diagnosis in flexible cystoscopy-a randomized study with focus on recurrence. Urology. 2020;137:91–6.
11. Pode D, Shapiro A, Wald M, Nativ O, Laufer M, Kaver I. Noninvasive detection of bladder cancer with the BTA stat test. J Urol. 1999;161(2):443–6.
12. Witjes JA, Morote J, Cornel EB, et al. Performance of the bladder EpiCheck™ methylation test for patients under surveillance for non-muscle-invasive bladder cancer: results of a multi-center, prospective, blinded clinical trial. Eur Urol Oncol. 2018;1(4):307–13.
13. de Bekker-Grob EW, van der Aa MN, Zwarthoff EC, et al. Non-muscle-invasive bladder cancer surveillance for which cystoscopy is partly replaced by microsatellite analysis of urine: a cost-effective alternative? BJU Int. 2009;104(1):41–7.
14. van der Aa MN, Steyerberg EW, Sen EF, et al. Patients' perceived burden of cystoscopic and urinary surveillance of bladder cancer: a randomized comparison. BJU Int. 2008;101(9):1106–10.
15. Babjuk M, Soukup V, Pesl M, et al. Urinary cytology and quantitative BTA and UBC tests in surveillance of patients with pTapT1 bladder urothelial carcinoma. Urology. 2008;71(4):718–22.
16. Smith AB, Daneshmand S, Patel S, et al. Patient-reported outcomes of blue-light flexible cystoscopy with hexaminolevulinate in the surveillance of bladder cancer: results from a prospective multicentre study. BJU Int. 2019;123(1):35–41.

Risk Stratification in Bladder Cancer

Urothelial tumours represent a spectrum of diseases with a range of prognoses [1]. Within each category of disease, more refined methods to determine prognosis and guide management, based on molecular staging, are under development [1]. These methods are aimed at optimizing the individual patient's likelihood of cure and chance for organ preservation [1]. For patients with more extensive disease, newer treatments typically involve combined-modality approaches using recently developed surgical procedures, or three-dimensional treatment planning for more precise delivery of radiation therapy [1]. While these are not appropriate in all cases, they do offer the promise of an improved quality of life and prolonged survival [1].

19.1   Accuracy of EORTC Risk Stratification

European Organization for Research and Treatment of Cancer (EORTC) risk tables only included 171 patients treated with bacillus Calmette-Guérin (BCG) for non-muscle-invasive bladder cancer (NMIBC) recurrence [2]. C-indices for progression were lower than c-indices reported previously [2]. Successful stratification of recurrence and progression probability at 1 and 5 years was achieved using the EORTC tables [2]. Model calibration showed lower risks of recurrence than those reported previously [2]. For progression, lower risks were found in higher-risk groups [2]. The EORTC model successfully stratified recurrence and progression risks [2].

19.2   EORTC Risk Stratification for MIBC Post Radical Cystectomy

May developed a risk stratification of muscle-invasive bladder cancer (MIBC) after radical cystectomy (RC) [3]. May compared the cancer-specific mortality (CSM) of primary MIBC and secondary MIBC in different risk groups according to the

S. S. Goonewardene et al., *Management of Muscle Invasive Bladder Cancer*, Management of Urology, https://doi.org/10.1007/978-3-030-57915-9_19

European Organisation for Research and Treatment of Cancer (EORTC) progression score [3]. CSM for patients with primary and secondary MIBC did not differ significantly [3]. Patients in SG2 with the highest risk for tumor stage progression at time of the first and last TURBT in non-MIBC showed a significantly higher CSM after RC compared with patients with low-to-intermediate risk and compared with patients in SG1 [3]. Risk stratification by the EORTC progression score can identify those at highest risk of CSM after progression to MIBC [3].

19.3   EORTC/CUETO Risk Stratification in Second TURBT

Applicability of European Organization for Research and Treatment of Cancer (EORTC) and Spanish Urological Club for Oncological Treatment (CUETO) models in NMIBC patients is under debate [4]. Zhang assessed the performance of EORTC and CUETO predictive models in NMIBC patients treated with second TUR [4]. Prior recurrence rate, grade, and second TUR pathology were independent prognostic factors for the risk of disease recurrence and progression [4]. The concordance index of the EORTC and the CUETO model was 0.563 and 0.516 for recurrence and 0.681 and 0.702 for progression, respectively [4]. The positive pathology after second TUR was significantly associated with risk of disease recurrence and progression [4]. EORTC and CUETO risk models estimated progression better than recurrence, especially with higher score groups [4].

19.4   Accuracy of EORTC and CUETO Scoring Systems

Choi aimed to confirm the utility of the European Organization for Research and Treatment of Cancer (EORTC) and the Spanish Urological Club for Oncological Treatment (CUETO) scoring systems, in non-muscle-invasive bladder cancer [5]. For risk of recurrence, with the EORTC model, all groups had statistically significant differences except between the group with a score of 0 and the group with a score of 1–4 [5]. With the CUETO model, all groups differed significantly [5]. For risk of progression, the EORTC model demonstrated significant differences between all groups except between the group with a score of 2–6 and the group with a score of 7–13 [5]. With the CUETO model, a significant difference was observed between the group with a score of 0 and the other groups [5]. The concordance index of the EORTC and CUETO models was 0.759 and 0.836 for recurrence and 0.704 and 0.745 for progression, respectively [5]. The area under the ROC curve for the EORTC and CUETO models was 0.832 and 0.894 for recurrence and 0.722 and 0.724 for progression, respectively [5].

Xylinas assessed the performance of these predictive tools in a large multicentre cohort of NMIBC patients [6]. Both tools exhibited a poor discrimination for disease recurrence and progression (0.597 and 0.662, and 0.523 and 0.616, respectively, for the EORTC and CUETO models) [6]. The EORTC tables overestimated the risk of disease recurrence and progression in high-risk patients [6]. The discrimination of the

EORTC tables was even lower in the subgroup of patients treated with BCG (0.554 and 0.576 for disease recurrence and progression, respectively) [6]. Conversely, the discrimination of the CUETO model increased in BCG-treated patients (0.597 and 0.645 for disease recurrence and progression, respectively) [6]. However, both models overestimated the risk of disease progression in high-risk patients [6].

Dalkilic compared the prediction accuracy of the European Organization for Research and Treatment of Cancer (EORTC) and the Spanish Urology Association for Oncological Treatment (CUETO) risk tables in all non-muscle invasive bladder cancer patients [7]. The recurrence rate was higher than in CUETO, and similar to EORTC [7]. The EORTC was determined to provide better discrimination than CUETO in the whole patient group and in those treated or not treated with BCG [7]. The concordance indices for these groups were 0.777, 0.705; 0.773, 0.669; and 0.823, 0.758, respectively [7]. The progression rate was similar in this study to the rate defined in both risk tables [7]. The discrimination power was similar in EORTC and CUETO for all the groups [7]. The concordance indices were 0.801, 0.881; 0.915, 0.930; and 0.832, 0.806, respectively [7].

19.5   EORTC vs. EAU Risk Stratification

Rieken characterized outcomes of TaT1 urothelial carcinoma of the bladder stratified by the European Association of Urology (EAU) categories and to compare them with European Organization for Research and Treatment of Cancer (EORTC) risk groups to assess the rate and effect of reclassification [8]. Of 5122 patients, 632 (12.3%), 2302 (45.0%), and 2188 (42.7%) were assigned to the low-, intermediate-, and high-risk EAU category, respectively [8]. Five hundred and sixteen (10.1%) experienced disease recurrence and progression, respectively [8]. In multivariable Cox-regression analyses, EAU intermediate- and high-risk categories were associated with a higher risk of disease recurrence (p < 0.001) and progression (p < 0.001) compared to low-risk patients [8]. Application of the EAU categories reclassified 1940 (37.9%) patients into a higher risk group for recurrence [8]. Likewise, 602 (11.8%) patients were reclassified to a higher and 278 (5.4%) to a lower risk group for progression [8].

Sakano validated the European Association of Urology (EAU) guidelines on risk group stratification to predict recurrence in Japanese patients with stage Ta and T1 bladder tumours [9]. Multivariate Cox proportional hazards regression analysis showed that the Eastern Cooperative Oncology Group performance status (ECOG PS), prior recurrence rate, number of tumours and T category were independent predictors of time to recurrence (p < 0.05) [9]. According to the EAU guidelines for predicting recurrence, the vast majority of Japanese patients were classified into intermediate risk [9]. The intermediate-risk patients were further divided into intermediate-low-risk and intermediate-high-risk subgroups, a significant difference in the recurrence-free survival rates was demonstrated (p < 0.001). It was also found that patients with high risk combined with intermediate-high risk had significantly poorer recurrence-free survival rates than those with low risk combined with intermediate-low risk (p < 0.001) [9].

19.6   Assessment of BCG Therapy Using the CUETO Risk Stratification Model

Bacillus Calmette-Guerin is the most effective therapy for non-muscle invasive bladder cancer [10]. Fernandez-Gomez developed a risk stratification model to provide accurate estimates of recurrence and progression probability after bacillus Calmette-Guerin [10]. A scoring system was calculated with a score of 0–16 for recurrence and 0–14 for progression [10]. Patients were categorized into four groups by score, and recurrence and progression probabilities were calculated in each group [10]. For recurrence the variables were gender, age, grade, tumour status, multiplicity and associated Tis [10]. For progression the variables were age, grade, tumour status, T category, multiplicity and associated Tis [10]. For recurrence calculated risks using Spanish Urological Club for Oncological Treatment tables were lower than those obtained with Sylvester tables [10].

19.7   AUA/SUO Guidelines in Bladder Cancer

Risk stratification should influence evaluation, treatment and surveillance [11]. The AUA/SUO guideline attempts to provide a clinical framework for the management of bladder cancer [11]. A risk-stratified approach categorizes patients into broad groups of low-, intermediate-, and high-risk. Importantly, the evaluation and treatment algorithm takes into account tumour characteristics and uniquely considers a patient's response to therapy [11]. This highlighted the intensity and scope of care for NMIBC should focus on patient, disease, and treatment response characteristics [11]. This guideline attempts to improve a clinician's ability to evaluate and treat each patient, but higher quality evidence in future trials will be essential to improve level of care for these patients [11].

Ravvaz evaluated the American Urological Association (AUA)/Society of Urologic Oncology (SUO) non-muscle invasive bladder cancer (NMIBC) risk model to predict recurrence and progression prior to death [12]. Patients <60 years old have a 40% greater probability of NMIBC recurrence versus death, whereas, patients ≥84 years old had a 12% greater probability of death prior to recurrence at 5 years [12]. The AUA/SUO NMIBC risk model provides similar predictive performance of recurrence and progression to previous NMIBC risk models such as EORTC, CUETO and NCCN [12].

19.8   EORTC Classification vs. AUA Guidelines for Bladder Cancer

Wang compared the applicability of European Organization for Research and Treatment of Cancer (EORTC) risk tables and American Urological Association (AUA) risk stratification in Chinese patients. Wang used EORTC risk tables to classify patients into three groups, depending on whether they suffered recurrence or progression after TURBT [13]. AUA risk stratification showed the same results [13]. Both classifications were suitable to predict recurrence and progression in Chinese patients [13]. However, for high-risk patients in both series, Kaplan-Meier curves showed significant differences between RFS levels ($p < 0.0001$, log-rank test) and between PFS levels ($p < 0.0001$, log-rank test). EORTC risk tables were stricter and AUA was more sensitive in assigning patients to a high-risk group [13].

References

1. Scher H, Bahnson R, Cohen S, Eisenberger M, Herr H, Kozlowski J, Lange P, Montie J, Pollack A, Raghaven D, Richie J, Shipley W. NCCN urothelial cancer practice guidelines. National Comprehensive Cancer Network. Oncology (Williston Park). 1998;12(7A):225–71.
2. Fernandez-Gomez J, Madero R, Solsona E, Unda M, Martinez-Piñeiro L, Ojea A, Portillo J, Montesinos M, Gonzalez M, Pertusa C, Rodriguez-Molina J, Camacho JE, Rabadan M, Astobieta A, Isorna S, Muntañola P, Gimeno A, Blas M, Martinez-Piñeiro JA, Club Urológico Español de Tratamiento Oncológico. The EORTC tables overestimate the risk of recurrence and progression in patients with non-muscle-invasive bladder cancer treated with bacillus Calmette-Guérin: external validation of the EORTC risk tables. Eur Urol. 2011;60(3):423–30.
3. May M, Burger M, Brookman-May S, Stief CG, Fritsche HM, Roigas J, Zacharias M, Bader M, Mandel P, Gilfrich C, Seitz M, Tilki D. EORTC progression score identifies patients at high risk of cancer-specific mortality after radical cystectomy for secondary muscle-invasive bladder cancer. Clin Genitourin Cancer. 2014;12(4):278–86.
4. Zhang G, Steinbach D, Grimm MO, Horstmann M. Utility of the EORTC risk tables and CUETO scoring model for predicting recurrence and progression in non-muscle-invasive bladder cancer patients treated with routine second transurethral resection. World J Urol. 2019;37:2699–705.
5. Choi SY, Ryu JH, Chang IH, Kim TH, Myung SC, Moon YT, Kim KD, Kim JW. Predicting recurrence and progression of non-muscle-invasive bladder cancer in Korean patients: a comparison of the EORTC and CUETO models. Korean J Urol. 2014;55(10):643–9.
6. Xylinas E, Kent M, Kluth L, Pycha A, Comploj E, Svatek RS, Lotan Y, Trinh QD, Karakiewicz PI, Holmang S, Scherr DS, Zerbib M, Vickers AJ, Shariat SF. Accuracy of the EORTC risk tables and of the CUETO scoring model to predict outcomes in non-muscle-invasive urothelial carcinoma of the bladder. Br J Cancer. 2013;109(6):1460–6.
7. Dalkilic A, Bayar G, Kilinc MF. A comparison of EORTC and CUETO risk tables in terms of the prediction of recurrence and progression in all non-muscle-invasive bladder cancer patients. Urol J. 2019;16(1):37–43.
8. Rieken M, Shariat SF, Kluth L, Crivelli JJ, Abufaraj M, Foerster B, Mari A, Ilijazi D, Karakiewicz PI, Babjuk M, Gönen M, Xylinas E. Comparison of the EORTC tables and the EAU categories for risk stratification of patients with nonmuscle-invasive bladder cancer. Urol Oncol. 2018;36(1):8.e17–24.
9. Sakano S, Matsuyama H, Takai K, Yoshihiro S, Kamiryo Y, Shirataki S, Kaneda Y, Hashimoto O, Joko K, Suga A, Yamamoto M, Hayashida S, Baba Y, Aoki A, Yamaguchi Uro-Oncology Group. Risk group stratification to predict recurrence after transurethral resection in Japanese patients with stage Ta and T1 bladder tumours: validation study on the European Association of Urology guidelines. BJU Int. 2011;107(10):1598–604.
10. Fernandez-Gomez J, Madero R, Solsona E, Unda M, Martinez-Piñeiro L, Gonzalez M, Portillo J, Ojea A, Pertusa C, Rodriguez-Molina J, Camacho JE, Rabadan M, Astobieta A, Montesinos M, Isorna S, Muntañola P, Gimeno A, Blas M, Martinez-Piñeiro JA. Predicting nonmuscle invasive bladder cancer recurrence and progression in patients treated with bacillus Calmette-Guerin: the CUETO scoring model. J Urol. 2009;182(5):2195–203.

11. Chang SS, Boorjian SA, Chou R, Clark PE, Daneshmand S, Konety BR, Pruthi R, Quale DZ, Ritch CR, Seigne JD, Skinner EC, Smith ND, McKiernan JM. Diagnosis and treatment of non-muscle invasive bladder Cancer: AUA/SUO guideline. J Urol. 2016;196(4):1021–9.
12. Ravvaz K, Weissert JA, Downs TM. American Urological Association non-muscle invasive bladder cancer risk model validation: should patient age be added to the risk model? J Urol. 2019;202:682–8.
13. Wang H, Ding W, Jiang G, Gou Y, Sun C, Chen Z, Xu K, Xia G. EORTC risk tables are more suitable for Chinese patients with nonmuscle-invasive bladder cancer than AUA risk stratification. Medicine (Baltimore). 2018;97(36):e12006.

Risk Prediction and Nomograms in Bladder Cancer

A systematic review relating to bladder cancer nomograms was conducted. This was to identify the bladder cancer and nomograms in muscle invasive disease. The search strategy aimed to identify all references related to bladder cancer AND screening. Search terms used were as follows: (Bladder cancer) AND (Nomograms). The following databases were screened from 1989 to June 2020:

- CINAHL
- MEDLINE (NHS Evidence)
- Cochrane
- AMed
- EMBASE
- PsychINFO
- SCOPUS
- Web of Science.

In addition, searches using Medical Subject Headings (MeSH) and keywords were conducted using Cochrane databases. Two UK-based experts in bladder cancer were consulted to identify any additional studies.

Studies were eligible for inclusion if they reported primary research focusing on bladder cancer and screening. Papers were included if published after 1984 and had to be in English. Studies that did not conform to this were excluded. Only primary research was included (Fig. 20.1). The overall aim was to identify bladder cancer risk factors and epidemiology in muscle invasive disease.

Abstracts were independently screened for eligibility by two reviewers and disagreements resolved through discussion or third-party opinion. Agreement level was calculated using Cohen's Kappa to test the intercoder reliability of this screening process. Cohens' Kappa allows comparison of inter-rater reliability between

© The Editor(s) (if applicable) and The Author(s), under exclusive license to
Springer Nature Switzerland AG 2021
S. S. Goonewardene et al., *Management of Muscle Invasive Bladder Cancer*,
Management of Urology, https://doi.org/10.1007/978-3-030-57915-9_20

papers using relative observed agreement. This also takes account of the comparison occurring by chance. The first reviewer agreed all 16 papers to be included, the second, agreed on 16. Cohens kappa was therefore 1.0.

Data extraction was piloted by the researcher and amended in consultation with the research team (author and two academic supervisors). Data collected included authors, year and country of publication, study aims, setting, intervention aims, number of participants, study design, intervention components and delivery methods, comparison groups and outcome measures, notes and follow-up questions for the authors. Studies were quality assessed using the PRISMA criteria for randomised controlled trials, Mays et al. [1, 2] for the action research and qualitative studies and the Critical Skills Appraisal programme for cohort studies. This was also applied to randomised controlled trials and qualitative studies.

The search identified 201 papers (Fig. 20.1). All 16 out of 201 mapped to the search terms and eligibility criteria. The current systematic reviews were examined to gain further knowledge about the subject. One hundred and eighty-five papers were excluded due to not conforming to eligibility criteria or adding to the evidence. Of the 16 papers left, relevant abstracts were identified and the full papers obtained (all of which were in English), to quality assure against search criteria. There was considerable heterogeneity of design among the included studies therefore a narrative review of the evidence was undertaken. There was significant heterogeneity within studies, including clinical topic, numbers, outcomes, as a result a narrative review was thought to be best. There were 16 cohort studies, with a moderate level of evidence. These were from a range of countries with minimal loss to follow-up. All participants were identified appropriately.

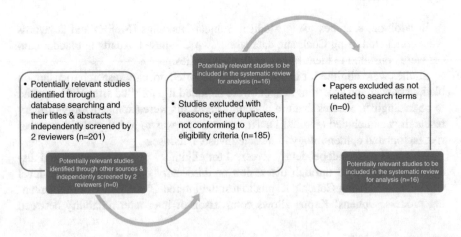

Fig. 20.1 Flow chart of studies identified through the systematic review. (Adapted from PRISMA)

20.1   Systematic Review Results

20.1.1 Molecular Markers in Bladder Cancer Risk

Huang investigated a hybrid nomogram with key demographic features and a multiplex urinary biomarker assay to identify risk of bladder cancer [3]. Area under the receiver operating characteristic curve (AUC) analyses revealed that demographic features alone predicted tumour burden with an accuracy of 0.806 [95% confidence interval (CI), 0.76–0.85], while biomarker data had an accuracy of 0.835 (95% CI, 0.80–0.87) [3]. The addition of molecular data into the nomogram improved the predictive performance to 0.891 (95% CI, 0.86–0.92) [3].

20.1.2 Preoperative Factors Predicting Risk

Yamada identified preoperative variables to predict major perioperative complications after RC and to develop a nomogram [4]. A multivariate model identified gender (OR: 1.63, p = 0.04), cardiovascular comorbidity (OR: 1.48, p = 0.03) and simultaneous nephroureterectomy (OR: 2.81, p = 0.01) as independent predictors [4]. Using these three variables, a nomogram was developed with the AUC of 0.58 [4]. Predictive performance demonstrated fair performance; but identified male, cardiovascular comorbidity and simultaneous nephroureterectomy as independent predictors of perioperative major complications [4].

20.1.3 Prediction of Lymph Node Metastasis

Wu developed and validate a radiomics nomogram for the preoperative prediction of lymph node (LN) metastasis in bladder cancer [5]. The radiomics signature, consisting of nine LN status-related features, achieved favourable prediction efficacy [5]. The radiomics nomogram, which incorporated the radiomics signature and CT-reported LN status, also showed good calibration and discrimination in the training set [AUC, 0.9262; 95% confidence interval (CI), 0.8657–0.9868] and the validation set (AUC, 0.8986; 95% CI, 0.7613–0.9901) [5]. The decision curve indicated the clinical usefulness of our nomogram [5]. Encouragingly, the nomogram also showed favourable discriminatory ability in the CT-reported LN-negative (cN0) subgroup (AUC, 0.8810; 95% CI, 0.8021–0.9598) [5].

Lu developed a prediction model in a training set from the TCGA-BLCA cohort including 196 bladder urothelial carcinoma samples with confirmed LN metastasis status [6]. Least absolute shrinkage and selection operator (LASSO) regression was harnessed for dimension reduction, feature selection, and LNM signature building [6]. Multivariable logistic regression was used to develop the prognostic model, incorporating the LNM signature, and a genomic mutation of MLL2, and was presented with a LNM nomogram [6]. The performance of the nomogram was assessed with respect to its calibration, discrimination, and clinical usefulness [6]. Predictors contained in the individualized prediction nomogram included the LNM signature and MLL2 mutation status [6]. The model demonstrated good discrimination, with an area under the curve (AUC) of 98.7% (85.3% for testing set) and good calibration with p = 0.973 (0.485 for testing set) in the Hosmer-Lemeshow goodness of fit test [6]. Decision curve analysis demonstrated that the LNM nomogram was clinically useful [6]. This study presents a pre-operative nomogram incorporating a LNM signature and a genomic mutation, which can be conveniently utilized to facilitate pre-operative individualized prediction of LN metastasis in patients with bladder urothelial carcinoma [6].

20.1.4 Nomogram to Predict Survival in Bladder Cancer

Zhang constructed a clinical nomogram to effectively predict bladder cancer survival [7]. Multivariate Cox regression analysis showed that age, sex, race, stage were independent predictors of BC survival [7]. A nomogram was constructed based on these factors [7]. The AUC for the 3- and the 5-year survival was 0.82 and 0.813, respectively [7]. The c-index for the TNM-based model was superior to that for the AJCC-TNM classification [7].

Yao assessed various treatment modalities using a primary cohort comprising 234 patients with clinicopathologically-confirmed BCa from 2004 to 2015 in the National Cancer Database [8]. For the original 169 patients considered in the model, the areas under the receiver operating characteristic curve (AUC) were 0.823 (95% CI 0.758–0.889, p < 0.001) and 0.854 (95% CI 0.785–0.924, p < 0.001) for 0.5- and 1-year overall survival respectively [8]. In the validation cohort, the nomogram displayed similar AUCs of 0.838 (95% CI 0.738–0.937, p < 0.001) and 0.809 (95% CI 0.680–0.939, p < 0.001), respectively [8]. The high and low risk groups had median survivals of 1.91 and 5.09 months for the training cohort and 1.68 and 8.05 months for the validation set, respectively (both p < 0.0001) [8].

Simone developed two nomograms predicting disease-free survival (DFS) and cancer-specific survival (CSS) and to externally validate them in multiple series [9]. Age, pathologic T stage, lymph-node density and extent of PLND were independent predictors of DFS and CSS (p < 0.05) [9]. Discrimination accuracies for DFS and CSS at 2, 5 and 8 years were 0.81, 0.8, 0.79 and 0.82, 0.81, 0.8, respectively, with a slight overestimation at calibration plots beyond 24 months [9]. In the external series, predictive accuracies for DFS and CSS at 2, 5 and 8 years were 0.83, 0.82, 0.82 and 0.85, 0.85, 0.83 for European centres; 0.73, 0.72, 0.71 and 0.80, 0.74, 0.68 for African series; 0.76, 0.74, 0.71 and 0.79, 0.76, 0.73 for American series [9].

Bandini provided a benchmark for predicting 1-year RFS in patients with cT2-4N0 MIBC [10]. The 1-year RFS rates were 67.9% (95% confidence interval [CI] 64–72) after no perioperative chemotherapy, 76.9% (95% CI 72–83%) after NAC, 77.8% (95% CI 71–85%) after AC, and 57% (95% CI 37–87) after NAC + AC. On multivariable analysis, positive surgical margins (p = 0.002), pT stage (p < 0.0001), and pN stage (p < 0.0001) were significantly associated with RFS, while NAC was not (p = 0.6) [10]. The model including all these factors yielded a c-index of 0.76 (95% CI 0.72–0.79), good calibration, and a high net benefit [10]. The 1-year RFS rates across nomogram tertiles were 90.5% (95% CI 87–94%), 73.4% (95% CI 68–79%), and 51.1% (95% CI 45–58%), respectively [10].

20.1.5 Prediction of Recurrence Risk

Xu developed and validate a nomogram based on radiomics and clinical predictors for personalized prediction of the first 2 years (TFTY) recurrence risk [11]. Preoperative MRI datasets of 71 BCa patients (34 recurrent) were collected, and divided into training (n = 50) and validation cohorts (n = 21) [11]. The nomogram developed by two independent predictors, MIS and Rad_Score, showed good performance in the training (accuracy 88%, AUC 0.915, p ≪ 0.01) and validation cohorts (accuracy 80.95%, AUC 0.838, p = 0.009) [11]. More benefit was observed by using the radiomics-clinical nomogram than using the radiomics or clinical model alone [11].

Brooks externally validated three previously published nomograms to predicting recurrence, and cancer specific and overall survival following radical cystectomy and pelvic lymph node dissection for urothelial carcinoma of the bladder [12]. At the time of analysis 34 patients had experienced recurrence, of whom 28 died of disease and 6 were currently alive with disease [12]. Discrimination at 2, 5 and 8 years was 0.776, 0.809 and 0.794 for recurrence, 0.822, 0.840 and 0.849 for cancer specific survival, and 0.812, 0.820 and 0.825, respectively, for overall survival [12].

Limited information is available about the pattern of relapse after perioperative chemotherapy with radical cystectomy (RC) vs. RC alone in muscle-invasive bladder cancer [13]. A total of 517 patients (47.8%) developed a relapse: 177 (16.4%) exclusive locoregional relapse [13]. In multivariable analyses, perioperative chemotherapy was associated with longer TTR_L (p < 0.001) [13]. Other factors were nonurothelial histology (p = 0.013), pT-stage (p < 0.001), and surgical margins (p < 0.001) [13]. The concordance index of the model was 0.681 (95% bootstrapped confidence interval, 0.666–0.716) [13]. Risk group categories were obtained according to nomogram tertiles. Despite, overall, observed locoregional RFS in the validation cohort exceeding predicted results, for high-risk patients (80 points or less, lowest nomogram tertile) observed 12-month RFS was similar between development and validation cohorts (60.1% and 66.6%) [13]. The study is limited by its retrospective nature [13].

Martini aimed at developing and validating a pre-cystectomy nomogram for the prediction of locally advanced urothelial carcinoma of the bladder (UCB) using clinicopathological parameters [14]. The distribution of tumour stages pT3/4, pN+ and pT3/4 and/or pN+ at RC was 44.2%, 27.6% and 50.4%, respectively [14]. Age (odds ratio (OR) 0.980; p < 0.001), advanced clinical tumor stage (cT3 vs. cTa, cTis, cT1; OR 3.367; p < 0.001), presence of hydronephrosis (OR 1.844; p = 0.043) and advanced tumour stage T3 and/or N+ at CT imaging (OR 4.378; p < 0.001) were independent predictors for pT3/4 and/or pN+ tumour stage [14]. The predictive accuracy of our nomogram for pT3/4 and/or pN+ at

RC was 77.5% [14]. DCA for predicting pT3/4 and/or pN+ at RC showed a clinical net benefit across all probability thresholds [14].

20.1.6 Postoperative Factors Affecting Survival

The outcome of bladder cancer after radical cystectomy is heterogeneous. Peng aimed to evaluate the prognostic value of HALP (hemoglobin, albumin, lymphocyte and platelet) and explore novel prognostic indexes for patients with bladder cancer after radical cystectomy [15]. In this retrospective study, 516 patients with bladder cancer after radical cystectomy were included [15]. The median follow-up was 37 months (2–99 months) [15]. Risk factors of decreased overall survival were older age, high TNM stage, high American Society of Anesthesiologists (ASA) grade and low HALP score [15]. The predictive accuracy was better with HALP-based nomogram than TNM stage (C-index 0.76 ± 0.039 vs. 0.708 ± 0.041) [15]. By combining ASA grade and HALP, we created a novel index-HALPA score and found it an independent risk factor for decreased survival (HALPA score = 1, HR 1.624, 95% CI 1.139–2.314, p = 0.007; HALPA score = 2, HR 3.471, 95% CI: 1.861–6.472, p < 0.001) [15]. The present study identified the prognostic value of HALP and provided a novel index HALPA score for bladder cancer after radical cystectomy [15].

20.1.7 Recurrence After Radical Cystectomy

Nakagawa aimed to identify prognostic clinicopathological factors and to create a nomogram able to predict overall survival (OS) for recurrence (Urothelial bladder cancer, UCB) after radical cystectomy (RC) [16]. Of the 306 patients, 268 died during follow-up with a median survival of 7 months (95% CI: 5.8–8.5) [16]. Post-recurrence chemotherapy was administered in 119 patients (38.9%) [16]. Multivariable analysis identified 9 independent predictors for OS; period of time from RC to recurrence (time-to-recurrence), symptomatic recurrence, liver metastasis, haemoglobin level, serum alkaline phosphatase level, serum lactate dehydrogenase level, serum C-reactive protein level, postrecurrence chemotherapy, and resection of metastasis [16]. A nomogram was formed with the following five variables to predict OS: time-to-recurrence, symptomatic recurrence, liver metastasis, albumin level, and alkaline phosphatase level [16].

Di Trapani developed a nomogram predicting the cancer-specific mortality (CSM) of patients who underwent RC for transitional BCa, evaluating the available clinical information and the NC [17]. Mean follow-up was 20.3 months [17]. The cohort had mainly pT2 disease (77.1%), and 19.4% had preoperative cisplatinum-based NC [17]. NC showed better CSS at UVA (p = 0.014) and MVA (odds ratio: 0.44; p = 0.043). Overall, the 3-year OS and the CSS rate were 69.3% and 79%, respective [17]. The nomogram developed to predict the 36-month CSM showed predictive accuracy of 67% [17].

References

1. Moher D, Liberati A, Tetzlaff J, Altman DG. "Preferred Reporting Items for Systematic Reviews and Meta-Analyses: The Prisma Statement." [In English]. BMJ (Online) 339, no. 7716 (08 Aug 2009):332–36.
2. Mays N, Pope C, Popay J. "Systematically Reviewing Qualitative and Quantitative Evidence to Inform Management and Policy-Making in the Health Field." [In English]. Journal of Health Services Research and Policy 10, no. SUPPL. 1 (July 2005):6–20.
3. Huang S, Kou L, Furuya H, et al. A nomogram derived by combination of demographic and biomarker data improves the noninvasive evaluation of patients at risk for bladder cancer. Cancer Epidemiol Biomark Prev. 2016;25(9):1361–6.
4. Yamada S, Osawa T, Abe T, et al. Hinyokika Kiyo. 2019;65(12):495–9.
5. Wu S, Zheng J, Li Y, et al. A radiomics nomogram for the preoperative prediction of lymph node metastasis in bladder cancer. Clin Cancer Res. 2017;23(22):6904–11.
6. Lu X, Wang Y, Jiang L, et al. A pre-operative nomogram for prediction of lymph node metastasis in bladder urothelial carcinoma. Front Oncol. 2019;9:488.
7. Zhang Y, Hong YK, Zhuang DW, He XJ, Lin ME. Bladder cancer survival nomogram: development and validation of a prediction tool, using the SEER and TCGA databases. Medicine (Baltimore). 2019;98(44):e17725.
8. Yao Z, Zheng Z, Ke W, et al. Prognostic nomogram for bladder cancer with brain metastases: a National Cancer Database analysis. J Transl Med. 2019;17(1):411.
9. Simone G, Bianchi M, Giannarelli D, et al. Development and external validation of nomograms predicting disease-free and cancer-specific survival after radical cystectomy. World J Urol. 2015;33(10):1419–28.
10. Bandini M, Briganti A, Plimack ER, et al. Modeling 1-year relapse-free survival after neoadjuvant chemotherapy and radical cystectomy in patients with clinical T2-4N0M0 urothelial bladder carcinoma: endpoints for phase 2 trials. Eur Urol Oncol. 2019;2(3):248–56.
11. Xu X, Wang H, Du P, et al. A predictive nomogram for individualized recurrence stratification of bladder cancer using multiparametric MRI and clinical risk factors. J Magn Reson Imaging. 2019;50(6):1893–904.
12. Brooks M, Godoy G, Sun M, Shariat SF, Amiel GE, Lerner SP. External validation of bladder cancer predictive nomograms for recurrence, cancer-free survival and overall survival following radical cystectomy. J Urol. 2016;195(2):283–9.
13. Necchi A, Pond GR, Moschini M, et al. Development of a prediction tool for exclusive locoregional recurrence after radical cystectomy in patients with muscle-invasive bladder cancer. Clin Genitourin Cancer. 2019;17(1):7–14.e3.
14. Martini T, Aziz A, Roghmann F, et al. Prediction of locally advanced urothelial carcinoma of the bladder using clinical parameters before radical cystectomy—a prospective multicenter study. Urol Int. 2016;96(1):57–64.
15. Peng D, Zhang CJ, Gong YQ, et al. Prognostic significance of HALP (hemoglobin, albumin, lymphocyte and platelet) in patients with bladder cancer after radical cystectomy. Sci Rep. 2018;8(1):794.
16. Nakagawa T, Taguchi S, Uemura Y, et al. Nomogram for predicting survival of postcystectomy recurrent urothelial carcinoma of the bladder. Urol Oncol. 2017;35(7):457.e15–21.
17. Di Trapani E, Sanchez-Salas R, Gandaglia G, et al. A nomogram predicting the cancer-specific mortality in patients eligible for radical cystectomy evaluating clinical data and neoadjuvant cisplatinum-based chemotherapy. World J Urol. 2016;34(2):207–13.

Preventative Measures for Those with High Risk MIBC

Each year, 430,000 people are diagnosed with bladder cancer. Due to the high recurrence rate of the disease, primary prevention is paramount [1].

21.1 Mediterranean Diet and Bladder Cancer Risk

Bravi examined the association between Mediterranean diet and bladder cancer [2]. The ORs of bladder cancer were 0.72 (95% confidence interval, CI, 0.54–0.98) for MDS of 4–5 and 0.66 (95% CI, 0.47–0.93) for MDS of 6–9 (p for trend = 0.02) compared to MDS = 0–3 [2]. Results were similar in strata of sex, age, and education. The risk was lower in never-smokers and pT1–pT4 bladder carcinomas [2]. Among individual components of the MDS, inverse associations for greater consumption of legumes, vegetables, and fish and risk of bladder cancer was associated [2]. The higher adherence to the Mediterranean diet was related to a lower risk of bladder cancer [2].

21.2 Risk Factors in Bladder Cancer: Preventative Measures

Al-Zalabani reviewed all meta-analyses on modifiable risk factors of primary bladder cancer [1]. Statistically significant associations were found for current (RR 3.14) or former (RR 1.83) cigarette smoking, pipe (RR 1.9) or cigar (RR 2.3) smoking, antioxidant supplementation (RR 1.52), obesity (RR 1.10), higher physical activity levels (RR 0.86), higher body levels of selenium (RR 0.61) and vitamin D (RR 0.75), and higher intakes of: processed meat (RR 1.22), vitamin A (RR 0.82), vitamin E (RR 0.82), folate (RR 0.84), fruit (RR 0.77), vegetables (RR 0.83), citrus fruit (RR 0.85), and cruciferous vegetables (RR 0.84) [1]. Finally, three occupations with the highest risk were tobacco workers (RR 1.72), dye workers (RR 1.58), and chimney sweeps (RR 1.53) [1]. Modification of lifestyle and occupational

S. S. Goonewardene et al., *Management of Muscle Invasive Bladder Cancer*, Management of Urology, https://doi.org/10.1007/978-3-030-57915-9_21

exposures can considerably reduce the bladder cancer burden [1]. While smoking remains one of the key risk factors, also several diet-related and occupational factors are very relevant [1].

21.3   Preventative Measures in Bladder Cancer: Impact of Vitamin A

Tang conducted a meta-analysis to investigate the quantitative effects of vitamin A on bladder cancer [3]. Twenty-five articles on dietary vitamin A or blood vitamin A were included according to the eligibility criteria [3]. The pooled risk estimates of bladder cancer were 0.82 (95% CI 0.65, 0.95) for total vitamin A intake, 0.88 (95% CI 0.73, 1.02) for retinol intake, and 0.64 (95% CI 0.38, 0.90) for blood retinol levels [3]. Tang found inverse associations between subtypes of carotenoids and bladder cancer risk [3]. The findings of this meta-analysis indicate that high vitamin A intake was associated with a lower risk of bladder cancer [3].

21.4   Prevention of Bladder Cancer: Fluid Intake

Michaud examined the relation between total fluid intake and the risk of bladder cancer [4]. Total daily fluid intake was inversely associated with the risk of bladder cancer; the multivariate relative risk was 0.51 (95% confidence interval, 0.32–0.80) for the highest quintile of total daily fluid intake (>2531 ml/day) as compared with the lowest quintile (<1290 ml/day) [4]. The consumption of water contributed to a lower risk (relative risk, 0.49, for 1440 ml/day vs. less than 240 ml/day), as did the consumption of other fluids (relative risk, 0.63 for greater than 1831 ml/day versus less than 735 ml/day) [4]. A high fluid intake is associated with a decreased risk of bladder cancer in men [4].

21.5   Mitomycin and BCG in Bladder Cancer Prevention

Mangiarotti compared intravesical BCG with intravesical mitomycin C chemotherapy in non-muscle invasive bladder cancer at intermediate risk of recurrence as a prospective randomised trial [5]. Half of the patients were free of recurrence respectively after mitomycin C (23/46) and BCG (23/46) treatment [5]. Recurrences after BCG presented in the first 6 month period (>50%) or after 3 years whereas early (less than 6 months) or long term (greater than 3 years) recurrences after MMC treatment were less frequent [5]. None progressed to muscle-invasive tumour or underwent cystectomy during the observation period [5]. Both MMC and BCG demonstrate efficacy in prolonging the time to recurrence with respect to the period of observation before treatment, so reducing the hospitalisation rate for TUR of the recurrent tumours, but no difference in the recurrence rates was observed between MMC and BCG as primary treatment [5].

21.6   Preventative Measures and Urethral Recurrence

Chan summarise the current literature on the diagnosis and management of urethral recurrence (UR) after radical cystectomy (RC), as UR after RC is rare but associated with high mortality [6]. Incidence of UR after RC ranges from 1% to 8% with most recurrences occurring within the first 2 years after surgery [6]. Increased risk of UR is associated with involvement of the prostate, tumour multifocality, bladder neck involvement, and cutaneous diversion [6]. The 5-year disease-specific survival after UR is reported to be between 0% and 83% [6]. Current literature suggests that urethral wash cytology may be useful in patients with intermediate- to high-risk of recurrence to enable early detection of non-invasive disease, which may be amenable to conservative therapy before urethrectomy [6].

21.7   BCG in Intermediate and High-Risk Disease

The optimal dose and duration of intravesical bacillus Calmette-Guérin (BCG) in the treatment of non-muscle-invasive bladder cancer (NMIBC) is controversial [7]. In an intention-to-treat analysis of 1355 patients with a median follow-up of 7.1 years, there were no significant differences in toxicity between 1/3 dose and full dose [7]. The null hypotheses of inferiority of the disease-free interval for both 1/3 dose and 1 year could not be rejected [7]. Oddens found that 1/3 dose-1 year is suboptimal compared with full dose-3 year (hazard ratio [HR]: 0.75; 95% confidence interval [CI], 0.59–0.94; p = 0.01) [7]. Intermediate-risk patients treated with full dose do not benefit from an additional 2 year of BCG [7]. In high-risk patients, 3 year is associated with a reduction in recurrence (HR: 1.61; 95% CI, 1.13–2.30; p = 0.009) but only when given at full dose [7].

References

1. Al-Zalabani AH, Stewart KF, Wesselius A, Schols AM, Zeegers MP. Modifiable risk factors for the prevention of bladder cancer: a systematic review of meta-analyses. Eur J Epidemiol. 2016;31(9):811–51.
2. Bravi F, Spei ME, Polesel J, Di Maso M, Montella M, Ferraroni M, Serraino D, Libra M, Negri E, La Vecchia C, Turati F. Mediterranean diet and bladder cancer risk in Italy. Nutrients. 2018;10(8). pii: E1061.
3. Tang JE, Wang RJ, Zhong H, Yu B, Chen Y. Vitamin A and risk of bladder cancer: a meta-analysis of epidemiological studies. World J Surg Oncol. 2014;12:130.
4. Michaud DS, Spiegelman D, Clinton SK, Rimm EB, Curhan GC, Willett WC, Giovannucci EL. Fluid intake and the risk of bladder cancer in men. N Engl J Med. 1999;340(18):1390–7.
5. Mangiarotti B, Trinchieri A, Del Nero A, Montanari E. A randomized prospective study of intravesical prophylaxis in non-muscle invasive bladder cancer at intermediate risk of recurrence: mitomycin chemotherapy vs BCG immunotherapy. Arch Ital Urol Androl. 2008;80(4):167–71.
6. Chan Y, Fisher P, Tilki D, Evans CP. Urethral recurrence after cystectomy: current preventative measures, diagnosis and management. BJU Int. 2016;117(4):563–9.
7. Oddens J, Brausi M, Sylvester R, Bono A, van de Beek C, van Andel G, Gontero P, Hoeltl W, Turkeri L, Marreaud S, Collette S, Oosterlinck W. Final results of an EORTC-GU cancers group randomized study of maintenance bacillus Calmette-Guérin in intermediate- and high-risk Ta, T1 papillary carcinoma of the urinary bladder: one-third dose versus full dose and 1 year versus 3 years of maintenance. Eur Urol. 2013;63(3):462–72.

Bladder Cancer Risk Post Pelvic Irradiation

22

Patients who have received prior pelvic irradiation may be at risk of bladder cancer. Radiotherapy-associated bladder carcinoma was found in 3.7% of 244 cases of advanced urothelial carcinoma [1].

22.1 Radiation Induced Bladder Cancer Post Cervical Cancer

Duncan had a 25-year experience with carcinoma of the uterine cervix who subsequently had bladder tumours is presented [2]. Of the 3091 patients treated 2674 had received radiotherapy and 8 suffered vesical malignancies of varied histopathological type 6 months to 20 years after irradiation [2]. This incidence rate is 299.9 per 100,000, which is 57.6 times that of the general female population [2].

Uyama reviewed two cases of radiation-induced bladder carcinoma which followed prior irradiation for cervical carcinoma [3]. From the late radiation change of the skin, it was estimated that the total dose of prior radiation might be 4000 rad or more [3]. Both had high-grade, high-stage transitional cell bladder carcinoma, and the former was with marked mucus-forming adenomatous metaplasia [3].

Saito reported four cases of urothelial carcinoma following pelvic irradiation for carcinomas of the cervix uteri (n = 3) and the ovary (n = 1). The urothelial carcinomas developed 26.8 (mean) years after radiotherapy and invaded the bladder in 3 patients and the ureter in 1 [4]. Despite radical surgery, the patients died of metastatic cancer [4].

22.2 Clinical Presentation of Bladder Cancer Post-pelvic Irradiation

Average age at diagnosis of the bladder tumour was 63.1 years, with a mean of 20.5 years between radiation treatment and diagnosis [1]. All nine patients presented with gross haematuria [1]. Eight patients had transitional cell carcinoma, 7/8 (87.5%) also had vascular or lymphatic invasion, and one was adenocarcinoma [1].

Post prostate radiation, patients presented at higher stage than expected from population-based studies of bladder cancer [5]. Patients and their physicians should be aware of such risks when choosing therapy for prostate cancer [5]. Haematuria following radiation therapy for prostate cancer should be investigated rather than being attributed to radiation-induced cystitis [5].

22.3 Survival Outcomes in Bladder Cancer Post Pelvic Irradiation

Quilty noted 11 women with bladder cancer have had previous pelvic irradiation [6]. The tumours were generally of high grade and advanced T-category. Prognosis was poor and only 32% survived for 1 year [6]. The interval observed between low dose pelvic irradiation and subsequent bladder cancer was longer than after high dose pelvic irradiation (mean interval of 30 years compared with 16.5 years) [6].

In a series by Sella, mean survival was 15.4 months (range 1–40 months), with a 55.5% 1-year disease-free survival after diagnosis [1]. Four patients died of bladder tumour, four were alive with no evidence of disease, and one was alive with metastasis [1].

22.4 Prior Irradiation for Prostate Cancer and Risk of Bladder Cancer

Prostate cancer is the most common cancer diagnosed in men and remains the second most lethal malignancy [5]. Prostate can be associated with secondary cancers [5]. The most common secondary malignancy is bladder carcinoma [5]. Shirodkar treated 44 patients with bladder cancer who had radiation therapy for prostate cancer [5]. At diagnosis, 60% had tumour, which invaded the bladder muscle (T2 or greater disease) [5]. The mean latency from radiation to diagnosis of bladder cancer was 5.5 years [5]. Radiation therapy for prostate cancer is associated with an increased risk of bladder cancer [5].

22.5 Management of Pelvic Irradiation Induced Bladder Cancer

Radiation exposure is an established risk factor for bladder cancer, however consensus is lacking on the survival characteristics of bladder cancer patients with a history of radiation therapy (RT) [7]. Krughoff compared the survival characteristics of patients with suspected radiation-induced second primary cancer (RISPC) of the bladder to those with de novo bladder cancer [7]. Twenty-nine patients with history of RT were matched with two controls each, resulting in a dataset of 87 observations in the event model [7]. Results from the Cox model indicate a significantly increased hazard ratio for death at 2.22 (p = 0.047, 95% CI: 1.015–4.860) given a history of prior radiation therapy [7]. In a small cohort, bladder cancer patients who underwent cystectomy had a significantly higher risk of death in the face of prior pelvic RT [7]. This effect was found to be independent of surgical complications, numerous established patient characteristics and comorbidities traditionally predictive of survival [7].

Ravi reviewed five cases of radiation-induced bladder cancer [8]. The first primary neoplasm was uterine cervical cancer in three patients, uterine endometrial cancer in one patient, and Hodgkin's disease in one patient [8]. All the bladder cancers were invasive [8]. The treatment modalities included anterior pelvic exenteration, partial cystectomy, reirradiation, including the use of intraoperative electron therapy in one patient, and TUR plus endoscopic Nd:YAG laser treatment in one patient [8]. Four patients are alive without disease at a mean follow-up period of 15 months from the diagnosis of bladder cancer [8].

References

1. Sella A, Dexeus FH, Chong C, Ro JY, Logothetis CJ. Radiation therapy-associated invasive bladder tumors. Urology. 1989;33(3):185–8.
2. Duncan RE, Bennett DW, Evans AT, Aron BS, Schellhas HF. Radiation-induced bladder tumors. J Urol. 1977;118(1 Pt 1):43–5.
3. Uyama T, Nakamura S, Moriwaki S. Radiation-induced bladder carcinoma. Urology. 1981;18(4):355–8.
4. Saito M, Kondo A, Kato T, Kobayashi M, Miyake K. Radiation-induced urothelial carcinoma. Urol Int. 1996;56(4):254–5.
5. Shirodkar SP, Kishore TA, Soloway MS. The risk and prophylactic management of bladder cancer after various forms of radiotherapy. Curr Opin Urol. 2009;19(5):500–3.
6. Quilty PM, Kerr GR. Bladder cancer following low or high dose pelvic irradiation. Clin Radiol. 1987;38(6):583–5.
7. Krughoff K, Lhungay TP, Barqawi Z, O'Donnell C, Kamat A, Wilson S. The prognostic value of previous irradiation on survival of bladder cancer patients. Bladder Cancer. 2015;1(2):171–9.
8. Ravi R. Second primary bladder cancer following pelvic irradiation for other malignancies. J Surg Oncol. 1993;54(1):60–3.

Part V
Management of MIBC

A Systematic Review on Bladder Preservation Strategies and MIBC

23.1 Research Methods

A systematic review relating to muscle invasive bladder cancer and bladder preservation was conducted. This was to identify the role of bladder preservation. The search strategy aimed to identify all references related to bladder cancer AND muscle invasive disease AND bladder preservation. Search terms used were as follows: (Bladder cancer) AND (muscle invasive disease) AND (Bladder Preservation). The following databases were screened from 1989 to June 2020:

- CINAHL
- MEDLINE (NHS Evidence)
- Cochrane
- AMed
- EMBASE
- PsychINFO
- SCOPUS
- Web of Science.

In addition, searches using Medical Subject Headings (MeSH) and keywords were conducted using Cochrane databases. Two UK-based experts in bladder cancer were consulted to identify any additional studies.

Studies were eligible for inclusion if they reported primary research focusing on muscle invasive bladder cancer and bladder preservation. Papers were included if published after 1984 and had to be in English. Studies that did not conform to this were excluded. Only primary research was included (Fig. 23.1).

Abstracts were independently screened for eligibility by two reviewers and disagreements resolved through discussion or third party opinion. Agreement level was calculated using Cohen's Kappa to test the intercoder reliability of this screening

© The Editor(s) (if applicable) and The Author(s), under exclusive license to
Springer Nature Switzerland AG 2021
S. S. Goonewardene et al., *Management of Muscle Invasive Bladder Cancer*,
Management of Urology, https://doi.org/10.1007/978-3-030-57915-9_23

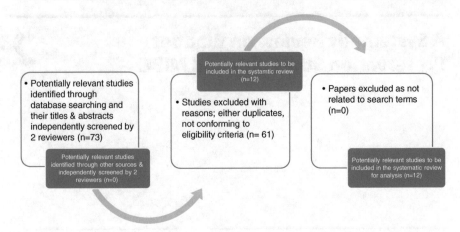

Fig. 23.1 Flow chart of studies identified through the systematic review. (Adapted from PRISMA)

process. Cohens' Kappa allows comparison of inter-rater reliability between papers using relative observed agreement. This also takes account of the comparison occurring by chance. The first reviewer agreed all 12 papers to be included, the second, agreed on 12.

Data extraction was piloted by the researcher and amended in consultation with the research team (author and two academic supervisors). Data collected included authors, year and country of publication, study aims, setting, intervention aims, number of participants, study design, intervention components and delivery methods, comparison groups and outcome measures, notes and follow-up questions for the authors. Studies were quality assessed using the PRISMA criteria for randomised controlled trials, Mays et al. [1, 2] for the action research and qualitative studies and the Critical Skills Appraisal programme for cohort studies. This was also applied to randomised controlled trials and qualitative studies.

The search identified 73 papers (Fig. 23.1). Twelve out of 73 mapped to the search terms and eligibility criteria. The current systematic reviews were examined to gain further knowledge about the subject. Sixty-one papers were excluded due to not conforming to eligibility criteria or adding to the evidence. Of the 12 papers left, relevant abstracts were identified and the full papers obtained (all of which were in English), to quality assure against search criteria. There was considerable heterogeneity of design among the included studies therefore a narrative review of the evidence was undertaken. There was significant heterogeneity within studies, including clinical topic, numbers, outcomes, as a result a narrative review was thought to be best. There were ten cohort studies, with a moderate level of evidence and two RCTs with a good level of evidence. These were from a range of countries with minimal loss to follow-up. All participants were identified appropriately.

23.2 Systematic Review Results

23.2.1 Tetramodal Bladder Preservation Therapy

Kijima evaluated the outcomes associated with selective tetramodal bladder-sparing therapy-resection of bladder tumour (TURBT), induction chemoradiotherapy (CRT), and consolidative partial cystectomy (PC) with pelvic lymph node dissection (PLND) [3]. MIBC remission was achieved in 121 patients (79%) after CRT, and 107 patients (69%) completed the tetramodal bladder-preservation protocol comprising consolidative PC with PLND [3]. The 5-year MIBC-RFS, CSS and OS rates in the 107 patients who completed the protocol were 97%, 93% and 91%, respectively [3]. Selective tetramodal bladder-preservation therapy, incorporating consolidative PC with PLND, yielded favourable oncological and functional outcomes in patients with MIBC [3].

23.2.2 Radical Cystectomy vs. Bladder Preservation in the Elderly

Radical cystectomy (RC) and radiochemotherapy (RCT) are curative options for muscle-invasive bladder cancer (MIBC) [4]. Boustani examined this in Patients aged 80 years old and above with T2-T4aN0-2M0-Mx MIBC were identified in the Retrospective International Study of Cancers of the Urothelial Tract (RISC) database [4]. Ninety-two patients underwent RC and 72 patients had RCT [4]. Median overall survival was 1.99 years (95% CI 1.17–2.76) after RC and 1.97 years (95% CI 1.35–2.64) after RCT (p = 0.73) [4]. Median progression-free survival (PFS) after RC and RCT were 1.25 years (95% CI 0.80–1.75) and 1.52 years (95% CI 1.01–2.04), respectively (p = 0.54) [4]. Only disease progression was significantly associated with worse OS (HR = 10.27 (95% CI 6.63–15.91), p < 0.0001) [4]. Treatment modality was not a prognostic factor [4]. RCT offers survival rates comparable to those observed with RC for patients aged ≥80 years [4].

23.2.3 Bladder Perseveration with Brachytherapy and External Beam Radiotherapy

Aluwini reported long-term results of a bladder preservation strategy for muscle-invasive bladder cancer (MIBC) using external beam radiation therapy and brachytherapy/interstitial radiation therapy (IRT) [5]. The LRFS rate was 80% and 73% at 5 and 10 years, respectively [5]. Salvage cystectomy-free survival at 5 and 10 years was 93% and 85% [5]. The 5- and 10-year overall survival rates were 65% and 46%, whereas cancer-specific survival at 5 and 10 years was 75% and 67% [5]. The distant metastases-free survival rate was 76% and 69% at 5 and 10 years [5]. Multivariate analysis revealed no independent predictors of LRFS [5]. Radiation

Therapy Oncology Group grade ≥3 late bladder and rectum toxicity were recorded in 11 patients (5.7%) and 2 patients (1%), respectively [5].

23.2.4 Survival Outcomes in Bladder Preservation Therapy for MIBC

Multiple prospective Radiation Therapy Oncology Group (RTOG) protocols have evaluated bladder-preserving combined-modality therapy (CMT) for muscle-invasive bladder cancer (MIBC), reserving cystectomy for salvage treatment [6]. Mak performed a pooled analysis of long-term outcomes in patients with MIBC enrolled across multiple studies [6]. The clinical T stage was T2 in 61%, T3 in 35%, and T4a in 4% of patients [6]. Complete response to CMT was documented in 69% of patients [6]. The 5- and 10-year OS rates were 57% and 36%, respectively, and the 5- and 10-year DSS rates were 71% and 65%, respectively [6]. The 5- and 10-year estimates of muscle-invasive LF, non-muscle-invasive LF, and DM were 13% and 14%, 31% and 36%, and 31% and 35%, respectively [6].

23.2.5 Patterns of Bladder Preservation Therapy

Trimodality bladder preservation therapy (BPT) in muscle invasive bladder cancer (MIBC) includes a maximal transurethral resection followed by concurrent chemoradiotherapy as an alternative to radical cystectomy (RC) in non-cystectomy candidates [7]. Rose described patterns of BPT and associated survival outcomes in MIBC [7]. Two hundred and sixty-five patients received BPT [7]. Compared with the 1447 patients who received RC, BPT patients were older, had poorer performance status, and had more comorbidities (p < 0.01 for all) [7]. Median overall survival (OS) was similar for patients treated with curative radiation doses in BPT and patients treated with RC (41 vs. 46 months, p = 0.33, respectively) [7]. Forty-five percent of BPT patients received concurrent chemotherapy with radiation [7]. The most common regimens included cisplatin alone (23%), carboplatin alone (22%), gemcitabine alone (10%), paclitaxel alone (9%), and 5-FU + mitomycin (5%) [7]. There were no significant differences in survival among chemotherapy regimens [7]. Only 10 patients (4% of BPT patients) underwent salvage cystectomy [7].

23.2.6 Bladder Preservation Rate

Huddart compared outcomes in neoadjuvant chemotherapy followed by radical cystectomy (RC) or selective bladder preservation (SBP) [8]. Definitive treatment [RC or radiotherapy (RT)] is determined by response to chemotherapy [8]. Trial recruitment was challenging and below the predefined target with 45 patients recruited in 30 months (25 RC; 20 SBP) [8]. Non-compliance with assigned treatment strategy was frequent, 6 of the 25 patients (24%) randomised to RC received RT [8]. Long-term bladder preservation rate was 11/15 (73%) in those who received RT per protocol [8]. OS survival was not significantly different between groups [8].

23.2.7 Paclitaxel, Trasuzumab with Irradiation After Transurethral Surgery

Bladder preservation therapy is an effective treatment for muscle-invasive urothelial carcinoma (UC) [9]. Michaelson treated noncystectomy candidates with daily radiation and weekly paclitaxel for 7 weeks [9]. Patients whose tumours showed her2/neu overexpression were additionally treated with weekly trastuzumab [9]. A total of 20 evaluable patients were treated in group 1 and 46 patients in group 2 [9]. Acute treatment-related adverse events (AEs) were observed in 7 of 20 patients in group 1 (35%) and 14 of 46 patients in group 2 (30.4%) [9]. Therapy was completed by 60% (group 1) and 74% (group 2) of patients [9]. Most incompletions were due to toxicity, and the majority of AEs were gastrointestinal [9]. Two other deaths (both in group 2) were unrelated to therapy [9]. No unexpected cardiac, hematologic, or other toxicities were observed [9]. The CR rate at 1 year was 72% for group 1 and 68% for group 2 [9].

23.2.8 Second TURBT in Bladder Preservation for MIBC

Suer evaluated a second TUR on disease-specific survival (DSS) and overall survival (OS) rates in muscle-invasive bladder cancer (MIBC) treated with MMT [10]. Suer assessed the data of 90 patients (stage T2–4, N0–1, M0 urothelial cancer) treated with MMT [10]. Patients with incomplete initial TURB were excluded. A total of 43 patients had a second TUR before starting radiochemotherapy of MMT (group 1), and 47 patients (group 2) were treated with MMT without having a second TUR [10]. The 5-year DSS rate was better in group 1 compared to group 2 (68% vs. 41%) (p = 0.046) [10]. The 5-year OS rates were 63.7% and 40.1% in groups 1 and 2, respectively (p = 0.054) [10]. Multivariate analysis revealed that second TUR, lymph node involvement, presence of hydronephrosis and tumour stage were independent prognostic factors for DSS [10].

23.2.9 Trimodal Chemotherapy with Cisplatin in Bladder Preservation

Open radical cystectomy (ORC) is currently the standard treatment for muscle-invasive bladder cancer (MIBC) without metastasis, while many patients with MIBC are not always appropriate candidates due to multiple comorbidities [11]. Nagao evaluated the bladder-preservation strategy compared to radical cystectomy [11]. Nagao retrospectively analysed the data of 50 patients with MIBC treated by trimodal chemoradiotherapy with cisplatin (CDDP-radiation) [11]. Transurethral resection of the bladder tumour (TURBT) was performed before treatment to confirm pathological stage $\geq$T2 [11]. Extensive TURBT was performed after chemoradiotherapy to evaluate the pathological response to treatment [11]. The 2- and 5-year progression-free survival, bladder-intact survival, cancer-specific survival, and overall survival (OS) rates after treatment were 70.8% and 63.9%, 64.0% and 49.8%, 86.7% and 71.8%, and 84.3% and 64.8%, respectively [11]. The 2- and 5-year OS rates after CDDP-R were 90.5% and 74.3%, respectively, and those after ORC were 71.8% and 59.9%, respectively, indicating a significant survival advantage conferred by CDDP-R over ORC ($p < 0.05$, HR 0.45, 95% CI 0.21–0.94) [11].

23.2.10   Grey Matter Relating to Systematic Review

Radical treatment for solid tumours has progressed to multimodal organ preservation strategies combining systemic and local treatments [12]. Trimodality bladder-preserving treatment (TMT) comprises transurethral resection of the bladder tumour, radiotherapy and radiosensitizing treatment, preserving the urinary bladder [12]. The choice of maintaining quality of life without a negative effect on the chances of cure and long-term survival is attractive [12]. In muscle-invasive bladder cancer (MIBC), the evidence shows comparable clinical outcomes between patients undergoing radical cystectomy and TMT [12]. Despite this evidence, many patients continue to be offered radical surgery as the standard-of-care treatment [12]. Improvements in radiotherapy techniques with adaptive radiotherapy and advances in imaging translate to increases in the accuracy of treatment delivery and reductions in long-term toxicities [12]. With the advent of novel biomarkers promising improved prediction of treatment response, stratification of patients for different treatments on the basis of tumour biology could soon be a reality [12]. The future of oncological treatment lies in personalized medicine with the combination of technological and biological advances leading to truly bespoke management for patients with MIBC [12].

References

1. Moher D, Liberati A, Tetzlaff J, Altman DG. "Preferred Reporting Items for Systematic Reviews and Meta-Analyses: The Prisma Statement." [In English]. BMJ (Online) 339, no. 7716 (08 Aug 2009):332–36.
2. Mays N, Pope C, Popay J. "Systematically Reviewing Qualitative and Quantitative Evidence to Inform Management and Policy-Making in the Health Field." [In English]. Journal of Health Services Research and Policy 10, no. SUPPL. 1 (July 2005):6–20.
3. Kijima T, Tanaka H, Koga F, Masuda H, Yoshida S, Yokoyama M, Ishioka J, Matsuoka Y, Saito K, Kihara K, Fujii Y. Selective tetramodal bladder-preservation therapy, incorporating induction chemoradiotherapy and consolidative partial cystectomy with pelvic lymph node dissection for muscle-invasive bladder cancer: oncological and functional outcomes of 107 patients. BJU Int. 2019;124(2):242–50.

4. Boustani J, Bertaut A, Galsky MD, Rosenberg JE, Bellmunt J, Powles T, Recine F, Harshman LC, Chowdhury S, Niegisch G, Yu EY, Pal SK, De Giorgi U, Crabb SJ, Caubet M, Balssa L, Milowsky MI, Ladoire S, Créhange G, Retrospective International Study of Cancers of the Urothelial Tract (RISC) Investigators. Radical cystectomy or bladder preservation with radiochemotherapy in elderly patients with muscle-invasive bladder cancer: Retrospective International Study of Cancers of the Urothelial Tract (RISC) Investigators. Acta Oncol. 2018;57(4):491–7.

5. Aluwini S, van Rooij PH, Kirkels WJ, Boormans JL, Kolkman-Deurloo IK, Wijnmaalen A. Bladder function preservation with brachytherapy, external beam radiation therapy, and limited surgery in bladder cancer patients: long-term results. Int J Radiat Oncol Biol Phys. 2014;90(1):241.

6. Mak RH, Hunt D, Shipley WU, Efstathiou JA, Tester WJ, Hagan MP, Kaufman DS, Heney NM, Zietman AL. Long-term outcomes in patients with muscle-invasive bladder cancer after selective bladder-preserving combined-modality therapy: a pooled analysis of Radiation Therapy Oncology Group protocols 8802, 8903, 9506, 9706, 9906, and 0233. J Clin Oncol. 2014;32(34):3801–9.

7. Rose TL, Deal AM, Ladoire S, Créhange G, Galsky MD, Rosenberg JE, Bellmunt J, Wimalasingham A, Wong YN, Harshman LC, Chowdhury S, Niegisch G, Liontos M, Yu EY, Pal SK, Chen RC, Wang AZ, Nielsen ME, Smith AB, Milowsky MI, Retrospective International Study of Cancers of the Urothelial Tract (RISC) Investigators. Patterns of bladder preservation therapy utilization for muscle-invasive bladder Cancer. Bladder Cancer. 2016;2(4):405–13.

8. Huddart RA, Birtle A, Maynard L, Beresford M, Blazeby J, Donovan J, Kelly JD, Kirkbank T, McLaren DB, Mead G, Moynihan C, Persad R, Scrase C, Lewis R, Hall E. Clinical and patient-reported outcomes of SPARE - a randomised feasibility study of selective bladder preservation versus radical cystectomy. BJU Int. 2017;120(5):639–50.

9. Michaelson MD, Hu C, Pham HT, Dahl DM, Lee-Wu C, Swanson GP, Vuky J, Lee RJ, Souhami L, Chang B, George A, Sandler H, Shipley W. A phase 1/2 trial of a combination of paclitaxel and trastuzumab with daily irradiation or paclitaxel alone with daily irradiation after transurethral surgery for noncystectomy candidates with muscle-invasive bladder Cancer (Trial NRG Oncology RTOG 0524). Int J Radiat Oncol Biol Phys. 2017;97(5):995–1001.

10. Suer E, Hamidi N, Gokce MI, Gulpinar O, Turkolmez K, Beduk Y, Baltaci S. Significance of second transurethral resection on patient outcomes in muscle-invasive bladder cancer patients treated with bladder-preserving multimodal therapy. World J Urol. 2016;34(6):847–51.

11. Nagao K, Hara T, Nishijima J, Shimizu K, Fujii N, Kobayashi K, Kawai Y, Inoue R, Yamamoto Y, Matsumoto H, Matsuyama H. The efficacy of trimodal chemoradiotherapy with cisplatin as a bladder-preserving strategy for the treatment of muscle-invasive bladder cancer. Urol Int. 2017;99(4):446–52.

12. Song YP, McWilliam A, Hoskin PJ, Choudhury A. Organ preservation in bladder cancer: an opportunity for truly personalized treatment. Nat Rev Urol. 2019;16:511–22.

Partial Cystectomy

24

Organ-sparing cystectomy remains an operation for a highly selected group that can offer similar oncologic outcomes but improved sexual function. Occult prostate cancer may occur even with screening but the majority is of clinical insignificance. Paramount to patient selection are oncologic concerns, but preoperative sexual function, age, performance status, and postoperative expectations must also be evaluated during patient selection. Improved diagnostic and surveillance tools may facilitate and improve patient selection in the future [1].

24.1 Predictive Factors in Partial Cystectomy

Ma identified predictive factors underlying recurrence and survival after partial cystectomy for pelvic lymph node-negative muscle-invasive bladder cancer (MIBC) (urothelial carcinoma) [2]. The 5-year overall survival (OS), cancer-specific survival (CSS) and recurrence-free survival (RFS) rates were 58%, 65% and 50%, respectively [2]. A total of 33 patients died of bladder cancer and 52 patients survived with intact bladder [2]. Of the 101 patients, 55 had no recurrence, 12 had non-muscle-invasive recurrence in the bladder that was treated successfully, and 34 had recurrence with advanced disease [2]. The multivariate analysis showed that prior history of urothelial carcinoma was associated with both CSS and RFS and weakly associated with OS; lymphovascular invasion (LVI) and ureteral reimplantation (UR) were associated with OS, CSS and RFS [2].

24.2 Partial Cystectomy Rate

Villavicencio evaluated a bladder preservation strategy in muscle-invasive bladder cancer (MIBC) or development of MIBC cancer due to progression [3]. The cancer-specific survival (CSS) was 80.8% [3]. Among the 39 patients with complete remission, 19 had invasive recurrence, CSS of 53.2%; by comparison, with pre-served bladders, CSS was 72.1% (p = 0.046) [3]. Predictive factors analysed were age, sex, tumour size >3 cm, grade, associated carcinoma in situ (CIS), number of tumours and number of previous recurrences [3]. In multivariate analysis only tumour size and CIS were significant predictive factors for progression after preser-vation [3]. Of the 6 patients with MIBC after NMIBC, 3 (50%) had no remission and underwent cystectomy and 15 patients (38.6%) had NMIBC recurrences during follow-up [3]. CIS and high-grade tumours were treated with bacillus Calmette-Guérin [3]. A bladder preservation rate of 81% and a CSS rate of 89% were obtained in the group with NMIBC recurrences [3].

24.3   Molecular Markers Allow Prediction of Survival in Bladder Preservation Strategies

Tanabe evaluated associations of Ki-67 expression with oncologic outcomes in muscle-invasive bladder cancer (MIBC) treated with chemoradiotherapy (CRT)-based bladder-sparing [4]. After induction CRT, 16 (17%) and 53 (56%) underwent partial cystectomy and RC, respectively, while the remaining 25 (27%) did not undergo cystectomy [4]. Successful bladder preservation was achieved in 34 patients (36%) [4]. Higher Ki-67 labeling index (LI) independently predicted CRT response clinically and pathologically [4]. Among the clinicopathologic variables available before CRT and cystectomy, high Ki-67 LI (≥20%) was independently associated with better cancer-specific survival (CSS) (5-year CSS rate, 78% vs. 46% for low Ki-67 LI; p = 0.019) [4]. The difference in CSS according to Ki-67 expression status was more remarkable in patients with cT3 disease (5-year CSS rate, 72% vs. 29%; p = 0.0098) [4].

24.4   Oncological Outcomes in Partial Cystectomy

Koga evaluated oncological outcomes of muscle-invasive bladder cancer (MIBC) who were treated with a selective bladder-sparing protocol consisting of induction low-dose chemoradiotherapy (LCRT) plus partial cystectomy (PC) with pelvic lymph node dissection [5]. Of the 183, 87 (48%) achieved a clinical complete response after LCRT and 65 (36%) met the PC criteria; 46 (25%) actually under-went PC, 86 (47%) had RC, and the remaining 51 (28%) had neither PC, nor RC [5]. Histological examination of the 46 PC specimens showed residual muscle-invasive disease in 3 (7%) [5]. Overall, 5-year overall survival and CSS rates were 64% and 71%, respectively (median follow-up for survivors of 45 months) [5]. In the 46 PC patients, neither MIBC, nor pelvic recurrence was observed; 5-year CSS and MRFS rates were both 100% [5]. In 13 non-PC patients with a complete response after LCRT and who met PC criteria but declined PC, 5-year CSS and MRFS rates were 74% and 81%, respectively; CSS and MRFS were significantly better in the PC group than in the non-PC group (p = 0.025 and 0.002, respectively) [5].

Ebbing evaluated outcomes and health-related quality of life (HR-QoL) in partial cystectomy (PC) for muscle-invasive bladder cancer (MIBC) [6]. Twenty-seven patients who underwent open PC for cT2 MIBC were included [6]. Estimated 5-year overall- and progression-free survival rates were 53.7% and 62.1% [6]. Five (18.5%) patients experienced local recurrence with MIBC [6]. Overall, the salvage cystectomy rate was 18.5% [6]. The 90-day mortality rate was 0% [6]. Significant risk factors for progression-free survival were vascular invasion (HR 5.33) and tumour multilocularity (HR 4.5) in the PC specimen, and a ureteric reimplantation during PC (HR 4.53) [6]. The rates of intraoperative complications, 30- and 90-day major complications were 7.4%, respectively and 14.8% for overall long-term complications [6]. Postoperatively, median (IQR) global health status and QoL in our PC cohort was 79.2 (52.1–97.9) [6]. Open PC can provide adequate cancer control of MIBC with good HR-QoL in highly selected cases [6]. Open PC can lead to long-term bladder preservation and shows an acceptable rate of severe perioperative complications, even in highly comorbid patients [6].

References

1. Avulova S, Chang SS. Role and indications of organ-sparing "radical" cystectomy: the importance of careful patient selection and counseling. Urol Clin North Am. 2018;45(2):199–214.
2. Ma B, Li H, Zhang C, Yang K, Qiao B, Zhang Z, Xu Y. Lymphovascular invasion, ureteral reimplantation and prior history of urothelial carcinoma are associated with poor prognosis after partial cystectomy for muscle-invasive bladder cancer with negative pelvic lymph nodes. Eur J Surg Oncol. 2013;39(10):1150–6.
3. Villavicencio H, Rodriguez Faba O, Palou J, Gausa L, Algaba F, Marcuello E. Bladder preservation strategy based on combined therapy in patients with muscle-invasive bladder cancer: management and results at long-term follow-up. Urol Int. 2010;85(3):281–6.
4. Tanabe K, Yoshida S, Koga F, Inoue M, Kobayashi S, Ishioka J, Tamura T, Sugawara E, Saito K, Akashi T, Fujii Y, Kihara K. High Ki-67 expression predicts favorable survival in muscle-invasive bladder cancer patients treated with chemoradiation-based bladder-sparing protocol. Clin Genitourin Cancer. 2015;13(4):e243–51.
5. Koga F, Kihara K, Yoshida S, Yokoyama M, Saito K, Masuda H, Fujii Y, Kawakami S. Selective bladder-sparing protocol consisting of induction low-dose chemoradiotherapy plus partial cystectomy with pelvic lymph node dissection against muscle-invasive bladder cancer: oncological outcomes of the initial 46 patients. BJU Int. 2012;109(6):860–6.
6. Ebbing J, Heckmann RC, Collins JW, Miller K, Erber B, Friedersdorff F, Fuller TF, Busch J, Seifert HH, Ardelt P, Wetterauer C, Hosseini A, Jentzmik F, Kempkensteffen C. Oncological outcomes, quality of life outcomes and complications of partial cystectomy for selected cases of muscle-invasive bladder cancer. Sci Rep. 2018;8(1):8360.

Vemana et al. [1] highlighted the role of chemotherapy in muscle invasive bladder cancer. What has been highlighted by the publication of these articles are the insufficient evidence for use of neoadjuvant chemotherapy. Neoadjuvant chemotherapy prior to radical treatment has been present for at least three decades. Despite local therapy with cystectomy and/or radical radiotherapy, the 5-year survival rate of patients with muscle invasive transitional cell carcinoma, is approximately 50% [2].

Radical cystectomy and pelvic lymphadenectomy have been the cornerstone treatment for muscle-invasive bladder cancer. Several phase III trials and meta-analyses have been published. In Europe combination chemotherapy, CMV (cisplatin, methotrexate and vinblastine) or no chemotherapy before local treatment, surgery or radiotherapy alone was examined. Four hundred and twenty-eight patients underwent cystectomy, the complete response rate (pT0) was higher in the chemotherapy arm (32% versus 12%). With a median follow-up of 8 years, there was a statistically significant 16% reduction in the risk of death corresponding to an increase in 10-year survival from 30% to 36% with CMV [3].

The South West Oncology Group (SWOG) study examined methotrexate-vinblastine-cisplatin plus doxorubicin (MVAC) vs. no chemotherapy before radical cystectomy. The pT0 response rate was higher in the chemotherapy arm (38% versus 15%). An overall survival improvement was reported (77 versus 46 months). These results correspond to a 33% greater risk of death in the cystectomy alone group. Survival benefit was related to complete pathological response. The 5-year survival of patients with pT0 at cystectomy (with or without MVAC) was 85% [4].

Potential disadvantages of NAC include less accurate staging, delay in curative surgery (risk greater if delay >12 weeks) if patient does not respond, toxicity from chemotherapy. Patients with disease progression on chemotherapy may have their benefit from surgery compromised. It is difficult to identify patients who would benefit from neoadjuvant chemotherapy. There has been very little research into this region. Although T2 and T3a patients, have an almost complete response, bladder preservation remains controversial.

© The Editor(s) (if applicable) and The Author(s), under exclusive license to
Springer Nature Switzerland AG 2021
S. S. Goonewardene et al., *Management of Muscle Invasive Bladder Cancer*,
Management of Urology, https://doi.org/10.1007/978-3-030-57915-9_25

Most recently, the LAMB study has been running, due to close in 2014 [5]. This used adjuvant lapatinib versus placebo in responders after successful first line chemotherapy, results are currently awaited. However, this did highlight difficulties with recruiting to a trial such as this.

In conclusion neoadjuvant chemotherapy followed by radical therapy is the gold standard for muscle invasive bladder tumours for patients sufficiently fit. As yet, this intervention has not been examined by NICE. However, there are many unanswered questions. The choice of neoadjuvant chemotherapy, whether MVAC, CMV or GC needs to be decided. However both its' cost effectiveness and clinical effectiveness remains to be evaluated in a prospective trial. Translational genomic and proteomic research needs to predict treatment response to different neoadjuvant chemotherapies needs to continue, to separate patients into responders or none responders based on genetic profile.

25.1 Health Related Quality of Life in the Elderly with Radical Cystectomies

Cerruto evaluated health-related quality of life (HR-QoL) outcomes in elderly patients with different type of urinary diversion (UD), ileal conduit (IC) and ileal orthotopic neobladder (IONB), after radical cystectomy (RC) [6]. At univariate analysis, at a mean follow-up of 60.91 ± 5.63 months, IONB results were favourable with regard to the following HR-QoL aspects: nausea and vomiting ($p = 0.045$), pain ($p = 0.049$), appetite loss ($p = 0.03$), constipation ($p = 0.000$), financial impact ($p = 0.012$) and cognitive functioning ($p = 0.000$) [6]. This last functional aspect was significantly worse in female patients ($p = 0.029$) [6]. Emotional functioning was significantly better in patients without long-term complications ($p = 0.016$) [6]. At multivariate analysis, male gender and IONB were independent predictors of better cognitive functioning, while long-term complications negatively affected emotional functioning [6].

Yang optimised the surgical procedures of laparoscopic radical cystectomy and urinary diversion for the elderly patients with bladder cancer, generalize operating technique, summarize clinical experiences [7]. Among 68 elderly patients with bladder cancer, 50 patients were male and 18 were female, the age of whom were (79 ± 4) (range 75–91) years old [7]. All the 68 operations were successfully performed without conversion to open surgery [7]. There were 26 cases receiving cutaneous ureterostomy, 34 cases receiving ileal conduit (intracorporeal for 16 cases and extracorporeal for 18 cases) and 8 cases receiving orthotopic ileal neobladder (intracorporeal for 4 cases and extracorporeal for 4 cases; Xing's technique for 4 cases, T-Pouch for 2 cases and Studer-Pouch for 2 cases) respectively [7]. Sixty patients received laparoscopic pelvic lymphadenectomy and the number of dissected lymph nodes was 17.1 ± 7.0. There were 46 cases with T stage greater than or equal to T2 (46/68, 67.6%), 4 cases of low grade (4/68, 5.9%) and 60 cases of high grade (60/68, 88.2%) [7]. The 5-year cancer specific survival rate and overall survival rate were 57% and 50% respectively [7]. There was significant difference between the preoperative and postoperative QOL (quality of life) score (56.0 ± 10.0 and 47.4 ± 5.8 respectively, p < 0.05) which indicated that the patients' postoperative quality of life was greatly improved [7].

The increasing life expectancy and the proportion of octogenarians make radical cystectomy (RC) more frequent in octogenarian patients with muscle invasive bladder cancer [8]. Garde analyzed overall survival and complications [8]. Thirty-three patients were included [8]. Their mean age was 81.9 ± 1.8 years [8]. There were 24 males (72.7%) [8]. The surgical risk was identified as follows: ASA II in 9 patients (27.3%), ASA III in 23 (69.7%) and ASA IV in 1 (3%) [8]. Concerning urinary diversion, 19 patients (57.6%) underwent ureteroileostomy and 14 (42.4%) bilateral cutaneous ureterostomy [8]. Average hospital length of stay was 19 days (14–30) [8]. TNM stage was T0 in 1 patient (3%), T1 in 4 (12.1%), T2 in 11 (33.3%), T3 in 13 (39.4%), T4 in 4 (12.1%), Nx in 9 (12%), N0 in 13 (39.4%), N1 in 3 (9.1%), and N2 in 5 (15.2%) [8]. The most frequent complications were pneumonia in 6 patients (18.2%) and surgical wound infection in 6 (18.2%) [8]. Lymphadenectomy did not involve a significant increase in complications [8]. Six patients (18.2%) died in the immediate postoperative period, 5 of whom from respiratory complications. The mean survival of the rest of the series was 24 months (range 15.1–32.8) [8].

The increasing life expectancy and the proportion of octogenarians make radical cystectomy (RC) more frequent in octogenarian patients with muscle invasive bladder cancer [8]. Garde analyzed overall survival and complications [8]. Thirty-three patients were included [8].

25.2   Bladder Preservation Therapy in the Elderly

Chen assessed the impacts of age, performance status, and clinical stage on advanced urothelial carcinoma of the bladder (UCB) in patients treated with different treatment modalities [9]. The median age of the patients was 74.0 years, and the mean survival interval was 31.5 months [9]. The 2-year OS was significantly different among the three modalities [RC > TURBT monotherapy, odds ratio (OR): 1.86, 95% CI: 1.17–2.96, p = 0.009; CRT > TURBT monotherapy, OR: 1.65, 95% CI: 1.06–2.57, p = 0.026] [9]. There were no significant differences in the 5- and 10-year OS rates between the three treatment modalities [9]. Those younger than 76 years receiving RC had a significantly better 2-year OS than those undergoing CRT and TURBT monotherapy (RC > TURBT monotherapy, OR: 2.38; 95% CI: 1.30–4.33, p = 0.005) [9]. The number and duration of re-hospitalizations were highest in the CRT group and lowest in the TURBT group [9].

25.3   Radiotherapy in Elderly Patients with MIBC

Aizawa evaluated the clinical results of external-beam radiotherapy (EBRT) for muscle-invasive bladder cancer (MIBC) in elderly patients [10]. The median overall survival (OS) and progression-free survival (PFS) were 14.7 months and 7.8 months, respectively [10]. The OS, cause-specific survival (CSS), and PFS rates at 1-year were 56.0%, 68.5%, and 40.0%, respectively [10]. The local progression-free rates (LPFR) at 6 months and 1 year were 89.3% and 59.5%, respectively [10]. Performance status 3 was a significantly unfavourable factor for OS, CSS, and progression-free survival; clinical N stage was a significantly unfavourable factor for progression-free survival; and lower irradiation dose ($\leq$50.4 Gy) was a significantly unfavourable factor for LPFR [10].

25.4 Grey Literature

Fonteyne reported on overall survival (OS), cancer specific survival (CSS), and morbidity after curative treatment in elderly patients, defined as age >70 year, with nonmetastatic MIBC and to compare this with the outcome of younger MIBC patients [11]. Forty-two articles were retrieved for review. No article directly addressed the use of geriatric assessment. OS and CSS worsen significantly with age both after radical cystectomy and radiotherapy regimens [11]. While POM significantly increases with age, morbidity seems comparable between younger and older patients [11].

Siddiqui reviewed the literature to investigate the factors influencing the choice of this diversion and its complications [12]. IC is the most common UD performed in elderly patients undergoing RC for bladder cancer [12]. Long-term studies looking at the change in renal function after UD report a universal decline in the glomerular filtration rate; however, this decline in renal function is the least for IC [12]. There is a significant morbidity of RC (20–56%), which can be attributed to patient factors, surgical technique and hospital volume [12]. Modern concepts of bowel preparation, postoperative nutrition, early enteral feeding and involvement of stoma therapists have helped improve the outcomes [12]. The quality of life is preserved, and in many including elderly, it may be improved with IC UD [12].

References

1. Vemana G, Nepple KG, Vetter J, et al. Defining the potential of neoadjuvant chemotherapy use as a quality indicator for bladder cancer care. J Urol. 2014;192(1):43–9.
2. Mead GM. Bladder cancer. Curr Opin Oncol. 1990;2:514–9.
3. International Collaboration of Trialists. International phase III trial assessing neoadjuvant cisplatin, methotrexate, and vinblastine chemotherapy for muscle-invasive bladder cancer: long-term results of the BA06 30894 trial. J Clin Oncol. 2011;29:2171–7.
4. Martinez-Pineiro JA, Leon JJ, Martin MG. Neoadjuvant cisplatinum in locally advanced urothelial bladder cancer: a prospective randomized study of the group CUETO. In: Splinter TAW, Scher HI, editors. Neoadjuvant chemotherapy in invasive bladder cancer. New York: Wiley-Liss; 1990. p. 95–103.
5. LAMB study, closed 2014, results pending.
6. Cerruto MA, D'Elia C, Siracusano S, Saleh O, Gacci M, Cacciamani G, De Marco V, Porcaro AB, Balzarro M, Niero M, Lonardi C, Iafrate M, Bassi P, Imbimbo C, Racioppi M, Talamini R, Ciciliato S, Serni S, Carini M, Verze P, Artibani W. Health-related quality of life after radical

cystectomy for bladder cancer in elderly patients with ileal orthotopic neobladder or ileal conduit: results from a multicentre cross-sectional study using validated questionnaires. Urol Int. 2018;100(3):346–52.

7. Yang FY, Wang WK, Liu S, Song LM, Xing NZ. Clinical experiences of laparoscopic radical cystectomy and urinary diversion in the elderly patients with bladder cancer. Zhonghua Yi Xue Za Zhi. 2019;99(14):1101–5.

8. Garde H, Ciappara M, Galante I, Fuentes Ferrer M, Gómez A, Blazquez J, Moreno J. Radical cystectomy in octogenarian patients: a difficult decision to take. Urol Int. 2015;94(4):390–3.

9. Chen CL, Liu CY, Cha TL, Hsu CY, Chou YC, Wu ST, Meng E, Sun GH, Yu DS, Tsao CW. Does radical cystectomy outperform other bladder preservative treatments in elderly patients with advanced bladder cancer? J Chin Med Assoc. 2015;78(8):469–74.

10. Aizawa R, Sakamoto M, Orito N, Kono M, Ogura M, Negoro Y, Sagoh T, Tsukahara K, Komatsu K, Noguchi M. The use of external-beam radiotherapy for muscle-invasive bladder cancer in elderly or medically-fragile patients. Anticancer Res. 2017;37(10):5761–6.

11. Fonteyne V, Ost P, Bellmunt J, Droz JP, Mongiat-Artus P, Inman B, Paillaud E, Saad F, Ploussard G. Curative treatment for muscle invasive bladder cancer in elderly patients: a systematic review. Eur Urol. 2018;73(1):40–50.

12. Siddiqui KM, Izawa JI. Ileal conduit: standard urinary diversion for elderly patients undergoing radical cystectomy. World J Urol. 2016;34(1):19–24.

Muscle Invasive Bladder Cancer and Neoadjuvant Chemotherapy

BLADDER cancer is the fifth most common cancer in the Western world, yet only seventh in the ranking of cancer related mortality [1]. Transitional cell carcinoma represents more than 90%. The majority are superficial disease but 40% will become muscle invasive [1]. This has different biological behaviour to superficial disease and is prognostically important due to the metastatic potential [2, 3]. Despite local therapy with cystectomy and/or radical radiotherapy, the 5-year survival rate of patients with muscle invasive transitional cell carcinoma, is approximately 50% [4–6]. Ten to 25% will occur in association with relapsed superficial bladder cancer [7]. Due to the poor prognostic rate and high death rate for muscle invasive urothelial tumours (only 60% of patients with T2, 50% with T3a, or 15% with T3b tumours will be alive at 5 year) more than surgery is required to improve prognostic outcomes [8]. Neoadjuvant chemotherapy has been used in management of muscle invasive bladder cancer. We aim to review management of bladder cancer, EAU and NICE guidance, with clinical and cost effectiveness of neoadjuvant disease.

26.1 The Rationale for Neoadjuvant Chemotherapy

Neoadjuvant chemotherapy treats subclinical disease and improves survival [9]. Theoretically, it uses systemic drugs prior to a local control procedure. Advantages of neoadjuvant chemotherapy include immediate treatment of micrometastatic disease, assessment of chemo-sensitivity of tumour response in vivo [7, 8], more effective delivery of chemotherapy before surgical disturbance, to allow bladder preservation, tumour down staging, to prevent tumour cells from settling, to reduce tumour size and to increase survival duration [8]. Criteria for neoadjuvant chemotherapy include, having a T2–T4a N0 tumour, in good general health (PS 0–1), with good renal function (creatinine clearance >50 ml/min), and age <70 year [10]. Radical cystectomy and pelvic lymphadenectomy have been the cornerstone treatment for muscle-invasive bladder cancer [11]. Despite negative preoperative staging, pelvic lymphadenectomy and cystectomy for bladder cancer reveal a high percentage of unsuspected nodal metastases (24%) that have a 25% chance for long-term survival [11]. Lymphadenectomy ensures a low pelvic recurrence rate even in lymph node-positive patients, and patients with locally advanced cancer have a 56% probability of 5-year recurrence-free survival [11].

26.2   Neoadjuvant Chemotherapy: Clinical Effectiveness

Initially cisplatin based therapy was used in the 1980s. This demonstrated a 60% response rate including 10% with a complete response [12]. This has also been shown in metastatic disease with 60% demonstrating clinically complete response [13]. The MVAC combination (methotrexate, vinblastine, doxorubicin and cisplatin) demonstrated an overall and progression free survival benefit over cisplatin alone [14, 15]. In the 1990s, a randomized trial comparing standard MVAC to GC (gemcitabine plus cisplatin). Both regimens showed nearly identical response rates and median survival rates [16].

Several phase III trials and meta-analyses have been published. In Europe combination chemotherapy, CMV (cisplatin, methotrexate and vinblastine) or no chemotherapy before local treatment, surgery or radiotherapy alone was examined. Four hundred and twenty-eight patients underwent cystectomy, the complete response rate (pT0) was higher in the chemotherapy arm (32% versus 12%). With a median follow-up of 8 years, there was a statistically significant 16% reduction in the risk of death corresponding to an increase in 10-year survival from 30% to 36% with CMV [17].

European Organisation for Research and Treatment of Cancer (EORTC) examined CMV [18]. Loco-regional treatment included cystectomy or radiotherapy. A survival increase of 5.5% for the chemotherapy group was demonstrated. The pT0 rate was 32% for patients who received a cystectomy (57%).

The South West Oncology Group (SWOG) study examined methotrexate-vinblastine-cisplatin plus doxorubicin (MVAC) vs. no chemotherapy before radical cystectomy. The pT0 response rate was higher in the chemotherapy arm (38% versus 15%). An overall survival improvement was reported (77 versus 46 months). These results correspond to a 33% greater risk of death in the cystectomy alone group. Survival benefit was related to complete pathological response. The 5-year survival of patients with pT0 at cystectomy (with or without MVAC) was 85% [19].

In the first Nordic cystectomy trial (NCT1) examined cisplatin-doxorubicin, plus 40 Gray irradiation and cystectomy vs. irradiation and cystectomy. The trial reported a small difference in a subgroup analysis of patients with T3–T4 disease. In a second Nordic cystectomy trial (NCT2), patients randomly received three cycles of cisplatin-methotrexate and leucovorin prior to cystectomy, or cystectomy alone [20]. The combined analysis of both demonstrated overall survival in favour of neoadjuvant treatment.

Efficacy of neoadjuvant chemotherapy is shown by the pT0 rate on cystectomy increasing from 15% to 35–45% [21]. Significant clinical effects including complete response are demonstrated in 50–60% with single agent cisplatin [22, 23].

During this time, tumour progression or metastases nearly never occur. It does not contribute to the morbidity or mortality outcomes. Combination chemotherapies also been tested as part of phase 2 trials [24]. MVAC demonstrated complete remission in 20–30%. The lower the stage, the better the outcome. Tumour downstaging occurred in 40–60%.

Seven small series examined gemcitabine-based regimens (gemcitabine and cisplatin) reported pT0 response rates ranging from 7% to 50% [24]. The literature review clearly supports the use of neoadjuvant chemotherapy by level I evidence demonstrating a survival benefit compared with surgery alone.

26.3   Meta-Analyses for Neoadjuvant Chemotherapy

Two main meta-analyses have been performed. The first used cisplatin-based chemotherapy. The overall survival improvement was 5% and risk reduction of death was 10% with neoadjuvant chemotherapy [20]. In the second, the 5-year survival rate improved from 45% to 50% in patients receiving cisplatin-based combination neoadjuvant chemotherapy [25]. The risk of death was reduced by 14% with an increase in specific survival of 9% [26].

The BC2001 trial looked at outcomes of chemo radiotherapy vs. radiotherapy alone [27]. At 2 years, rates of locoregional disease-free survival were 67% in the chemo radiotherapy group and 54% in the radiotherapy group. Five-year rates of overall survival were 48% (95% CI, 40–55) in the chemo radiotherapy group and 35% in the radiotherapy group. However, Grade 3 or 4 adverse events were slightly more common in the chemo radiotherapy group than in the radiotherapy group during treatment. Results of this trial have led some to surmise that chemoradiotherapy is equivalent to cystectomy with neoadjuvant chemotherapy but no head to head comparison has been. A randomised controlled trial between surgery and chemoradiotherapy is unlikely largely because urologists still regard cystectomy as a gold standard and select fitter patients for surgery.

26.4   Disadvantages of Neoadjuvant Chemotherapy

Potential disadvantages of NAC include less accurate staging, delay in curative surgery (risk greater if delay >12 weeks) if patient does not respond, toxicity from chemotherapy. Patients with disease progression on chemotherapy will not benefit from surgery. The ability to identify patients who would benefit from preoperative treatment is a major issue, however very little has been investigated in this region. The difficulty with neoadjuvant trials, are that the patients have already under gone tumour resection and are having adjuvant rather than neoadjuvant therapy. Neoadjuvant chemotherapy is not preventive for progression of disease. Although T2 and T3a patients, have an almost complete response, bladder preservation remains controversial. Cases may be inadequately clinical staged resulting in tumour invasion.

Absence of residual tumour does not mean the patient has been cured. Patient survival after resection has not yet been compared in a randomised trial with survival after cystectomy. Several factors are favourable indications for bladder preservation: clinical stage, tumour size (<3 cm), absence of a palpable mass, and a single lesion [5].

26.5   Targeted Therapies and Bladder Preservation

Preliminary data with antiangiogenic agents such as bevacizumab or sunitinib combined with chemotherapy suggest an absence of improvement in pT0 response rates as compared to historical data with chemotherapy alone [28]. However, further results are required. Furthermore, predictive biomarkers are urgently needed in order to determine responses from neoadjuvant chemotherapy.

Interestingly, several trials [29–32] evaluated neoadjuvant chemotherapy associated with radiotherapy alone or combined with chemotherapy, dose-dense MVAC, or gemcitabine and cisplatin (GC). Survival varied from 48% to 63% at 5 years [29–31]. The proportion of bladders left in place at 5 year is >40% [32, 33]. A bladder sparing option could use neoadjuvant chemotherapy in combination with a high-quality transurethral bladder resection in complete responders.

Even though neoadjuvant chemotherapy for this cohort has become the gold standard, it has never been evaluated by NICE.

26.6   Evaluation of 'QUALYs'

NICE use a standard and internationally recognised method to compare different drugs and measure their clinical effectiveness: the quality-adjusted life years measurement (the 'QALY') [48]. A QALY gives an idea of how many extra months or years of life of a reasonable quality a person might gain as a result of treatment and show much the drug or treatment costs per QALY. This is the cost of using the drugs to provide a year of the best quality of life available Cost effectiveness is expressed as '£ per QALY' [48]. Generally, however, if a treatment costs more than £20,000–30,000 per QALY, then it would not be considered cost effective.

Few studies, if any have been conducted into cost effectiveness of neoadjuvant chemotherapy. One American study examined mean total cost of treatment during follow-up for radical cystectomy vs. cost of neoadjuvant chemotherapy [34]. These were £26,317 and £32,111, respectively. The absolute increase in cost of therapy for patients receiving NAC compared to RC alone was £5959. The increased cost per additional QALY gained for patients receiving NAC was £6330.

26.7   Benefits vs. Risks of Neoadjuvant Chemotherapy

From the literature review, the benefits of neoadjuvant chemotherapy for muscle invasive bladder cancer are wide ranging. This includes a greatly improved response rate including compete response and improved survival rate. Potential disadvantages of NAC include less accurate staging, delay in curative surgery (risk greater if delay >12 weeks) in none-responders and a well-known fact that none responders will fare worse later on.

In conclusion neoadjuvant chemotherapy followed by radical therapy is the gold standard for muscle invasive bladder tumours for patients sufficiently fit despite cost effectiveness. As yet, this intervention has not been examined by NICE. However, there are many unanswered questions. The choice of neoadjuvant chemotherapy, whether MVAC CMV or GC needs to be decided. However, its efficacy remains to be evaluated in a prospective trial. Translational genomic and proteomic research needs to predict treatment response to different neoadjuvant chemotherapies needs to continue, to separate patients into responders or none responders based on genetic profile.

26.8   Controversies in Clinical Effectiveness of Neoadjuvant Chemotherapy

Data from randomized trials did not show any morbidity difference after neoadjuvant treatment [35, 36]. Even randomized trials did not demonstrate statistical survival benefit despite the prolongation of disease free interval [37–39]. These early reports were criticized due to single agent chemotherapy regimen used, and insufficient number of patients enrolled.

A randomised trial [40] has compared outcomes after cystectomy plus adjuvant MVAC with pre- and postoperative MVAC. No differences were found between the groups. In intention-to-treat analyses, 81 patients (58%) were in remission with a median follow-up of 6.8 year. Again, the study design and small number of inclusions prevent us from concluding the differences in outcome.

Other combinations e.g. cyclophosphamide, fluorouracil and methotrexate for T3 disease, did not demonstrated any significant effect [35]. Methotrexate has been used as part of a clinical trial [36]. No survival benefit was observed. Single agent cisplatin has also been trialled followed by radical radiotherapy. However, trials closed prematurely, due to poor patient recruitment. Separate and meta-analysis have failed to show any benefit [41].

Another study, similar to the SWOG one, is the Italian GUONE trial [41]. Patients were randomized to M-VAC before cystectomy, or cystectomy alone. The trial was closed early because failed to achieve any difference in survival. This is a small trial in which no difference in survival was observed (62% vs. 68%). Another Italian trial substituted doxorubicin with epirubicin and studied the neoadjuvant M-VEC regimen plus cystectomy versus cystectomy alone [42, 43]. Again, no difference in survival was observed.

Several other published randomized trials of neoadjuvant chemotherapy [44–46] have failed to show survival difference, mostly because in order to detect a 10% survival benefit of investigational chemotherapy arm over standard therapy, a randomized trial requires approximately 1000 patients.

A single-centre randomized trial of five cycles of MVAC chemotherapy, given either as two neoadjuvant and three post-operative cycles, or five cycles of adjuvant therapy has recently been published [21]. One hundred and forty patients with T3b or T4a were enrolled. Significant difference in overall survival was not observed between the two arms. A disadvantage of this trial was that no observation-only arm was included.

References

 1. Dirix LY, Van Oosterom AT. Neoadjuvant and adjuvant therapy for invasive bladder tumours. Eur J Cancer. 1991;27:330–3.
 2. Raghavan D, Shipley WU, Garnick MB. Biology and management of bladder cancer. N Engl J Med. 1990;322:1129–38.
 3. Younes M, Sussman J, True LD. The usefulness of the level of the muscularis mucosae in the staging of invasive transitional cell carcinoma of the urinary bladder. Cancer. 1990;66:543–8.
 4. Mead GM. Bladder cancer. Curr Opin Oncol. 1990;2:514–9.
 5. Raghavan D, Shipley WU, Hall RR, Richie JP. Biology and management of invasive bladder cancer. In: Raghavan D, Scher HI, Leibel SA, Lange PH, editors. Principles and practice of genitourinary oncology. Philadelphia: Lippincott-Ravel; 1997. p. 281–98.
 6. Ghonheim MA, El-Mekresh MM, Mokhtar AA, Gomha MA, El-Baz MA, El-Attar IA. A predictive model of survival after radical cystectomy for carcinoma of the bladder. BJU Int. 2000;85:811–6.
 7. Pectasides D, Pectasides M, Nikolao M. Adjuvant and neoadjuvant chemotherapy in muscle invasive bladder cancer: literature review. Eur Urol. 2005;48:60–8.
 8. Houe N, Pourquie P, Beuzeboc P. Review of neoadjuvant and adjuvant chemotherapy, muscle-invasive bladder cancer. Eur Urol. 2011;2011(Suppl):e10–20.
 9. Pouessel D, Mongiat-Artus P, Culine S. Neoadjuvant chemotherapy in muscle-invasive bladder cancer: ready for prime time? Crit Rev Oncol Hematol. 2013;85:288–94.
10. Teramukai S, Nishiyama H, Matsui Y, Ogawa O, Fukushima M. Evaluation for surrogacy of end points by using data from observational studies: tumor downstaging for evaluating neoadjuvant chemotherapy in invasive bladder cancer. Clin Cancer Res. 2006;12:139–43.
11. Madersbacher S, Hochreiter W, Burkhard F, Thalmann GN, Danuser H, Markwalder R, Studer UE. Radical cystectomy for bladder cancer today–a homogeneous series without neoadjuvant therapy. J Clin Oncol. 2003 Feb 15;21(4):690–6.
12. Raghavan D, Pearson B, Duval P, et al. Initial intravenous cisplatinum therapy: improved management for invasive high risk bladder cancer. J Urol. 1985;133:399–402.
13. Meyers FJ, Palmer JM, Freiha FS, et al. The fate of the bladder in patients with metastatic bladder cancer treated with cisplatin, methotrexate and vinblastine: a Northern California Oncology Group study. J Urol. 1985;134:1118–21.
14. Logothetis CJ, Dexeus FH, Finn L. A prospective randomized trial comparing MVAC and CISCA chemotherapy for patients with metastatic urothelial tumors. J Clin Oncol. 1990;8:1050–5.
15. Loehrer PJ Sr, Einhorn LH, Elson PJ. A randomized comparison of cisplatin alone or in combination with methotrexate, vinblastine, and doxorubicin in patients with metastatic urothelial carcinoma: a cooperative group study. J Clin Oncol. 1992;10:1066–73.
16. Von der Maase H, Senegelov L, Roberts JT, et al. Long-term survival results of a randomized trial comparing gemcitabine plus cisplatin, with methotrexate, vinblastine, doxorubicin, plus cisplatin in patients with bladder cancer. J Clin Oncol. 2005;23:4602–8.
17. International Collaboration of Trialists. International phase III trial assessing neoadjuvant cisplatin, methotrexate, and vinblastine chemotherapy for muscle-invasive bladder cancer: long-term results of the BA06 30894 trial. J Clin Oncol. 2011;29:2171–7.

18. International Collaboration of Trialists. Neoadjuvant cisplatin, methotrexate, and vinblastine chemotherapy for muscle-invasive bladder cancer: a randomised controlled trial. Lancet. 1999;354:533–40.

19. Martinez-Pineiro JA, Leon JJ, Martin MG. Neoadjuvant cisplatinum in locally advanced urothelial bladder cancer: a prospective randomized study of the group CUETO. In: Splinter TAW, Scher HI, editors. Neoadjuvant chemotherapy in invasive bladder cancer. New York: Wiley-Liss; 1990. p. 95–103.

20. Winquist E, Kirchner TS, Segal R, Chin J, Lukka H. Neoadjuvant chemotherapy for transitional cell carcinoma of the bladder: a systematic review and meta-analysis. J Urol. 2004;171:561–9.

21. Sternberg CN, Pansadoro V, Calabro F, et al. Can patient selection for bladder preservation be based on response to chemotherapy? Cancer. 2003;97:1644–52.

22. Fagg SL, Dawson-Edwards P, Hughes MA, et al. Cis-diamminedichloroplatinum (DDP) as initial treatment of invasive bladder cancer. Br J Urol. 1984;56:299–300.

23. Raghavan D, Grundy R, Greenaway TM. Pre-emptive (neoadjuvant) chemotherapy prior to radical radiotherapy for fit septuagenarians with bladder cancer: age itself is not a contraindication. Br J Urol. 1988;62:154–9.

24. Scher H, Herr H, Sternberg C, et al. M-VAC (methotrexate, vinblastin, doxorubicin and cisplatin) and bladder preservation. In: Splinter TAW, Scher HI, editors. Neoadjuvant chemotherapy in invasive bladder cancer. New York: Wiley-Liss; 1990. p. 179–86.

25. Advanced Bladder Cancer Meta-Analysis Collaboration. Neoadjuvant chemotherapy in invasive bladder cancer: a systematic review and metaanalysis. Lancet. 2003;361:1927–34.

26. Smith DC, Mackler NJ, Dunn RL, et al. Phase II trial of paclitaxel, carboplatin and gemcitabine in patients with locally advanced carcinoma of the bladder. J Urol. 2008;180:2384–8.

27. James ND, Hussein S, Hall P, Tremlett J, Rawlings C, Crundwell R, Sizer B, Sreenivasan T, Hendron C, Lewis R, Waters R, Huddart RA. Radiotherapy with or without chemotherapy in muscle-invasive bladder cancer. N Engl J Med. 2012;366:1478–89.

28. Balar AV, Iyer G, Apolo AB, et al. Phase II trial of neoadjuvant gemcitabine and cisplatin with sunitinib in patients with muscle-invasive bladder cancer. J Clin Oncol. 2012;30(Suppl):Abstract 4581.

29. Housset M, Dufour B, Maulard-Durdux C, Chretien Y, Mejean A. Concomitant fluorouracil (5-FU)-cisplatin (CDDP) and bifractionated split course radiation therapy (BSCRT) for invasive bladder cancer [abstract 1139]. Proc Am Soc Clin Oncol. 1997;16:319a.

30. Kaufman DS, Shipley WU, Griffin PP, et al. Selective bladder preservation by combination treatment of invasive bladder cancer. N Engl J Med. 1993;329:1377–82.

31. Rodel C, Grabenbauer GG, Kuhn R, et al. Combined-modality treatment and selective organ preservation in invasive bladder cancer: long-term results. J Clin Oncol. 2002;20:3061–71.

32. Herr HW. Outcome of patients who refuse cystectomy after receiving neoadjuvant chemotherapy for muscle-invasive bladder cancer. Eur Urol. 2008;54:126–32.

33. Heidenreich A. Muscle-invasive urothelial carcinoma of the bladder: neoadjuvant chemotherapy enables organ-preserving therapy in carefully selected patients. Eur Urol. 2008;54:21–3.

34. Scosyrev E, Ely BW, Messing EM, et al. Do mixed histological features affect survival from neoadjuvant platinum-based combination chemotherapy in patients with locally advanced bladder cancer? A secondary analysis of Southwest Oncology Group – directed Intergroup Study (S8710). BJU Int. 2010;108:693–700.

35. Kaye SB, MacFarlane JR, McHattie I, Hart AJL. Chemotherapy before radiotherapy for T3 bladder cancer. A pilot study. Br J Urol. 1985;57:434–7.

36. Shearer RJ, Chilvers CED, Bloom HGJ. Adjuvant chemotherapy in T3 carcinoma of the bladder. A prospective trial: preliminary report. J Urol. 1988;62:558–64.

37. Martinez-Pineiro JA, Martin MG, Arocena F, Flores N, Roncero CR, Portillo JA, et al. Neoadjuvant cisplatin chemotherapy before radical cystectomy in invasive transitional cell carcinoma of the bladder: a prospective randomized phase III study. J Urol. 1995;153:964–73.

38. Wallace MA, Raghavan D, Kelly KA, Sandeman TF, Conn IG, Teriana N, et al. Neo-adjuvant (pre-emptive) cisplatin therapy in invasive transitional cell carcinoma of the bladder. Br J Urol. 1991;67:608–15.

39. Ghersi D, Stewart LA, Parmar MKB, Coppin C, Martinez-Pineiro J, Raghavan D, et al., Advanced Bladder Cancer Overview Collaboration. Does neoadjuvant cisplatin-based chemotherapy improve the survival of patients with locally advanced bladder cancer: a metaanalysis of individual patient data from randomized clinical trials. Br J Urol. 1995;75:206–13.
40. Millikan R, Dinney C, Swanson D, et al. Integrated therapy for locally advanced bladder cancer: final report of a randomized trial of cystectomy plus adjuvant M-VAC versus cystectomy with both preoperative and postoperative M-VAC. J Clin Oncol. 2001;19:4005–13.
41. Wallace MA, Raghavan D, Kelly KA, Sandeman TF, Conn IG, Teriana N, et al. Neo-adjuvant (pre-emptive) cisplatin therapy in invasive transitional cell carcinoma of the bladder. Br J Urol (1991) 67:608–15.
42. Cortesi E. Neoadjuvant treatment for locally advanced bladder cancer: a randomized prospective clinical trial. Meeting abstract;1995.
43. Malmstrom PU, Rintala E, Wahlqvist R, Hellstrom P, Hellsten S, Hannisdal E. Five year follow-up of a prospective trial of radical cystectomy and neoadjuvant chemotherapy: Nordic Cystectomy Trial I. The Nordic Cooperative Bladder Cancer Study Group. J Urol. 1996;155:1903–6.
44. Sengelov L, von der Maase H, Lundbeck F, Barlebo H, Colstrup H, Engelholm SA, et al. Neoadjuvant chemotherapy with cisplatin and methotrexate in patients with muscle invasive bladder tumours. Acta Oncol. 2002;41:447–56.
45. Shipley WU, Winter KA, Kaufman DS, Lee WR, Heney NM, Tester BJ, et al. Phase III trial of neoadjuvant chemotherapy in patients with invasive bladder cancer treated with elective bladder preservation by combined radiation therapy and chemotherapy: initial results of Radiation Therapy Oncology Group 89-03. J Clin Oncol. 1998;16:3576–83.
46. Parmar MK. Neoadjuvant chemotherapy in invasive bladder cancer. Trial design. Prog Clin Biol Res. 1990;353:1115–8.

Trimodal Therapy in Bladder Cancer 27

Trimodal therapy (TMT) is considered the most effective bladder-sparing approach for muscle-invasive urothelial carcinoma of the bladder (MIBC) and an alternative to radical cystectomy [1]. TMT consists of a maximal resection of the bladder, followed by a concurrent radiotherapy and chemotherapy, limiting salvage radical cystectomy to non-responder tumours or muscle-invasive recurrence [1]. In large population studies, less than 6% of the patients with nonmetastatic MIBC receive a chemoradiation therapy and this rate is stable. A growing body of evidence exists that TMT provides good oncologic outcomes with low morbidity when compared with radical cystectomy [1]. TMT requires, however, a close follow-up because of the high risk of local recurrence and salvage radical cystectomy in up to 30% of the patients [1]. Salvage radical cystectomy can be performed with adequate results but does not offer the same opportunity of reconstruction and functional outcomes than primary radical cystectomy. Although radical cystectomy is still the treatment of reference for most of the patients with localized MIBC, TMT represents a reasonable alternative in highly selected patients [1]. Any firm conclusion on the equivalence or superiority of one treatment to the other is still limited by the lack of randomized controlled trials and the heterogeneity of the available literature. Future studies and multidisciplinary approach are mandatory to optimize the patient selection and regimen of TMT.

Lee et al., retrospectively reviewed the efficacy and organ preservation experience for muscle-invasive bladder cancer by trimodality therapy [2]. Complete response (CR) rate assessed 3 month after CCRT was 78.1% [2]. Ten patients (20%) had local recurrence after initial CR (n = 50), 3 of them were superficial recurrence. One patient underwent radical cystectomy after recurrence [2]. The overall 5-year bladder intact survival was 49.0% (95% CI, 35.5–62.5%). Acute toxicities were limited to grade 1–2. One patient developed late grade 3 GU toxicity.

This suggests that trimodality bladder-sparing approach without NAC or dose-intensification could be well-tolerated with a high CR rate and bladder preserving rate for muscle-invasive bladder cancer [2].

© The Editor(s) (if applicable) and The Author(s), under exclusive license to
Springer Nature Switzerland AG 2021
S. S. Goonewardene et al., *Management of Muscle Invasive Bladder Cancer*,
Management of Urology, https://doi.org/10.1007/978-3-030-57915-9_27

Aims of bladder preservation in muscle-invasive bladder cancer (MIBC) are to offer a quality-of-life advantage and avoid potential morbidity or mortality of radical cystectomy (RC) without compromising oncologic outcomes [3]. Because of the lack of a completed randomised controlled trial, oncologic equivalence of bladder preservation modality treatments compared with RC remains unknown. The 5-year cancer-specific survival and overall survival rates range from 50% to 82% and from 36% to 74%, respectively, with salvage cystectomy rates of 25–30% [3]. There are no definitive data to support the benefit of using of neoadjuvant or adjuvant chemotherapy. Critical to good outcomes is proper patient selection [3]. The best cancers eligible for bladder preservation are those with low-volume T2 disease without hydronephrosis or extensive carcinoma in situ. A growing body of accumulated data suggests that bladder preservation with TMT leads to acceptable outcomes and therefore may be considered a reasonable treatment option in well-selected patients [3]. Treatment based on a combination of resection, chemotherapy, and radiotherapy as bladder-sparing strategies may be considered as a reasonable treatment option in properly selected patients.

While radical cystectomy (RC) with pelvic lymph node dissection (PLND) represents the accepted gold standard for the treatment of muscle-invasive bladder cancer, this treatment approach is associated with significant morbidity [4]. As such, bladder preservation strategies are often utilized in patients who are either deemed medically unfit due to significant comorbidities or whom decline management with RC and PLND secondary to its associated morbidity. In a select group of patients, meeting strict criteria, bladder preservation approaches may be employed with curative intent [4]. Trimodal therapy, consisting of complete transurethral resection of bladder tumor (TURBT), chemotherapy, and radiation therapy has demonstrated durable oncologic control and long-term survival.

Takaoka retrospectively elucidated the oncological outcomes, prognostic factors and toxicities of proton beam therapy in trimodal bladder-preserving therapy for muscle-invasive bladder cancer at our institution [5]. Bladder-preserving therapy with proton beam therapy was well tolerated and achieved a favourable mortality rate [5]. Tumour multiplicity and tumour size were important risk factors for progression.

Purpose Multidisciplinary management improves complex treatment decision making in cancer care, but its impact for bladder cancer (BC) has not been documented [6]. Although radical cystectomy (RC) currently is viewed as the standard of care for muscle-invasive bladder cancer (MIBC), radiotherapy-based, bladder-sparing trimodal therapy (TMT) that combines transurethral resection of bladder tumour, chemotherapy for radiation sensitization, and external beam radiotherapy has emerged as a valid treatment option [6]. In the setting of a MDBCC, TMT yielded survival outcomes similar to those of matched patients who underwent RC. Appropriately selected patients with MIBC should be offered the opportunity to discuss various treatment options, including organ-sparing TMT.

Radical cystectomy is the guidelines-recommended treatment of muscle-invasive bladder cancer, but a resurgence of trimodal therapy has occurred [7]. Williams et al., compared the survival outcomes and costs between trimodal therapy and radical cystectomy in older adults with muscle-invasive bladder cancer [7]. Trimodal therapy was associated with significantly decreased overall survival and cancer-specific survival as well as $335 million in excess spending in 2011 [7]. These findings have important health policy implications regarding the appropriate use of high value-based care among older adults with invasive bladder cancer who are candidates for either radical cystectomy or trimodal therapy.

References

1. Mathieu R, Lucca I, Klatte T, Babjuk M, Shariat SF. Trimodal therapy for invasive bladder cancer: is it really equal to radical cystectomy? Curr Opin Urol. 2015;25(5):476–82.
2. Lee CY, Yang KL, Ko HL, Huang RY, Tsai PP, Chen MT, Lin YC, Hwang TI, Juang GD, Chi KH. Trimodality bladder-sparing approach without neoadjuvant chemotherapy for node-negative localized muscle-invasive urinary bladder cancer resulted in comparable cystectomy-free survival. Radiat Oncol. 2014;9:213.
3. Ploussard G, Daneshmand S, Efstathiou JA, Herr HW, James ND, Rödel CM, Shariat SF, Shipley WU, Sternberg CN, Thalmann GN, Kassouf W. Critical analysis of bladder sparing with trimodal therapy in muscle-invasive bladder cancer: a systematic review. Eur Urol. 2014;66(1):120–37.
4. Russell CM, Lebastchi AH, Borza T, Spratt DE, Morgan TM. The role of transurethral resection in trimodal therapy for muscle-invasive bladder cancer. Bladder Cancer. 2016;2(4):381–94.
5. Takaoka EI, Miyazaki J, Ishikawa H, Kawai K, Kimura T, Ishitsuka R, Kojima T, Kanuma R, Takizawa D, Okumura T, Sakurai H, Nishiyama H. Long-term single-institute experience with trimodal bladder-preserving therapy with proton beam therapy for muscle-invasive bladder cancer. Jpn J Clin Oncol. 2017;47(1):67–73.
6. Kulkarni GS, Hermanns T, Wei Y, Bhindi B, Satkunasivam R, Athanasopoulos P, Bostrom PJ, Kuk C, Li K, Templeton AJ, Sridhar SS, van der Kwast TH, Chung P, Bristow RG, Milosevic M, Warde P, Fleshner NE, Jewett MAS, Bashir S, Zlotta AR. Propensity score analysis of radical cystectomy versus bladder-sparing trimodal therapy in the setting of a multidisciplinary bladder cancer clinic. J Clin Oncol. 2017;35(20):2299–305.
7. Williams SB, Shan Y, Jazzar U, Mehta HB, Baillargeon JG, Huo J, Senagore AJ, Orihuela E, Tyler DS, Swanson TA, Kamat AM. Comparing survival outcomes and costs associated with radical cystectomy and trimodal therapy for older adults with muscle-invasive bladder cancer. JAMA Surg. 2018;153:881.

Trimodal Therapy: A Systematic Review—Is It Really Better than Radical Therapy?

28

A systematic review relating to trimodal therapy and muscle invasive bladder cancer was conducted. The search strategy aimed to identify all references related to bladder cancer AND trimodal therapy. Search terms used were as follows: (Bladder cancer) AND (trimodal therapy). The following databases were screened from 1989 to June 2019:

- CINAHL
- MEDLINE (NHS Evidence)
- Cochrane
- AMed
- EMBASE
- PsychINFO
- SCOPUS
- Web of Science.

In addition, searches using Medical Subject Headings (MeSH) and keywords were conducted using Cochrane databases. Two UK-based experts in bladder cancer were consulted to identify any additional studies.

Studies were eligible for inclusion if they reported primary research focusing on bladder cancer and screening. Papers were included if published after 1984 and had to be in English. Studies that did not conform to this were excluded. Only primary research was included. The overall aim was to identify the role and components of Trimodal therapy in Bladder Cancer.

Abstracts were independently screened for eligibility by two reviewers and disagreements resolved through discussion or third party opinion (Fig. 28.1). Agreement level was calculated using Cohen's Kappa to test the intercoder reliability of this screening process. Cohens' Kappa allows comparison of inter-rater reliability between papers using relative observed agreement. This also takes account

© The Editor(s) (if applicable) and The Author(s), under exclusive license to
Springer Nature Switzerland AG 2021
S. S. Goonewardene et al., *Management of Muscle Invasive Bladder Cancer*,
Management of Urology, https://doi.org/10.1007/978-3-030-57915-9_28

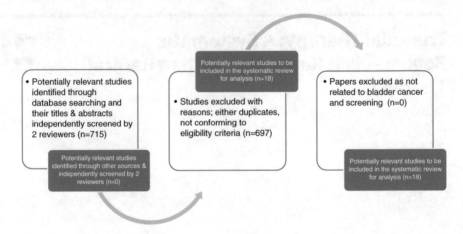

Fig. 28.1 Flow chart of studies identified through the systematic review. (Adapted from PRISMA)

of the comparison occurring by chance. The first reviewer agreed all 43 papers to be included, the second, agreed on 43.

Data extraction was piloted by the researcher and amended in consultation with the research team (author and two academic supervisors). Data collected included authors, year and country of publication, study aims, setting, intervention aims, number of participants, study design, intervention components and delivery methods, comparison groups and outcome measures, notes and follow-up questions for the authors. Studies were quality assessed using the PRISMA criteria for randomised controlled trials, Mays et al. [1, 2] for the action research and qualitative studies and the Critical Skills Appraisal programme for cohort studies. This was also applied to randomised controlled trials and qualitative studies.

28.1   Trimodal Chemotherapy

Open radical cystectomy (ORC) is currently the standard treatment for muscle-invasive bladder cancer (MIBC) without metastasis, while many patients with MIBC are not always appropriate candidates due to multiple comorbidities [3]. Nagao, evaluated the bladder-preservation strategy and compared the results with those obtained by ORC [3]. The data of 50 patients with MIBC was retrospectively collated including those treated by trimodal chemoradiotherapy with cisplatin (CDDP-radiation [CDDP-R]). Transurethral resection of the bladder tumor (TURBT) was performed before treatment to confirm pathological stage ≥T2. Extensive TURBT was performed after chemoradiotherapy to evaluate the pathological response to treatment [3]. The 2- and 5-year progression-free survival, bladder-intact survival, cancer-specific survival, and overall survival (OS) rates after treatment were 70.8% and 63.9%, 64.0% and 49.8%, 86.7% and 71.8%, and 84.3% and 64.8%, respectively [3]. The 2- and 5-year OS rates after CDDP-R were

90.5% and 74.3%, respectively, and those after ORC were 71.8% and 59.9%, respectively, indicating a significant survival advantage conferred by CDDP-R over ORC (p < 0.05, HR 0.45, 95% CI 0.21–0.94) [3]. In selected patients, CDDP-R for MIBC may provide comparative oncological outcomes as ORC.

28.2 Efficacy of 5FU as Part of Trimodal Therapy

Organ preservation has been investigated in patients with muscle-invasive bladder carcinoma over the past decades as an alternative to radical cystectomy [4]. The majority of studies reported that trimodal schedules, including transurethral resection of bladder tumour (TURB), radiotherapy (RT), and chemotherapy, are a feasible and safe organ-sparing approach without deferring the survival probability [4]. Danesi et al. [4] evaluated the long-term results of a schedule of concurrent cisplatin and 5-fluorouracil (5-FU) administered as protracted intravenous infusions (PVI) during hyperfractionated radiotherapy (HFRT) with organ-sparing intent in patients with infiltrating transitional cell carcinoma of the bladder (TCCB) [4]. Seventy-seven patients with a classification of T2–T4aN0M0 TCCB were enrolled in the current study. After a complete TURB and bladder mapping, 42 of 77 patients underwent 2 cycles of induction chemotherapy [4]. Seventy-two patients were evaluable for response: 65 achieved a CR (90.3%) and 7 (9.7%) achieved a partial response. No significant difference was observed for the different prognostic factors with the exception of stage of disease (T2 [95.7%] vs. T3–T4a [80.0%]; p = 0.04) [4]. The observed toxicity, mainly hematologic, was higher among the patients who received induction chemotherapy compared with the patients who did not receive induction chemotherapy, even though the difference was not statistically significant. After a median follow-up of 82.2 months (range, 30–138 months), 44 of 65 (57.1%) patients who achieved a CR were alive [4]. Of these 44 patients, 33 had tumour-free bladders. The 5-year overall, bladder-intact, tumour-specific, disease-free, and cystectomy-free survival rates for all 77 patients were 58.5%, 46.6%, 75.0%, 53.5%, and 76.1%, respectively. No associations were observed in overall and tumour-specific survival with different prognostic factors [4]. Combined treatment appeared to provide high response rates and can be offered as an alternative option to radical cystectomy in selected patients who refuse or are unsuitable for surgery.

28.3 Outcomes from Trimodal Therapy for MIBC

Seisen performed an observational cohort study to examine the comparative effectiveness of these two definitive treatments [5]. Within the National Cancer Data Base (2004–2011), 1257 were identified (9.8%) and 11,586 (90.2%) patients who received TMT and RC, respectively. Inverse probability of treatment weighting (IPTW)-adjusted Kaplan-Meier analysis showed that median overall survival (OS) was similar between the TMT (40 months, 95% confidence interval [CI] 34–46) and RC groups (43 months 95% CI 41–45; p = 0.3) [5]. TMT was generally associated with worse long-term OS compared to RC for muscle-invasive bladder cancer. However, the survival benefit of RC should be weighed against the risks of surgery, especially in older patients [5]. These results are preliminary and emphasize the need for a randomized controlled trial to compare TMT versus RC.

Although radical cystectomy (RC) is considered as the standard therapy for muscle-invasive bladder cancer (MIBC), trimodal therapy (TMT) combining transurethral resection of the tumor with radiotherapy and chemotherapy is increasingly recommended as an alternative approach for bladder preservation [6]. Kim compared the clinical outcomes between RC and TMT using propensity score matching with 50 patients in the RC arm and 29 patients in the TMT arm [6]. With respective median follow-up periods of 23 and 32 months for the RC and TMT groups, 5-year distant metastasis-free survival (58% vs. 67%), overall survival (56% vs. 57%), and cancer-specific survival (69% vs. 63%) rates between the RC and TMT groups, respectively, were similar [6]. However, the 5-year local recurrence-free survival was significantly better in the RC group than in the TMT group (74% vs. 35%). Following TMT, acute grade 3 hematological (n = 2) and late grade 3 genitourinary (n = 1) toxicities were reported [6]. These findings demonstrated that oncological outcomes of TMT were comparable with those of RC, except for poorer local control. Large-scale, randomized trials are warranted to confirm the findings of the present retrospective comparison and to guide toward best treatment options.

Organ preservation has been investigated in patients (p) with infiltrating transitional cell carcinoma (TCC) of the bladder over the past decade as an alternative to radical cystectomy. Cobo examined a trimodal schedule study, including transurethral resection of bladder tumor (TURB), neoadjuvant chemotherapy and concomitant radiochemotherapy (RTC) [7]. Cobo included 28 men and 1 women (median age 63, range 39–72 years) with PS (ECOG) 0–1 [7]. The stage was: 21 p T2; 6 p T3a; and 2 p T3b. Toxicity was higher in CMV compared with Gem-Cis: grade (3/4) neutropenia 4/15 (26%) vs. 1/14 (7%); febrile neutropenia 3/15 (20%) vs. 1/14 (7%); grade (3/4) thrombocytopenia 2/15 (13%) vs. 1/14 (7%) [7]. Toxicities with concomitant RCT were low-moderate: urocystitis (26%) and enteritis (18%). A complete histologic response after induction RCT occurred in 25 patients (86%) [7]. After a median follow-up of 69.4 months (range: 8–97.7), there were 8 deaths, with a overall survival of 72%. Furthermore 14 of 29 p (48%) were alive with intact bladder, and median survival time with intact bladder was 63.6 months (50.1–77.2); were predictive of best outcome T2 stage vs. T3 (p < 0.0001), and complete histologic resection in initial TURB vs. residual tumor (p = 0.0004) [7]. Combined treatment provide high response rates and can be offered as an alternative option to radical cystectomy in selected patients with TCC. Patients with T2 stage and complete histologic resection in initial TURB had the best outcome.

Sabaa evaluated the 5-year results of the following trimodal therapy for treatment of some selected cases of muscle invasive bladder cancer [8]. Sabaa et al. conducted a prospective study, with 104 patients with transitional cell carcinoma (TCC) (T2 and T3a, N0, M0). All patients received adjuvant chemo-radiotherapy

(CRT) in the form of gemcitabine and cisplatin and conventional radiotherapy after the maximum resection of their tumours [8]. Two weeks later, all cases had radiologic and cystoscopic evaluation. The patients who showed no evidence of the bladder tumours [complete response (CR)] went on to complete the CRT, while those with recurrent invasive tumours did not receive any more CRT and were assigned to have salvage cystectomy [8]. Thereafter, all patients were subjected to a regular follow-up. This trimodal therapy was well tolerated in most of cases with no severe acute toxicities. Complete response was achieved in 78.8% of cases after the initial CRT, and tumour grade was found to be the most significant risk factor to predict this response (p = 0.004). With a median follow-up of 71 months for patients with initial CR, 16.2% of cases showed muscle invasive recurrences, and multifocality was the only significant risk factor for their development (p = 0.003) [8]. Meanwhile, superficial recurrences were detected in 8.1% of cases with initial CR and were successfully treated with transurethral resection and intravesical bacillus Calmette-Guerin (BCG). On the other hand, we reported distant metastasis in 24.3% of patients with initial CR, and tumour grade, stage and multifocality were the most significant risk factors for this complication (p = 0.002, 0.031, 0.006) [8]. No cases of contracted bladder or late gastrointestinal complications were demonstrated in this series. The 5-year overall survival rate for patients with initial CR was 67.6%, and for all the patients in this study it was 59.4%.

This trimodal therapy can be considered as a treatment option for patients with localized muscle invasive TCC. The best candidates for such therapy are those with solitary T2, low grade tumours that are amenable to complete transurethral resection.

Williams compared the survival outcomes and costs between trimodal therapy and radical cystectomy in older adults with muscle-invasive bladder cancer [9]. This population-based cohort study used data from the Surveillance, Epidemiology, and End Results-Medicare linked database. A total of 3200 older adults (aged ≥66 years) with clinical stage T2 to T4a bladder cancer were included. Patients who received radical cystectomy underwent either only surgery or surgery in combination with radiotherapy or chemotherapy [9]. Patients who received trimodal therapy underwent transurethral resection of the bladder followed by radiotherapy and chemotherapy [9]. Of the 3200 patients who met the inclusion criteria, 2048 (64.0%) were men and 1152 (36.0%) were women, with a mean (SD) age of 75.8 (6.0) years. After propensity score matching, 687 patients (21.5%) underwent trimodal therapy and 687 patients (21.5%) underwent radical cystectomy [9]. Patients who underwent trimodal therapy had significantly decreased overall survival (hazard ratio [HR], 1.49; 95% CI, 1.31–1.69) and cancer-specific survival (HR, 1.55; 95% CI, 1.32–1.83) [9]. Trimodal therapy was associated with significantly decreased overall survival and cancer-specific survival [9]. These findings have important health policy implications regarding the appropriate use of high value-based care among older adults with invasive bladder cancer who are candidates for either radical cystectomy or trimodal therapy.

28.4   Trimodal Therapy in the Elderly

Radical cystectomy is the guidelines-recommended treatment of muscle-invasive bladder cancer, but a resurgence of trimodal therapy has occurred [9]. Williams compared the survival outcomes and costs between trimodal therapy and radical cystectomy in older adults with muscle-invasive bladder cancer [9]. Of the 3200 patients who met the inclusion criteria, 2048 (64.0%) were men and 1152 (36.0%) were women, with a mean (SD) age of 75.8 (6.0) years. After propensity score matching, 687 patients (21.5%) underwent trimodal therapy and 687 patients (21.5%) underwent radical cystectomy [9]. Patients who underwent trimodal therapy had significantly decreased overall survival (hazard ratio [HR], 1.49; 95% CI, 1.31–1.69) and cancer-specific survival (HR, 1.55; 95% CI, 1.32–1.83).

28.5   Trimodal Therapy and Radical Cystectomy

Multidisciplinary management improves complex treatment decision making in cancer care, but its impact for bladder cancer (BC) has not been documented [10]. Kulkarni compared data from patients treated in a multidisciplinary bladder cancer clinic (MDBCC) from 2008 to 2013 were reviewed retrospectively [10]. A total of 112 patients with MIBC were included after matching (56 who had been treated with TMT, and 56 who underwent RC) [10]. The median age was 68.0 years, and 29.5% had stage cT3/cT4 disease. At a median follow-up of 4.51 years, there were 20 deaths (35.7%) in the RC group (13 as a result of BC) and 22 deaths (39.3%) in the TMT group (13 as a result of BC) [10]. The 5-year DSS rate was 73.2% and 76.6% in the RC and TMT groups, respectively (p = 0.49). Salvage cystectomy was performed in 6 (10.7%) of 56 patients who received TMT [10]. In the setting of a MDBCC, TMT yielded survival outcomes similar to those of matched patients who underwent RC [10]. Appropriately selected patients with MIBC should be offered the opportunity to discuss various treatment options, including organ-sparing TMT.

Maarouf evaluate the efficacy of a bladder preservation multimodality protocol for patients with operable carcinoma invading bladder muscle [11]. Out of 33 eligible patients, were included. Trimodal therapy was well tolerated in most of cases, with no severe acute toxicities. After 12 months of follow-up, a complete response was achieved in 39.3% and a partial response in 7.1%, with an overall response rate of 46.4% [11]. By the end of the first year, disease-free survival was reported in 39.3%, whereas 25% were still alive with their disease, giving an overall survival of 64.3% for all patients who maintained their intact, well-functioning bladders [11]. Stage and completeness of transurethral resection of bladder tumour were the most important predictors of response and survival. T2 lesions had complete and partial response rates of 69.2% and 23%, respectively, whereas T3 lesions had rates of 40% and 13.3%, respectively (p = 0.001). The response rate in complete TURBT was 82.6% vs. 20% with cystoscopic biopsy only (p = 0.001). In addition, disease-free survival was 72.7% in T2 patients and 27.3% in T3 patients (p = 0.001) [11]. In the present study, bladder preservation protocol with MVAC and radical radiotherapy achieved suboptimal response rates at 1 year in patients with localized TCC invading bladder muscle. Patients with solitary T2 lesions that are amenable to complete TURBT achieved the best response rates. Longer follow-up is needed to verify these results. Patients with localized disease should be encouraged for radical cystectomy, which achieved better results.

28.6   Proton Beam Therapy in Trimodal Therapy

Takaoka et al. [12] retrospectively elucidated the oncological outcomes, prognostic factors and toxicities of proton beam therapy in trimodal bladder-preserving therapy for muscle-invasive bladder cancer at our institution [12]. The patients' median age was 65 (range 36–85) years. The median follow-up period was 3.4 (range 0.6–19.5) years [12]. The 5-year cumulative overall survival rate, progression-free survival rate and time to progression rate were 82%, 77%, and 82%, respectively. In univariate and multivariate analyses, tumor multiplicity and tumor size ($\geq$5 cm) were significant and independent factors associated with progression (hazard ratio 3.5, 95% confidence interval 1.1–12; hazard ratio 5.0, 95% confidence interval 1.3–17; $p < 0.05$ for all) [12]. As for toxicity, 26 (18%) patients had grade 3–4 acute hematologic toxicities and 2 (3%) patients had grade 3 late genitourinary toxicity. No patient had to discontinue the treatment due to acute toxicity [12]. The bladder-preserving therapy with proton beam therapy was well tolerated and achieved a favorable mortality rate. Tumor multiplicity and tumor size were important risk factors for progression. These findings indicate that this therapy can be an effective treatment option for selected muscle-invasive bladder cancer patients [12].

28.7   Reviews Related to Trimodal Therapy for MIBC

Garcia-Perdomo et al. [13] determined the effectiveness and harms of bladder-preserving trimodal therapy (TMT) as a first-line treatment versus radical cystectomy (RC) plus radical pelvic lymphadenectomy in the treatment of muscle-invasive bladder cancer in terms of overall survival [13]. There were 2682 records with the search strategies and, finally, 11 studies were included in the quantitative analysis. The summary HR for OS was 1.06 95% CI (0.85–1.31) $I^2 = 77\%$, showing no statistical difference [13]. Regarding cancer-specific survival, the summary HR was 1.23 95% CI (1.04–1.46) $I^2 = 14\%$. On the other side, for the progression-free survival, the summary HR was 1.11 95% CI (0.63–1.95) $I^2 = 78\%$. Only one study described HR for adverse events (1.37 95% CI 1.16–1.59) [13]. There were no differences in overall survival and progression-free survival between these two interventions.

Fahmy analysed the oncological long-term outcomes of trimodal therapy (TMT) and radical cystectomy (RC) for the treatment of muscle-invasive bladder cancer (BC) with or without neoadjuvant chemotherapy (NAC) [14]. The mean 10-year OS was 30.9% for TMT and 35.1% for RC ($p = 0.32$). The mean 10-year DSS was 50.9% for

TMT and 57.8% for RC (p = 0.26). NAC was administered before therapy to 453 (13.3%) of 3402 patients treated with TMT and 812 (3.0%) of 27,867 patients treated with RC (p < 0.001) [14]. Complete response (CR) was achieved in 1545 (75.3%) of 2051 evaluable patients treated with TMT. A 5-year OS, DSS, and RFS after CR were 66.9%, 78.3%, and 52.5%, respectively [14]. The survival outcomes of patients after TMT and RC for MIBC were comparable. Patients who experienced downstaging after NAC and RC exhibited improved survival compared to patients treated with RC only [14]. Best survival outcomes after TMT are associated with CR to this approach [14].

Trimodal therapy (TMT) is considered the most effective bladder-sparing approach for muscle-invasive urothelial carcinoma of the bladder (MIBC) and an alternative to radical cystectomy. Mathieu et al. [15] reviewed the current knowledge on the equiva-lence of TMT and radical cystectomy based on the recent literature. TMT consists of a maximal transurethral resection of the bladder, followed by a concurrent radiother-apy and chemotherapy, limiting salvage radical cystectomy to non-responder tumours or muscle-invasive recurrence [15]. In large population studies, less than 6% of the patients with nonmetastatic MIBC receive a chemoradiation therapy and this rate is stable. A growing body of evidence exists that TMT provides good oncologic out-comes with low morbidity when compared with radical cystectomy [15]. TMT requires, however, a close follow-up because of the high risk of local recurrence and salvage radical cystectomy in up to 30% of the patients. Salvage radical cystectomy can be performed with adequate results but does not offer the same opportunity of reconstruction and functional outcomes than primary radical cystectomy [15].

Aims of bladder preservation in muscle-invasive bladder cancer (MIBC) are to offer a quality-of-life advantage and avoid potential morbidity or mortality of radi-cal cystectomy (RC) without compromising oncologic outcomes [16]. Because of the lack of a completed randomised controlled trial, oncologic equivalence of blad-der preservation modality treatments compared with RC remains unknown [16]. Optimal bladder-preservation treatment includes a safe transurethral resection of the bladder tumour as complete as possible followed by radiation therapy (RT) with concurrent radiosensitising chemotherapy. A standard radiation schedule includes external-beam RT to the bladder and limited pelvic lymph nodes to an initial dose of 40 Gy, with a boost to the whole bladder to 54 Gy and a further tumour boost to a total dose of 64–65 Gy [16]. Radiosensitising chemotherapy with phase 3 trial evidence in support exists for cisplatin and mitomycin C plus 5-fluorouracil. A cys-toscopic assessment with systematic rebiopsy should be performed at TMT comple-tion or early after TMT induction. Thus, nonresponders are identified early to promptly offer salvage RC [16]. The 5-year cancer-specific survival and overall survival rates range from 50% to 82% and from 36% to 74%, respectively, with salvage cystectomy rates of 25–30%. There are no definitive data to support the benefit of using of neoadjuvant or adjuvant chemotherapy. Critical to good out-comes is proper patient selection. The best cancers eligible for bladder preservation are those with low-volume T2 disease without hydronephrosis or extensive carci-noma in situ [16]. A growing body of accumulated data suggests that bladder pres-ervation with TMT leads to acceptable outcomes and therefore may be considered a reasonable treatment option in well-selected patients [17].

References

1. Moher D, Liberati A, Tetzlaff J, Altman DG. "Preferred Reporting Items for Systematic Reviews and Meta-Analyses: The Prisma Statement." [In English]. BMJ (Online) 339, no. 7716 (08 Aug 2009):332–36.
2. Mays N, Pope C, Popay J. "Systematically Reviewing Qualitative and Quantitative Evidence to Inform Management and Policy-Making in the Health Field." [In English]. Journal of Health Services Research and Policy 10, no. SUPPL. 1 (July 2005):6–20.
3. Nagao K, Hara T, Nishijima J, Shimizu K, Fujii N, Kobayashi K, Kawai Y, Inoue R, Yamamoto Y, Matsumoto H, Matsuyama H. The efficacy of trimodal chemoradiotherapy with cisplatin as a bladder-preserving strategy for the treatment of muscle-invasive bladder cancer. Urol Int. 2017;99(4):446–52.
4. Danesi DT, Arcangeli G, Cruciani E, Altavista P, Mecozzi A, Saracino B, Orefici F. Conservative treatment of invasive bladder carcinoma by transurethral resection, protracted intravenous infusion chemotherapy, and hyperfractionated radiotherapy: long term results. Cancer. 2004;101(11):2540–8.
5. Seisen T, Sun M, Lipsitz SR, Abdollah F, Leow JJ, Menon M, Preston MA, Harshman LC, Kibel AS, Nguyen PL, Bellmunt J, Choueiri TK, Trinh QD. Comparative effectiveness of trimodal therapy versus radical cystectomy for localized muscle-invasive urothelial carcinoma of the bladder. Eur Urol. 2017;72(4):483–7.
6. Kim YJ, Byun SJ, Ahn H, Kim CS, Hong BS, Yoo S, Lee JL, Kim YS. Comparison of outcomes between trimodal therapy and radical cystectomy in muscle-invasive bladder cancer: a propensity score matching analysis. Oncotarget. 2017;8(40):68996–9004.
7. Cobo M, Delgado R, Gil S, Herruzo I, Baena V, Carabante F, Moreno P, Ruiz JL, Bretón JJ, Del Rosal JM, Fuentes C, Moreno P, García E, Villar E, Contreras J, Alés I, Benavides M. Conservative treatment with transurethral resection, neoadjuvant chemotherapy followed by radiochemotherapy in stage T2–3 transitional bladder cancer. Clin Transl Oncol. 2006;8(12):903–11.
8. Sabaa MA, El-Gamal OM, Abo-Elenen M, Khanam A. Combined modality treatment with bladder preservation for muscle invasive bladder cancer. Urol Oncol. 2010;28(1):14–20.
9. Williams SB, Shan Y, Jazzar U, Mehta HB, Baillargeon JG, Huo J, Senagore AJ, Orihuela E, Tyler DS, Swanson TA, Kamat AM. Comparing survival outcomes and costs associated with radical cystectomy and trimodal therapy for older adults with muscle-invasive bladder cancer. JAMA Surg. 2018;153:881.
10. Kulkarni GS, Hermanns T, Wei Y, Bhindi B, Satkunasivam R, Athanasopoulos P, Bostrom PJ, Kuk C, Li K, Templeton AJ, Sridhar SS, van der Kwast TH, Chung P, Bristow RG, Milosevic M, Warde P, Fleshner NE, Jewett MAS, Bashir S, Zlotta AR. Propensity score analysis of radical cystectomy versus bladder-sparing trimodal therapy in the setting of a multidisciplinary bladder cancer clinic. J Clin Oncol. 2017;35(20):2299–305.
11. Maarouf AM, Khalil S, Salem EA, ElAdl M, Nawar N, Zaiton F. Bladder preservation multimodality therapy as an alternative to radical cystectomy for treatment of muscle invasive bladder cancer. BJU Int. 2011;107(10):1605–10.
12. Takaoka EI, Miyazaki J, Ishikawa H, Kawai K, Kimura T, Ishitsuka R, Kojima T, Kanuma R, Takizawa D, Okumura T, Sakurai H, Nishiyama H. Long-term single-institute experience with trimodal bladder-preserving therapy with proton beam therapy for muscle-invasive bladder cancer. Jpn J Clin Oncol. 2017;47(1):67–73.
13. García-Perdomo HA, Montes-Cardona CE, Guacheta M, Castillo DF, Reis LO. Muscle-invasive bladder cancer organ-preserving therapy: systematic review and meta-analysis. World J Urol. 2018;36:1997–2008.
14. Fahmy O, Khairul-Asri MG, Schubert T, Renninger M, Malek R, Kübler H, Stenzl A, Gakis G. A systematic review and meta-analysis on the oncological long-term outcomes after trimodality therapy and radical cystectomy with or without neoadjuvant chemotherapy for muscle-invasive bladder cancer. Urol Oncol. 2018;36(2):43–53.

15. Mathieu R, Lucca I, Klatte T, Babjuk M, Shariat SF. Trimodal therapy for invasive bladder cancer: is it really equal to radical cystectomy? Curr Opin Urol. 2015;25(5):476–82.
16. Ploussard G, Daneshmand S, Efstathiou JA, Herr HW, James ND, Rödel CM, Shariat SF, Shipley WU, Sternberg CN, Thalmann GN, Kassouf W. Critical analysis of bladder sparing with trimodal therapy in muscle-invasive bladder cancer: a systematic review. Eur Urol. 2014;66(1):120–37.
17. Smith ZL, Christodouleas JP, Keefe SM, Malkowicz SB, Guzzo TJ. Bladder preservation in the treatment of muscle-invasive bladder cancer (MIBC): a review of the literature and a practical approach to therapy. BJU Int. 2013;112(1):13–25.

Part VI

Radical Cystectomy

Radical Cystectomy Outcomes

29

The current 'gold standard' for radical cystectomy remains open radical cystectomy [1]. RARC has lagged behind robot-assisted prostatectomy in terms of adoption and perceived patient benefit, but there are indications that this is now changing [1]. Radical cystectomy is complex surgery with several important outcome measures, including oncological and functional outcomes, complication rates, patient recovery and cost implications [1].

Given that the urologist has a major influence on outcomes of radical cystectomy, it is of interest to patients, trainees, urologists and administrators to understand the provider characteristics associated with favourable outcomes [2]. Bhindi et al. assessed associations between various surgeon characteristics and long-term oncologic outcomes for patients undergoing radical cystectomy for bladder cancer. While radical cystectomy volume, experience and uro-oncology fellowship are all likely important, subspecialized focus in bladder cancer was independently associated with improved long-term oncologic outcomes [2]. Our data support disease site differentiation among uro-oncologists at large institutions.

Although open radical cystectomy (ORC) is still the standard approach, laparoscopic radical cystectomy (LRC) and robot-assisted radical cystectomy (RARC) are increasingly performed [3]. Oncologic and functional data from RARC remain immature, and longer-term prospective studies are needed. Conclusive long-term survival outcomes for RARC were limited, although oncologic outcomes up to 5 years were similar to those reported for ORC performed [3]. Although open radical cystectomy (RC) is still regarded as the standard treatment for muscle-invasive bladder cancer, laparoscopic and robot-assisted RCs are becoming more popular performed [3]. Templates of lymph node dissection, lymph node yields, and positive surgical margin rates are acceptable with robot-assisted RC. Although definitive comparisons with open RC with respect to oncologic or functional outcomes are lacking, early results appear comparable performed [3].

S. S. Goonewardene et al., *Management of Muscle Invasive Bladder Cancer*, Management of Urology, https://doi.org/10.1007/978-3-030-57915-9_29

Although open radical cystectomy (ORC) is still the standard approach, laparoscopic radical cystectomy (LRC) and robot-assisted radical cystectomy (RARC) have gained popularity [4]. Comparing RARC and ORC, cumulative analyses demonstrated shorter operative time for ORC, whereas blood loss and in-hospital stay were better with RARC (all p values <0.003). Moreover, 90-day complication rates of any-grade and 90-day grade 3 complication rates were lower for RARC (all p values <0.04), whereas high-grade complication and mortality rates were similar [4].

RARC can be performed safely with acceptable perioperative outcome, although complications are common. Although open radical cystectomy (RC) is still regarded as a standard treatment for muscle-invasive bladder cancer, laparoscopic and robot-assisted RC are becoming more popular. Robotic RC can be safely performed with acceptably low risk of blood loss, transfusion, and intraoperative complications; however, as for open RC, the risk of postoperative complications is high, including a substantial risk of major complication and reoperation.

Stein et al. looked at outcomes from radical cystectomy [5]. Patients with nonorgan-confined (P3b, P4), lymph node-negative tumours demonstrated a significantly higher probability of recurrence compared with those with organ-confined bladder cancers (p < 0.001). The 5- and 10-year recurrence-free survival for P3b tumours was 62% and 61%, and for P4 tumours was 50% and 45%, respectively. A total of 246 patients (24%) had lymph node tumour involvement [5]. The 5- and 10-year recurrence-free survival for these patients was 35%, and 34%, respectively, which was significantly lower than for patients without lymph node involvement (p < 0.001) [5]. Patients could also be stratified by the number of lymph nodes involved and by the extent of the primary bladder tumour (p stage).

May et al. examined how the survival rates for patients with muscle-invasive bladder carcinoma are influenced by the tumour stage at initial presentation [6]. This study examined the clinical course of 452 patients who underwent radical cystectomy for bladder carcinoma from 1992 to 2004. Patients with superficial bladder carcinoma with tumour progression to muscle invasion do not have a better prognosis after radical cystectomy than patients presenting initially with muscle-invasive bladder carcinoma [6]. Survival rates in this group can only be improved by singling out patients on the basis of risk factors at an earlier stage and carrying out cystectomy.

References

1. Collins JW, Wiklund NP. Totally intracorporeal robot-assisted radical cystectomy: optimizing total outcomes. BJU Int. 2014;114(3):326–33.
2. Bhindi B, Yu J, Kuk C, Sridhar SS, Hamilton RJ, Finelli A, Jewett MA, Evans A, Fleshner NE, Zlotta AR, Kulkarni GS. The importance of surgeon characteristics on impacting oncologic outcomes for patients undergoing radical cystectomy. J Urol. 2014;192(3):714–9.

3. Yuh B, Wilson T, Bochner B, Chan K, Palou J, Stenzl A, Montorsi F, Thalmann G, Guru K, Catto JW, Wiklund PN, Novara G. Systematic review and cumulative analysis of oncologic and functional outcomes after robot-assisted radical cystectomy. Eur Urol. 2015;67(3):402–22.
4. Novara G, Catto JW, Wilson T, Annerstedt M, Chan K, Murphy DG, Motttrie A, Peabody JO, Skinner EC, Wiklund PN, Guru KA, Yuh B. Systematic review and cumulative analysis of perioperative outcomes and complications after robot-assisted radical cystectomy. Eur Urol. 2015;67(3):376–401.
5. Stein JP, Lieskovsky G, Cote R, et al. Radical cystectomy in the treatment of invasive bladder cancer: long-term results in 1,054 patients. J Clin Oncol. 2001;19(3):666–75.
6. May M, Braun KP, Richter W, Helke C, Vogler H, Hoschke B, Siegsmund M. [Radical cystectomy in the treatment of bladder cancer always in due time?]. Urologe A. 2007;46(8):913–9.

Zhao et al. study whether extraperitoneal radical cystectomy (EORC) accelerates the postoperative recovery of bowel function compared with laparoscopic radical cystectomy (LRC) [1].

All the patients with bladder cancer who underwent EORC or LRC with an ileal conduit by a single surgeon were reviewed [1]. No significant differences were noted in blood transfusion requirements, interval to flatus or liquid intake, or opioid dosage [1]. There were no positive surgical margins in either group, and no significant differences were observed in the lymph node count (p = 0.112). No significant differences were seen between the LRC and EORC groups in the 3-year overall, cancer-specific, or cancer-free survival rates [1]. EORC resulted in a POI rate similar to that of LRC, despite factors favouring LRC. Our results suggest that extraperitoneal LRC could improve the perioperative outcomes.

Yasui et al. [2] explored the oncological outcomes of 3-port laparoscopic radical cystectomy (LRC) compared to open radical cystectomy (ORC) in patients older than 75 years. Both groups had comparable preoperative characteristics. A significantly longer operating time (p = 0.0002) and less estimated blood loss (p = 0.021) were observed in the LRC group compared to the ORC group. Infection and ileus were the most common early complications after surgery [2]. ORC suffered from more postoperative infection (22.2% vs. 0.0%, p = 0.054) and ileus (25.0% vs. 12.5%, p = 0.521) than the LRC group (not significant).

Kanno et al. [3] described initial experience of laparoscopic radical cystectomy compared to open radical cystectomy (ORC) [3]. Characteristics were similar in LRC and ORC groups except for ASA score. Operating time during LRC was longer but complication rate of LRC was lower than that of ORC [3]. In addition, pathological stage or outcomes were similar in both groups and there were no significant difference between LRC and ORC groups in terms of overall and recurrence free survival rate [3]. As for learning curve of LRC, operating time and blood loss tended to decrease with increased experience. These results indicate that LRC

© The Editor(s) (if applicable) and The Author(s), under exclusive license to
Springer Nature Switzerland AG 2021
S. S. Goonewardene et al., *Management of Muscle Invasive Bladder Cancer*,
Management of Urology, https://doi.org/10.1007/978-3-030-57915-9_30

could be performed safely with decreased complication rate and similar oncological outcomes compared to ORC.

Yong compared the morbidity, mortality, oncological results and quality of life between laparoscopic radical cystectomy (LRC) and open radical cystectomy (ORC) in the elderly patients over 75 years old [4]. This study confirmed that LRC could achieve similar tumour treatment efficacy compared to ORC, with fewer perioperative complications and less blood loss [4]. LRC should be considered as the primary intervention for patients aged over 75 years old with muscle invasive bladder cancer or non-muscle invasive bladder cancer with high risk factors.

Laparoscopic radical cystectomy (LRC) is increasingly being used for muscle-invasive bladder cancer. A prospective randomised controlled clinical trial comparing LRC vs. ORC in patients undergoing radical cystectomy for bladder cancer was conducted [5]. Thirty-five patients were eligible for final analysis in each group. Significant differences were noted in operative time, estimated blood loss (EBL), blood transfusion rate, analgesic requirement, and time to resumption of oral intake. No significant differences were noted in the length of hospital stay, complication rate, lymph node yield (14.1 ± 6.3 for LRC and 15.2 ± 5.9 for ORC), positive surgical margin rate, postoperative pathology, or recurrence rate (7 for LRC and 8 for ORC) [5]. The 5-year recurrence-free survival with laparoscopic vs. ORC was 78.5% vs. 70.9%, respectively (p = 0.773). The overall survival with laparoscopic vs. ORC was 73.8% vs. 67.4%, respectively (p = 0.511). Lin et al. [5] demonstrated that LRC is superior to ORC in perioperative outcomes, including EBL, blood transfusion rate, and analgesic requirement. There were no major difference in oncologic outcomes. The number of patients is too small to allow for a final conclusion.

The role of minimally invasive radical cystectomy as opposed to open surgery for bladder cancer is not yet established. Khan et al. [6] present comparative outcomes of open, laparoscopic and robotic-assisted radical cystectomy. RARC took longer than LRC and ORC. Patients were about 30 times more likely to have a transfusion if they had ORC than if they had RARC (p < 0.0001) and about eight times more likely to have a transfusion if they had LRC compared with RARC (p < 0.006) [6]. Patients were four times more likely to have a transfusion if they had ORC as compared with LRC (p < 0.007). Patients were four times more likely to have complications if they had ORC than RARC (p = 0.006) and about three times more likely to have complications with LRC than with RARC (p = 0.02) [6]. Hospital stay was mean 19 days after ORC, 16 days after LRC and 10 days after RARC.

Despite study limitations, RARC had the lowest transfusion and complication rates and the shortest length of stay, although taking the longest to perform [6].

Radical cystectomy is the standard method for treatment of muscle-invasive and locally advanced bladder cancer. Less invasive approaches such as totally laparoscopic radical cystectomy and robotic cystectomy. However despite significant improvements in surgical techniques the overall occurrence of perioperative complications is still high. Nosov et al., analysed the literature data and compared of this data with respect to perioperative complications after radical cystectomy and oncological outcomes [7]. In most of the studies, operating time during laparoscopic cystectomy was longer than that of open approach. Despite that, there was no influence of type of surgery on intraoperative complications. Major complication rates were similar between all groups. However laparoscopic cystectomy had lower rate of minor complications compared to open cystectomy [7]. Laparoscopic cystectomy is safe and associated with lower blood loss, decreased postoperative ileus and lower length of stay compared with open radical cystectomy. Laparoscopic surgery for bladder cancer decreased minor complications (mainly due to lower bleeding and gastrointestinal complication rate) and had no impact on major complications [7]. Moreover, if performed following the oncologic principles of open surgery, results suggest LRC is safe and determines good cancer control compared with open surgery [7].

Open radical cystectomy (ORC) and urinary diversion in bladder cancer (BCa) are associated with significant perioperative complication risk [8]. Bochner, compared perioperative complications between robot-assisted radical cystectomy (RARC) and ORC techniques.

A prospective randomized controlled trial was conducted during 2010 and 2013 in BCa patients scheduled for definitive treatment by radical cystectomy (RC), pelvic lymph node dissection (PLND), and urinary diversion. Patients were randomized to ORC/PLND or RARC/PLND, both with open urinary diversion [8]. The trial enrolled 124 patients, of whom 118 were randomized and underwent RC/PLND. The rate of complications within 90 days after surgery for the open group versus the robotic group and found no significant difference between the two groups [8].

Musch et al. [9], evaluated early postoperative morbidity in patients undergoing either robot-assisted (RARC) or open radical cystectomy (ORC) for bladder cancer. A total of 100 patients underwent RARC and 42 underwent ORC (between October 2007 and July 2009) as treatment for bladder cancer. Data on the peri-operative course were collected prospectively RARC group and the ORC group [9]. A significant reduction in early postoperative morbidity was associated with the robotic approach. Despite more serious comorbidities and a 30-day longer follow-up in the RARC group, the RARC group experienced fewer postoperative complications than those in the ORC group [9]. Major complications, in particular, were less frequent after RARC.

References

1. Zhao J, Zeng S, Zhang Z, Zhou T, Yang B, Song R, Sun Y, Xu C. Laparoscopic radical cystectomy versus extraperitoneal radical cystectomy: is the extraperitoneal technique rewarding? Clin Genitourin Cancer. 2015;13(4):e271–7.
2. Yasui T, Tozawa K, Ando R, Hamakawa T, Iwatsuki S, Taguchi K, Kobayashi D, Naiki T, Mizuno K, Okada A, Umemoto Y, Kawai N, Sasaki S, Hayashi Y, Kohri K. Laparoscopic versus open radical cystectomy for patients older than 75 years: a single-center comparative analysis. Asian Pac J Cancer Prev. 2015;16(15):6353–8.
3. Kanno T, Matsuda A, Sakamoto H, Nishiyama R, Oida T, Okada T, Akao T, Yamada H. [Treatment outcome of laparoscopic radical cystectomy at a single institution]. Nihon Hinyokika Gakkai Zasshi. 2013;104(5):651–6.

4. Yong C, Daihui C, Bo Z. Laparoscopic versus open radical cystectomy for patients with bladder cancer over 75-year-old: a prospective randomized controlled trial. Oncotarget. 2017;8(16):26565–72.

5. Lin T, Fan X, Zhang C, Xu K, Liu H, Zhang J, Jiang C, Huang H, Han J, Yao Y, et al. A prospective randomised controlled trial of laparoscopic vs open radical cystectomy for bladder cancer: perioperative and oncologic outcomes with 5-year follow-up. Br J Cancer. 2014;110(4):842–9.

6. Khan MS, Challacombe B, Elhage O, Rimington P, Coker B, Murphy D, Grieve A, Dasgupta P. A dual-centre, cohort comparison of open, laparoscopic and robotic-assisted radical cystectomy. Int J Clin Pract. 2012;66(7):656–62.

7. Nosov AK, Reva SA, Dzhalilov IB, Petrov SB. [Laparoscopic and open radical cystectomy for bladder cancer]. Vopr Onkol. 2015;61(3):352–61.

8. Bochner BH, Dalbagni G, Sjoberg DD, Silberstein J, Keren Paz GE, Donat SM, Coleman JA, Mathew S, Vickers A, Schnorr GC, Feuerstein MA, Rapkin B, Parra RO, Herr HW, Laudone VP. Comparing open radical cystectomy and robot-assisted laparoscopic radical cystectomy: a randomized clinical trial. Eur Urol. 2015;67(6):1042–50.

9. Musch M, Janowski M, Steves A, Roggenbuck U, Boergers A, Davoudi Y, Loewen H, Groeben H, Kroepfl D. Comparison of early postoperative morbidity after robot-assisted and open radical cystectomy: results of a prospective observational study. BJU Int. 2014;113(3):458–67.

A Systematic Review on Radical Cystectomy: Laparoscopic vs. Open vs. Robotic

31

31.1 Research Methods

A systematic review relating to muscle invasive bladder cancer and laparoscopic vs. open vs. robotic surgery was conducted. This was to identify the outcomes. The search strategy aimed to identify all references related to bladder cancer AND muscle invasive disease AND bladder preservation. Search terms used were as follows: (Radical cystectomy) AND (Laparoscopic) AND (Open) AND (Robotic). The following databases were screened from 1989 to June 2020:

- CINAHL
- MEDLINE (NHS Evidence)
- Cochrane
- AMed
- EMBASE
- PsychINFO
- SCOPUS
- Web of Science

In addition, searches using Medical Subject Headings (MeSH) and keywords were conducted using Cochrane databases. Two UK-based experts in bladder cancer were consulted to identify any additional studies.

Studies were eligible for inclusion if they reported primary research focusing on muscle invasive bladder cancer and bladder preservation. Papers were included if published after 1984 and had to be in English. Studies that did not conform to this were excluded. Only primary research was included (Fig. 31.1).

Abstracts were independently screened for eligibility by two reviewers and disagreements resolved through discussion or third party opinion. Agreement level was calculated using Cohen's Kappa to test the intercoder reliability of this screening process. Cohens' Kappa allows comparison of inter-rater reliability between papers

© The Editor(s) (if applicable) and The Author(s), under exclusive license to
Springer Nature Switzerland AG 2021
S. S. Goonewardene et al., *Management of Muscle Invasive Bladder Cancer*,
Management of Urology, https://doi.org/10.1007/978-3-030-57915-9_31

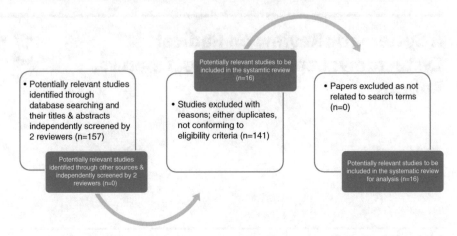

Fig. 31.1   Flow chart of studies identified through the systematic review. (Adapted from PRISMA)

using relative observed agreement. This also takes account of the comparison occurring by chance. The first reviewer agreed all 16 papers to be included, the second, agreed on 16.

Data extraction was piloted by the researcher and amended in consultation with the research team (author and two academic supervisors). Data collected included authors, year and country of publication, study aims, setting, intervention aims, number of participants, study design, intervention components and delivery methods, comparison groups and outcome measures, notes and follow-up questions for the authors. Studies were quality assessed using the PRISMA criteria for randomised controlled trials, Mays et al. [1, 2] for the action research and qualitative studies and the Critical Skills Appraisal programme for cohort studies. This was also applied to randomised controlled trials and qualitative studies.

The search identified 157 papers (Fig. 31.1). One hundred and fifty-seven mapped to the search terms and eligibility criteria. The current systematic reviews were examined to gain further knowledge about the subject. One hundred and forty-one papers were excluded due to not conforming to eligibility criteria or adding to the evidence. Of the 16 papers left, relevant abstracts were identified and the full papers obtained (all of which were in English), to quality assure against search criteria. There was considerable heterogeneity of design among the included studies therefore a narrative review of the evidence was undertaken. There was significant heterogeneity within studies, including clinical topic, numbers, outcomes, as a result a narrative review was thought to be best. There were 14 cohort studies, with a moderate level of evidence and two RCTs with a good level of evidence. These were from a range of countries with minimal loss to follow-up. All participants were identified appropriately.

31.2   Complication Rate Robotic vs. Open Cystectomy

Niegisch assessed the surgical and oncological outcome of robot-assisted radical cystectomy (RARC) compared with open radical cystectomy (ORC) [3]. RARC patients had significantly less blood loss (RARC: 300 [interquartile range: 200–500] ml; perioperative transfusion rate: 0 [IQR: 0–2] red packed blood cells [RPBCs]; ORC: 800 [IQR: 500–1200] ml, p < 0.01; transfusion rate: 3 [IQR: 2–4] RPBCs, p < 0.01), and hospital stay of RARC patients was reduced by 20% (RARC: 13 [IQR: 9–17] days, ORC: 16 [IQR: 13–21] days, p < 0.01) [3]. No differences between patients undergoing RARC or ORC were observed [3].

Although robot-assisted laparoscopic radical cystectomy (RARC) was first reported in 2003 and has gained popularity, comparisons with open radical cystectomy (ORC) are limited to reports from high-volume referral centers [4]. Yu compared population-based perioperative outcomes and costs of ORC and RARC [4]. Yu identified 1444 ORCs and 224 RARCs [4]. Women were less likely to undergo RARC than ORC (9.8% compared with 15.5%, p = 0.048), and 95.7% of RARCs and 73.9% of ORCs were performed at teaching hospitals (p < 0.001) [4]. In adjusted analyses, subjects undergoing RARC compared with ORC experienced fewer inpatient complications (49.1% and 63.8%, p = 0.035) and fewer deaths (0% and 2.5%, p < 0.001) [4]. RARC compared with ORC was associated with lower parenteral nutrition use (6.4% and 13.3%, p = 0.046); however, there was no difference in length of stay [4].

Kader compared perioperative morbidity and oncological outcomes of robot-assisted laparoscopic radical cystectomy (RARC) to open RC (ORC) at a single institution [5]. Patients in both groups had comparable preoperative characteristics. The overall and major complication (Clavien ≥3) rates were lower for RARC patients at 35% vs. 57% (p = 0.001) and 10% vs. 22% (p = 0.019), respectively [5]. There were no significant differences between groups for pathological outcomes, including stage, number of nodes harvested or positive margin rates [5].

Parekh conducted a pilot prospective randomized trial evaluating perioperative outcomes and oncologic efficacy of open vs. robotic assisted laparoscopic radical cystectomy for consecutive patients was performed [6]. There were no significant differences between oncologic outcomes of positive margins (5% each, p = 0.50) or number of lymph nodes removed for open radical cystectomy (23, IQR 15–28) vs. robotic assisted laparoscopic radical cystectomy (11, IQR 8.75–21.5) groups (p = 0.135) [6]. The robotic assisted laparoscopic radical cystectomy group (400 ml, IQR 300–762.5) was noted to have decreased estimated blood loss compared to the open radical cystectomy group (800 ml, IQR 400–1100) and trended toward a decreased rate of excessive length of stay (greater than 5 days) (65% vs. 90%, p = 0.11) compared to the open radical cystectomy group [6]. The robotic group also trended toward fewer transfusions (40% vs. 50%, p = 0.26) [6].

Nix reported results on a prospective randomized trial of open versus robotic-assisted laparoscopic radical cystectomy on perioperative outcomes, complications, and short-term narcotic usage [7]. Significant differences were noted in operating room time, estimated blood loss, time to flatus, time to bowel movement, and use of inpatient morphine sulfate equivalents [7]. There was no significant difference regarding overall complication rate or hospital stay [7]. On surgical pathology, in the robotic group 14 patients had pT2 disease or higher; 3 patients had pT3/T4 disease; and 4 patients had node-positive disease [7]. In the open group, eight patients had pT2 disease or higher; five patients had pT3/T4 disease; and seven patients had node-positive disease [7]. The mean number of LNs removed was 19 in the robotic group versus 18 in the open group [7].

Bochner compared cancer outcomes in BCa patients managed with ORC or robotic-assisted radical cystectomy (RARC) [8]. The trial randomized 118 patients who underwent RC/PLND and urinary diversion [8]. Sixty were randomized to RARC and 58 to ORC [8]. Four RARC-assigned patients refused randomization and received ORC; however, an intention to treat analysis was performed [8]. No differences were observed in recurrence (hazard ratio [HR]: 1.27; 95% confidence interval [CI]: 0.69–2.36; p = 0.4) or cancer-specific survival (p = 0.4) [8]. No difference in overall survival was observed (p = 0.8). However, the pattern of first recurrence demonstrated a nonstatistically significant increase in metastatic sites for those undergoing ORC (sub-HR [sHR]: 2.21; 95% CI: 0.96–5.12; p = 0.064) and a greater number of local/abdominal sites in the RARC-treated patients (sHR: 0.34; 95% CI: 0.12–0.93; p = 0.035) [8].

Tostivint compared ORC and RARC with totally intracorporal (IC) orthotopic neobladder (ONB) reconstruction, in terms of perioperative outcomes, morbidity, functional results and quality of life (Qol) [9]. Operative time was longer in RARC group (median 360 vs. 300 min; p < 0.001) but length of stay was 5 days shorter (median 12 vs. 17 days; p < 0.05) [9]. Patients in RARC group had less blood transfusion (0% vs. 23.6%; p < 0.05), but a higher rate of uretero-ileal anastomosis stenosis and eventration at long term (respectively 25.5% vs. 3.6% and 23% vs. 2%; p < 0.05) [9].

31.3   Laparoscopic vs. Open Radical Cystectomy with Prior Abdominal Surgery

Wei investigated the feasibility, peri-operative and oncologic outcomes of laparoscopic radical cystectomy (LRC) vs. open radical cystectomy in prior abdominal surgery (PAS) [10]. Estimated blood loss (EBL) was higher in patients with PAS undergoing ORC compared to those with no PAS (p = 0.008) [10]. However, there was no significant difference of EBL among patients undergoing LRC with or without PAS (p = 0.896) [10]. Patients with PAS undergoing ORC and ileal conduit had a higher vascular injury rate (p = 0.017) [10]. Comparing patients with PAS performed by LRC and ORC, the number of patients with the vascular injury was higher in ORC groups regardless of the type of diversion (ileal conduit, p = 0.001, cutaneous ureterostomy, p = 0.025) [10].

31.4   Laparoscopic vs. Open Cystectomy Outcomes

Haber evaluated the outcomes of these two techniques with a focus on perioperative outcomes and associated morbidity [11]. Of the 54 patients, 17 underwent a pure laparoscopic (group 1, 8 conduit and 9 neobladder) and 37 underwent an open-assisted laparoscopic (group 2, 18 conduit and 19 neobladder) procedure [11]. No significant differences were noted between the groups in patient age, comorbidities, or pathologic stage of malignancy [11]. Group 2 was superior with regard to operative time, blood loss, transfusion rate, time to oral intake, time to ambulation, and postoperative complications ($p < 0.05$ for all comparisons) [11]. Anastomotic leak, bowel obstruction, or sepsis requiring reexploration developed in 5 patients (29%) in group 1 and 4 patients (11%) in group 2. A "learning curve" was observed for both procedures, but it was particularly steep for the pure laparoscopic technique, and this approach was eventually abandoned [11].

31.5   Robotic Cystectomy vs. Laparoscopic Cystectomy Outcomes

Tesishima evaluated perioperative outcomes in initial experiences of robot-assisted laparoscopic radical cystectomy (RARC) in comparison with those of laparoscopic radical cystectomy (LRC) for muscle-invasive or high-risk non-muscle-invasive bladder cancer [12]. Robot-assisted procedures were completed in all cases without conversion to open surgery [12]. The median time of pneumoperitoneum was 252 min, and the median blood loss was 340 ml [12]. No severe complications were observed. Perioperative outcomes did not significantly differ between RARC and LRC [12]. Although two cases of troubles in uretero-conduit anastomosis sites were observed after LRC, no patients experienced postoperative complication related to urinary diversion after RARC [12].

31.6   Recurrence After Open and Robotic Radical Cystectomy

The median follow-up time for patients without recurrence was 30 months (interquartile range [IQR] 5–72) for ORC and 23 months (IQR 9–48) for RARC ($p = 0.6$) [13]. Within 2 years of surgery, there was no large difference in the number of local recurrences between ORC and RARC patients (15/65 [23%] vs. 24/136 [18%]), and the distribution of local recurrences was similar between the two groups [13]. Similarly, the number of distant recurrences did not differ between the groups (26/73 [36%] vs. 43/147 [29%]). However, there were distinct patterns of distant recurrence [13]. Extrapelvic lymph node locations were more frequent for RARC than ORC (10/43 [23%] vs. 4/26 [15%]) [13]. Furthermore, peritoneal carcinomatosis was found in 9/43 (21%) RARC patients compared to 2/26 (8%) ORC patients [13].

31.7   Robotic vs. Laparoscopic Radical Cystectomy in Elderly Patients

Guillotreau compared the perioperative outcomes of laparoscopic/robotic radical cystectomy (LRRC) for urothelial cancer of bladder (UCB) between elderly ($\geq$70 years) and younger (<70 years) patients [14]. Ileal conduit-type diversion was favored in the older vs. younger group, 84% vs. 36%, respectively [14]. Overall conversion rate to open procedures was 4% in both groups [14]. Perioperative complication rate was not significantly different between the younger and older patients [14]. Positive margin rate was 5% in both groups [14]. The 5-year OS for older and younger patients was 75% and 87%, respectively (p = 0.03), and the 5-year CSS for the two groups was 51% and 54%, respectively (p = 0.7) [14].

31.8   Robotic vs. Laparoscopic High Extended Pelvic Lymph Node Dissection

Desai described the robotic and laparoscopic technique and the short-term outcomes of high extended pelvic LND (PLND) up to the inferior mesenteric artery (IMA) during RC [15]. All 15 procedures were technically successful without need for conversion to open surgery [15]. Median operative time was 6.7 h, estimated blood loss was 500 ml, and three patients (21%) required blood transfusion. Median nodal yield in the entire cohort was 31 (range: 15–78) [15]. The IMA group had more nodes retrieved (median: 42.5) compared with the aortic bifurcation group (median: 20.5) [15]. Histopathology confirmed nodal metastases in four patients (27%), including three patients in the IMA group and one patient in the aortic bifurcation group [15]. Perioperative complications were recorded in six cases (40%) [15]. During a median follow-up of 13 months, no patient developed local or systemic recurrence [15].

31.9   Open vs. Laparoscopic vs. Robotic Cystectomy

Khan present comparative outcomes of open, laparoscopic and robotic-assisted radical cystectomy [16]. RARC took longer than LRC and ORC [16]. Patients were about 30 times more likely to have a transfusion if they had ORC than if they had RARC (p < 0.0001) and about eight times more likely to have a transfusion if they had LRC compared with RARC (p < 0.006) [16]. Patients were four times more likely to have a transfusion if they had ORC as compared with LRC (p < 0.007) [16]. Patients were four times more likely to have complications if they had ORC than RARC (p = 0.006) and about three times more likely to have complications with LRC than with RARC (p = 0.02) [16]. Hospital stay was mean 19 days after ORC, 16 days after LRC and 10 days after RARC [16].

Kim investigated oncological outcomes in patients with muscle-invasive bladder cancer who underwent open radical cystectomy (ORC), laparoscopic radical cystectomy (LRC), or robot-assisted radical cystectomy (RARC) [17]. The median patient age for ORC, LRC, and RARC groups was 68.0 (interquartile range [IQR]: 60.0–73.0), 65.0 (IQR: 62.8–74.0), and 61.5 (IQR: 54.8–72.0) years, respectively (p = 0.017), and the median follow-up duration was 27.9 (IQR: 14.7–47.9), 28.8 (IQR: 15.7–41.8), and 32.0 (IQR: 15.5–45.4) months, respectively (p = 0.955) [17]. There was no significant difference in RFS, CSS, and OS according to the surgical approach (p = 0.253, p = 0.431, and p = 0.527, respectively) [17]. Subgroup analysis revealed that RFS, CSS, and OS were not significantly different in both subgroups with stage ≤pT2 or ≥pT3 [17]. Multivariable Cox regression analyses showed that the surgical approach was not a significant predictor of RFS, CSS, and OS [17].

Matsumoto compared the perioperative outcomes of patients with bladder cancer according to three different procedures: robot-assisted laparoscopic radical cystectomy (RALC), laparoscopic radical cystectomy (LRC), and open radical cystectomy (ORC) [18]. EBL was less for RALC than for other procedures (p = 0.0004). No blood transfusions were performed for RALC, but ORC required significant blood transfusions (p = 0.003) [18]. Operative time, laparoscopic time, intraoperative anesthesia, and postoperative anesthesia did not differ among the groups. High-grade adverse events were only seen for ORC [18].

References

1. Moher D, Liberati A, Tetzlaff J, Altman DG. "Preferred Reporting Items for Systematic Reviews and Meta-Analyses: The Prisma Statement." [In English]. BMJ (Online) 339, no. 7716 (08 Aug 2009):332–36.
2. Mays N, Pope C, Popay J. "Systematically Reviewing Qualitative and Quantitative Evidence to Inform Management and Policy-Making in the Health Field." [In English]. Journal of Health Services Research and Policy 10, no. SUPPL. 1 (July 2005):6–20.
3. Niegisch G, Albers P, Rabenalt R. Perioperative complications and oncological safety of robot-assisted (RARC) vs. open radical cystectomy (ORC). Urol Oncol. 2014;32(7):966–74.
4. Yu HY, Hevelone ND, Lipsitz SR, Kowalczyk KJ, Nguyen PL, Choueiri TK, Kibel AS, Hu JC. Comparative analysis of outcomes and costs following open radical cystectomy versus robot-assisted laparoscopic radical cystectomy: results from the US Nationwide Inpatient Sample. Eur Urol. 2012;61(6):1239–44.
5. Kader AK, Richards KA, Krane LS, Pettus JA, Smith JJ, Hemal AK. Robot-assisted laparoscopic vs open radical cystectomy: comparison of complications and perioperative oncological outcomes in 200 patients. BJU Int. 2013;112(4):E290–4.
6. Parekh DJ, Messer J, Fitzgerald J, Ercole B, Svatek R. Prospective randomized controlled trial of robotic versus open radical cystectomy for bladder cancer: perioperative and pathologic results. J Urol. 2013;189(2):474–9.
7. Nix J, Smith A, Kurpad R, Nielsen ME, Wallen EM, Pruthi RS. Prospective randomized controlled trial of robotic versus open radical cystectomy for bladder cancer: perioperative and pathologic results. Eur Urol. 2010;57(2):196–201.
8. Bochner BH, Dalbagni G, Marzouk KH, Sjoberg DD, Lee J, Donat SM, Coleman JA, Vickers A, Herr HW, Laudone VP. Randomized trial comparing open radical cystectomy and robot-assisted laparoscopic radical cystectomy: oncologic outcomes. Eur Urol. 2018;74(4):465–71.
9. Tostivint V, Roumiguié M, Cabarrou B, Verhoest G, Gas J, Coloby P, Soulié M, Thoulouzan M, Beauval JB. Orthotopic neobladder reconstruction for bladder cancer: robotic-assisted versus open-radical cystectomy for perioperative outcomes, functional results and quality of life. Prog Urol. 2019;29(8–9):440–8.

10. Wei X, Lu J, Siddiqui KM, Li F, Zhuang Q, Yang W, Hu Z, Chen Z, Song X, Wang S, Ye Z. Does previous abdominal surgery adversely affect perioperative and oncologic outcomes of laparoscopic radical cystectomy? World J Surg Oncol. 2018;16(1):10.
11. Haber GP, Campbell SC, Colombo JR Jr, Fergany AF, Aron M, Kaouk J, Gill IS. Perioperative outcomes with laparoscopic radical cystectomy: "pure laparoscopic" and "open-assisted laparoscopic" approaches. Urology. 2007;70(5):910–5.
12. Teishima J, Hieda K, Inoue S, Goto K, Ikeda K, Ohara S, Kobayashi K, Kajiwara M, Matsubara A. Comparison of initial experiences of robot-assisted radical cystectomy with those of laparoscopic for bladder cancer. Innovations (Phila). 2014;9(4):322–6.
13. Nguyen DP, Al Hussein Al Awamlh B, Wu X, O'Malley P, Inoyatov IM, Ayangbesan A, Faltas BM, Christos PJ, Scherr DS. Recurrence patterns after open and robot-assisted radical cystectomy for bladder cancer. Eur Urol. 2015;68(3):399–405.
14. Guillotreau J, Miocinovic R, Gamé X, Forest S, Malavaud B, Kaouk J, Rischmann P, Haber GP. Outcomes of laparoscopic and robotic radical cystectomy in the elderly patients. Urology. 2012;79(3):585–90.
15. Desai MM, Berger AK, Brandina RR, Zehnder P, Simmons M, Aron M, Skinner EC, Gill IS. Robotic and laparoscopic high extended pelvic lymph node dissection during radical cystectomy: technique and outcomes. Eur Urol. 2012;61(2):350–5.
16. Khan MS, Challacombe B, Elhage O, Rimington P, Coker B, Murphy D, Grieve A, Dasgupta P. A dual-centre, cohort comparison of open, laparoscopic and robotic-assisted radical cystectomy. Int J Clin Pract. 2012;66(7):656–62.
17. Kim TH, Sung HH, Jeon HG, Seo SI, Jeon SS, Lee HM, Choi HY, Jeong BC. Oncological outcomes in patients treated with radical cystectomy for bladder cancer: comparison between open, laparoscopic, and robot-assisted approaches. J Endourol. 2016;30(7):783–91.
18. Matsumoto K, Tabata KI, Hirayama T, Shimura S, Nishi M, Ishii D, Fujita T, Iwamura M. Robot-assisted laparoscopic radical cystectomy is a safe and effective procedure for patients with bladder cancer compared to laparoscopic and open surgery: Perioperative outcomes of a single-center experience. Asian J Surg. 2019;42(1):189–96.

Prostate Sparing Cystectomy: A Systematic Review

32

32.1 Research Methods

A systematic review relating to muscle invasive bladder cancer and prostate sparing cystectomy was conducted. This was to identify whether prostate sparing cystectomy has a role in this cohort. The search strategy aimed to identify all references related to bladder cancer AND muscle invasive disease AND radical cystectomy AND prostate sparing. Search terms used were as follows: (Bladder cancer) AND (muscle invasive disease) AND (prostate preservation). The following databases were screened from 1989 to June 2020:

- CINAHL
- MEDLINE (NHS Evidence)
- Cochrane
- AMed
- EMBASE
- PsychINFO
- SCOPUS
- Web of Science

In addition, searches using Medical Subject Headings (MeSH) and keywords were conducted using Cochrane databases. Two UK-based experts in bladder cancer were consulted to identify any additional studies.

Studies were eligible for inclusion if they reported primary research focusing on muscle invasive bladder cancer and prostate preservation. Papers were included if published after 1984 and had to be in English. Studies that did not conform to this were excluded. Only primary research was included (Fig. 32.1).

Abstracts were independently screened for eligibility by two reviewers and disagreements resolved through discussion or third party opinion. Agreement level was calculated using Cohen's Kappa to test the intercoder reliability of this screening

S. S. Goonewardene et al., *Management of Muscle Invasive Bladder Cancer*, Management of Urology, https://doi.org/10.1007/978-3-030-57915-9_32

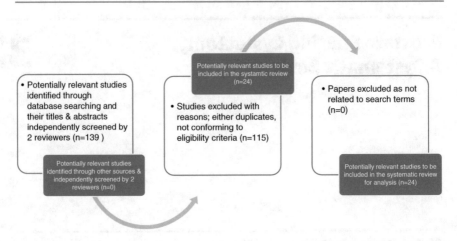

Fig. 32.1 Flow chart of studies identified through the systematic review. (Adapted from PRISMA)

process. Cohens' Kappa allows comparison of inter-rater reliability between papers using relative observed agreement. This also takes account of the comparison occurring by chance. The first reviewer agreed all 24 papers to be included, the second, agreed on 24.

Data extraction was piloted by the researcher and amended in consultation with the research team (author and two academic supervisors). Data collected included authors, year and country of publication, study aims, setting, intervention aims, number of participants, study design, intervention components and delivery methods, comparison groups and outcome measures, notes and follow-up questions for the authors. Studies were quality assessed using the PRISMA criteria for randomised controlled trials, Mays et al. [1, 2] for the action research and qualitative studies and the Critical Skills Appraisal programme for cohort studies. This was also applied to randomised controlled trials and qualitative studies.

The search identified 139 papers (Fig. 32.1). Twenty-four mapped to the search terms and eligibility criteria. The current systematic reviews were examined to gain further knowledge about the subject. One hundred and thirty-nine papers were excluded due to not conforming to eligibility criteria or adding to the evidence. Of the 24 papers left, relevant abstracts were identified and the full papers obtained (all of which were in English), to quality assure against search criteria. There was considerable heterogeneity of design among the included studies therefore a narrative review of the evidence was undertaken. There was significant heterogeneity within studies, including clinical topic, numbers, outcomes, as a result a narrative review was thought to be best. There were 24 cohort studies, with a moderate level of evidence and no RCTS. These were from a range of countries with minimal loss to follow-up. All participants were identified appropriately.

32.2   Systematic Review: Results

32.2.1   A Modification of Technique: Prostate Sparing Cystectomy

Rivas introduced a modified technique of laparoscopic radical cystectomy in which the prostatic capsule is spared in bladder cancer [3]. This study includes 20 patients selected by clinical analysis and imaging criteria operated on using laparoscopic radical cystectomy with prostate capsule sparing [3]. No patient had bladder cancer recurrence [3]. Only one patient died of disease progression, as the pathological findings was a pT3 pN1 Mx [3]. No patients had prostate cancer recurrence [3]. Satisfactory daytime and night-time continence was achieved [3]. Ninety percent of patients have sexual function preserved [3].

Colombo evaluated oncologic and functional outcomes of three different surgical procedures of nerve-sparing radical cystectomy (NS-RC): nerve-sparing cysto-vesicle prostatectomy (NS-CVP), capsule-sparing cystectomy (CS-C) and seminal-sparing cysto-prostatectomy (SS-CP) [4]. Overall, 90 patients underwent NS-RC, 35 (38.9%) of whom received a NS-CVP, while 36 (40%) and 19 (21.1%) underwent capsule CS-C and SS-CP, respectively [4]. No difference was registered comparing oncologic outcomes of the three different techniques; however, two local recurrences after CS-C were attributed to the surgical technique [4]. Complete postoperative daytime and night-time urinary continence (UC) at 24 and 48 months was achieved in 94.4% and 74.4% and in 88.8% and 84.4% of cases, respectively [4]. CS-C showed both the best UC and sexual function preservation rate at early follow-up (24 months) [4]. Overall, a satisfactory post-operative erectile function (IIEF-5 $\geq$22) was proved in 57 (68.6%) and 54 (65.0%) patients at 24 and 48 months, respectively [4]. Significant difference was found when comparing sexual function preservation rate of NS-CVP (28.5%) to that of CS-C (91.6%) and SS-CP (84.2%) [4].

32.2.2   Seminal Sparing Cystectomy

Muto demonstrated the oncologic and functional results of seminal-sparing cystectomy (SSC) in with bladder cancer (BC) and to describe the evolution of our surgical technique over a 20-year period [5]. After a mean follow-up of 102 months, 81 patients (89%) were alive, and 10 patients (11%) had died (8 of disease progression) [5]. Early and late complication rates were 25% and 24%, respectively [5]. Complete daytime continence was obtained in 87 patients (95.6%), and night-time continence was achieved in 34 patients (37%) [5]. In the ICP group, stricture of the prostatic fossa affected 7 patients (11%), whereas no neobladder-urethral anastomosis stricture was noticed in the EIUA group. Normal erectile function was preserved in 87 patients (95.6%) [5].

Botto evaluated the oncological outcome and functional results of prostate-sparing cystectomy (PSC), proposed for treating bladder cancer, used since

1999 in our institution in an attempt to preserve male sexuality and to increase continence after cystectomy [6]. Eight patients were excluded from PSC because they had TCC (seven) or prostate adenocarcinoma (one) [6]. After a mean follow-up of 26 months, seven patients (21%) had a recurrence; one developed a local recurrence, there were widespread metastases in six (18%), and five had histologically confirmed organ-confined tumour (T1-2N0M0) [6]. Rates for daytime and night-time continence were 90% and 85%, and in 29 patients potency was unchanged [6].

Ong reviewed the functional and oncologic outcomes of seminal vesicle and prostate capsule sparing cystectomy combined with ileal orthotopic bladder substitution [7]. At 6 months 25 of the 30 evaluable patients (83%) had daytime continence and 13 of 30 (43%) had nighttime continence [7]. At last followup (median 18 months) 27 of 29 evaluable patients (93%) had daytime continence and 19 of 29 (66%) had nighttime continence [7]. In terms of postoperative potency 15 of 19 evaluable patients (79%) remained potent, 9 with oral medications [7]. There was pelvic recurrence in 1 patient (3%), distant metastases developed in 4 (13%) and 1 (3%) died of metastatic transitional cell carcinoma [7].

32.2.3 Oncological Outcomes of Prostate Sparing Cystectomy

Voskuilen assessed long-term functional and oncologic outcomes of prostate sparing cystectomy (PSC) as a sexuality-preserving alternative to radical surgery [8]. One hundred and eighty-five patients (cTa-3N0M0) with a mean age of 57 years were included [8]. Five-year OS was 71% and 5-year cumulative incidence of recurrence was 31% [8]. Twenty patients (10.8%) had a loco-regional recurrence, two recurrences were in the PU [8]. During follow-up, prostate cancer was detected in six patients (3.2%) [8]. Erectile function was preserved in 86.1% of patients, complete daytime and nighttime continence in 95.6% and 70.2%, respectively [8].

Horenblas reported the initial results of modified cystectomy in males and females meant to preserve all sexual function, called sexuality preserving cystectomy and neobladder [9]. Ten males and 3 females 38 to 71 years old were enrolled in this protocol [9]. Two patients died of widespread metastasis without local recurrence [9]. In 1 case prostate cancer developed 5 years after sexuality preserving cystectomy and neobladder, which was treated with external radiation therapy [9]. Erection was normal in 7 men with antegrade ejaculation in 5 and vaginal lubrication was reported to be normal in all women [9]. Daytime continence was achieved in 9 of the 10 males and 2 of the 3 females, while nighttime continence was achieved in 7 and 2, respectively [9]. One woman and 3 men perform intermittent catheterization because of post-void residual urine after voiding [9]. Postoperatively a vaginal fistula and ureteral stenosis developed in 1 case each [9].

32.2.4   Risk of Prostate/Urothelial Cancer in Prostate Sparing Cystectomy

Weizer evaluated the risk of urothelial and prostate cancer undergoing radical cystoprostatectomy [10]. Fifty-seven percent had cancer involving the prostate at radical cystoprostatectomy [10]. There were 9 patients (26%) with urothelial carcinoma involving the prostate; only prostatic urethral biopsy identified these patients before radical cystoprostatectomy [10]. Prostate adenocarcinoma was evident in 16 of 35 (47%) patients, with a majority involving the prostate peripheral zone/capsule (43%) [10]. There were 4 patients (11%) who had clinically significant prostate cancer (Gleason sum >6 or tumour volume >0.5 cm) [10]. Patients with prostate cancer were significantly older than patients without prostate cancer (p = 0.01) [10].

Nieuwenhuijzen describes the functional outcome on erectile function, continence and voiding, and local and distant cancer recurrence rates in 44 patients after sexuality preserving cystectomy and neobladder (prostate sparing cystectomy) [11]. Thirteen (30%) patients died of cancer [11]. All 13 experienced widespread disease, which was combined with a pelvic recurrence (pelvic recurrence rate 6.9%) in 3 [11]. The 3-year survival according to pathological stage was 86% for pT2N0 or lower, 63% pT3N0 and 39% for node positive tumours (any T/N positive) [11]. Prostate cancer was diagnosed in 1 patient 5 years after treatment, and recurrent carcinoma in situ in the prostatic urethra in a different patient [11].

Komyakov determined the incidence of spreading bladder transitional cell carcinoma and primary adenocarcinoma to the prostate in patients with bladder cancer undergoing radical cystectomy [12]. The spread of transitional cell cancer of the bladder to the prostate occurred in 50 (15.2%) patients [12]. Twelve (3.6%) patients were found to have primary prostate adenocarcinoma. Clinically significant prostate cancer was diagnosed in 4 (33.3%) patients [12].

Ruffion estimated the frequency and characteristics of prostatic lesions discovered incidentally in radical cystoprostatectomy specimens and determine detection factors of prostate cancer preoperatively [13]. The overall incidence of prostate cancer discovered incidentally in radical cystoprostatectomy specimens was 51%, of which 29% were microcancers (volume less than 0.5 cm^3) and 22% were significantly larger (volume 0.5 cm^3 or more) [13]. The mean Gleason score was 6. Of the tumours, 24% could be considered "clinically nonsignificant" (less than 0.5 cm^3 and Gleason score less than 7) [13]. The mean preoperative PSA level was 4.13 ± 1.36 ng/ml. Of 66 patients with a PSA level of less than 4 ng/ml (mean PSA 1.5 ± 0.8) and a normal digital rectal examination before surgery, 50% had prostate cancer, of which 69% were microcancers [13].

Abdelhady reviewed the incidence, histopathological features and clinical outcomes of patients with incidental prostate cancer found in radical cystoprostatectomy (RCP) specimens excised for bladder cancer, to determine if these cancers affected the follow-up strategy and if prostate-sparing cystectomy would be appropriate for these patients [14]. In all, 217 men had RCP for TCC; 13 were excluded from the study due to a preoperative diagnosis or clinical suspicion of prostate cancer, and 58 (28%) were found to have incidental prostate cancer [14]. Of these prostate cancers, 20% were of Gleason score ≥ 7 and two patients developed local and metastatic prostate cancer recurrences [14].

Gakis analysed retrospectively the clinicopathological features of incidental prostate cancer in patients undergoing radical cystoprostatovesiculectomy (RCP) for invasive bladder cancer, as recent studies suggest that prostatic apex-sparing surgery in patients undergoing RCP improves urinary continence and erectile function after surgery, but in those with incidental prostate cancer, leaving the apical region endangers the oncological outcome [15]. Of the 95 patients, 26 had incidental prostate cancer (mean age 68 years, range 53–80) on definitive histological examination [15]. Involvement of the apex was histologically confirmed in seven of the 26 patients (27%), including four with significant prostate cancer (p = 0.039) [15]. Preserving the apex of the prostate to decrease morbidity after RCP carried a 7.3% risk (7 of 95 patients) of leaving significant cancer in the residual prostatic tissue [15].

32.2.5 Functional Outcomes Post Prostate Sparing Cystectomy

Nour assessed the functional results and to evaluate the oncological outcome after PSC, to judge the value of this technique [16]. The final functional results were assessed at 1 year, with daytime continence achieved in 22 patients (95%) and nocturnal leak in four (13%) [16]. At 1 year, 18 patients (83%) reported having erections on sexual stimulation. The median follow-up was 43 months, with an overall incidence of recurrence of 30% and a median time to metastasis of 30 months [16]. At 36 months, the overall survival rate was 81%, with a tumour-free survival rate of 70% [16].

Meinhardt assessed the sexual functions in patients in need of a cystectomy [17]. Storage and voiding strongly resembled the patterns reported in neobladder patients with the anastomosis directly to the urethra [17]. Four of the 24 males needed to perform clean intermittent catheterisation (CIC) [17]. All but one patient had daytime continence [17]. Three patients needed a pad at night [17]. Five patients had erectile dysfunction, of whom two responded well to sildenafil treatment, one had good rigiscan measured nightly erectile function and one had poor erections prior to the operation [17]. Half of the patients had antegrade ejaculation, two patients reported sometimes antegrade and sometimes retrograde ejaculation [17].

Sèbe evaluate cystectomy with preservation of the prostate in the treatment of bladder tumours [18]. The morbidity is not worsened [18]. The functional results were globally improved, especially in terms of erectile function [18]. In terms of cancer control, local recurrences were not more frequent, but metastatic recurrence rates appeared to be higher [18].

Complete daytime and night-time continence was achieved in 95.3% and 74.4%, respectively [11]. Incontinence during day and night could be managed by 1 pad per day/night in 4.7% and 20.9%, respectively, while 4.7% needed more than 1 pad per night [11]. Erectile function could be determined in 40 patients, and potency was maintained in 77.5%, impaired in 12.5% and absent in 10% [11].

Chen compared health-related quality of life and oncological and functional outcomes on erectile function, continence, and voiding function among bladder patients who underwent orthotopic neobladder reconstruction after prostate-sparing cystectomy (PSC) and conventional radical cystoprostatectomy (CRC) [19]. There were better physical and social functioning scales, less fatigue symptoms, better IIEF (16 versus 3.7, $p = 0.01$), and less self-catheterization rate (33% versus 89%, $p = 0.006$) in the PSC group [19]. The oncologic outcomes were the same between two groups [19].

32.2.6 Erectile Function after Prostate Sparing Cystectomy

Davila reviewed the long-term results in patients treated with either total or partial prostate-sparing cystectomy (TPSC or PASC), focusing on erectile function (EF), as en-bloc radical cystectomy (RC) with or without urethrectomy has been the method of choice for managing invasive bladder carcinoma, but has inherent risks of subsequent urinary incontinence and erectile dysfunction, with a marked effect on quality of life, especially in younger patients [20]. The EF domain score was 20 after PASC and 30 after TPSC; mild to moderate ED in the PASC group vs. normal erectile function in the TPSC group [20]. After transurethral resection of the bladder tumours (TURBT) 10 of 14 in the PASC group were T1 or T2a, and in the TPSC group, five of six were T2a and one patient was T2b [20]. From the cystectomy specimen, in the PASC group eight were understaged compared with the TURBT specimen (T2b/T4a vs. T1/T2a), while in the TPSC group there was understaging two (T3a vs. T2a/T2b); this was significantly different (p < 0.05) [20]. There was recurrence of urothelial carcinoma in 1 of 15 and 1 of 6 after PASC and TPSC, respectively [20].

Terrone described the original surgical technique of supra-ampullar cystectomy associated with ileal neobladder [21]. Out of 28 patients 6 died of bladder cancer (all with metastases, 2 also with local recurrence); 4 out of the 22 patients who were free of disease at follow-up died of other causes [21]. Potency was preserved in 26 patients (92.8%), reporting satisfactory sexual intercourses; 15 patients (53.5%) also maintained antegrade ejaculation allowing procreation in 3 cases [21]. In one patient the orthotopic neobladder according to Camey I was converted into an ileal conduit because of the excessive capacity of the reservoir, high post-void residual and recurrent pyelonephritis [21]. Of the remaining 27 patients 16 showed both daytime and nighttime urinary continence (average interval between micturitions = 3 h), 6 were continent during the day and 5 performed self-intermittent catheterization [21].

Salen presented a novel technique of radical cystectomy with preservation of the vas deferens only is described aimed at preservation of sexual function [22]. There was no mortality [22]. All patients were free of the disease (no local or distant recurrence) at the last follow-up [22]. All patients reported adequate sexual function with normal erections and satisfactory intercourse similar to that reported before surgery [22]. Two patients maintained antegrade ejaculation allowing procreation in one case [22].

Thorstenson describes the functional outcome after cystectomy with a prostatic capsule- and seminal-sparing approach [23]. During the follow-up period (mean 72 months, range 33–129) five patients developed metastases and died of bladder cancer [23]. Four men were diagnosed with concomitant prostate cancer [23]. Complete day-time continence was reported in 17/20 (85%) patients [23]. Complete nocturnal continence was seen in 10/20 (50%) men [23]. A total of 20/21 (95%) were sexually active following prostate-sparing cystectomy [23].

32.2.7 Post-operative Complications After Prostate Sparing Cystectomy

Gou reviewed laparoscopic radical cystectomy with preservation of the neurovascular bundles and partial prostate for the treatment of bladder cancer [24]. All patients underwent laparoscopic resection without requiring a traditional open procedure [24]. After removal of the urinary catheter, all patients had a daytime urinary continence; six had a short period of night-time urinary incontinence [24]. Most patients reported a strong desire for sexual activity and were able to complete sexual intercourse without auxiliary measures at 3 months postoperatively [24]. Grade-3 complications developed in 2 patients graded by the classification of Clavien system [24]. One patient was diagnosed with pelvic recurrence 16 months postoperatively [24].

Dall'Oglio reported orthotopic ileal neobladder after radical cystectomy with prostatic adenomectomy with regard to urinary continence, sexual outcome and disease control [25]. Daytime and nighttime urinary continence after 48 h was 47 and 14%, respectively [25]. After 2, 6 and 12 months, these rates were 74% and 16%, 85% and 26%, and 94% and 31%, respectively [25]. Sexual intercourse was achieved in 69% of patients [25]. Overall survival rate was 68%, and cancer-specific survival rate was 73% [25]. Overall survival rates according to pathologic stage for pT0, pT1, pT2 and pT3 were 100%, 60%, 71% and 57%, and cancer-specific survival were 100%, 80%, 71% and 57%, respectively [25].

Akbulut reported with robot-assisted laparoscopic neurovascular bundle (NVB) sparing radical cystoprostatectomy (RALRC), bilateral extended lymph node dissection (BELND) with intracorporeal Studer pouch construction for invasive bladder cancer [26]. Surgical margins were negative in all patients [26]. Postoperative pathologic stages were: pT(0) (n = 2), pT(1) (n = 1), pT(2a) (n = 2), pT(2b) (n = 2), pT(3a) (n = 4), and pT(4a) (n = 1) [26]. Positive LNs and incidental prostate cancer were detected in five and three patients, respectively [26]. Perioperative death rate was zero. Right external iliac vein injury occurred in one patient during the performance of BELND; surgery was converted to an open procedure and the injury was repaired [26]. Colonic fistula developed in one patient at postoperative day 40; the patient died from cardiac disease at day 60 [26]. At a mean follow-up of

7.1 ± 2.3 months, three patients died from metastatic disease [26]. Of the available seven patients, six were fully continent and one had mild daytime incontinence [26].

32.2.8 Grey Literature Relating to Systematic Review

There are a limited number of studies addressing prostate capsule or prostate sparing cystectomy [27]. All are retrospective, non-comparative and not uniform in terms of patient selection and technique [27]. Long-term follow-up is lacking [27]. The incidence of synchronous and or metachronous prostate cancer and TCC of the prostatic urethra is lower than that found in conventional cystoprostatectomy [27]. This is likely due to pre-operative patient selection, restricting the procedure to those with no evidence of prostatic involvement by either disease[27]. The local recurrence rate is 5%, comparable to standard cystoprostatectomy [27]. Recurrence free and overall survival rates are comparable [27].

Hautmann conducted a systematic review [28]. Although a local recurrence rate of 7 of 252 patients is to be expected in this combined series the distant failure rate of 34 of 252 patients is at least twice as high as expected for the given series of superficial or organ-confined TCC [28]. The observed distant failure rate of sexuality-preserving cystectomy in this potentially lethal disease is more than 5% higher as compared with standard radical cystectomy [28]. The precise underlying mechanism of this unexpected pattern of failure following sexuality-sparing cystectomy is not fully understood [28]. Furthermore, surgeons considering procedures that preserve a portion of the prostatic urethra, the prostatic capsule, or the entire prostate should recognize a 6% risk of significant prostatic cancer in any residual tissue, and the potential risk of urethral tumor involvement with TCC [28]. Daytime continence following radical versus sexuality-sparing cystectomy is identical [28]. The continuous intermittent catheterization rate following sexuality-sparing cystectomy, however, seems to be higher than after standard cystectomy [28]. The only advantage sexuality-preserving cystectomy has is indeed preservation of these functions in a much higher percentage than following standard or nerve-sparing cystectomy [28]. This is at the cost of radicality, however, and results in a 10–15% higher oncologic failure rate [28].

References

1. Moher D, Liberati A, Tetzlaff J, Altman DG. "Preferred Reporting Items for Systematic Reviews and Meta-Analyses: The Prisma Statement." [In English]. BMJ (Online) 339, no. 7716 (08 Aug 2009):332–36.
2. Mays N, Pope C, Popay J. "Systematically Reviewing Qualitative and Quantitative Evidence to Inform Management and Policy-Making in the Health Field." [In English]. Journal of Health Services Research and Policy 10, no. SUPPL. 1 (July 2005):6–20.

3. Rivas JG, Gregorio SA, Gómez ÁT, Alvarez-Maestro M, Sebastián JD, Ledo JC. Laparoscopic radical cystectomy with prostate capsule sparing. Initial experience. Cent Eur J Urol. 2016;69(1):25–31.
4. Colombo R, Pellucchi F, Moschini M, Gallina A, Bertini R, Salonia A, Rigatti P, Montorsi F. Fifteen-year single-centre experience with three different surgical procedures of nerve-sparing cystectomy in selected organ-confined bladder cancer patients. World J Urol. 2015;33(10):1389–95.
5. Muto G, Collura D, Rosso R, Giacobbe A, Muto GL, Castelli E. Seminal-sparing cystectomy: technical evolution and results over a 20-year period. Urology. 2014;83(4):856–61.
6. Botto H, Sebe P, Molinie V, Herve JM, Yonneau L, Lebret T. Prostatic capsule- and seminal-sparing cystectomy for bladder carcinoma: initial results for selected patients. BJU Int. 2004;94(7):1021–5.
7. Ong CH, Schmitt M, Thalmann GN, Studer UE. Individualized seminal vesicle sparing cystoprostatectomy combined with ileal orthotopic bladder substitution achieves good functional results. J Urol. 2010;183(4):1337–41.
8. Voskuilen CS, Fransen van de Putte EE, Pérez-Reggeti JI, van Werkhoven E, Mertens LS, van Rhijn BWG, Saad M, Bex A, Cathelineau X, van der Poel HG, Horenblas S, Sanchez-Salas R, Meijer RP. Prostate sparing cystectomy for bladder cancer: a two-center study. Eur J Surg Oncol. 2018;44(9):1446–52.
9. Horenblas S, Meinhardt W, Ijzerman W, Moonen LF. Sexuality preserving cystectomy and neobladder: initial results. J Urol. 2001;166(3):837–40.
10. Weizer AZ, Shah RB, Lee CT, Gilbert SM, Daignault S, Montie JE, Wood DP Jr. Evaluation of the prostate peripheral zone/capsule in patients undergoing radical cystoprostatectomy: defining risk with prostate capsule sparing cystectomy. Urol Oncol. 2007;25(6):460–4.
11. Nieuwenhuijzen JA, Meinhardt W, Horenblas S. Clinical outcomes after sexuality preserving cystectomy and neobladder (prostate sparing cystectomy) in 44 patients. J Urol. 2005;173(4):1314–7.
12. Komyakov BK, Sergeev AV, Fadeev VA, Ismailov KI, Ulyanov AY, Shmelev AY, Onoshko MV. [Concomitant oncopathological changes in the prostate of urinary bladder cancer patients undergoing radical cystoprostateectomy]. Urologiia. 2017;(4):42–45.
13. Ruffion A, Manel A, Massoud W, Decaussin M, Berger N, Paparel P, Morel-Journel N, Lopez JG, Champetier D, Devonec M, Perrin P. Preservation of prostate during radical cystectomy: evaluation of prevalence of prostate cancer associated with bladder cancer. Urology. 2005;65(4):703–7.
14. Abdelhady M, Abusamra A, Pautler SE, Chin JL, Izawa JI. Clinically significant prostate cancer found incidentally in radical cystoprostatectomy specimens. BJU Int. 2007;99(2):326–9. Epub 2006 Oct 9.
15. Gakis G, Schilling D, Bedke J, Sievert KD, Stenzl A. Incidental prostate cancer at radical cystoprostatectomy: implications for apex-sparing surgery. BJU Int. 2010;105(4):468–71.
16. Nour H, Abdelrazak O, Wishahy M, Elkatib S, Botto H. Prostate-sparing cystectomy: potential functional advantages and objective oncological risks; a case series and review. Arab J Urol. 2011;9(2):107–12.
17. Meinhardt W, Horenblas S. Sexuality preserving cystectomy and neobladder (SPCN): functional results of a neobladder anastomosed to the prostate. Eur Urol. 2003;43(6):646–50.
18. Sèbe P, Traxer O, Cussenot O, Haab F, Thibault P, Gattegno B. [Cystectomy with preservation of the prostate in the treatment of bladder tumours: anatomical basis, surgical techniques, indications and results]. Prog Urol. 2003;13(6):1279–1285.
19. Chen PY, Chiang PH. Comparisons of quality of life and functional and oncological outcomes after orthotopic neobladder reconstruction: prostate-sparing cystectomy versus conventional radical cystoprostatectomy. Biomed Res Int. 2017;2017:1983428.
20. Davila HH, Weber T, Burday D, Thurman S, Carrion R, Salup R, Lockhart JL. Total or partial prostate sparing cystectomy for invasive bladder cancer: long-term implications on erectile function. BJU Int. 2007;100(5):1026–9. Epub 2007 Sept 14.

21. Terrone C, Cracco C, Scarpa RM, Rossetti SR. Supra-ampullar cystectomy with preservation of sexual function and ileal orthotopic reservoir for bladder tumor: twenty years of experience. Eur Urol. 2004;46(2):264–9; discussion 269–70.
22. Salem HK. Radical cystectomy with preservation of sexual function and fertility in patients with transitional cell carcinoma of the bladder: new technique. Int J Urol. 2007;14(4):294–8; discussion 299.
23. Thorstenson A, O'Connor RC, Ahonen R, Jonsson MN, Wijkstrom H, Akre O, Hosseini A, Wiklund NP, Henningsohn L. Clinical outcome following prostatic capsule- and seminal-sparing cystectomy for bladder cancer in 25 men. Scand J Urol Nephrol. 2009;43(2):127–32.
24. Gou X, Wang M, He WY, Liu CD, Deng YZ, Ren K, Chen Y. Laparoscopic radical cystectomy for bladder cancer with prostatic and neurovascular sparing: initial experience. Int Urol Nephrol. 2012;44(3):787–92.
25. Dall'Oglio MF, Antunes AA, Crippa A, Nesrallah AJ, Srougi M. Long-term outcomes of radical cystectomy with preservation of prostatic capsule. Int Urol Nephrol. 2010;42(4):951–7.
26. Akbulut Z, Canda AE, Ozcan MF, Atmaca AF, Ozdemir AT, Balbay MD. Robot-assisted laparoscopic nerve-sparing radical cystoprostatectomy with bilateral extended lymph node dissection and intracorporeal studer pouch construction: outcomes of first 12 cases. J Endourol. 2011;25(9):1469–79.
27. Klotz L. Prostate capsule sparing radical cystectomy: oncologic safety and clinical outcome. Ther Adv Urol. 2009;1(1):43–50.
28. Hautmann RE, Stein JP. Neobladder with prostatic capsule and seminal-sparing cystectomy for bladder cancer: a step in the wrong direction. Urol Clin N Am. 2005;32(2):177–85.

A Systematic Review on Nerve Sparing Cystoprostatectomy

33

33.1 Research Methods

A systematic review relating to muscle invasive bladder cancer and nerve sparing cystoprostatectomy was conducted. The search strategy aimed to identify all references related to bladder cancer AND muscle invasive disease AND radical cystectomy AND nerve sparing. Search terms used were as follows: (Bladder cancer) AND (muscle invasive disease) AND (nerve sparing). The following databases were screened from 1989 to June 2020:

- CINAHL
- MEDLINE (NHS Evidence)
- Cochrane
- AMed
- EMBASE
- PsychINFO
- SCOPUS
- Web of Science

In addition, searches using Medical Subject Headings (MeSH) and keywords were conducted using Cochrane databases. Two UK-based experts in bladder cancer were consulted to identify any additional studies.

Studies were eligible for inclusion if they reported primary research focusing on muscle invasive bladder cancer and nerve sparing. Papers were included if published after 1984 and had to be in English. Studies that did not conform to this were excluded. Only primary research was included (Fig. 33.1).

Abstracts were independently screened for eligibility by two reviewers and disagreements resolved through discussion or third party opinion. Agreement level was calculated using Cohen's Kappa to test the intercoder reliability of this screening

S. S. Goonewardene et al., *Management of Muscle Invasive Bladder Cancer*, Management of Urology, https://doi.org/10.1007/978-3-030-57915-9_33

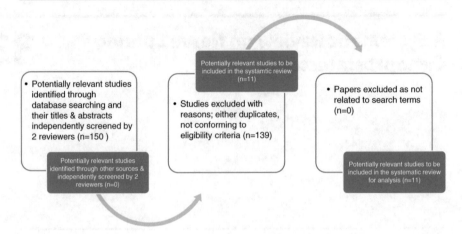

Fig. 33.1   Flow chart of studies identified through the systematic review. (Adapted from PRISMA)

process. Cohens' Kappa allows comparison of inter-rater reliability between papers using relative observed agreement. This also takes account of the comparison occurring by chance. The first reviewer agreed all 11 papers to be included, the second, agreed on 11.

Data extraction was piloted by the researcher and amended in consultation with the research team (author and two academic supervisors). Data collected included authors, year and country of publication, study aims, setting, intervention aims, number of participants, study design, intervention components and delivery methods, comparison groups and outcome measures, notes and follow-up questions for the authors. Studies were quality assessed using the PRISMA criteria for randomised controlled trials, Mays et al. [1, 2] for the action research and qualitative studies and the Critical Skills Appraisal programme for cohort studies. This was also applied to randomised controlled trials and qualitative studies.

The search identified 139 papers (Fig. 33.1). Eleven of 139 mapped to the search terms and eligibility criteria. The current systematic reviews were examined to gain further knowledge about the subject. One hundred and thirty-nine papers were excluded due to not conforming to eligibility criteria or adding to the evidence. Of the 11 papers left, relevant abstracts were identified and the full papers obtained (all of which were in English), to quality assure against search criteria. There was considerable heterogeneity of design among the included studies therefore a narrative review of the evidence was undertaken. There was significant heterogeneity within studies, including clinical topic, numbers, outcomes, as a result a narrative review was thought to be best. There were 9 cohort studies, with a moderate level of evidence and two trials with a good level of evidence. These were from a range of countries with minimal loss to follow-up. All participants were identified appropriately.

33.2 Outcomes of Nerve-Sparing in Radical Cystectomy

Saad evaluated oncological and functional outcomes of nerve sparing cystoprosta-tectomy (NSCP) [3]. The 5-year cancer-specific survival was 90% for the PCSC group and 78% for the NSCP group (p = 0.055) [3]. Thirteen percent and 21% patients had Clavien ≥III complications in the PCSC and NSCP groups, respec-tively (p = 0.2) [3]. At 3 months after surgery, 54 (90%) and 24 (51%) patients reported full recovery of daytime urinary continence in the PCSC and NSCP groups, respectively (p < 0.001); and for erectile function recovery, 32 (53%) and four (9%) patients in the PCSC group and in the NSCP group were respectively potent without any treatment (p < 0.001) [3].

Schoenberg reviewed this technique to ascertain survival and local recurrence rates [4]. The disease-specific 10-year survival rate for all stages of bladder cancer treated was 69% and the 10-year survival rate free of local recurrence was 94% [4]. Recovery of sexual function following nerve sparing cystectomy correlated with patient age: 62% in men 40–49 years old, 47% in men 50–59 years old, 43% in men 60–69 years old and 20% in men 70–79 years old [4].

Brendler examined 76 men underwent nerve-sparing radical cystoprostatectomy [5]. Of the 76 patients 2 (2.6%) had positive surgical margins (dome of the bladder and left ureter) and neither had positive margins at the site of nerve-sparing modifi-cations [5]. Of 3 patients (3.9%) who had local recurrence none had positive surgi-cal margins [5]. The 5-year actuarial local recurrence rate is 7.5%. Thirteen of 76 patients (17%) died of transitional cell carcinoma and 7 (9%) died of other causes, while 53 (70%) are alive without evidence of disease [5]. The 5-year actuarial sur-vival rates are 64% over-all, 68% without disease and 78% disease-specific [5].

33.3 Post-operative Complications in Nerve Sparing Prostatectomy

Nyame described outcomes of robotic-assisted nerve-sparing cystoprostatectomy with prostatic apex preservation and orthotopic ileal conduit urinary diversion in young men undergoing robotic-assisted radical cystectomy (RARC) for the man-agement of urothelial carcinoma [6]. Two patients experienced grade II complica-tions postoperatively [6]. Pathologic assessment demonstrated negative surgical margins in all 3 cases [6]. With mean follow-up time of 28.2 months, 2 out of 3 patients are free from disease recurrence [6]. All patients report daytime urinary continence with no pad usage and potency without the need for phosphodiesterase-5 inhibitors [6].

Menon developed a technique of nerve-sparing robot-assisted radical cystopros-tatectomy (RRCP) in muscle invasive bladder cancer [7]. RRCP was carried out in 14 men and three women by the primary surgeon (M.M.) [7]. The form of urinary reconstruction was ileal conduit in three, a W-pouch with a serosal-lined tunnel in 10, a double-chimney or a T-pouch with a serosal-lined tunnel in two each [7]. The mean blood loss was <150 ml [7]. The number of lymph nodes removed was 4–27, with one patient having N1 disease. The margins of resection were free of tumour in all patients [7].

33.4 Radical Cystectomy and Nerve Sparing in Women

Bhatta Dhar describes a surgical technique of cystectomy and orthotopic urinary diversion in female patients [8]. An improved understanding of the anatomic neurovascular and fascial planes related to the rhabdosphincter has identified elements needed for orthotopic diversion in female patients [8]. The technique of en bloc anterior exenteration includes the anterior portion of the vagina; however, preservation of the rhabdosphincter and its autonomic nerve supply necessitates specific modifications of the standard operation [8].

Stenzl developed refinements for cystectomy and subsequent intestine to urethra anastomosis to improve outcomes in women with anterior exenteration and orthotopic neobladder to the urethra [9]. Optimal postoperative results may be obtained by preserving the entire lateral vaginal walls, performing nerve sparing dissection of the bladder neck and proximal urethra, removing 1 cm [9]. Proximal urethra en bloc with the cystectomy specimen and using additional attachments of the anastomosed intestinal pouch to surrounding pelvic structures [9]. Patients achieved day and night continence after 6 months, mean pouch volume was 580 cc (range 450–750) and residual volumes ranged from 0 to 150 cc. No tumour recurred after 6–17 months [9].

33.5 Nerve Sparing in Either Gender

Lane reported the technique and early outcomes of nerve-sparing laparoscopic radical cystectomy with continent orthotopic ileal neobladder in selected male and female patients with bladder cancer [10]. No patient required blood transfusion, and one had a postoperative complication [10]. All patients were free of recurrence at a median follow-up of 30 months [10]. At 12 months, nocturnal and daytime continence was preserved in 100% and 75% of patients, respectively [10]. Sexual function was preserved in the female patient and 2 of the 4 male patients [10].

33.6 Nerve Sparing Radical Cystectomy and Impact on Continence

Furrer analysed urinary continence after radical cystectomy (RC) and orthotopic bladder substitution (OBS) with attempted nerve-sparing (NS) status [11]. Of 180 patients, attempted NS status was 0 in 24 (13%), unilateral in 100 (56%), and bilateral in 56 (31%) [11]. One hundred and sixty (89%) patients were continent during daytime and 124 (69%) during night-time [11]. In multivariable analysis, any degree of attempted NS was significantly associated with daytime continence (odds ratio [OR] 2.08, 95% confidence interval [CI] 1.05–4.11; p = 0.04) [11]. Correspondingly, any attempted NS was significantly associated with night-time continence (OR 2.51, 95% CI 1.08–5.85; p = 0.03) [11]. Recovery of erectile function at 5 years was also significantly associated with attempted NS (p < 0.001) [11].

Kessler assessed factors influencing urinary continence and erectile function after radical cystoprostatectomy and ileal orthotopic bladder substitution [12]. In univariate analysis, attempted nerve sparing and age younger than 65 years were significantly associated with better daytime (p = 0.002 and p = 0.007, respectively) and night-time continence (p = 0.036 and p = 0.005, respectively) [12]. In multivariate analysis the rate of daytime continence was significantly higher in patients with attempted nerve sparing (hazards ratio [HR] 1.4, 95% confidence interval [CI] 1.05–1.87) and night-time continence was significantly better in patients younger than 65 years (HR 1.39, 95% CI 1.07–1.8) [12]. Daytime continence was significantly better (p < 0.0001) and achieved more quickly than night-time continence (p < 0.0001) [12]. The time to daytime continence was shorter with attempted nerve sparing (p = 0.012) [12]. In multivariate analysis erectile function recovered significantly more often with attempted nerve sparing (HR 2.59, 95% CI 1.24–5.39) and in those younger than 65 years (HR 2.98, 95% CI 1.83–4.85) [12].

33.7   Nerve Sparing Cystectomy and Impact on Orthotopic Neobladder

Asgari compared the erectile function after radical cystoprostatectomy (RCP) in either an ileal conduit urinary diversion or orthotropic ileal neobladder substitution [13]. Postoperatively the EF and SD domains deteriorated significantly in both groups, but in a small proportion submitted to ileal neobladder they gradually improved with time (p = 0.006) [13]. At 12-month postoperative period, 4 (9.8%) and 14 (35.0%) patients in ileal conduit and ileal neobladder groups were able to achieve erections hard enough for vaginal penetration and maintained their erection to completion of intercourse, respectively (p = 0.006) [13]. Among patients in the ileal conduit and ileal neobladder groups, additional 4 (9.8%) and 7 (17.1%) patients were able to get some erection, but were unable to maintain their erection to completion of intercourse (p = 0.02) [13]. At 12-month follow up period 24.4% of the ileal conduit and 45.0% of the ileal neobladder patients rated their sexual desire very high or high (p = 0.01) [13].

33.8   Prostate Sparing vs. Nerve Sparing Cystectomy

Prostate capsule sparing and nerve sparing cystectomies are alternative procedures for bladder cancer with decreased morbidity while achieving cancer control [14]. Urinary function at 12 months decreased by 13 and 28 points in the prostate capsule and nerve sparing groups, respectively (p = 0.10) [14]. Sexual function followed a similar pattern (p = 0.06) [14]. There was no difference in recurrence-free, metasta-sis-free or overall survival (each p > 0.05). The rate of incidentally detected prostate cancer was similar (p = 0.15) [14].

33.9   Outcomes in Nerve Sparing Cystectomy

Asimakopoulos describes nerve and seminal vesicle sparing robot-assisted radical cystectomy with an orthotopic neobladder with outcomes [15]. A global rate of 30% early and 32.5% late complications was observed [15]. However, the grade III or higher complication rate was low in both settings at 2.5% and 5%, respectively [15]. There was 1 cancer related death 23 months after surgery [15]. Of the 40 patients 30 (75%) gained daytime continence (0 pad) within 1 month postoperatively [15]. The 12-month nocturnal continence rate was 72.5% (29 of 40 patients). Mean preopera-tive IIEF-6 (International Index of Erectile Function-6) score was 24.4 [15]. Erectile function returned to normal, defined as an IIEF-6 score greater than 17, in 31 of 40 patients (77.5%) within 3 months while 29 of 40 patients (72.5%) returned to the preoperative IIEF-6 score within 12 months [15].

Miyao examined recovery of sexual function (erectile function and frequency of sexual intercourse) over time after cystoprostatectomy [16]. Forty-nine consecutive patients with clinically localized prostate cancer and muscle-invasive bladder can-cer were treated [16]. The recovery rates of erectile function were 49% at 3 years and 79% at 5 years [16]. For recovery of sexual intercourse the rates were 36% at 3 years and 57% at 5 years [16]. Multivariate analysis revealed that the preoperative NPT value was the only independent factor which significantly affected the recov-ery of erectile function [16].

33.10   Penile Rehabilitation in Cystoprostatectomy

Mosbah compared early vs. late penile rehabilitation in patients with nerve-sparing (NS) radical cystoprostatectomy based on a prospective randomized trial [17]. At final evaluation, a significant improvement was found in the EF, the intercourse satisfaction and overall satisfaction domains (p = 0.02, 0.03, and 0.02, respectively) in group I compared with group II [17]. Regarding PDU findings, significant improvement in end-diastolic velocity was elicited in the early rehabilitation group compared with the pre-treatment value (p = 0.03) with no significant difference between both groups [17].

Haberman evaluated the effects on the potency of a bilateral cavernosal nerve-sparing approach to robot-assisted radical cystectomy (RARC) in a preoperatively potent population [18]. Postoperatively, 13 (45%) patients had documented erec-tions sufficient for penetration with or without the use of phosphodiesterase 5 inhibitors [18]. Additional 6 (21%) were potent with intracavernosal injections (ICI), and the remaining 10 (34%) failed ICI usage, had on-going medical issues, or lost interest in sexual activity [18]. With univariate analysis, no significant difference was found between those who recovered erections and those who did not on a wide range of demographic, operative, and perioperative factors, including age, comorbidities, operative time, or pathologic stage [18]. Despite neurovascular bundle preservation, there was no local cancer recurrence and no positive soft tissue margins [18].

33.11 High Risk Bladder Cancer and Nerve Sparing Radical Cystectomy

Puppo reported the oncological and functional results of potency sparing cystectomy with intrafascial prostatectomy for high risk, superficial bladder cancer [19]. One patient died of disease progression and 1 died of an unrelated cause [19]. Of the 37 patients 35 (95%) were free of tumour [19]. Daily continence was achieved in 36 patients (97.2%) and night-time continence was achieved in 35 (95%) [19]. Two patients (5%) needed clean intermittent catheterization [19]. A total of 35 patients (95%) stated that they maintained erectile function, including 28 (76%) without oral drugs [19]. A significant decrease in the median International Index of Erectile Function score from baseline was noted 2 years after surgery (25 vs. 21) [19]. A total of 32 patients (86%) had an International Index of Erectile Function score of greater than 17 at 2 years after cystectomy [19].

References

1. Moher D, Liberati A, Tetzlaff J, Altman DG. "Preferred Reporting Items for Systematic Reviews and Meta-Analyses: The Prisma Statement." [In English]. BMJ (Online) 339, no. 7716 (08 Aug 2009):332–36.
2. Mays N, Pope C, Popay J. "Systematically Reviewing Qualitative and Quantitative Evidence to Inform Management and Policy-Making in the Health Field." [In English]. Journal of Health Services Research and Policy 10, no. SUPPL. 1 (July 2005):6–20.
3. Saad M, Moschini M, Stabile A, Macek P, Lanz C, Prapotnich D, Rozet F, Cathala N, Mombet A, Sanchez-Salas R, Cathelineau X. Long-term functional and oncological outcomes of nerve-sparing and prostate capsule-sparing cystectomy: a single-centre experience. BJU Int. 2020;125:253–9.
4. Schoenberg MP, Walsh PC, Breazeale DR, Marshall FF, Mostwin JL, Brendler CB. Local recurrence and survival following nerve sparing radical cystoprostatectomy for bladder cancer: 10-year followup. J Urol. 1996;155(2):490–4.
5. Brendler CB, Steinberg GD, Marshall FF, Mostwin JL, Walsh PC. Local recurrence and survival following nerve-sparing radical cystoprostatectomy. J Urol. 1990;144(5):1137–40; discussion 1140–1.
6. Nyame YA, Zargar H, Ramirez D, Ganesan V, Babbar P, Villers A, Haber GP. Robotic-assisted laparoscopic bilateral nerve sparing and apex preserving cystoprostatectomy in young men with bladder cancer. Urology. 2016;94:259–64.
7. Menon M, Hemal AK, Tewari A, Shrivastava A, Shoma AM, El-Tabey NA, Shaaban A, Abol-Enein H, Ghoneim MA. Nerve-sparing robot-assisted radical cystoprostatectomy and urinary diversion. BJU Int. 2003;92(3):232–6.

8. Bhatta Dhar N, Kessler TM, Mills RD, Burkhard F, Studer UE. Nerve-sparing radical cystectomy and orthotopic bladder replacement in female patients. Eur Urol. 2007;52(4):1006–14. Epub 2007 Mar 5.
9. Stenzl A, Colleselli K, Poisel S, Feichtinger H, Pontasch H, Bartsch G. Rationale and technique of nerve sparing radical cystectomy before an orthotopic neobladder procedure in women. J Urol. 1995;154(6):2044–9.
10. Lane BR, Finelli A, Moinzadeh A, Sharp DS, Ukimura O, Kaouk JH, Gill IS. Nerve-sparing laparoscopic radical cystectomy: technique and initial outcomes. Urology. 2006;68(4):778–83.
11. Furrer MA, Studer UE, Gross T, Burkhard FC, Thalmann GN, Nguyen DP. Nerve-sparing radical cystectomy has a beneficial impact on urinary continence after orthotopic bladder substitution, which becomes even more apparent over time. BJU Int. 2018;121(6):935–44.
12. Kessler TM, Burkhard FC, Perimenis P, Danuser H, Thalmann GN, Hochreiter WW, Studer UE. Attempted nerve sparing surgery and age have a significant effect on urinary continence and erectile function after radical cystoprostatectomy and ileal orthotopic bladder substitution. J Urol. 2004;172(4 Pt 1):1323–7.
13. Asgari MA, Safarinejad MR, Shakhssalim N, Soleimani M, Shahabi A, Amini E. Sexual function after non-nerve-sparing radical cystoprostatectomy: a comparison between ileal conduit urinary diversion and orthotopic ileal neobladder substitution. Int Braz J Urol. 2013;39(4):474–83.
14. Jacobs BL, Daignault S, Lee CT, Hafez KS, Montgomery JS, Montie JE, Humrich JE, Hollenbeck BK, Wood DP Jr, Weizer AZ. Prostate capsule sparing versus nerve sparing radical cystectomy for bladder cancer: results of a randomized, controlled trial. J Urol. 2015;193(1):64–70.
15. Asimakopoulos AD, Campagna A, Gakis G, Corona Montes VE, Piechaud T, Hoepffner JL, Mugnier C, Gaston R. Nerve sparing, robot-assisted radical cystectomy with intracorporeal bladder substitution in the male. J Urol. 2016;196(5):1549–57.
16. Miyao N, Adachi H, Sato Y, Horita H, Takahashi A, Masumori N, Kitamura H, Tsukamoto T. Recovery of sexual function after nerve-sparing radical prostatectomy or cystectomy. Int J Urol. 2001;8(4):158–64.
17. Mosbah A, El Bahnasawy M, Osman Y, Hekal IA, Abou-Beih E, Shaaban A. Early versus late rehabilitation of erectile function after nerve-sparing radical cystoprostatectomy: a prospective randomized study. J Sex Med. 2011;8(7):2106–11.
18. Haberman K, Wittig K, Yuh B, Ruel N, Lau C, Wilson TG, Chan KG. The effect of nerve-sparing robot-assisted radical cystoprostatectomy on erectile function in a preoperatively potent population. J Endourol. 2014;28(11):1352–6.
19. Puppo P, Introini C, Bertolotto F, Naselli A. Potency preserving cystectomy with intrafascial prostatectomy for high risk superficial bladder cancer. J Urol. 2008;179(5):1727–32; discussion 1732.

Robotic Radical Cystectomy and Lymph Node Dissection: What Are the New Ways Forward?

34

Robotic radical cystectomy has developed significantly over the past 10 years, from extracorporeal stoma formation to intracorporeal stoma formation. However, the next question arises, as to how can advance lymph node dissections.

With the increasing use of laparoscopic and robotic radical cystectomy (RARC), there are perceived concerns about the adequacy of lymph node dissection (LND) [1]. High extended LND during laparoscopic or robotic RARC is technically feasible [2]. RARC with intra corporeal urinary diversion is feasible with acceptable oncological outcome and excellent lymph node count provided an extended LND is performed [3].

It has been demonstrated that a correct lymphadenectomy in radical surgery of bladder leads to an increase in disease specific survival; removing more lymph nodes prolongs survival [4]. Robotic surgery allows a correct dissection of all the tissue around the pelvic vessels and adequate dissection around vessels [5]. Extended lymph node dissection using the robotic platform has demonstrated comparable lymph node yield compared to the open approach, with no added morbidity [6]. Robot-assisted laparoscopic surgery is a safe and effective procedure with acceptable morbidity and good oncologic results from the viewpoint of LND, especially LND [5]. The robot-assisted LND is easily reproducible and simple to perform, achieving a good lymph node yield with low complication rate [7]. Findings from the prior year suggest that—in high-volume centres—lymph node dissection for urologic cancers is equivalent between open and minimally invasive techniques in lymph node yield and short-term to medium-term oncologic results.

Adequate lymphadenectomy in the setting of radical cystectomy has been proven to be an independent predictor for disease-free survival in patients with muscle-invasive bladder cancer [8]. Robot-assisted radical cystectomy has evolved to become an accepted alternative to the standard open technique [8]. A robotic approach facilitates the mobilization of the iliac vessels and lymphatic package away from the pelvic wall, through an avascular plane that gives access to the obturator nerve and the endopelvic lymphnodes without encountering the branches of

S. S. Goonewardene et al., *Management of Muscle Invasive Bladder Cancer*, Management of Urology, https://doi.org/10.1007/978-3-030-57915-9_34

the internal iliac vessels [8]. LND and cystectomy can achieve acceptable oncologic results. The S model gives the surgeon greater access to the higher lymph node zones [9].

However to advance lymph node dissection in conjunction with robotic surgery, it is important to examine other cancers [10]. Preoperative lymphoscintigraphy is used to map the lymphatic drainage patterns and sentinel lymph nodes in patients with head and neck malignancy. It is often challenging to localise the lymph node sites accurately on planar imaging and hybrid SPECT/CT imaging improves accurate localization by reliably showing sentinel nodes relative to important anatomical structures [10]. During surgery, a portable Gamma camera, with adapted counter, can be used in place of a scintilation counter for intraoperative sentinel node localization by mapping on to presurgical SPECT/CT images [10]. This would be one method that would allow the surgeon to correctly identify cancer carrying nodes, as opposed to conducting an extended LND dissection [11]. This method of sentinel node biopsy has been examined in breast cancer and been found to avoid unnecessary clearance.

Non-sentinel nodes (non-SNs) are often taken during the Sentinel Node (SN) procedure. The total number of lymph nodes taken can vary and on occasions many are harvested which may cause morbidity. Taking non-SNs was of clinical significance in five cases where the SN was negative and the non-SN was positive. However, this involved taking and examining non-SNs which is expensive, time consuming and could lead to increase morbidity.

The most recent development, especially with the Da Vinci Xi, is the novel use of near-infrared fluorescence (NIRF) imaging without contrast agents, like indocyanine green, to identify areas of interest during robot-assisted laparoscopic surgery. This technique enabled more precise identification of important areas and successful completion of robotic surgery. If this technique is taken forward, it could potentially be used to identify areas of interest within the pelvis when conducting a cystectomy.

In conclusion, surgical skills and technique are still key to reducing morbidity from lymph node dissection. However, other developments in the field such as sentinel node biopsy and use of indocyannine green can take this further forward.

References

1. Desai MM, Berger AK, Brandina RR, Zehnder P, Simmons M, Aron M, et al. Robotic and laparoscopic high extended pelvic lymph node dissection during radical cystectomy: technique and outcomes. Eur Urol. 2012;61(2):350–5.
2. Desai MM, de Abreu AL, Goh AC, Fairey A, Berger A, Leslie S, et al. Robotic intracorporeal urinary diversion: technical details to improve time efficiency. J Endourol. 2014;28(11):1320–7.
3. Jonsson MN, Schumacher MC, Hosseini A, Adding C, Nilsson A, Carlsson S, et al. Oncological outcome after robot-assisted radical cystectomy with intracorporeal urinary diversion technique. Eur Urol Suppl. 2011;10(2):273–4.

4. Palou J, Breda A, Gausa L, Gaya JM, Rodriguez-Faba O, Villavicencio HM. Lymphadenectomy at the time of robotassisted radical cystectomy: procedure and performance. J Endourol. 2010;24:A357.

5. Volpe A, Ploumidis A, Gan M, De Naeyer G, Ficarra V, Mottrie A. Robot-assisted pelvic lymph node dissection during radical cystectomy. The OLV Vattikuti Robotic Surgery Institute technique. Eur Urol Suppl. 2014;13(1):eV72.

6. Seung CK, Sung GK, Choi H, Young HK, Jeong GL, Je JK, et al. The feasibility of robot-assisted laparoscopic radical cystectomy with pelvic lymphadenectomy: from the viewpoint of extended pelvic lymphadenectomy. Korean J Urol. 2009;50(9):870–8.

7. Prasad SM, Shalhav AL. Comparative effectiveness of minimally invasive versus open lymphadenectomy in urological cancers. Curr Opin Urol. 2013;23(1):57–64.

8. Mansour AM, Abol-Enein H, Manoharan M. Exploring the marcille triangle during robot-assisted pelvic lymphadenectomy for bladder cancer: replicating the open surgical technique. J Endourol. 2013;27:A308–A9.

9. Davis JW, Dasgupta P. A case-mix-adjusted comparison of early oncological outcomes of open and robotic prostatectomy performed by experienced high volume surgeons. BJU Int. 2013;111(2):184–5.

10. Connelly J, Gnanasegaran G, Schilling C, McGurk M. 99mTc-Nanocolloid SPECT/CT and a portable gamma camera for image-guided sentinel node biopsy in head and neck malignancy: science & practice. Nucl Med Commun. 2013;34(4):386.

11. French R, Kurup V. Targetted axillary node sampling—is there a role in the era of sentinel node biopsy? Eur J Surg Oncol. 2012;38(5):426.

A Systematic Review on RARC and LND

35.1 Research Methods

A systematic review relating to muscle invasive bladder cancer, robotic cystectomy and lymphadenectomy was conducted. The search strategy aimed to identify all references related to bladder cancer AND muscle invasive disease AND Robotic Surgery AND Lymphadenectomy. Search terms used were as follows: (Bladder cancer) AND (muscle invasive disease) AND (Robotic Surgery) AND (Lymphadenectomy). The following databases were screened from 1989 to June 2020:

- CINAHL
- MEDLINE (NHS Evidence)
- Cochrane
- AMed
- EMBASE
- PsychINFO
- SCOPUS
- Web of Science

In addition, searches using Medical Subject Headings (MeSH) and keywords were conducted using Cochrane databases. Two UK-based experts in bladder cancer were consulted to identify any additional studies.

Studies were eligible for inclusion if they reported primary research focusing on muscle invasive bladder cancer and nerve sparing. Papers were included if published after 1984 and had to be in English. Studies that did not conform to this were excluded. Only primary research was included (Fig. 35.1).

Abstracts were independently screened for eligibility by two reviewers and disagreements resolved through discussion or third party opinion. Agreement level was calculated using Cohen's Kappa to test the intercoder reliability of this screening

© The Editor(s) (if applicable) and The Author(s), under exclusive license to
Springer Nature Switzerland AG 2021
S. S. Goonewardene et al., *Management of Muscle Invasive Bladder Cancer*,
Management of Urology, https://doi.org/10.1007/978-3-030-57915-9_35

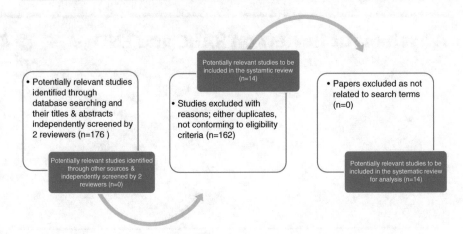

Fig. 35.1 Flow chart of studies identified through the systematic review. (Adapted from PRISMA)

process. Cohens' Kappa allows comparison of inter-rater reliability between papers using relative observed agreement. This also takes account of the comparison occurring by chance. The first reviewer agreed all 14 papers to be included, the second, agreed on 14.

Data extraction was piloted by the researcher and amended in consultation with the research team (author and two academic supervisors). Data collected included authors, year and country of publication, study aims, setting, intervention aims, number of participants, study design, intervention components and delivery methods, comparison groups and outcome measures, notes and follow-up questions for the authors. Studies were quality assessed using the PRISMA criteria for randomised controlled trials, Mays et al. [1, 2] for the action research and qualitative studies and the Critical Skills Appraisal programme for cohort studies. This was also applied to randomised controlled trials and qualitative studies.

The search identified 176 papers (Fig. 35.1). Fourteen mapped to the search terms and eligibility criteria. The current systematic reviews were examined to gain further knowledge about the subject. One hundred and sixty-two papers were excluded due to not conforming to eligibility criteria or adding to the evidence. Of the 14 papers left, relevant abstracts were identified and the full papers obtained (all of which were in English), to quality assure against search criteria. There was considerable heterogeneity of design among the included studies therefore a narrative review of the evidence was undertaken. There was significant heterogeneity within studies, including clinical topic, numbers, outcomes, as a result a narrative review was thought to be best. There were 12 cohort studies, with a moderate level of evidence and 2 controlled trials with a good level of evidence. These were from a range of countries with minimal loss to follow-up. All participants were identified appropriately.

35.2 Robotic RARC and LND

Kang reported short-term retrospective perioperative and pathologic outcomes of the first robot-assisted radical cystectomy (RARC) series in Korea [3]. Among the 104 patients, 60 had an ileal conduit and 44 had an orthotopic neobladder [3]. The mean total operative time was 554 min, and the mean blood loss was 526 ml [3]. The time to flatus and bowel movement was about 3 days, and the time until hospital discharge was about 18 days [3]. The mean number of lymph nodes removed were 18, and 10 patients had node metastatic disease on final pathologic evaluation [3]. Postoperative complications occurred in 28 (26.9%) patients [3].

35.3 Post-operative Complications from LND

Guru reported on 20 consecutive patients underwent robot-assisted radical cystectomy, pelvic lymph node dissection, and open urinary diversion for operable bladder cancer from October 2005 to June 2006 [4]. The mean operative time was 197 min for robot-assisted radical cystectomy, 44 min for pelvic lymph node dissection, and 133 min for urinary diversion [4]. The mean blood loss was 555 ml [4]. One case was converted to an open procedure because of the patient's inability to tolerate the Trendelenburg position [4]. Two patients had major complications [4]. One patient had positive vaginal margins and 9 of 26 nodes were positive [4]. Four patients had incidental prostate cancer [4].

Kasraeian reviewed robot-assisted laparoscopic cystoprostatectomy (RALCP) with extended pelvic lymphadenectomy (epLAD) and intracorporeal enterourethral anastomosis (IEUA) [5]. Median total operative time was 270 min (range 210–330): 60 min, bilateral epLAD; 90 min, RALCP; 60 min, open enterocystoplasty; 60 min (range 45–90), IEUA. Median blood loss was 400 ml (range 200–900 ml) [5]. All surgical margins were negative [5]. Median number of lymph nodes removed was 11 (range 4–21) [5]. Postoperative complications were noted in three patients and included urinoma (n = 1), pyelonephritis (n = 1), and hematoma (n = 1) [5].

Pruthi reviewed robotic-assisted laparoscopic pelvic lymphadenectomy in cystectomy [6]. Twenty-eight patients underwent a standard dissection with a mean number of lymph nodes removed of 19 (range 8–33) [6]. Extended lymph node dissection has been performed in 22 patients with a mean of 30 lymph nodes removed (range 12–39) [6]. No surgical complications have occurred related to the lymphadenectomy [6].

35.4 Extended Pelvic Lymphadenopathy in RARC

Marshall evaluated the incidence of, and predictors for, extended lymphnode dissection (LND) in patients undergoing robot-assisted radical cystectomy (RARC) for bladder cancer, as extended LND is critical for the treatment of bladder cancer but the role of minimally invasive surgery for extended LND has not been well-defined in a multi-institutional setting [7]. In all, 445 (58%) patients underwent extended LND. Among all patients, a median (range) of 18 (0–74) LNs were examined [7]. High-volume institutions ($\geq$100 cases) had a higher mean LN yield (23 vs. 15, p < 0.001) [7]. On univariable analysis, surgeon volume, institutional volume, and sequential case number were associated with likelihood of undergoing extended LND [7]. On multivariable analysis, surgeon volume [odds ratio (OR) 3.46, 95% confidence interval (CI) 2.37–5.06, p < 0.001] and institution volume [OR 2.65, 95% CI 1.47–4.78, p = 0.001] were associated with undergoing extended LND [7].

Woods evaluated perioperative and pathologic outcomes of patients undergoing robot-assisted extended pelvic lymphadenectomy for bladder cancer [8]. There was a total of 27 patients, and all procedures were completed laparoscopically; all urinary diversions were constructed extracorporeally in RARC patients [8]. The mean total operative time was 400 min, and mean blood loss was 277 ml [8]. All patients had transitional-cell carcinoma in the bladder cancer group [8]. The mean total lymph node count for the RARC group was 12.3 (range 7–20) [8]. There were no intraoperative complications, and 9 (33%) patients experienced postoperative complications [8].

35.5   Standard Lymphadenectomy in RARC

Gamboa reviewed standard PLND and its perioperative outcomes with robot-assisted laparoscopic radical cystectomy (RARC) [9]. A total of 41 patients were included in the study: 30 men and 11 women with a mean age of 69.7 years (range 49–85) and a mean body mass index of 26.9 (range 19.5–43.7) [9]. The median total operative time was 497.77 min (320–805) [9]. The mean estimated blood loss was 253.66 ml (range 50–700) [9]. The transfusion rate was 44% (18 out of 41) ranging from 0 to 4 units (median 0 units of blood) [9]. The mean total number of lymph nodes retrieved was 25.07 (range 4–68) [9]. Nodal metastases were seen in 14.63% (6/41). Rate of positive surgical margin was 4.87% (2/41) [9]. The median length of hospital stay was 8 days (5–37) [9]. The median duration of nasogastric tube, time to ambulation, first clear liquid intake, passage of colonic gas, time to bowel movement, and start of solid food intake were 1 (0–5), 2 (1–7), 3 (2–10), 4 (1–6), 5 (2–11) and 6 days (3–24), respectively [9].

35.6   Robotic Lymphadenectomy with the Da Vinci S

Hemal reports their experience with radical cystectomy (RRC) for bladder cancer using the four-arm da Vinci® S(TM) robot (Intuitive Surgical, Sunnyvale, CA, USA) [10]. The mean operative time was 12, 148, 44, and 126 min for docking, cystectomy, lymphadenectomy, and urinary diversion, respectively [10]. Median blood loss was 200 ml [10]. Mean hospital stay was 9.2 days [10]. Surgical margins were negative in all the patients [10]. The mean number of nodes removed was 12 (4–19) [10]. Histopathology revealed transitional cell carcinoma in all the patients (pT2a-1, pT2b-3, pT3a-2) [10].

35.7   Robotic vs. Open Lympadenectomy

Richards analysed the pelvic lymph node dissection (PLND) and margin status using a standard technique in the first 35 patients undergoing robot-assisted radical cystectomy (RARC) [11]. There was no significant difference between the ORC and RARC group in regards to patient characteristics, tumour stage (43% ORC and 40% RARC having pT3/pT4 disease), and node status (29% N+ in each group) [11]. The median total lymph node yield was similar, with 15 (interquartile range [IQR] 11, 22) in the ORC group and 16 (IQR 11, 24) in the RARC group (p = 0.5) [11]. One patient who underwent RARC had a positive margin compared with 3 patients in the ORC group [11].

Davis determined the fraction of lymph nodes yielded by robot assisted pelvic lymph node dissection [12]. The median yield of robot assisted and second look open pelvic lymph node dissection was 43 (range 19–63) and 4 (range 0–8), respectively, for an overall robot assisted yield of 93% [12]. Of second look open pelvic lymph node dissections 67% were clear of residual tissue, 13% had tissue without lymph nodes and 20% had 1 or more lymph nodes [12]. Median operative time for robot assisted pelvic lymph node dissection was 117 min [12]. Concurrently open radical cystectomy without required multiple lymph node specimen submission yielded a median 24 nodes [12].

Lavery reported experience with robot-assisted extended pelvic lymphnode dissection (ePLND) using a standardized open template [13]. The mean (range) and median length of hospital stay were 3.4 (3–7) days and 3 days, respectively [13]. The mean (range) nodal yield was 41.8 (18–67) nodes, with greater than 25 nodes in 13 patients [13]. Three patients were found to have nodal positivity [13]. Of the fifteen patients, four received neoadjuvant chemotherapy [13]. Two patients were re-admitted for postoperative complications within 30 days [13]. There were no complications directly resulting from the ePLND [13].

Abaza compared extended lymphnode dissection in 120 open and 35 robotic cystectomy cases [14]. The mean ± SD node count in the open group was 36.9 ± 14.8 (range 11–87) and in the robotic group the mean yield was 37.5 ± 13.2 (range 18–64). Only 12 of 120 open (10%) and 2 of 35 robotic (6%) cases had fewer than 20 nodes [14]. A total of 36 open (30%) and 12 robotic (34%) cases were node positive [14]. Open extended lymphnode dissection identified 80% and 90% confidence of accurate staging as pN0 when obtaining 23 and 27 nodes, respectively [14]. A node count of 23 or 27 was achieved in 87% and 77% of open cases, and in 91% and 83% of robotic cases, respectively [14]. Of patients with open surgery 36% received neoadjuvant chemotherapy compared to 31% of those with robotic surgery [14].

35.8   Robotic vs. Laparoscopic Lymphadenectomy for Radical Cystectomy

Desai describes the robotic and laparoscopic technique and the short-term outcomes of high extended pelvic LND (PLND) up to the inferior mesenteric artery (IMA) during RC [15]. Desai performed robotic extended PLND with the proximal extent up to the IMA or aortic bifurcation [15]. All 15 procedures were technically successful without need for conversion to open surgery [15]. Median operative time was 6.7 h, estimated blood loss was 500 ml, and three patients (21%) required blood transfusion. Median nodal yield in the entire cohort was 31 (range: 15–78) [15]. The IMA group had more nodes retrieved (median: 42.5) compared with the aortic bifurcation group (median: 20.5) [15]. Histopathology confirmed nodal metastases in four patients (27%), including three patients in the IMA group and one patient in the aortic bifurcation group [15]. Perioperative complications were recorded in six cases (40%) [15]. During a median follow-up of 13 months, no patient developed local or systemic recurrence [15]. Limitations of the study include its retrospective design and small cohort of patients [15].

35.9   Grey Literature Relating to Review

Recent investigations have demonstrated a clinical benefit to performance of an extended PLND, including all lymphatic tissue to the level of the aortic bifurcation [16]. Recent studies have demonstrated increased recurrence-free survival and overall survival rates in patients undergoing radical cystectomy with extended PLND, even in cases of pathologically lymph node negative disease [16]. The growing use of minimally invasive techniques has prompted interest in robotic radical cystectomy and extended PLND, and recent reports have demonstrated the feasibility of this technique [16].

References

1. Moher D, Liberati A, Tetzlaff J, Altman DG. "Preferred Reporting Items for Systematic Reviews and Meta-Analyses: The Prisma Statement." [In English]. BMJ (Online) 339, no. 7716 (08 Aug 2009):332–36.
2. Mays N, Pope C, Popay J. "Systematically Reviewing Qualitative and Quantitative Evidence to Inform Management and Policy-Making in the Health Field." [In English]. Journal of Health Services Research and Policy 10, no. SUPPL. 1 (July 2005):6–20.
3. Kang SG, Kang SH, Lee YG, Rha KH, Jeong BC, Ko YH, Lee HM, Seo SI, Kwon TG, Park SC, Jung SI, Sung GT, Kim HH. Robot-assisted radical cystectomy and pelvic lymph node dissection: a multi-institutional study from Korea. J Endourol. 2010;24(9):1435–40.
4. Guru KA, Kim HL, Piacente PM, Mohler JL. Robot-assisted radical cystectomy and pelvic lymph node dissection: initial experience at Roswell Park Cancer Institute. Urology. 2007;69(3):469–74.
5. Kasraeian A, Barret E, Cathelineau X, Rozet F, Galiano M, Sanchez-Salas R, Vallancien G. Robot-assisted laparoscopic cystoprostatectomy with extended pelvic lymphadenec-

tomy, extracorporeal enterocystoplasty, and intracorporeal enterourethral anastomosis: initial Montsouris experience. J Endourol. 2010;24(3):409–13.

6. Pruthi RS, Wallen EM. Robotic-assisted laparoscopic pelvic lymphadenectomy for bladder cancer: a surgical atlas. J Laparoendosc Adv Surg Tech A. 2009;19(1):71–4.

7. Marshall SJ, Hayn MH, Stegemann AP, Agarwal PK, Badani KK, Balbay MD, Dasgupta P, Hemal AK, Hollenbeck BK, Kibel AS, Menon M, Mottrie A, Nepple K, Pattaras JG, Peabody JO, Poulakis V, Pruthi RS, Palou Redorta J, Rha KH, Richstone L, Schanne F, Scherr DS, Siemer S, Stöckle M, Wallen EM, Weizer AZ, Wiklund P, Wilson T, Woods M, Guru KA. Impact of surgeon and volume on extended lymphadenectomy at the time of robot-assisted radical cystectomy: results from the International Robotic Cystectomy Consortium (IRCC). BJU Int. 2013;111(7):1075–80.

8. Woods M, Thomas R, Davis R, Andrews PE, Ferrigni RG, Cheng J, Castle EP. Robot-assisted extended pelvic lymphadenectomy. J Endourol. 2008;22(6):1297–302.

9. Gamboa AJ, Young JL, Dash A, Abraham JB, Box GN, Ornstein DK. Pelvic lymphnode dissection and outcome of robot-assisted radical cystectomy for bladder carcinoma. J Robot Surg. 2009;3(1):7–12.

10. Hemal AK, Kolla SB, Wadhwa P. First case series of robotic radical cystoprostatectomy, bilateral pelvic lymphadenectomy, and urinary diversion with the da Vinci S system. J Robot Surg. 2008;2(1):35–40.

11. Richards KA, Hemal AK, Kader AK, Pettus JA. Robot assisted laparoscopic pelvic lymphadenectomy at the time of radical cystectomy rivals that of open surgery: single institution report. Urology. 2010;76(6):1400–4.

12. Davis JW, Gaston K, Anderson R, Dinney CP, Grossman HB, Munsell MF, Kamat AM. Robot assisted extended pelvic lymphadenectomy at radical cystectomy: lymph node yield compared with second look open dissection. J Urol. 2011;185(1):79–83.

13. Lavery HJ, Martinez-Suarez HJ, Abaza R. Robotic extended pelvic lymphadenectomy for bladder cancer with increased nodal yield. BJU Int. 2011;107(11):1802–5.

14. Abaza R, Dangle PP, Gong MC, Bahnson RR, Pohar KS. Quality of lymphadenectomy is equivalent with robotic and open cystectomy using an extended template. J Urol. 2012;187(4):1200–4.

15. Desai MM, Berger AK, Brandina RR, Zehnder P, Simmons M, Aron M, Skinner EC, Gill IS. Robotic and laparoscopic high extended pelvic lymph node dissection during radical cystectomy: technique and outcomes. Eur Urol. 2012;61(2):350–5.

16. Dorin RP, Skinner EC. Extended lymphadenectomy in bladder cancer. Curr Opin Urol. 2010;20(5):414–20.

Robotic Cystectomy and Sentinel Node Mapping

36

Early detection greatly improves the chances of survival from bladder cancer. More recently ICG use has been reported in robotic surgery, which review in the context of bladder cancer.

ICG allows visualization of malignant lesions in human bladder carcinoma ex vivo [1]. Accurate targeting of bladder lesions was achieved with a sensitivity of 97%. Specificity is 100%, but reduced to 80% if targeting of necrotic tissue from previous transurethral resections or chemotherapy are considered as false positives [1]. The ICG marked high-grade urothelial carcinomas, both muscle invasive and non-muscle invasive. Carcinoma in situ was accurately diagnosed in 11 cases, whereas only four cases were seen using white light, so imaging with the ICG offers improved early diagnosis of bladder cancers and may also enable new treatment alternatives [1]. This demonstrates use of florescence as part of endoscopic tumour management.

Unlike other cancers, the Sentinel Lymph Node (SLN) procedure in bladder cancer requires special attention to the injection technique [2]. The aim of this study was to assess feasibility and to optimize tracer injection technique for SLN mapping in bladder cancer patients using NIR fluorescence imaging [2]. ICG conjugated to albumin was first administrated serosally (n = 5), and subsequently mucosally by cystoscopic injection (n = 15). In the last cohort of 12 patients treated with cystoscopic injection, the bladder was kept filled with saline for at least 15 min [2]. Fluorescent lymph nodes were observed only in the patient group with cystoscopic injection of ICG. Filling of the bladder post-injection was of added value to promote drainage of ICG to the lymph nodes, and in 11 of these 12 patients (92%) one or more NIR fluorescent lymph nodes were identified [2]. This demonstrates value of fluorescence imaging for SLN identification in bladder cancer.

This was further confirmed by Inoue et al. [3]. In total, 12 candidates for radical cystectomy and pelvic lymph node dissection (PLND) were included in this study. After an indocyanine green (ICG) solution was injected into the bladder during radical cystectomy, lymphatic vessels draining from the bladder were analyzed using a

FN system [3]. A lymphatic pathway along inferior vesical vessels to internal iliac LNs was clearly illustrated in 7 cases. Under in-vivo probing, the fluorescence intensity of internal iliac nodes was greater than that of external iliac or obturator nodes. Under ex-vivo probing, the fluorescence intensity of internal iliac and obturator nodes was greater than that of external iliac nodes [3]. This demonstrates a FN system after injecting ICG during a radical cystectomy operation is a safe approach to lymphatic channel draining from the bladder.

Manny and Hemal [4] reviewed 10 patients with clinically localized high-grade bladder cancer. Bladder tumour marking and identification of sentinel drainage were achieved in 9 of 10 (90%) patients [4]. The area of bladder tumour was identified at a median of 15 min after injection, whereas sentinel drainage was visualized at a median of 30 min. Mesenteric angiography was successful in 8 of 8 (100%) patients at a median time of <1 min after intravenous injection and enabled identification of bowel arcades before intracorporeal bowel stapling [4]. This demonstrates using combined cystoscopic and intravenous injection of ICG is safe and feasible.

In conclusion, use of sentinel node mapping as part of bladder cancer therapy is safe and effective.

References

1. Golijanin J, Amin A, Moshnikova A, Brito JM, Tran TY, Adochite RC, Andreev GO, Crawford T, Engelman DM, Andreev OA, Reshetnyak YK, Golijanin D. Targeted imaging of urothelium carcinoma in human bladders by an ICG pHLIP peptide ex vivo. Proc Natl Acad Sci U S A. 2016;113:11829–34.
2. Schaafsma BE, Verbeek FP, Elzevier HW, Tummers QR, Van Der Vorst JR, Frangioni JV, Van De Velde CJ, Pelger RC, Vahrmeijer AL. Optimization of sentinel lymph node mapping in bladder cancer using near-infrared fluorescence imaging. J Surg Oncol. 2014;110:845–50.
3. Inoue S, Shiina H, Mitsui Y, Yasumoto H, Matsubara A, Igawa M. Identification of lymphatic pathway involved in the spread of bladder cancer: evidence obtained from fluorescence navigation with intraoperatively injected indocyanine green. Can Urol Assoc J. 2013;7:E322–8.
4. Manny TB, Hemal AK. Fluorescence-enhanced robotic radical cystectomy using unconjugated indocyanine green for pelvic lymphangiography, tumor marking, and mesenteric angiography: the initial clinical experience. Urology. 2014;83:824–9.

MIBC and Radical Cystectomy in the Elderly: A Systematic Review

37

37.1   Research Methods

A systematic review relating to muscle invasive bladder cancer and radical cystectomy in the elderly was conducted. This was to identify whether radical cystectomy has a role in this cohort. The search strategy aimed to identify all references related to bladder cancer AND muscle invasive disease AND radical cystectomy AND elderly. Search terms used were as follows: (Bladder cancer) AND (muscle invasive disease) AND (radical cystectomy) AND (elderly). The following databases were screened from 1989 to June 2020:

- CINAHL
- MEDLINE (NHS Evidence)
- Cochrane
- AMed
- EMBASE
- PsychINFO
- SCOPUS
- Web of Science

In addition, searches using Medical Subject Headings (MeSH) and keywords were conducted using Cochrane databases. Two UK-based experts in bladder cancer were consulted to identify any additional studies.

Studies were eligible for inclusion if they reported primary research focusing on muscle invasive bladder cancer and bladder preservation. Papers were included if published after 1984 and had to be in English. Studies that did not conform to this were excluded. Only primary research was included (Fig. 37.1).

© The Editor(s) (if applicable) and The Author(s), under exclusive license to
Springer Nature Switzerland AG 2021
S. S. Goonewardene et al., *Management of Muscle Invasive Bladder Cancer*,
Management of Urology, https://doi.org/10.1007/978-3-030-57915-9_37

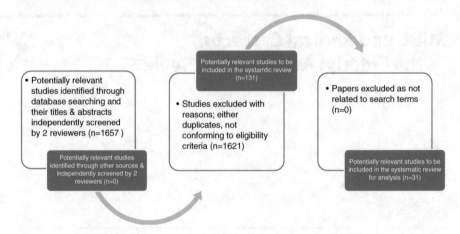

Fig. 37.1   Flow chart of studies identified through the systematic review. (Adapted from PRISMA)

Abstracts were independently screened for eligibility by two reviewers and disagreements resolved through discussion or third party opinion. Agreement level was calculated using Cohen's Kappa to test the intercoder reliability of this screening process. Cohens' Kappa allows comparison of inter-rater reliability between papers using relative observed agreement. This also takes account of the comparison occurring by chance. The first reviewer agreed all 31 papers to be included, the second, agreed on 31.

Data extraction was piloted by the researcher and amended in consultation with the research team (author and two academic supervisors). Data collected included authors, year and country of publication, study aims, setting, intervention aims, number of participants, study design, intervention components and delivery methods, comparison groups and outcome measures, notes and follow-up questions for the authors. Studies were quality assessed using the PRISMA criteria for randomised controlled trials, Mays et al. [1, 2] for the action research and qualitative studies and the Critical Skills Appraisal programme for cohort studies. This was also applied to randomised controlled trials and qualitative studies.

The search identified 1657 papers (Fig. 37.1). Thirty-one mapped to the search terms and eligibility criteria. The current systematic reviews were examined to gain further knowledge about the subject. One thousand six hundred and thirty-one papers were excluded due to not conforming to eligibility criteria or adding to the evidence. Of the 31 papers left, relevant abstracts were identified and the full papers obtained (all of which were in English), to quality assure against search criteria. There was considerable heterogeneity of design among the included studies therefore a narrative review of the evidence was undertaken. There was significant heterogeneity within studies, including clinical topic, numbers, outcomes, as a result a narrative review was thought to be best. There were 31 cohort studies, with a moderate level of evidence and no RCTS. These were from a range of countries with minimal loss to follow-up. All participants were identified appropriately.

37.2 Systematic Review Results

37.2.1 Prognostic Factors in Elderly Patients

Dehayni assessed prognostic impact of age on the carcinological prognosis of invasive-muscle-bladder cancer treated by total cystectomy [3]. The patients were divided into two groups: patients under 65 years of age = 150 cases (group 1), patients aged 65 years and over = 195 cases (group 2) [3]. The 3-year survival rates for patients according to the age groups were 88% and 64% respectively, end the recurrence-free survival 66% and 28% [3]. When age was analysed as a categorical variable, was associated with hydronephrosis (p = 0.001), advanced pathological stage (p = 0.034), high grade (p = 0.026), nodal involvement (p = 0.011) and lymphovascular invasion (p = 0.008) [3]. The multivariate Cox model analysis showed that hydronephrosis and pathological stage was prognostic factors of survival (p = 0.012 and p = 0.035, respectively). Higher age is significantly associated with the risk of pathologically advanced disease and poorer global survival [3].

37.2.2 Mortality Rate in Elderly undergoing Cystectomy

Soulie evaluated the morbidity of radical cystectomy for invasive bladder cancer in select patients older than 75 years using recent data from 2 academic hospitals [4]. The perioperative mortality rate was 2.7% [4]. The intraoperative, early and late postoperative complication rates were 38.4%, 46.5% and 16.4%, respectively [4]. Three reoperations (4.1%) were necessary [4]. The most common early complications were pyelonephritis in 12.3% of cases, disorientation in 10.9%, pneumonia in 8.2% and prolonged ileus in 12.3% [4]. The most common late complications were ureteroileal anastomotic stenosis in 5 cases and hernia in [4]. At a median followup of 14.4 months (range 6–74) the overall mortality rate was 31.5 [4]. Hospital stay was significantly higher in patients with complications [4].

Morgan sought to better identify patients at substantial risk for postoperative mortality [5]. Of the 220 patients 28 (12.7%) died within 90 days of surgery [5]. Older age (HR 2.30, 95% CI 1.22–4.32) and lower preoperative albumin (HR 2.50, 95% CI 1.40–4.45) were significant predictors of 90-day mortality [5]. Morgan developed a nomogram based on patient age, clinical stage, Charlson comorbidity index and albumin to predict the likelihood of 90-day mortality with 75% accuracy. Internal validation showed a bootstrap adjusted concordance index of 71% [5].

March Villalba analysed perioperative outcomes in muscle-invasive bladder neoplasm treated with radical cystectomy [6]. There was no difference between both age groups about: time of surgery, intraoperative complications (<70 = 21.8%, ≥70 = 31.6%), postoperative mortality (<70 = 3.6%, ≥70 = 8.8%), minor (<70 = 18.2%, ≥70 = 26.3%) and major medical postoperative complications (<70 = 7.3%, ≥70 = 8.8%), late outcomes as cancer-specific morbidity-mortality and actuarial overall survival stratified by patient age [6]. The rate of major postoperative complications (<70 = 23.6%, ≥70 = 43.9%) as well as the mean length of hospital stay (<70 = 10.2, ≥70 = 15.2 days) differed significantly between the two age groups [6]. Age and cardiovascular risk factors were independent predictive factors of mayor postoperative complications [6].

March Villalba analysed the differences about perioperative and later outcomes between ages of patients with muscle-invasive bladder neoplasm treated with radical cystectomy [6]. There was no difference between both age groups about: time of surgery, intraoperative complications (<70 = 21.8%, ≥70 = 31.6%), postoperative mortality (<70 = 3.6%, ≥70 = 8.8%), minor (<70 = 18.2%, ≥70 = 26.3%) and major medical postoperative complications (<70 = 7.3%, ≥70 = 8.8%), late outcomes as cancer-specific morbidity-mortality and a overall survival according to patient age [6]. The rate of major postoperative complications (<70 = 23.6%, ≥70 = 43.9%) and mean length of hospital stay (<70 = 10.2, ≥70 = 15.2 days) differed significantly between the two age groups [6]. Age and cardiovascular risk factors were independent predictive factors of mayor postoperative complications [6].

Farnham determined the long-term benefit and survival outcomes after radical cystectomy in the elderly, high operative risk patient [7]. Of 382 patients undergoing cystectomy, 38 patients with transitional cell carcinoma were elderly, high perioperative risk patients [age ≥75 years and American Society of Anesthesiologists (ASA) classification ≥3] [7]. No patient died in the early perioperative period [7]. Of the patients with ≤pT2B pathology, 9/27 (33%) are alive and are disease-free [7]. There are 2/11 patients (18%) with ≥pT3 pathology still alive with 1 of those patients (pT4a) alive with disease 34 months after radical cystectomy [7]. Kaplan-Meier survival curves demonstrate that patients with organ confined disease (≤pT2B) had a significantly longer mean overall survival than patients with non-organ confined disease (≥pT3): 31 months vs. 18 months, p = 0.046. Cause of death was known in 17 patients, with the majority (14/17) because of bladder cancer [7].

Radical cystectomy bears a considerable perioperative mortality risk particularly in elderly patients [8]. In this study, predictors of perioperative and long-term competing (non-bladder cancer) mortality in elderly patients selected for radical cystectomy were assessed [8]. Whereas Charlson score and the American Society of Anesthesiologists (ASA) physical status classification (but not age) were independent predictors of 90-day mortality in younger patients, only age predicted 90-day mortality in patients aged 80 years or older (odds ratio per year 1.24, p = 0.0422) [8]. Unlike in their younger counterparts, neither age nor Charlson score or ASA classification were predictors of long-term competing mortality in patients aged 80 years or older (hazard ratios 1.07–1.10, p values 0.21–0.77) [8].

De Groote evaluated perioperative morbidity and mortality rate, in patients older than 80 years undergoing robot-assisted radical cystectomy (RARC) [9]. Of 155 consecutive patients, 22 (14.2%) patients were 80 years or older [9]. Octogenarians did not significantly differ from younger patients in ASA score (p = 0.4) and Charlson comorbidity index (p = 0.4) [9]. Prevalence of any grade and high-grade complications was similar in both groups (all p ≥ 0.6) [9]. Older patients had a significantly higher pathologic tumor grade (p = 0.04) and a lower use of pelvic lymphadenectomy (p < 0.001) [9]. No perioperative mortality rate was recorded within

90 days from surgery [9]. Elderly patients had a similar risk of 3-year oncologic recurrence after surgery compared with their younger counterparts (odds ratio [OR] 1.63; p = 0.2) [9]. Conversely, the risk of cancer-specific mortality rate was significantly higher (OR 2.78; p = 0.02) [9].

37.2.3 Type of Reconstruction in the Elderly

Saika compared the health-related quality of life of elderly patients after radical cystectomy for bladder cancer in urinary diversion groups: ileal conduit, ureterocutaneostomy, or orthotopic urinary reservoir [10]. Fifty-six patients had undergone constructions for ileal conduit diversion, 31 for ureterocutaneostomy, and 22 for orthotopic urinary reservoir (OUR) [10]. Regardless of the type of urinary diversion, the majority of patients reported having good overall quality of life [10]. No significant differences among urinary diversion subgroups were found in any quality of life area in the QLQ-C30 questionnaire [10]. More patients in the OUR subgroup felt disappointment than those in the ileal conduit or cutaneostomy sub-groups. Patient demands and expectations may be so different from the results that the details of each urinary diversion method should be explained thoroughly [10]. OUR construction could be a candidate even for elderly patients [10].

Saika compared the clinical and functional results of radical cystectomy and urinary reconstructions performed on 19 elderly bladder cancer patients over 75 years old to those on 22 younger patients to determine whether age was one of the critical points for the application of this type of surgery [11]. Bladder substitution was performed after cystectomy using either the Hautmann, Studer or Reddy procedure in 9 of the 19 elderly patients [11]. Urinary diversion was performed after cystectomy using ileal conduit and ureterocutaneostomy procedures in the rest of the patients [11]. On the other hand, bladder substitutions were performed in 11; urinary diversions with continent urinary reservoir in 6 and with ileal conduit in 4 of the 22 younger patients [11]. Neither prolongation of the operation time, nor increase in the amount of bleeding or prolongation of hospital stay was observed in elderly compared with younger patients. In elderly patients, the average operation time of radical cystectomy with bladder substitution was slightly longer than that of total cystectomy with ileal conduit or ureterocutaneostomy [11]. There were no peri-operative deaths, and early post-operative complications were observed in 3 of 9 cases of the bladder substitution, in 4 of 10 cases of ileal conduit or ureterocutaneostomy [11]. Five cases of bladder substitution maintained their comfortable voiding urine comfortably, while 4 had dysuria and/or urinary incontinence [11]. Overall, late complications occurred in 10 of the elderly patients [11]. The rate and types of complications in the elderly patients were not different from those in the younger patients [11]. The cause-specific survival rate and overall survival rates of the elderly patients were similar to those of the younger patients [11].

Age is an established risk factor for developing bladder cancer and is associated with increased stage and worse treatment outcomes [12]. Furthermore, elderly patients who require radical cystectomy are more likely to undergo an incontinent urinary diversion compared with younger patients [12]. While age was shown to be a risk factor for complications following orthotopic neobladder, similar complication rates were reported between those who received either an orthotopic neobladder or ileal conduit when compared within age groups [12]. Additionally, in properly selected elderly patients, similar outcomes and quality of life can be expected when compared with younger patients [12].

37.2.4 Open Radical Cystectomy

Wuethrich reported results in patients >75 years of age who underwent open radical cystectomy (RC) and urinary diversion [13]. Thirty five of the 224 patients (17%) received an OBS, 178 of the 224 patients (78%) an IC, and 11 of the 224 patients (5%) an UCST [13]. The 90-day complication rate was 54.3% in the OBS (major: Clavien grade 3–5: 22.9%, minor: Clavien Grade 1–2: 31.4%), 56.7% in the IC (major: 27%, minor: 29.8%), and 63.6% in the UCST group (major: 36.4%, minor: 27.3%); p = 0.001 [13]. The 90-day mortality was 0% in the OBS group, 13% in the IC group, and 10% in the UCST group (p = 0.077) [13]. Overall and cancer-specific survivals were 90 and 98, 47 and 91, and 11 and 12 months for OBS, IC, and UCST, respectively [13]. In OBS patients, daytime continence was considered as dry in 66% and humid in 20% of patients. Night-time continence was dry in 46% and humid 26% of patients [13].

37.2.5 Laparoscopic Radical Series in Elderly

Hermans compare outcome of laparoscopic radical cystectomy (LRC) with ileal conduit in 22 elderly (≥75 years) versus 51 younger (<75 years) patients [14]. Median operative time (340 versus 341 min) and estimated blood loss (<500 versus >500 ml) did not differ between groups [14]. Median total hospital stay was 12.0 versus 14.0 days for younger and elderly patients [14]. Grade I–II 90-day complication rate was higher for elderly patients (68% versus 43%, p = 0.05) [14]. Grade III–V 90 day complication rate was equal for both groups (23% versus 29%, p = 0.557). Ninety day mortality rate was higher for elderly patients (14% versus 4%, p = 0.157) [14]. Estimated overall and cancer-specific survival at 5 years was 46% versus 35% and 64% versus 64% for younger and elderly patients respectively [14].

37.2.6 National Trends in Cystectomy Figures for the Elderly

Roghmann examined national trends of radical cystectomy (RC) for urothelial carcinoma of urinary bladder in octogenarian patients and to assess the rates of adverse outcomes [15]. Of 12,274 RC patients, 1605 were ≥80 years (13.1%) [15]. The RC rates in octogenarians increased significantly from 9.9% in 1998 to 13.7% in 2007

[15]. After propensity score matching, the inpatient mortality rate was higher in octogenarians (4.6% vs. 2.6%, p < 0.001) [15]. In multivariable analyses, octogenarians were at increased risk of blood transfusions (OR: 1.30) and postoperative complications (OR: 1.22) [15].

37.2.7 Robotic vs. Open Radical Cystectomy in Elderly

Richards compared robot-assisted radical cystectomy (RARC) and ORC in elderly patients [16]. Complete median operative times for RARC was 461 (interquartile range [IQR] 331, 554) vs. 370 min for ORC (IQR 294, 460) (p = 0.056); however, median blood loss for RARC was 275 ml (IQR 150, 450) vs. 600 ml for ORC (IQR 500, 1925) [16]. The median hospital stay for RARC was 7 days (IQR 5, 8) vs. 14.5 days for ORC (IQR 8, 22) (p < 0.001) [16]. The major complication (Clavien ≥III) rate for RARC was 10% compared with 35% for ORC (p = 0.024) [16]. There were two positive margins in the ORC group compared with one in the RARC group with median LN yields of 15 nodes (IQR 11, 22) and 17 nodes (IQR 10, 25) (p = 0.560) respectively [16].

37.2.8 Extraperitoneal vs. Transperitoneal Laparoscopic Approaches

Feng reported extraperitoneal laparoscopic radical cystectomy (ELRC) and compared with transperitoneal laparoscopic radical cystectomy (TLRC) in the treatment of selected elderly [17]. A significantly shorter time to exsufflation (p = 0.026) and liquid intake (p = 0.035) were observed in the ELRC group compared with the TLRC group [17]. The incidence of postoperative ileus in the ELRC group was lower than the TLRC group (0% vs. 9.5%) [17], yet this was non-significant. The removed lymph node number in the ELRC group was significantly lower than the TLRC group (p < 0.001) [17]. No significant differences were observed between the two groups in the overall and cancer-free survival rates (p > 0.05) [17].

37.2.9 Younger vs. Older Patients for Radical Cystectomy

Coward reported experience with robotic radical cystectomy as applied to an older patient population with regard to perioperative measures and pathologic outcomes [18]. A robotic approach to radical cystectomy for bladder cancer have recently been described, but its application in an older patient population, which is often the case in bladder cancer and cystectomy [18]. The younger versus older patients had a lower American Society of Anesthesiologists score (2.6 vs. 3.0; p < 0.001), greater body mass index (28.2 vs. 26.1; p = 0.008), and longer operating room time (4.8 vs. 4.4 h; p = 0.015). No differences were observed between the 2 groups in blood loss, time to discharge, or complication rate [18]. Also, no significant differences were found in the surgical pathologic findings, including the organ-confined rate (62% vs. 71%) and lymph node yield (19.5 vs. 18.1) [18].

37.2.10   Risks and Benefits of Pelvic Lymphadenectomy in the Elderly

Grabbert analysed the influence of PLND on survival rates and complication rates in a selected group of elderly patients with a minimum age of 80 years [19]. In univariate analysis of the data, there was not a significant impact of PLND on CSS ($p = 0.606$), OS ($p = 0.979$) or PFS ($p = 0.883$) [19]. Also in multivariate analysis of the data, PLND was not identified as an independent prognostic parameter on survival rates of patients undergoing RC, neither for CSS ($p = 0.912$) nor OS ($p = 0.618$) or PFS ($p = 0.900$) [19].

37.2.11   Outcomes in Elderly Patients

Lance reviewed the outcome of 33 patients age 80 years or older treated with radical cystectomy and ileal conduit urinary diversion [20]. Five patients received neoadjuvant chemotherapy, and 2 had salvage cystectomy after failure of external beam radiation therapy [20]. Twenty-seven complications occurred in 20 patients (60.6%), of which 17 were minor (63%) and 10 were major (37%) [20]. There was no difference in the rate of complications in patients receiving neoadjuvant treatment compared to the group treated with cystectomy alone [20].

Berger assessed perioperative complications and 90-day mortality of radical cystectomy (RC) in elderly patients with muscle-invasive bladder cancer (MIBC) [21]. Urinary diversion with the use of bowel was performed in 79.5% and ureterocutaneostomy in 20.5%, with a higher proportion in the ≥80 cohort (32.2% vs. 14%; $p = 0.001$). Forty-one point four percent had an uneventful postoperative course (Clavien grade 0) and 26.6% developed severe complications (Clavien grade III–V) [21]. In a multivariable regression analysis, the Charlson comorbidity index (odds ratio 1.5 per unit increase; $p < 0.001$) and the body mass index (odds ratio 1.13/kg/m^2 increase; $p = 0.015$) were predictors for the development of complications [21]. The 90-day mortality rate was 9% and the independent correlates thereof were the development of severe medical complications ($p = 0.004$), the American Society of Anesthesiologists (ASA) score ($p = 0.03$) and age ($p = 0.005$) [21].

Winters compared perioperative surgical outcomes in elderly patients undergoing robotic vs. open radical cystectomy (RC) [22]. Eighty-seven patients >75 years of age underwent cystectomy for MIBC (58 open, 29 robotic) [22]. Mean age was 79.6 (±3.2) and 79.2 (±3.5) for open and robotic groups, respectively ($p = 0.64$) [22]. There were no significant differences in baseline comorbidities, clinical or pathologic stage, or use of neoadjuvant chemotherapy [22]. The mean number of lymph nodes removed was similar ($p = 0.08$) [22]. Robotic cystectomy had significantly longer mean OR times (p < 0.001) [22]. On multivariate analyses, robotic surgery was associated with 389 cc less EBL (95% CI 547 to 230, p < 0.001) and a 1.5-day-shortened LOS (95% CI 2.9 to 0.2, p = 0.02) compared with open surgery [22]. There were no significant differences in surgical complications or 90-day readmission rates between the two groups [22].

Haden compare surgical complications following radical cystectomy in septuagenarians and octogenarians [23]. 28.8% (n = 493) were 80 years and older, while 71.2% (n = 1217) were between 70 and 79 years old [23]. Operative time (338.4 vs. 307.2 min, p = 0.0001) and the length of stay (11.9 vs. 10.4 days, p = 0.0016) were higher in the octogenarian group [23]. The intra- and postoperative transfusion rates, reoperative rates, wound dehiscence rates, and pneumonia, sepsis, and myocardial infarction rates were similar between the two groups [23]. The wound infection rate (7.3% vs. 4.1%, p = 0.01) was higher in the septuagenarians and mortality rate (4.3% vs. 2.3%, p = 0.04) was higher in the octogenarian group [23].

37.2.12 Pathology of Elderly Patients Undergoing Radical Cystectomy

Horovitz reviewed a large group of patients from two major tertiary care academic institutions [24]. Pathological specimens were reviewed by dedicated genitourinary pathologists, including those recovered from peripheral hospitals. Compared with younger patients (age ≤79 years), elderly patients (age ≥80 years) had higher American Society of Anesthesiologists scores (p < 0.001), a greater number of lymph nodes removed during surgical dissection (p < 0.001), and underwent less adjuvant treatment (p < 0.001) [24]. Choice of urinary diversion differed among the groups, with ileal conduit being used for all patients ≥80 years (p < 0.001) [24]. No differences were noted between age groups with respect to RFS (p = 0.3), DSS (p = 0.4) or OAS (p = 0.4) [24].

37.2.13 Post-operative Outcomes in Younger and Older Patients

Cusano compared peri-postoperative complication rates following robotic urologic surgery in elderly and younger patients [25]. 97.5% and 2.5% of patients were ≤74 or ≥75 years old, respectively [25]. Cystectomies, partial nephrectomies and prostatectomies accounted for 3.5%, 9.5% and 87.1% of surgeries, respectively [25]. Within cystectomy, nephrectomy and prostatectomy groups, 24.4%, 12.5% and 0.6% patients were ≥75 years old [25]. Within each surgical type, elderly patients had significantly elevated CCI scores [25]. Length of stay was significantly prolonged in elderly patients undergoing partial nephrectomy or prostatectomy [25]. In elderlycystectomy, partial nephrectomy and prostatectomy patients, 36.7%, 14.3% and 5.9% suffered ≥1 Clavien grade 3–5 complication, respectively [25]. Major complications were not significantly different between age groups [25]. A qualitatively similar pattern was observed regarding Clavien grade 1–2 complications [25].

Chang determined the safety of radical cystectomy in elderly patients at high risk [26]. Median age of the 44 patients was 77.5 years (range 75–87) [26]. American Society of Anesthesiologists class was 3 in 40 patients and 4 in 4 [26]. Postoperatively 31 of the 44 patients (70%) were transferred directly to the general urology floor, while cardiac monitoring was required postoperatively in 30% [26]. Nine of these patients were transferred to a step-down unit and the remaining 4 required surgical intensive care unit admission[26]. Minor and major complications developed in 10 (22.7%) and 2 (4.5%) cases, respectively [26]. No patients died in the perioperative period and 4 patients were hospitalized within 6 months of discharge [26].

Tilki reported experience with morbidity of radical cystectomy in patients over 75 years compared to younger patients [27]. Eighty-five of 326 patients (26%) were ≥75 years (75–95) old. ASA score was equal 3 or greater in 51% of patients ≥75 years and 32% of patients <75 years [27]. Ileal conduit was performed in 83% of patients ≥75, 16% received an ileal neobladder compared to 46% and 51%, respectively, in patients <75 [27]. A total of 33 patients (39%) in the older patient group received blood transfusions intraoperatively compared to 76 patients (32%) in the younger age group [27]. In 6 patients ≥75 years (7.1%) and 17 patients <75 (7.1%) open surgical revision was necessary, perioperative complication rate was 22% and 21%, respectively [27]. The most common complications were wound dehiscence (5.9% vs. 7.5%), infections (4.7% vs. 4.6%), and pulmonary embolism (3.5% vs. 2.1%). Perioperative mortality was 1.2% (1 patient) in the elderly versus 0.4% (1 patient) in the younger age group [27].

Zattoni evaluated perioperative outcomes and early survival in a series of octogenarians who underwent radical cystectomy (RC) and urinary diversion for bladder cancer [28]. Ileal conduit (IC) was performed in 21/44 (48%) cases, cutaneous ureterostomy (CU) in 20/44 (45%), and no urinary diversion was required for 3 (7%) dialytic patients [28]. Median EBL was 700 ml (IQR 500–1000) and 23 (52%) patients required blood transfusion [28]. Overall complications were recorded in 29 (66%) patients, with major complications observed in 12 (27%), with death occurring in 1 [28]. No differences in complications were observed between IC and CU. The 2-year OS estimate was 62.5% [28].

37.2.14   Survival Benefit Younger vs. Older Patients: Radical Cystectomy

Chamie determined whether the survival benefit achieved with radical cystectomy (RC, the reference standard for treating muscle-invasive bladder cancer) in younger patients justifies its use in octogenarians [29]. In all, 8034 patients had RC and 2773 radiotherapy; RC was the primary method of treatment in all age groups except for octogenarians [29]. Those who had RC had a sizeable overall survival advantage in all age groups, except for the octogenarians (18 vs. 15 months) [29]. This small survival advantage improved only slightly (23 vs. 15 months) when excluding patients having nodal or distant metastasis [29]. The octogenarians who have RC with a limited pelvic lymph node dissection or RC alone receive little (16 vs. 15 months) or no survival benefit [29]. However, cancer-specific survival was significantly higher in those who had RC, including octogenarians [29].

References

1. Moher D, Liberati A, Tetzlaff J, Altman DG. "Preferred Reporting Items for Systematic Reviews and Meta-Analyses: The Prisma Statement." [In English]. BMJ (Online) 339, no. 7716 (08 Aug 2009):332–36.
2. Mays N, Pope C, Popay J. "Systematically Reviewing Qualitative and Quantitative Evidence to Inform Management and Policy-Making in the Health Field." [In English]. Journal of Health Services Research and Policy 10, no. SUPPL. 1 (July 2005):6–20.
3. Dehayni Y, Tetou M, Khdach Y, Janane A, Alami M, Ameur A. [Prognostic of older age for patients with invasive-muscle-bladder cancer and treated by radical cystectomy]. Prog Urol. 2018;28(3):166–72.
4. Soulié M, Straub M, Gamé X, Seguin P, De Petriconi R, Plante P, Hautmann RE. A multicenter study of the morbidity of radical cystectomy in select elderly patients with bladder cancer. J Urol. 2002 Mar;167(3):1325–8.
5. Morgan TM, Keegan KA, Barocas DA, Ruhotina N, Phillips SE, Chang SS, Penson DF, Clark PE, Smith JA Jr, Cookson MS. Predicting the probability of 90-day survival of elderly patients with bladder cancer treated with radical cystectomy. J Urol. 2011;186(3):829–34.
6. March Villalba JA, Martínez Jabaloyas JM, Pastor Hernández F, Günthner Stefan FJ, Rodríguez Navarro R, Chuan Nuez P. [Radical cystectomy as a muscle-invasive bladder cancer treatment in elderly patients]. Actas Urol Esp 2008;32(7):696-704.
7. Farnham SB, Cookson MS, Alberts G, Smith JA Jr, Chang SS. Benefit of radical cystectomy in the elderly patient with significant co-morbidities. Urol Oncol. 2004;22(3):178–81.
8. Froehner M, Koch R, Hübler M, Heberling U, Novotny V, Zastrow S, Hakenberg OW, Wirth MP. Predicting 90-day and long-term mortality in octogenarians undergoing radical cystectomy. BMC Urol. 2018;18(1):91.
9. De Groote R, Gandaglia G, Geurts N, Goossens M, Pauwels E, D'Hondt F, Gratzke C, Fossati N, De Naeyer G, Schatteman P, Carpentier P, Novara G, Mottrie A. Robot-assisted radical cystectomy for bladder cancer in octogenarians. J Endourol. 2016;30(7):792–8.
10. Saika T, Arata R, Tsushima T, Nasu Y, Suyama B, Takeda K, Ebara S, Manabe D, Kobayashi T, Tanimoto R, Kumon H, Okayama Urological Research Group. Health-related quality of life after radical cystectomy for bladder cancer in elderly patients with an ileal conduit, ureterocutaneostomy, or orthotopic urinary reservoir: a comparative questionnaire survey. Acta Med Okayama. 2007;61(4):199–203.
11. Saika T, Manabe D, Suyama B. Clinical study of radical cystectomy and urinary reconstruction in elderly patients with bladder cancer. Hinyokika Kiyo. 1999;45(1):19–23.
12. Hugen CM, Daneshmand S. Orthotopic urinary diversion in the elderly. World J Urol. 2016;34(1):13–8.
13. Wuethrich PY, Vidal A, Burkhard FC. There is a place for radical cystectomy and urinary diversion, including orthotopic bladder substitution, in patients aged 75 and older: results of a retrospective observational analysis from a high-volume center. Urol Oncol. 2016;34(2):58.e19–27.
14. Hermans TJ, Fossion LM, Verhoeven R, Horenblas S. Laparoscopic radical cystectomy in the elderly—results of a single center LRC only series. Int Braz J Urol. 2016;42(6):1099–108.
15. Roghmann F, Sukumar S, Ravi P, Trinh VQ, Meskawi M, Ghani KR, Sammon JD, Friedman AA, Peabody JO, Menon M, Noldus J, Karakiewicz PI, Sun M, Trinh QD. Radical cystectomy in the elderly: national trends and disparities in perioperative outcomes and quality of care. Urol Int. 2014;92(1):27–34.

16. Richards KA, Kader AK, Otto R, Pettus JA, Smith JJ 3rd, Hemal AK. Is robot-assisted radical cystectomy justified in the elderly? A comparison of robotic versus open radical cystectomy for bladder cancer in elderly ≥75 years old. J Endourol. 2012;26(10):1301–6.

17. Feng L, Song J, Wu M, Tian Y, Zhang D. Extraperitoneal versus transperitoneal laparoscopic radical cystectomy for selected elderly bladder cancer patients: a single center experience. Int Braz J Urol. 2016;42(4):655–62.

18. Coward RM, Smith A, Raynor M, Nielsen M, Wallen EM, Pruthi RS. Feasibility and outcomes of robotic-assisted laparoscopic radical cystectomy for bladder cancer in older patients. Urology. 2011;77(5):1111–4.

19. Grabbert M, Grimm T, Buchner A, Kretschmer A, Apfelbeck M, Schulz G, Jokisch F, Schneevoigt BS, Stief CG, Karl A. Risks and benefits of pelvic lymphadenectomy in octogenarians undergoing radical cystectomy due to urothelial carcinoma of the bladder. Int Urol Nephrol. 2017;49(12):2137–42.

20. Lance RS, Dinney CP, Swanson D, Babaian RJ, Pisters LL, Palmer LJ, Grossman HB. Radical cystectomy for invasive bladder cancer in the octogenarian. Oncol Rep. 2001;8(4):723–6.

21. Berger I, Martini T, Wehrberger C, Comploj E, Ponholzer A, Wolfgang M, Breinl E, Dunzinger M, Hofbauer J, Höltl W, Jeschke K, Krause S, Kugler W, Pauer W, Rauchenwald M, Pycha A, Madersbacher S. Perioperative complications and 90-day mortality of radical cystectomy in the elderly (75+): a retrospective, multicentre study. Urol Int. 2014;93(3):296–302.

22. Winters BR, Bremjit PJ, Gore JL, Lin DW, Ellis WJ, Dalkin BL, Porter MP, Harper JD, Wright JL. Preliminary comparative effectiveness of robotic versus open radical cystectomy in elderly patients. J Endourol. 2016;30(2):212–7.

23. Haden TD, Prunty MC, Jones AB, Deroche CB, Murray KS, Pokala N. Comparative perioperative outcomes in septuagenarians and octogenarians undergoing radical cystectomy for bladder cancer-do outcomes differ? Eur Urol Focus. 2018;4(6):895–9.

24. Horovitz D, Turker P, Bostrom PJ, Mirtti T, Nurmi M, Kuk C, Kulkarni G, Fleshner NE, Finelli A, Jewett MA, Zlotta AR. Does patient age affect survival after radical cystectomy? BJU Int. 2012;110(11 Pt B):E486–93.

25. Cusano A, Haddock P, Staff I, Jackson M, Abarzua-Cabezas F, Dorin R, Meraney A, Wagner J, Shichman S, Kesler S. Surgical complications associated with robotic urologic procedures in elderly patients. Can J Urol. 2015;22(1):7607–13.

26. Chang SS, Alberts G, Cookson MS, Smith JA Jr. Radical cystectomy is safe in elderly patients at high risk. J Urol. 2001;166(3):938–41.

27. Tilki D, Zaak D, Trottmann M, Buchner A, Ekiz Y, Gerwens N, Schlenker B, Karl A, Walther S, Bastian PJ, Gratzke C, Tritschler S, Knüchel-Clarke R, Ergün S, Stief CG, Reich O, Seitz M. Radical cystectomy in the elderly patient: a contemporary comparison of perioperative complications in a single institution series. World J Urol. 2010;28(4):445–50.

28. Zattoni F, Palumbo V, Giannarini G, Crestani A, Kungulli A, Novara G, Zattoni F, Ficarra V. Perioperative outcomes and early survival in octogenarians who underwent radical cystectomy for bladder cancer. Urol Int. 2018;100(1):13–7.

29. Chamie K, Hu B, Devere White RW, Ellison LM. Cystectomy in the elderly: does the survival benefit in younger patients translate to the octogenarians? BJU Int. 2008;102(3):284–90.

Female Outcomes in Bladder Cancer

38

38.1 Research Methods

A systematic review relating to muscle invasive bladder cancer, radical cystectomy and renal transplant was conducted. This was to identify whether outcomes from renal transplant patients in this cohort. The search strategy aimed to identify all references related to radical cystectomy AND renal transplant. Search terms used were as follows: (Radical Cystectomy) AND (Female outcomes). The following databases were screened from 1989 to June 2020:

- CINAHL
- MEDLINE (NHS Evidence)
- Cochrane
- AMed
- EMBASE
- PsychINFO
- SCOPUS
- Web of Science

In addition, searches using Medical Subject Headings (MeSH) and keywords were conducted using Cochrane databases. Two UK-based experts in bladder cancer were consulted to identify any additional studies.

Studies were eligible for inclusion if they reported primary research focusing on muscle invasive bladder cancer and nerve sparing. Papers were included if published after 1984 and had to be in English. Studies that did not conform to this were excluded. Due to the paucity of studies, all study types were included, including case series and case reports (Fig. 38.1).

Abstracts were independently screened for eligibility by two reviewers and disagreements resolved through discussion or third party opinion. Agreement level was calculated using Cohen's Kappa to test the intercoder reliability of this screening

S. S. Goonewardene et al., *Management of Muscle Invasive Bladder Cancer*,
Management of Urology, https://doi.org/10.1007/978-3-030-57915-9_38

process. Cohens' Kappa allows comparison of inter-rater reliability between papers using relative observed agreement. This also takes account of the comparison occurring by chance. The first reviewer agreed all 19 papers to be included, the second, agreed on 19.

Data extraction was piloted by the researcher and amended in consultation with the research team (author and two academic supervisors). Data collected included authors, year and country of publication, study aims, setting, intervention aims, number of participants, study design, intervention components and delivery methods, comparison groups and outcome measures, notes and follow-up questions for the authors. Studies were quality assessed using the PRISMA criteria for randomised controlled trials, Mays et al. [1, 2] for the action research and qualitative studies and the Critical Skills Appraisal programme for cohort studies. This was also applied to randomised controlled trials and qualitative studies.

The search identified 300 papers (Fig. 38.1). Nineteen mapped to the search terms and eligibility criteria. The current systematic reviews were examined to gain further knowledge about the subject. Two hundred and eighty papers were excluded due to not conforming to eligibility criteria or adding to the evidence. Of the 19 papers left, relevant abstracts were identified and the full papers obtained (all of which were in English), to quality assure against search criteria. There was considerable heterogeneity of design among the included studies therefore a narrative review of the evidence was undertaken. There was significant heterogeneity within studies, including clinical topic, numbers, outcomes, as a result a narrative review was thought to be best. There were 20 cohort studies, with a moderate level of evidence. These were from a range of countries with minimal loss to follow-up. All participants were identified appropriately.

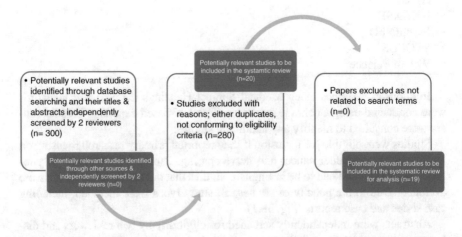

Fig. 38.1 Flow chart of studies identified through the systematic review. (Adapted from PRISMA)

38.2   Prognostic Factors in Female Bladder Cancer

Paulou evaluated prognostic factors after adjuvant intravesical BCG immunotherapy in T1G3 NMIBC and long-term follow-up [3]. Sixty-five patients (44.5%) had recurrence, 25 patients (17.1%) had progression, and 18 patients (12.3%) died because of bladder cancer [3]. Female gender and presence of CIS in the prostatic urethra were associated with an increased risk of recurrence (p = 0.0003, HR: 2.53), progression (p = 0.001, HR: 3.59), and death due to bladder cancer (p = 0.004, HR: 3.53) [3].

The impact of gender on the staging and prognosis of urothelial carcinoma of the bladder (UCB) is insufficiently understood [4]. Female patients were older at the time of RC (p = 0.033) and had higher rates of pathologic stage T3/T4 disease (p < 0.001) [4]. In univariable, but not in multivariable analysis, female gender was associated with a higher risk of DR (p = 0.022 and p = 0.11, respectively) [4]. Female gender was an independent predictor for CSM (p = 0.004) [4]. Kluth did not find a significant interaction between gender and stage, nodal metastasis, or LVI (all p values >0.05) [4].

Dabi confirm gender specific differences in pathologic factors and survival rates of urothelial bladder cancer patients treated with radical cystectomy [5]. As part of a retrospective study 701 patients were treated with radical cystectomy and pelvic lymphadenectomy [5].

Dabi collected data on 553 males (78.9%) and 148 females (21.1%) [5]. One hundred and sixty-three patients (23.3%) had recurrence of their tumour and 127 (18.1%) died from their disease [5]. In multivariable Cox regression analyses, female gender was independently associated with disease recurrence (RR: 1.73; 95% CI 1.22–2.47; p = 0.02) and cancer-specific mortality (RR = 2.50, 95% CI = 1.71–3.68; p < 0.001). Dabi confirmed female gender to be an independent negative prognosis factor for patients following a radical cystectomy and lymphadenectomy for an invasive muscle bladder cancer [5].

Soave analysed gender-specific outcomes in a homogenous, contemporary radical cystectomy (RC) cohort [6]. Compared to men, women were more likely to have advanced tumour stages (p = 0.017), nodal metastasis (p = 0.047) and received more frequently adjuvant chemotherapy (p = 0.009) [6]. There was no statistical difference in disease recurrence, cancer-specific mortality and overall survival between the genders [6]. In stage-adjusted analyses, only women with non-invasive UCB were more likely to die of UCB compared to the male counterparts (p = 0.013) [6]. In gender-specific multivariable analyses that adjusted for standard clinicopathologic features, pathologic tumour stage was an independent predictor for disease recurrence (p-values ≤0.047) and cancer-specific mortality (p-values ≤0.049), respectively [6].

38.3   Postoperative Complications in Female Gender for Cystectomy

Abdi evaluated if female sex is associated with postoperative SSI and if experiencing an SSI was associated with subsequent adverse events [7]. The primary outcome was development of a SSI (superficial, deep, or organ/abdominal space) within 30 days of surgery [7]. A total of 9275 radical cystectomy patients met the inclusion criteria. SSI occurred in 1277 (13.7%) patients, 308 (16.4%) females and 969 (13.1%) males (odds ratio = 1.27; 95% confidence interval 1.10–1.47; p = 0.009) [7]. Infections were superficial in 150 (8.0%) females versus 410 (5.5%) males (p < 0.0001), deep in 40 (2.1%) females versus 114 (1.5%) males (p = 0.07), and organ/abdominal space in 118 (6.2%) females versus 445 (6.0%) males (p = 0.66) [7]. On multivariable analysis, female sex was independently associated with SSI (odds ratio = 1.21 confidence interval 1.01–1.43 p = 0.03) [7]. Females who experience SSI had higher probability of developing other complications including wound dehiscence, septic shock, and need for reoperation (all p < 0.05) [7].

Lin presented their experience and results of laparoscopic radical cystectomy (LRC) with orthotopic ileal neobladder in female patients with bladder carcinoma [8]. Postoperative complications included uretero-pouch anastomotic stricture in 1 patient and pouch-vaginal fistula in 1 patient [8]. One patient had occasional daytime urinary incontinence and 2 had night-time incontinence [8]. Two patients who had undergone hysterectomy and ovariectomy had voiding difficulties after 1 year, which was treated by intermittent self-catheterization [8]. Surgical margins were tumor free for all patients [8]. One patient had bone metastasis and died 11 months after the operation [8].

38.4   Survival Outcomes in Female Bladder Cancer

Keck assessed female gender as a possible prognostic factor in bladder cancer treated with transurethral resection (TURBT) and radio- (RT) or radiochemotherapy (RCT) [9]. After a follow-up of 5 years, female sex demonstrated a hazard ratio (HR) of 1.79 (95% CI 1.24–2.57) for OS; for CSS, the HR was 2.4 (95% CI 1.52–3.80) [9]. Sex was an adverse prognosticator of both OS and CSS independent from age at diagnosis, cT stage, grading, concurrent cis, LVI, focality, therapy response, resection status and therapy mode [9]. Kaplan-Meier analysis showed significantly reduced OS of women compared with men, with a median survival of 2.3 years for female patients and 5.1 years for male patients (p = 0.045, log-rank test) [9]. The estimated median CSS was 7.1 years for female patients and 12.7 years for male patients (p = 0.11, log-rank test) [9].

Anreassen assessed gender-specific differences in survival [10]. Risk rates were significantly higher for women than men, particularly for muscle-invasive cancers [10]. Thereafter, risk rates appeared to be higher in men [10]. Adverse T-Stage distribution in women explained half of the unfavourable survival difference in female patients 2 years after diagnosis [10].

May assessed the impact of detailed clinical and histopathological criteria on gender-dependent cancer-specific survival (CSS) in a large consecutive series of patients following radical cystectomy (RCE) for muscle-invasive bladder cancer (MIBC) [11]. Among clinical and histopathological parameters, only type of urinary diversion differed between men and women [11]. In univariable analysis, CSS did not differ between genders [11]. In multivariable Cox-regression analysis, advanced pT-stage (HR = 2.12; p < 0.001), lymphovascular invasion (LVI) (HR = 3.47; p < 0.001), time interval between diagnosis of MIBC and RCE exceeding 90 days (HR = 2.07; p < 0.001) and female gender (HR = 1.35; p = 0.048) were related to reduced CSS [11]. In separate multivariable Cox-models for time period of surgery, age ≤55 years (HR = 3.00; p = 0.022), presence of LVI (HR = 1.45; p = 0.031) and female gender were associated with independent reduced CSS [11].

Fifty-nine cases of bladder cancer were reviewed retrospectively [12]. Women had lower odds of being diagnosed with superficial disease (OR = 0.24, 95% CI, 0.06–0.94) and a higher incidence of a cancer-specific death (OR = 2.7, 95% CI) [12]. The poor outcome and high incidence of bladder cancer cases among women is intriguing [12]. Overall, primary care utilization, comorbidities, and social factors did not seem to influence stage or death as an outcome [12]. The significantly elevated prevalence of smoking among women in this community, increased age at diagnosis, and possible environmental influences may play a role [12].

Heberling investigated a large single center sample with long-term follow-up in order to determine the relationship between gender and outcome [13]. Female patients were older, healthier, less frequently current smokers and had more extravesical tumours [13]. In the multivariate analyses, female gender was an independent predictor of (lower) non-bladder cancer (competing) mortality (hazards ratio [HR] 0.68, 95% CI 0.49–0.95, p = 0.0248) but no predictor of bladder cancer-specific mortality (HR in the full model 1.20, 95% CI 0.94–1.54, p = 0.15) [13]. Gender was no predictor of the receipt of adjuvant cisplatin-based chemotherapy [13].

Messer determined the association of gender with outcome after radical cystectomy for patients with bladder cancer [14]. The study comprised 4296 patients, including 890 women (21%) [14]. The median follow-up duration was 31.5 months for all patients. Disease recurred in 1430 patients (33.9%) (36.8% of women and 33.1% of men) at a median of 11 months after surgery [14]. Death from any cause was observed in 46.0% of men and 50.1% of women [14]. Cancer-specific death was observed in 33.0% of women and 27.2% of men [14]. Multivariable regression with competing risk found that female gender was associated with an increased risk for disease recurrence and cancer-specific mortality (hazard ratio, 1.27; 95% confidence interval, 1.108–1.465; p = 0.007) compared with male gender [14]. Important limitations include the inability to account for additional potential confounders, such as differences in environmental exposures, treatment selection, and histologic subtypes between men and women [14].

38.5   Urethral Sparing Cystectomy

Stenzl reviewed experience in urethra-sparing cystectomy in women undergoing subsequent orthotopic lower-urinary-tract reconstruction with regard to the anatomy of the remnant urethra, patient selection, refinements of the surgical technique, the patients' outcome with respect to the underlying disease, the risk for tumour recurrence, and postoperative urodynamics [15]. Thirty carefully selected female patients underwent orthotopic reconstruction of the lower urinary tract [15]. Surgical variations emerging from the first learning curve, including nerve-sparing anterior exenteration, vaginal reconstruction, omental support of the neobladder floor, and ureterointestinal anastomosis, were applied in 21 patients with lower-urinary-tract reconstruction [15]. Of 24 patients followed for more than 6 months, 21 (87.5%) are continent at daytime, 19 (79%) have nocturnal continence, and only 1 (4%) requires self-catheterization; 3 patients with urinary retention were successfully treated for obstructed ileal valves [15]. After a follow-up period of 2–41 (mean 15.4) months one patient each developed local recurrence (uterine adenosarcoma) after 13 months and distant metastasis transitional-cell cancer of the bladder after 3 months; all other patients are currently free of disease [15]. Urethra-sparing surgery has established itself in selected women with bladder cancer [15]. Refinements in the technique of radical cystectomy and orthotopic creation of a neobladder to the urethra may improve the continence, spontaneous micturition, and surgical oncological outcome of these patients [15].

38.6   Survival Outcomes in T4 Bladder Cancer in Females

Kaushik evaluated the association of gender with survival following radical cystectomy (RC) for patients with pT4 bladder cancer [16]. A total of 7 women and 30 men with pT4 tumour received perioperative chemotherapy [16]. Twenty seven patients experienced local recurrence (LR) and 120 died, including 90 who died from bladder cancer [16]. Women with pT4 tumour trended to have higher 5-year recurrence-free survival (72% vs. 59%; p = 0.83), cancer-specific survival (31% vs. 17%; p = 0.50), and overall survival (19% vs. 11%; p = 0.33), although these differences did not reach statistical significance [16]. On multivariate analysis, moreover, gender was not significantly associated with LR (HR 0.96; p = 0.93), cancer-specific mortality (HR 1.05; p = 0.87), or all-cause mortality (ACM) (HR 1.14; p = 0.58) [16]. Poor ECOG performance status and pN+ disease were associated with an increased risk of ACM, while removal of a greater number of lymph nodes was associated with decreased ACM [16].

38.7   Health Related Quality of Life in Female Patients Post Radical Cystectomy

Siracusano evaluated bladder-specific long-term HR-QoL after radical cystectomy and ileal conduit [17]. Siracusano demonstrated women who underwent IC presented greater problems than men in cognitive functioning as well in future perspective [17]. Nevertheless, men undergoing IC had more problems in sexual functioning than women (all $p < 0.05$) [17]. Female patients presented a greater burden than male patients in cognitive functioning as well in future perspective, but lower concerns with regard to sexual function [17].

Zahran evaluated HRQOL in women after RC and orthotopic neobladder (ONB) versus ileal loop conduit (IC) and to assess the impact of urinary continence [18]. ONB group included 22 continent women, 35 with NI and 27 in CUR and on CIC [18]. There were no statistically significant differences between ONB and IC groups in all domains of the two questionnaires [18]. However, continent women showed statistically significant better most of EORTC-QLQ-C30 scales and emotional well-being, functional well-being, bladder cancer subscale and FACT-Bl total Score ($p < 0.05$) than IC group [18]. Similarly, women in CUR showed statistically significant better global health and physical functioning EORTC-QLQ-C30 scores (p values = 0.0001, 0.01) and all domains of FACT-Bl [18]. On the other hand, women with NI showed statistically significant lower values in all domains of the EORTC-QLQ-C30 and FACT-Bl than IC group [18].

38.8   Urethral Recurrence in Female Bladder Cancer

Hrbáček reviewed urethral recurrence (UR) after radical cystectomy (RC) for muscle-invasivebladder cancer with orthotopic neobladder in women have rarely been addressed in the literature [20]. The primary bladder tumours in the 12 patients were urothelial carcinoma in 8 patients, squamous cell carcinoma and adenocarcinoma in 1 patient each, and mixed histology in 2 patients [20]. Three patients (25%) had lymph node-positive disease at RC [20]. The median time from RC to the detection of UR was 8 months (range 4–55) [20]. Eight recurrences manifested with clinical symptoms and 4 were detected during follow-up or during a diagnostic work-up for clinical symptoms caused by distant metastases [20]. Treatment modalities were surgery, chemotherapy, radiotherapy, and bacillus Calmette-Guérin urethral instillations[20]. Nine patients died of cancer. The median survival after the diagnosis of UR was 6 months [20].

38.9   Female Sexual Dysfunction After Radical Cystectomy and Neobladder Construction

Bhatt focused on the impact of neurovascular preservation after radical cystectomy and neobladder construction [19]. Bhatt assessed female sexuality in 13 patients after orthotopic cystectomy using a standardized questionnaire, Female Sexual Function Index (FSFI). Six patients had undergone nerve-sparing cystectomy and seven had undergone contemporary non-nerve-sparing cystectomy [19]. In the nerve-sparing group (mean age 55.9 years), the baseline and 12-month postoperative scores showed a minimal decline in results, with a total mean FSFI score of 24.5 versus 22.3, respectively [19]. In analysing each of the six domains, no significant decline or difference was observed [19]. Conversely, in the non-nerve-sparing group (mean age 56.7 years), a significant decline or difference was found in the 12-month total mean FSFI scores between the baseline and postoperative FSFI scores (25.0 versus 11.0, respectively) [19]. In the non-nerve-sparing group, 6 of 7 patients ultimately discontinued sexual intercourse [19].

38.10   Reviews Related to the Systematic Review

Urethra-sparing cystectomy in women and orthotopic urinary diversion can be performed safely in appropriately selected women with invasive bladder cancer [21]. Excellent oncological outcomes can be expected with a minimal risk of urethral recurrence in case of negative frozen section of the proximal urethra [21]. Orthotopic neobladder diversion offers excellent clinical and functional results, and should be the diversion of choice in most women following cystectomy [21]. Female sexual dysfunction can be avoided in patients who received neurovascular preservation, although quality of life declined in women who had undergone non-nerve-sparing radical cystectomy [21].

Extensive knowledge about pelvic anatomy and nerve-sparing surgical techniques in men is well understood from studies about prostate anatomy and nerve-sparing prostatectomy [22]. However, anatomical and surgical details of sexual-sparing RC in women needs further characterization [22]. Several questionnaires are used to investigate sexuality after RC, but a standardized approach is still missing [22]. Therapeutic options are available to treat sexual dysfunction, but limited studies have been conducted to specifically address the post-RC population [22].

Zahran evaluated the impact of radical cystectomy and urinary diversion on female sexual function [23]. From the resulting 117 articles, 11 studies were finally included in the systematic review, with a total of 361 women [23]. Loss of sexual desire and orgasm disorders were the most frequently reported (49% and 39%) [23]. Dyspareunia and vaginal lubrication disorders were reported in 25% and 9.5%, respectively [23]. The incidence of sexual dysfunction was 10% in 30 patients receiving genital- or nerve-sparing cystectomy vs. 59% receiving conventional cystectomy [23].

Liu performed a first meta-analysis on the association between female gender and cancer-specific death risk after radical cystectomy [24]. A total of 17 studies were included in the meta-analysis with a total population of 27,912 patients [24]. Female gender was associated with a worse survival outcome (pooled HR 1.20; 95% CI 1.09–1.32) compared with male gender after radical cystectomy [24]. Subgroup analysis found the correlation was significant in North American and European studies (HR 1.17, 95% CI 1.02–1.32 and HR 1.34, 95% CI 1.19–1.51, respectively) and studies from larger size of samples (HR 1.24, 95% CI 1.11–1.38) [24].

Surgical techniques to spare female reproductive organs at the time of radical cystectomy [reproductive organ-sparing radical cystectomy (ROSRC)] improve quality of life regarding sexual and urinary function [25]. The literature provides small cohorts with intermediate-term follow-up to support oncologic safety, and thus ROSRC must continue to be evaluated with long-term studies [25]. Pertinent techniques for ROSRC are described based on underlying anatomic principles [25]. Lastly, studies on the potential sexual and urinary functional advantages are promising, but must be evaluated in light of the excellent baseline functional characteristics of those selected for inclusion [25]. ROSRC appears to provide measurable benefits to sexual and urinary function. However, the magnitude of these benefits is unclear and the selection of appropriate candidates requires further prospective study vis-a-vis oncologic control. ROSRC must be adopted cautiously until further data are available [25].

References

1. Moher D, Liberati A, Tetzlaff J, Altman DG. "Preferred Reporting Items for Systematic Reviews and Meta-Analyses: The Prisma Statement." [In English]. BMJ (Online) 339, no. 7716 (08 Aug 2009):332–36.
2. Mays N, Pope C, Popay J. "Systematically Reviewing Qualitative and Quantitative Evidence to Inform Management and Policy-Making in the Health Field." [In English]. Journal of Health Services Research and Policy 10, no. SUPPL. 1 (July 2005):6–20.
3. Palou J, Sylvester RJ, Faba OR, Parada R, Peña JA, Algaba F, Villavicencio H. Female gender and carcinoma in situ in the prostatic urethra are prognostic factors for recurrence, progression, and disease-specific mortality in T1G3 bladder cancer patients treated with bacillus Calmette-Guérin. Eur Urol. 2012;62(1):118–25.
4. Kluth LA, Rieken M, Xylinas E, Kent M, Rink M, Rouprêt M, Sharifi N, Jamzadeh A, Kassouf W, Kaushik D, Boorjian SA, Roghmann F, Noldus J, Masson-Lecomte A, Vordos D, Ikeda M, Matsumoto K, Hagiwara M, Kikuchi E, Fradet Y, Izawa J, Rendon R, Fairey A, Lotan Y, Bachmann A, Zerbib M, Fisch M, Scherr DS, Vickers A, Shariat SF. Gender-specific differences in clinicopathologic outcomes following radical cystectomy: an international multi-institutional study of more than 8000 patients. Eur Urol. 2014;66(5):913–9.
5. Dabi Y, Rouscoff Y, Delongchamps NB, Sibony M, Saighi D, Zerbib M, Peyraumore M, Xylinas E. Negative prognostic impact of female gender on oncological outcomes following radical cystectomy. Prog Urol. 2016;26(2):83–8.
6. Soave A, Dahlem R, Hansen J, Weisbach L, Minner S, Engel O, Kluth LA, Chun FK, Shariat SF, Fisch M, Rink M. Gender-specific outcomes of bladder cancer patients: a stage-specific analysis in a contemporary, homogenous radical cystectomy cohort. Eur J Surg Oncol. 2015;41(3):368–77.
7. Abdi H, Elzayat E, Cagiannos I, Lavallée LT, Cnossen S, Flaman AS, Mallick R, Morash C, Breau RH. Female radical cystectomy patients have a higher risk of surgical site infections. Urol Oncol. 2018;36(9):400.e1–5.

8. Lin TX, Zhang CX, Xu KW, Huang H, Jiang C, Han JL, Yao YS, Guo ZH, Xie WL, Yin XB, Huang J. Laparoscopic radical cystectomy with orthotopic ileal neobladder in the female: report of 14 cases. Chin Med J. 2008;121(10):923–6.

9. Keck B, Ott OJ, Häberle L, Kunath F, Weiss C, Rödel C, Sauer R, Fietkau R, Wullich B, Krause FS. Female sex is an independent risk factor for reduced overall survival in bladder cancer patients treated by transurethral resection and radio- or radiochemotherapy. World J Urol. 2013;31(5):1023–8.

10. Andreassen BK, Grimsrud TK, Haug ES. Bladder cancer survival: women better off in the long run. Eur J Cancer. 2018;95:52–8.

11. May M, Stief C, Brookman-May S, Otto W, Gilfrich C, Roigas J, Zacharias M, Wieland WF, Fritsche HM, Hofstädter F, Burger M. Gender-dependent cancer-specific survival following radical cystectomy. World J Urol. 2012;30(5):707–13.

12. Hoke GP, Stone BA, Klein L, Williams KN. The influence of gender on incidence and outcome of patients with bladder cancer in Harlem. J Natl Med Assoc. 1999;91(3):144–8.

13. Heberling U, Koch R, Hübler M, Baretton GB, Hakenberg OW, Wirth MP, Froehner M. Gender and mortality after radical cystectomy: competing risk analysis. Urol Int. 2018;101(3):293–9.

14. Messer JC, Shariat SF, Dinney CP, Novara G, Fradet Y, Kassouf W, Karakiewicz PI, Fritsche HM, Izawa J, Lotan Y, Skinner EC, Tilki D, Ficarra V, Volkmer BG, Isbarn H, Wei C, Lerner SP, Curiel TJ, Kamat AM, Svatek RS. Female gender is associated with a worse survival after radical cystectomy for urothelial carcinoma of the bladder: a competing risk analysis. Urology. 2014;83(4):863–7.

15. Stenzl A, Colleselli K, Bartsch G. Update of urethra-sparing approaches in cystectomy in women. World J Urol. 1997;15(2):134–8.

16. Kaushik D, Frank I, Eisenberg MS, Cheville JC, Tarrell R, Thapa P, Thompson RH, Boorjian SA. Gender-specific survival following radical cystectomy for pT4 bladder cancer. World J Urol. 2014;32(6):1433–9.

17. Siracusano S, D'Elia C, Cerruto MA, Saleh O, Serni S, Gacci M, Ciciliato S, Simonato A, Porcaro A, De Marco V, Talamini R, Toffoli L, Visalli F, Niero M, Lonardi C, Imbimbo C, Verze P, Mirone V, Racioppi M, Iafrate M, Cacciamani G, Marchi D, Bassi P, Artibani W. Quality of life in patients with bladder Cancer undergoing ileal conduit: a comparison of women *versus* men. In Vivo. 2018;32(1):139–43.

18. Zahran MH, Taha DE, Harraz AM, Zidan EM, El-Bilsha MA, Tharwat M, El Hefnawy AS, Ali-El-Dein B. Health related quality of life after radical cystectomy in women: orthotopic neobladder versus ileal loop conduit and impact of incontinence. Minerva Urol Nefrol. 2017;69(3):262–70.

19. Bhatt A, Nandipati K, Dhar N, Ulchaker J, Jones S, Rackley R, Zippe C. Neurovascular preservation in orthotopic cystectomy: impact on female sexual function. Urology. 2006 Apr;67(4):742–5. https://doi.org/10.1016/j.urology.2005.10.015. Epub 2006 Mar 29. PMID: 16566975.

20. Hrbáček J, Macek P, Ali-El-Dein B, Thalmann GN, Stenzl A, Babjuk M, Shaaban AA, Gakis G. Treatment and outcomes of urethral recurrence of urinary bladder cancer in women after radical cystectomy and orthotopic neobladder: a series of 12 cases. Urol Int. 2015;94(1):45–9.

21. Kübler H, Gschwend JE. Ileal neobladder in women with bladder cancer: cancer control and functional aspects. Curr Opin Urol. 2011;21(6):478–82.

22. Pederzoli F, Campbell JD, Matsui H, Sopko NA, Bivalacqua TJ. Surgical factors associated with male and female sexual dysfunction after radical cystectomy: what do we know and how can we improve outcomes? Sex Med Rev. 2018;6(3):469–81.

23. Zahran MH, Fahmy O, El-Hefnawy AS, Ali-El-Dein B. Female sexual dysfunction post radical cystectomy and urinary diversion. Climacteric. 2016;19(6):546–50.

24. Liu S, Yang T, Na R, Hu M, Zhang L, Fu Y, Jiang H, Ding Q. The impact of female gender on bladder cancer-specific death risk after radical cystectomy: a meta-analysis of 27,912 patients. Int Urol Nephrol. 2015;47(6):951–8.

25. Niver BE, Daneshmand S, Satkunasivam R. Female reproductive organ-sparing radical cystectomy: contemporary indications, techniques and outcomes. Curr Opin Urol. 2015;25(2):105–10.

Part VII

Radical Radiotherapy

MIBC Radical Radiotherapy

39

39.1   Research Methods

A systematic review relating to muscle invasive bladder cancer and nerve sparing cystoprostatectomy was conducted. This was to identify whether radical cystectomy has a role in this cohort. The search strategy aimed to identify all references related to bladder cancer AND muscle invasive disease AND radical radiotherapy. Search terms used were as follows: (Bladder cancer) AND (muscle invasive disease) AND (radical radiotherapy). The following databases were screened from 1989 to June 2020:

- CINAHL
- MEDLINE (NHS Evidence)
- Cochrane
- AMed
- EMBASE
- PsychINFO
- SCOPUS
- Web of Science

In addition, searches using Medical Subject Headings (MeSH) and keywords were conducted using Cochrane databases. Two UK-based experts in bladder cancer were consulted to identify any additional studies.

Studies were eligible for inclusion if they reported primary research focusing on muscle invasive bladder cancer and nerve sparing. Papers were included if published after 1984 and had to be in English. Studies that did not conform to this were excluded. Only primary research was included (Fig. 39.1).

Abstracts were independently screened for eligibility by two reviewers and disagreements resolved through discussion or third party opinion. Agreement level was calculated using Cohen's Kappa to test the intercoder reliability of this screening

© The Editor(s) (if applicable) and The Author(s), under exclusive license to
Springer Nature Switzerland AG 2021
S. S. Goonewardene et al., *Management of Muscle Invasive Bladder Cancer*,
Management of Urology, https://doi.org/10.1007/978-3-030-57915-9_39

process. Cohens' Kappa allows comparison of inter-rater reliability between papers using relative observed agreement. This also takes account of the comparison occurring by chance. The first reviewer agreed all 15 papers to be included, the second, agreed on 15.

Data extraction was piloted by the researcher and amended in consultation with the research team (author and two academic supervisors). Data collected included authors, year and country of publication, study aims, setting, intervention aims, number of participants, study design, intervention components and delivery methods, comparison groups and outcome measures, notes and follow-up questions for the authors. Studies were quality assessed using the PRISMA criteria for randomised controlled trials, Mays et al. [1, 2] for the action research and qualitative studies and the Critical Skills Appraisal programme for cohort studies. This was also applied to randomised controlled trials and qualitative studies.

The search identified 79 papers (Fig. 39.1). Fifteen mapped to the search terms and eligibility criteria. The current systematic reviews were examined to gain further knowledge about the subject. Seventy-nine papers were excluded due to not conforming to eligibility criteria or adding to the evidence. Of the 15 papers left, relevant abstracts were identified and the full papers obtained (all of which were in English), to quality assure against search criteria. There was considerable heterogeneity of design among the included studies therefore a narrative review of the evidence was undertaken. There was significant heterogeneity within studies, including clinical topic, numbers, outcomes, as a result a narrative review was thought to be best. There were 15 cohort studies, with a moderate level of evidence and two trials with a good level of evidence. These were from a range of countries with minimal loss to follow-up. All participants were identified appropriately.

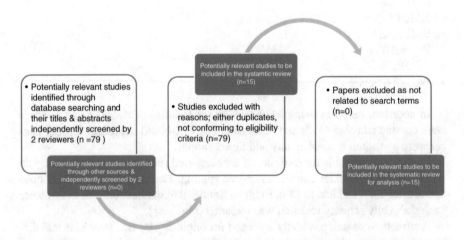

Fig. 39.1 Flow chart of studies identified through the systematic review. (Adapted from PRISMA)

39.2 Overall Survival for Radical Radiotherapy

D'Rummo investigated the association between facility radiotherapy (RT) case volume and overall survival (OS) for patients with MIBC who received bladder-preserving RT, and the relationship with adherence to National Comprehensive Cancer Network (NCCN) guidelines for bladder preservation [3]. There were 7562 patients included [3]. No differences in age, Charlson-Deyo score, T stage, or node-positive rates were observed between groups [3]. HVFs exhibited greater compliance with NCCN guidelines for bladder preservation (p < 0.0001) [3]. Treatment at an HVF was associated with the improved OS for all patients (p = 0.001) and for the subset of patients receiving NCCN-recommended RT doses (p = 0.0081) [3].

Wang explored the effect of radical TURBT combing with concomitant chemoradiotherapy for muscle-invasive bladder cancer (MIBC) [4]. The overall survival (OS) rate of trimodality therapy (TMT) group was 64.3%, cancer specific survival (CSS) rate was 78.6%. And the OS rate of RC group was 66.7%, CSS rate was 82.2% [4]. There was no statistical difference between two groups. The life quality of TMT group was better than that of RC group [4].

Lendínez-Cano reviewed bladder-sparing treatment with TURB ± Chemotherapy + Radiotherapy to selected patients as an alternative [5]. Fourteen patients remained disease free (46.6%), 10 had recurrent non-muscle invasive bladder cancer (33%). 81.3% complete clinical response. Seventy-one percent of bladder preserved at 5-years [5]. Overall, 5-years survival rate was 79% and 85% cancer-specific survival rate [5].

39.3 Chemoradiation vs. Radical Cystectomy for MIBC

Ritch compared survival outcome between chemoradiation therapy (CRT) and radical cystectomy (RC) for muscle-invasive bladder cancer (MIBC) [6]. In all, 8379 (6606 RC and 1773 CRT) patients met the inclusion criteria and 1683 patients in each group were propensity matched [6]. On multivariable extended Cox analysis, significant predictors of decreased OS were age, Charlson-Deyo Comorbidity score of 1, Charlson-Deyo Comorbidity score of 2, stage cT3-4, and urothelial histology [6]. CRT was associated with decreased mortality at year 1 (hazard ratio [HR] 0.84, 95% confidence interval [CI] 0.74–0.96; p = 0.01), but at 2 years (HR 1.4, 95% CI 1.2–1.6; p < 0.001) and 3 years onward (HR 1.5, 95% CI 1.2–1.8; p < 0.001) CRT was associated with increased mortality [6]. The 5-year OS was greater for RC than for CRT (38% vs. 30%, p = 0.004) [6].

39.4 Trimodal Therapy vs. Cystectomy

Kim compared the clinical outcomes between RC and trimodal therapy (TMT) using propensity score matching with 50 patients in the RC arm and 29 patients in the TMT arm [7]. With respective median follow-up periods of 23 and 32 months for the RC and TMT groups, 5-year distant metastasis-free survival (58% vs. 67%), overall survival (56% vs. 57%), and cancer-specific survival (69% *vs.* 63%) rates between the RC and TMT groups, respectively, were similar [7]. However, the 5-year local recurrence-free survival was significantly better in the RC group than in the TMT group (74% *vs.* 35%). Following TMT, acute grade 3 haematological ($n = 2$) and late grade 3 genitourinary ($n = 1$) toxicities were reported [7]. These findings demonstrated that oncological outcomes of TMT were comparable with those of RC, except for poorer local control. Large-scale, randomized trials are warranted to confirm the findings of the present retrospective comparison and to guide toward best treatment options [7].

Gerardi assessed the feasibility, toxicity profile, and tumour outcome of an organ preservation curative approach in non-metastatic muscle-invasive bladder cancer [8]. None of the patients developed severe urinary or intestinal acute toxicity [8]. In 10 patients with a follow-up >6 months, no cases of severe late toxicity were observed [8]. Response evaluated in 12 patients included complete response and stable disease in 11 patients (92%), and one patient (8%), respectively [8]. At the time of data analysis (March 2016), 10 patients (77%) are alive with no evidence of disease, two patients (15%) died for other reasons, and one patient has suspicious persistent local disease [8]. The trimodality approach, including maximal TURBT, radiotherapy, and chemotherapy for muscle-invasive bladder cancer, is well-tolerated and might be considered a valid and feasible option in fit patients who refuse radical cystectomy [8].

Kulkarni compared the oncologic outcomes between patients treated with RC or TMT by using a propensity score matched-cohort analysis [9]. The median age was 68.0 years, and 29.5% had stage cT3/cT4 disease [9]. At a median follow-up of 4.51 years, there were 20 deaths (35.7%) in the RC group (13 as a result of BC) and 22 deaths (39.3%) in the TMT group (13 as a result of BC) [9]. The 5-year DSS rate was 73.2% and 76.6% in the RC and TMT groups, respectively ($p = 0.49$) [9]. Salvage cystectomy was performed in 6 (10.7%) of 56 patients who received TMT [9].

39.5   Radiochemotherapy vs. Radical Cystectomy

Boustani examined both radical cystectomy (RC) and radiochemotherapy (RCT) in elderly patients [10]. Ninety-two patients underwent RC and 72 patients had RCT [10]. Median OS was 1.99 years (95% CI 1.17–2.76) after RC and 1.97 years (95% CI 1.35–2.64) after RCT ($p = 0.73$) [10]. Median progression-free survival (PFS) after RC and RCT were 1.25 years (95% CI 0.80–1.75) and 1.52 years (95% CI 1.01–2.04), respectively ($p = 0.54$) [10]. In multivariate analyses, only disease progression was significantly associated with worse OS (HR = 10.27 (95% CI 6.63–15.91), $p < 0.0001$) [10]. Treatment modality was not a prognostic factor [10].

39.6 Radiochemotherapy in the Elderly

Christodoulou evaluated concurrent radical radiotherapy with gemcitabine radio-sensitisation (GemX) in elderly patients versus bladder carbogen and nicotinamide (BCON) as a phase III trial [11]. Elderly patients had worse performance status (p = 0.020) and co-morbidities (p = 0.030) [11]. A similar proportion of patients received planned dose radiotherapy in both groups (p = 0.260), although fewer elderly patients received all four cycles of concurrent chemotherapy (p = 0.017) due to toxicity [11]. For OS, age had some prognostic power; HR 1.04 (95% CI 1.00–1.08; p = 0.068) [11]. Overall survival and LPFS in elderly patients were comparable between CON and GemX (HR 1.13, 95% CI 0.69–1.85; p = 0.616 and HR 0.85, 95% CI 0.41–1.74; p = 0.659 respectively) [11].

Varughese examined contemporary UK radiotherapy practice for the management of muscle invasive bladder cancer (MIBC) against published national guidance [12]. Sixty-nine percent (41/59) of UK radiotherapy centres completed a detailed questionnaire for 508 patients [12]. The median age was 78 years and 64% (n = 323 patients) had stage II or III disease [12]. Treatment intent was radical in 54% (n = 275). From transurethral resection of the bladder tumour, patients waited 57 days before starting neoadjuvant chemotherapy (NAC) (interquartile range 46–72 days) [12]. Patients who had radical radiotherapy as their first definitive treatment waited a median of 82 days (interquartile range 62–105 days) [12]. NAC was considered in 66% (n = 182) of all radical cases and given in 43% (n = 119) [12]. Concurrent radiosensitisation (CRT) was considered for 53% (n = 146) and delivered in 40% (n = 109) of patients [12]. The most common fractionation was 55 Gy/20 fractions/4 weeks in 49% (n = 134) for radical patients and 36 Gy/6 fractions/6 weeks in 25% (n = 57) for palliative patients [12].

Maebayashi examined whether the feasibility of concurrent use of intra-arterial chemotherapy (IAC) can be assessed using both treatment results of RT for MIBC in elderly patients and the G8 Screening Tool [13]. The overall median G8 score was 12 (range = 9–15), with scores of 13 (range = 12–15) in the IACRT group and 10 (range = 9–11) in the RT-alone group [13]. The G8 score was 12 or more in all patients in the IACRT group. The 2- and 5-year overall survival rates were 80% and 66.7% in the IACRT group [13]. The 1- and 2-year survival rates in the RT-alone group were 50% and 25%, respectively. Regarding late adverse events, only one patient experienced grade 2 genitourinary toxicity [13].

Wujanto reviewed the outcomes of older patients treated with RT with or without concurrent chemotherapy (CRT) [14]. The 2- and 5-year OS was 64% and 44%, respectively [14]. The 2- and 5-year RFS was 68% and 49%, respectively [14]. Median RFS was 34 months (range 8–121 months) [14]. Univariate analysis showed that performance status (0–1 vs. 2–3; HR 2.7, 95% CI 1.07–6.8, p = 0.035) and International Society of Geriatric Oncology (SIOG) group (≤2 vs. >2; HR 3.23, 95% CI 1.12–8.64, p = 0.019) were significantly associated with increased hazard for death [14]. One patient (2%) had grade 3 cystitis [14].

39.7   GU Toxicity from Radical Radiotherapy

Nowak-Sadzikowska evaluated the clinical outcome and toxicity of the treatment of muscle-invasive bladder cancer (MIBC) that combined transurethral resection of bladder tumour (TURB) with "concomitant boost" radiotherapy delivered over a shortened overall treatment time of 5 weeks, with or without concurrent chemotherapy [15]. Acute genitourinary toxicity of G3 was scored in 3/73 (4%) patients [15]. Late gastrointestinal toxicity higher than G2 and genitourinary higher than G3 were not reported [15]. Complete remission was achieved in 48/73 (66%), partial remission in 17/73 (23%), and stabilization disease in 8/73 (11%) patients [15]. Three- and five-year overall, disease specific and invasive locoregional disease-free survival rates were 65% and 52%, 70% and 59%, 52% and 43%, respectively [15].

McPherson evaluated TURBT and chemoradiotherapy without salvage cystectomy in medically inoperable octogenarian patients [16]. Mean overall survival (OS) was 20.7 months (IQR 12.75–23.25), while mean recurrence-free survival (RFS) was 13.75 months (IQR 3.75–16.5) [16]. Patients receiving HD radiotherapy showed improved OS and local RFS (LRFS) without significant differences in Grade 3–4 toxicities [16]. Univariate Cox regression identified hydronephrosis as a predictor of worse OS and local recurrence and HD radiotherapy as a predictor of improved OS and local recurrence rates [16].

39.8   Grey Matter

Fonteyne reported on overall survival (OS), cancer specific survival (CSS), and morbidity after curative treatment in elderly patients, defined as age >70 year, with nonmetastatic MIBC and to compare this with the outcome of younger MIBC patients [17]. Forty-two articles were retrieved for review [17]. No article directly addressed the use of geriatric assessment [17]. OS and CSS worsen significantly with age both after radical cystectomy and radiotherapy regimens [17]. While POM significantly increases with age, morbidity seems comparable between younger and older patients [17].

McAlpine evaluated the efficacy and safety of radiotherapy preoperatively or postoperatively for patients with MIBC receiving cystectomy compared to cystectomy alone [18]. There was a non-statistically significant improvement in overall survival for patients who received neo-adjuvant radiotherapy and cystectomy [18]. At 3 and 5 years, the odds ratios were 1.23 (95% confidence interval [CI] 0.72–2.09) and 1.26 (95% CI 0.76–2.09), respectively, in favour of neoadjuvant radiotherapy [18]. Subgroup analyses including higher doses of radiotherapy showed greater effect on survival [18].

References

1. Moher D, Liberati A, Tetzlaff J, Altman DG. "Preferred Reporting Items for Systematic Reviews and Meta-Analyses: The Prisma Statement." [In English]. BMJ (Online) 339, no. 7716 (08 Aug 2009):332–36.
2. Mays N, Pope C, Popay J. "Systematically Reviewing Qualitative and Quantitative Evidence to Inform Management and Policy-Making in the Health Field." [In English]. Journal of Health Services Research and Policy 10, no. SUPPL. 1 (July 2005):6–20.
3. D'Rummo KA, TenNapel MJ, Shen X. The impact of radiotherapy facility volume on the survival and guideline concordance of patients with muscle-invasive bladder cancer receiving bladder-preservation therapy. Am J Clin Oncol. 2019;42(9):705–10.
4. Wang JF, Zhou XF, Fang DB, Wu ZM, Ding ZS, Chen X, Liu NB. [The effect of tri-modality therapy on the treatment of muscle-invasive bladder cancer]. Zhonghua Yi Xue Za Zhi. 2018;98(20):1614–6.
5. Lendínez-Cano G, Rico-López J, Moreno S, Fernández Parra E, González-Almeida C, Camacho Martínez E. Elective bladder-sparing treatment for muscle invasive bladder cancer. Actas Urol Esp. 2014;38(1):7–13.
6. Ritch CR, Balise R, Prakash NS, Alonzo D, Almengo K, Alameddine M, Venkatramani V, Punnen S, Parekh DJ, Gonzalgo ML. Propensity matched comparative analysis of survival following chemoradiation or radical cystectomy for muscle-invasive bladder cancer. BJU Int. 2018;121(5):745–51.
7. Kim YJ, Byun SJ, Ahn H, Kim CS, Hong BS, Yoo S, Lee JL, Kim YS. Comparison of outcomes between trimodal therapy and radical cystectomy in muscle-invasive bladder cancer: a propensity score matching analysis. Oncotarget. 2017;8(40):68996–9004.
8. Gerardi MA, Jereczek-Fossa BA, Zerini D, Surgo A, Dicuonzo S, Spoto R, Fodor C, Verri E, Rocca MC, Nolè F, Muto M, Ferro M, Musi G, Bottero D, Matei DV, De Cobelli O, Orecchia R. Bladder preservation in non-metastatic muscle-invasive bladder cancer (MIBC): a single-institution experience. Ecancermedicalscience. 2016;10:657.
9. Kulkarni GS, Hermanns T, Wei Y, Bhindi B, Satkunasivam R, Athanasopoulos P, Bostrom PJ, Kuk C, Li K, Templeton AJ, Sridhar SS, van der Kwast TH, Chung P, Bristow RG, Milosevic M, Warde P, Fleshner NE, Jewett MAS, Bashir S, Zlotta AR. Propensity score analysis of radical cystectomy versus bladder-sparing trimodal therapy in the setting of a multidisciplinary bladder cancer clinic. J Clin Oncol. 2017;35(20):2299–305.
10. Boustani J, Bertaut A, Galsky MD, Rosenberg JE, Bellmunt J, Powles T, Recine F, Harshman LC, Chowdhury S, Niegisch G, Yu EY, Pal SK, De Giorgi U, Crabb SJ, Caubet M, Balssa L, Milowsky MI, Ladoire S, Créhange G, Retrospective International Study of Cancers of the Urothelial Tract (RISC) Investigators. Radical cystectomy or bladder preservation with radiochemotherapy in elderly patients with muscle-invasive bladder cancer: Retrospective International Study of Cancers of the Urothelial Tract (RISC) Investigators. Acta Oncol. 2018;57(4):491–7.
11. Christodoulou M, Reeves KJ, Hodgson C, Zeniou A, Slevin F, Kennedy J, Hoskin PJ, Henry A, Choudhury A. Outcomes of radiosensitisation in elderly patients with advanced bladder cancer. Radiother Oncol. 2018;129(3):499–506.
12. Varughese M, Treece S, Drinkwater KJ. Radiotherapy management of muscle invasive bladder cancer: evaluation of a national cohort. Clin Oncol (R Coll Radiol). 2019;31(9):637–45.
13. Maebayashi T, Ishibashi N, Aizawa T, Sakaguchi M, Sato K, Matsui T, Yamaguchi K, Takahashi S. Radiotherapy for muscle-invasive bladder Cancer in very elderly patients. Anticancer Res. 2016;36(9):4763–9.
14. Wujanto C, Tey J, Chia D, Ho F, Ooi KH, Wong AS, Soon YY, Lim K. Radical radiotherapy in older patients with muscle invasive bladder cancer. J Geriatr Oncol. 2019;10(2):292–7.

15. Nowak-Sadzikowska J, Skóra T, Szyszka-Charewicz B, Jakubowicz J. Muscle-invasive bladder cancer treated with TURB followed by concomitant boost with small reduction of radiotherapy field with or without of chemotherapy. Rep Pract Oncol Radiother. 2016;21(1):31–6.

16. McPherson VA, Rodrigues G, Bauman G, Winquist E, Chin J, Izawa J, Potvin K, Ernst S, Venkatesan V, Sexton T, Ahmad B, Power N. Chemoradiotherapy in octogenarians as primary treatment for muscle-invasive bladder cancer. Can Urol Assoc J. 2017;11(1–2):24–30.

17. Fonteyne V, Ost P, Bellmunt J, Droz JP, Mongiat-Artus P, Inman B, Paillaud E, Saad F, Ploussard G. Curative treatment for muscle invasive bladder cancer in elderly patients: a systematic review. Eur Urol. 2018;73(1):40–50.

18. Mcalpine K, Fergusson DA, Breau RH, Reynolds LF, Shorr R, Morgan SC, Eapen L, Cagiannos I, Morash C, Lavallée LT. Radiotherapy with radical cystectomy for bladder cancer: a systematic review and meta-analysis. Can Urol Assoc J. 2018;12(10):351–60.

The Robotic Approach to Redo Surgery

40

Robotic radical cystectomy is a common operation. Ileal conduits are the most commonly performed diversion following radical cystectomy with acceptable morbidity. It also has the lowest reoperation rates as compared to continent diversion. The question arises, if diversion has to be conducted, as redo surgery, is the robotic approach best?

With new robotic platforms, robotic surgery is advancing. Applications of robotic surgery in urology are rapidly expanding. These include single docking abilities and access from the kidney to the prostate without having to change patient position [1]. Emerging robotic platforms are being developed to improve performance of a wider variety of urologic interventions [2]. At the start of any learning curve, the complication rate can be high. Robotics improve safety outcomes and approaches to previously inaccessible areas. Can revision surgery be done safely robotically by the inexperienced surgeon?

Robotic surgery has been used with success for ileal conduit revision with repair of ureteral stenosis. Five trocars can be used for the 4 arms of the Si da Vinci robot in a 4-arm approach. Estimated blood loss was minimal (50 ml) [1]. There were no perioperative complications after this procedure. At 3 months of follow-up, the patient remained complication-free [1]. This demonstrated redo surgery is not an easy procedure due to postoperative adhesions and anatomical distortion. Robotic surgery is precise for dissection of adhesions and robotic suturing [1]. Re-do surgery using a robot, which is a complicated procedure is the way forward.

Application of robotic surgery has also been used to manage a robotic cystectomy with conduit diversion [3]. A ureteroileal anastomotic stricture was treated robotically. A robotic ureteroileal anastomosis revision was performed through three robotic ports (12, 8, 8 mm) at a new site on the conduit using interrupted sutures with bowel mucosal eversion [3]. There has been no recurrence of stricture after 6 months.

Again, this demonstrates successful use of robotics in complication revision. Even though the learning curve can be difficult for a surgeon, totally intracorporeal

S. S. Goonewardene et al., *Management of Muscle Invasive Bladder Cancer*, Management of Urology, https://doi.org/10.1007/978-3-030-57915-9_40

RARC with intracorporeal neobladder is a complex procedure, but it can be performed safely, with a structured approach, at a high-volume established robotic surgery centre without compromising perioperative and pathological outcomes during the learning curve for surgeons [4, 5].

Postoperative bleeding is a known risk of any surgery. Although this risk is recognized, there is limited characterization of the rate of this occurrence in laparoscopic and robotic surgery [6]. Bleeding requiring re-operation is a recognized rare complication of minimally invasive surgery, even in experienced hands. None of the patients post robotic prostatectomy required transfusion [6]. All reoperations occurred within the first 24 h postoperatively and indications for reoperation included hemodynamic instability in all cases, but this can be conducted robotically with success.

It has been demonstrated that robotic surgery is clearly an advantage technique (easy manoeuvring, comfortable and ergonomic position for the surgeon, 3D visualization and short learning curve) [7]. Robotic revision surgery is a challenging but feasible procedure in well-selected patients. Appropriate trocar and patient positioning is crucial to facilitate this surgery. Adhesiolysis can also be conducted robotically, with the advantage of extended instruments for greater access. This minimally invasive procedure is facilitated by the use of the robotic platform and advances in robotic technology. An experienced robotic team and mentor can impact the learning curve of a new surgeon in the same centre resulting in decreased complication rates [4].

References

1. Merseburger AS, Herrmann TR, Shariat SF, Kyriazis I, Nagele U, Traxer O, Liatsikos EN; European Association of Urology. EAU guidelines on robotic and singlesite surgery in urology. Eur Urol. 2013 Aug;64(2):277–91.
2. Ouzaid I, Diaz E, Autorino R, Samarasekera D, Ganesan V, Stein R, et al. Ileal conduit revision and ureteral stenosis repair: robot assisted laparoscopic technique. J Endourol. 2013;27:A439.
3. Herrell SD, Webster R, Simaan N. Future robotic platforms in urologic surgery: recent developments. Curr Opin Urol. 2014;24(1):118–26.
4. Abaza R. Robotic ureteroileal anastomosis revision. J Endourol. 2009;23:A386.
5. Collins JW, Wiklund NP. Totally intracorporeal robot-assisted radical cystectomy: optimizing total outcomes. BJU Int. 2014;114(3):326–33.
6. Kreshover J, Richstone L, Kavoussi L. Acute bleeding requiring re-operation in minimally invasive urologic surgery. J Endourol. 2014;28:A11.
7. Villavicencio Mavrich H, Esquena S, Palou Redorta J, Gomez Ruciz JJ. Robotic radical prostatectomy: overview of our learning curve [Spanish]. Actas Urologicas Espanolas. 2007;31(6):587–92.

Secondary Pelvic Malignancies and Bladder Cancer

41

There have been a number of articles recently on secondary pelvic malignancies [1]. With the advent of robotic surgery, and new platforms, many changes have come into place. However, what can be done differently to allow improved outcomes?

Robotic radical cystectomy (RARC) is one of the hardest robotic operations a urological surgeon conducts. Robotic surgery has made operations for pelvic oncology considerably better, yet if there is any prior therapy, this makes the operation a lot harder. Techniques for radical cystectomy and reconstruction have evolved over the past 10 years, yet the data for robotic vs. open cystectomy is still lacking [2].

Robot-assisted surgery offers the same results as in open surgery in a minimally invasive fashion with better vision, allowing very meticulous and precise handling [3]. A robot-assisted RARC with total intracorporeal ileal conduit represents a feasible, reproducible and safe operative technique [1]. This was highlighted by Luchey et al., as being important in salvage or secondary pelvic malignancies [1]. Many reconstructive procedures supported by sound evidence [2]. But what are the new advances in robotic surgery, what are the other techniques that can be used to advance robotic radical cystectomy and reconstruction further and minimise poor oncological outcomes?

Evolutions in technique often mean limited incisions. Robotic-assisted laparoscopic radical cystectomy with a modified Pfannenstiel incision has been used successfully [4]. Whilst a completely intracorporeal procedure is a technically difficult and time-consuming procedure, it does allow minimal incisions to be made. Technically, the incision provides good exposure, facilitating reconstruction, can be used for specimen retrieval, and heals better with a cosmetic scar [5]. This has improved patient outcomes as a result. This was also highlighted by Luchey et al., minimal access is a way forward, but as with robotics, precision and meticulous tissue handling also are key [1].

Robotic surgery has also opened up the field for older patients. This cohort are less likely to be treated with radical surgery compared to younger patients [6]. Yet RARC is feasible and safe for older patients. Despite a higher prevalence of

S. S. Goonewardene et al., *Management of Muscle Invasive Bladder Cancer*, Management of Urology, https://doi.org/10.1007/978-3-030-57915-9_41

comorbidities in octogenarians, RARC with ileal conduit can provide similar disease control and survival outcomes with risks of major perioperative morbidity comparable to those in younger patients [6]. Luchey et al. look at secondary malignancies, and whilst the outcomes are not as promising as operating on a virgin abdomen, they are nonetheless promising [1].

This has furthermore become enhanced when dealing with salvage therapy or a secondary surgery. Luchey et al. highlighted how surgical treatment for a secondary pelvic cancer can give less optimistic outcomes [1]. RARC after pelvic radiation is complicated by impaired wound healing potentially predisposing to stricture, wound breakdown, and other late complications [7], yet for salvage therapy good outcomes with robotic techniques can be obtained.

Clearly, one of the factors supporting RARC and good outcomes, is use and development of robotic techniques, clearly highlighted by Luchey et al. [1]. Robotics is here to stay, especially in cases of secondary pelvic malignancy.

References

1. Luchey AM, Lin H-Y, Yue B, Agarwal G, Gilbert SM, Lockhart J, et al. Implications of definitive prostate cancer therapy on soft tissue margins and survival in patients undergoing radical cystectomy for bladder urothelial cancer. J Urol. 2015;194(5):1220–5.
2. Challacombe B, Dasgupta P. Reconstruction of the lower urinary tract by laparoscopic and robotic surgery. Curr Opin Urol. 2007;17(6):390–5.
3. Thuer D, Mottrie A, Buffi N, Koliakos N, De Naeyer G, Carpentier P, et al. Total intracorporeal robot-assisted ileal conduit. Urologe—Ausgabe A. 2011;50:153.
4. Jonsson MN, Schumacher MC, Hosseini A, Adding C, Nilsson A, Carlsson S, et al. Oncological outcome after robot-assisted radical cystectomy with intracorporeal urinary diversion technique. Eur Urol Suppl. 2011;10(2):273–4.
5. Manoharan M, Katkoori D, Kishore TA, Antebie E. Robotic-assisted radical cystectomy and orthotopic ileal neobladder using a modified pfannenstiel incision. Urology. 2011;77(2):491–3.
6. Charles Osterberg E, Ramasamy R, Greenwood E, Dubin J, Ng CK, Lee RK, et al. Robotic radical cystectomy is feasible and safe in the treatment of adequately selected octogenarians. J Urol. 2011;1:e196.
7. Eisenberg M, Dorin R, Bartsch G, Cai J, Miranda G, Skinner E. Cystectomy after high dose pelvic radiation: does type of urinary diversion affect late complications? J Urol. 2010;1:e297.

Robotic Radical Cystectomy: Technical Tips and Tricks

42

Robot-assisted laparoscopic radical cystectomy (RARC) has proven to reduce morbidity after cystectomy [1]. Many centres initially were conducting robot assisted laparoscopic radical cystectomy with extracorporeal urinary diversion [1]. Things have evolved so urinary diversion is being performed intracorporeally along with radical cystectomy [1]. This covers technical tips and tricks that can make one of the most difficult operations in urology easier.

The robotic cystectomy is performed via a six-port transperitoneal approach [2]. To gain access to the peritoneum, a Hassan technique or open technique can be used to obtain intraperitoneal access [3]. A 12-mm camera port is inserted, and pneumoperitoneum is achieved. Three 8-mm robotic ports and a 12-mm assistant port are placed in the "W" configuration under direct visualization [3]. There are minor alterations to this technique, including using hybrid ports. The patient is placed in the steep Trendelenberg position and the robot is docked [2].

A standard approach to the procedure would be to start with bilateral classical lymph node dissection followed by ureter dissection [4]. One of the most important steps of RARC and ileal conduit formation, is adequate mobilisation of the ureters, to avoid tension free anastomosis. In practice, these can be difficult to identify. Each ureter must be mobilized, and the left ureter taken beneath the sigmoid colon [5]. As part of this, frozen section can also be used to confirm the presence of no recurrence of tumor. Each ureter would be spatulated and anastomosis completed over a double-J stent using two running 4-0 Vicryl sutures [5].

The left ureter is mobilised under the descending colon with the aid of the 30° telescope [6]. The third arm positioned on the patient's right side is used to place tension on the ureters caudally telescope [6]. Lateral dissection included identification and clipping of individual branches from internal iliac artery to bladder and identification of endopelvic fascia [4]. Posterior dissection included opening of both peritoneum and denonvilliers fascia [4]. Then both the ureters were clipped and divided followed by ligation of bilateral posterolateral vascular pedicles [4]. The dorsal venous complex is then oversewn and the pressure goes up to 20.

© The Editor(s) (if applicable) and The Author(s), under exclusive license to
Springer Nature Switzerland AG 2021
S. S. Goonewardene et al., *Management of Muscle Invasive Bladder Cancer*,
Management of Urology, https://doi.org/10.1007/978-3-030-57915-9_42

In women, posterior dissection is conducted with the aid of a malleable retractor placed under the cervix [2]. Intraoperatively, a stay suture lifts the uterus [7]. This allows manipulation and precise dissection. The anterior dissection of the bladder is then performed, followed by en-bloc removal of the bladder, urethra, and uterus [3]. After the division of the suspensory ligament of the ovary and the supporting ligaments of the uterus, the ureters are identified and dissected free [8]. The vaginal cuff was then closed using V-lock stitch, and an extended lymph node dissection was performed [7]. This can be a procedure with complications, but with an appropriate multidisciplinary team, these can be reduced.

To mobilise the bladder, lateral dissection of the bladder is performed until the pubic bone and endopelvic fascia are visualized [7]. Both pedicles of the bladder are dissected, clipped and divided [8]. The bladder is detached from the anterior abdominal wall and the endopelvic fascia is opened [8].

To form the ileal conduit, isolation of at least 15 cm of ileum needs to occur [9] if using the extracorporeal technique. With time robotic surgeons are becoming more familiar with intracorporeal urinary diversion especially ileal conduit [10]. As part of this procedure, patients need retroperitoneal transfer of left ureter to the right side, beneath the sigmoid colon [11]. Ileal conduit urinary diversion including isolation of the ileal loop and bilateral stented uretero-ileal anastomosis in end to side fashion and restoration of bowel continuity, should all be performed intracorporeally [11].

The ureters are spatulated and joined in side to side Bricker fashion with redundant distal ureter excised [6]. Isolation of the caecum or terminal Ileum is performed with the forceps of the surgical assistant and double fenestrated robotic graspers to prevent bowel injury [6]. The left hand of the assistant and grasper of the robot are used to position the ileum in a side by side fashion to staple together [6]. Two sequential staple are deplounsyed to ensure good bowel patency and is also used to close the open end of the ileum [6]. The ileal staple line is oversewn with a 2-0 vicryl as well as tension reducing stitch is placed at the point of the bowel anastomosis [6].

For the ileal–ureteric reconstruction, the third Robotic arm is again placed on the Infant feeding catheters and caudal traction placed on the ureter [6]. Ureteric–ileal anastomosis (Wallace or Bricker) is performed on the end of the Ileum [6]. The Ureteric anastomosis is placed under the descending colon and peritoneum placed over it to reduce leakage or fistula formation [6]. The distal cutaneous Ileal reconstruction is performed as per open technique and extracted as much as possible via the right Robotic arm site if possible [6].

This procedure is a successfully oncological procedure, however, the outcomes from robotic cystectomy, as an improvement over open remain to be seen.

References

1. Pushkar P, Taneja R, Sharma MK. Total intracorporeal robot-assisted laparoscopic radical cystectomy with ileal conduit (bricker) urinary diversion. Indian J Urol. 2015;31:S102.
2. Alexandrov A, Kassabov B, Buse S. Robot-assisted intracorporeal radical cystectomy, lymph node dissection, and fully intracorporeal ileal conduit reconstruction. Eur Urol Suppl. 2011;10(8):559.
3. Nyame Y, Babbar P, Greene D, Shoshtari HZ, Krishnamurthi V, Haber GP. Robotic anterior pelvic exenteration with intracorporeal ileal conduit in a patient with history of kidney pancreas transplantation. J Urol. 2015;1:e718.
4. Singh P, Dogra PN, Saini A. Robot assisted laparoscopic radical cystectomy: a minimal invasive approach for bladder cancer. Indian J Urol. 2014;30:S55.
5. Carneiro A, Dovirak O, Kaplan J, Chang P, Wagner AA. Robot-assisted ureteroileal reimplantation for post-cystectomy anastomotic stricture. J Urol. 2015;1:e848.
6. Raz O, Arianayagam M, Varol C. Intracorporeal ileal conduit reconstruction following robotic radical cystectomy. Video highlight of technique. BJU Int. 2014;113:141.
7. Ploumidis A, Volpe A, Ficarra V, Mottrie A. Robot-assisted radical cystectomy for female patients. The OLV Vattikuti Robotic Surgery Institute technique. Eur Urol Suppl. 2014;13(1):eV16.
8. Ploumidis A, Gan M, De Naeyer G, Schatteman P, Volpe A, Mottrie A. Robot-assisted radical cystectomy for female patients. The O.L.V. vattikuti robotic surgery institute technique. J Endourol. 2013;27:A307–A8.
9. Thyavihally Y, Patil A, Dharmadhikari N, Gulavani N, Rao H, Pednekar A. Urinary diversion after radical cystectomy-our initial experience comparing outcomes of extracorporeal and intracorporeal technique. Eur Urol Suppl. 2014;13(3):40.
10. Yang CK, Ou YC, Huang CF. Preliminary experience of robotic assisted radical cystectomy with total intracorporeal urinary diversion in VGHTC, Taiwan. J Endourol. 2014;28:A70.
11. Goel A, Gupta A, Khanna S, Vashishtha S, Rawal S. Surgical technique of staplerless total intracorporeal robot assisted laparoscopic ileal conduit for transitional cell carcinoma of bladder. J Urol. 2014;1:e551–e2.

A Focus on Robotic Intracorporeal Neobladder Formation

43

There are a number of issues as no difference in outcomes between open and robotic cystectomies that have been noted. A complete minimally invasive approach shows consistent advantages compared with open radical cystectomy [1]. The lower complications rates, and shorter length of stay all contribute towards better functional and oncological outcomes [2].

Whilst minimally invasive surgery contributes to better post-operative recovery, so does pre-operative patient fitness. Very often, patients do not undergo cardiopulmonary exercise testing as part of their management regime. As yet this has not undergone trial testing.

However, this is one part of patient care that needs to be addressed. Surgeon experience, especially with the publication of surgeon outcomes, is now becoming a more important topic than ever. Prior open experience in these cases is often invaluable. However, with todays' training programmes, it is harder and harder to get open surgical experience, as so much operating has become robotic. The development of a robotic surgical curriculum and training of trainees must take this into account.

An experienced team, both surgeon, trainee and assistant are required to work in harmony together. This is what makes the difference giving shorter lengths of stay, lower complication rates and better outcomes [3]. Additionally, it is better to be an experienced robotic prostatectomist, prior to conducting robotic cystectomies and neobladder.

The only limiting factor for robotic cystectomies becoming widespread, is cost. At the end of the day, care should be patient centred, not cost centred.

© The Editor(s) (if applicable) and The Author(s), under exclusive license to Springer Nature Switzerland AG 2021
S. S. Goonewardene et al., *Management of Muscle Invasive Bladder Cancer*,
Management of Urology, https://doi.org/10.1007/978-3-030-57915-9_43

References

1. Collins JW, Tyritzis S, Nyberg T, Schumacher MC, Laurin O, Adding C, Jonsson M, Khazaeli D, Steineck G, Wiklund P, Hosseini A. Robot-assisted radical cystectomy (RARC) with intracorporeal neobladder—what is the effect of the learning curve on outcomes? BJU Int. 2014;113(1):100–7.
2. Desai MM, Gill IS, de Castro Abreu AL, Hosseini A, Nyberg T, Adding C, Laurin O, Collins J, Miranda G, Goh AC, Aron M, Wiklund P. Robotic intracorporeal orthotopic neobladder during radical cystectomy in 132 patients. J Urol. 2014;192(6):1734–40.
3. Collins JW, Wiklund NP. Totally intracorporeal robot-assisted radical cystectomy: optimizing total outcomes. BJU Int. 2014;114(3):326–33.

Orthotopic Neobladders vs. Ileal Conduits

44

A wide body of literature exists on orthotopic neobladders (ONB) vs. ileal conduits (IC). This is a really important topic, and one which needs to be addressed. These are significant articles, as they highlight ONB is better than IC in terms of physical functioning, role functioning, social functioning, global health status/QoL and financial expenditure-all central to survivorship care. ONB reconstruction provides better QoL outcomes than does IC urinary diversion [1]. This is more so when topics like this may even be considered censured in some parts of the world.

The problem is two-fold. Firstly, the age of the new bladder cancer diagnoses are getting younger and younger. This is especially related to campaigns by the government, regarding haematuria and increased awareness. This population that are very often sexually active. As a result, the majority of patients may not want an ileal conduit and bag attached. In contrast to that, even the older more active population may not want this option.

If a patient does have an ONB, it immediately saves on cost of stoma care, stoma bags and all the accessories that go with it [2]. Given the number of patients undergoing cystectomy, this is a considerable figure. Due to the cost of the tariff for an ONB and ileal conduit being the same in the NHS, more centres would opt to do IC. This is due to the fact it is a shorter operation, when compared with the ONB, which can be up to five hours long. With waiting list and breach pressures on all teams, this seems to be the logical option, however, it may not give the best outcome to the patient. Added to that, if trainees are being trained predominately to do IC, then again ONB will fall by the wayside, with yet another generation of young urologists opting for IC.

Firstly the DoH needs to reconsider the tariff for ONB vs. IC given that ONB is a far longer procedure and that significant savings are made on stoma care. Secondly, trainees need to be trained on both procedures. Thirdly, the option of ONB should be made available to patients, should they require it, instead of IC alone.

© The Editor(s) (if applicable) and The Author(s), under exclusive license to
Springer Nature Switzerland AG 2021
S. S. Goonewardene et al., *Management of Muscle Invasive Bladder Cancer*,
Management of Urology, https://doi.org/10.1007/978-3-030-57915-9_44

References

1. Singh V, Yadav R, Sinha RJ, Gupta DK. Prospective comparison of quality-of-life outcomes between ileal conduit urinary diversion and orthotopic neobladder reconstruction after radical cystectomy: a statistical model. BJU Int. 2014;113:726–32.
2. Studer UE. Life is good with orthotopic bladder substitutes! BJU Int. 2014;113:686–7.

The Role of Enhanced Recovery in Robotic Cystectomy

45

There have been a number of articles recently examining pain within enhanced recovery. This clearly highlighted patients on an enhanced recovery pathway after open surgery have a number of factors contributing to their recovery [1, 2]. This included significantly less opioid analgesics, possibly contributing to decreased postoperative ileus and shorter length of hospital stay. In todays' world, the focus seems to be on robotic surgery as the driving force behind shorter recovery periods and day case surgery [3]. However, whilst appropriate patient selection may be true in prostate surgery, the same cannot be said of robotic cystectomy. With a far wider resectional area and greater stress response, appropriate patient selection beforehand and support afterwards is key to good patient outcomes.

ERAS studies have shown objective parameters that can improve peri-op outcomes [4]. However, a survey has shown significant individual differences in peri-op management of bladder cancer with the majority of urologists using personal experience as a primary guide [4].

The key to successful post-operative recovery with robotic cystectomy is preoperative, intraoperative, and postoperative care advances with implementation of cystectomy enhanced recovery pathways [5]. This is a novel way to reduce length of stay and overall complications within 90 days of cystectomy without increasing readmissions or complications as demonstrated by Xu et al. [2]. A well designed pathway in combination with robotic surgery can dramatically improve complications and length of stay compared to the national standards [6].

The pathway starts pre-operatively, with assessment of the patient using cardiopulmonary exercise testing. The use of cardiopulmonary exercise testing is gaining popularity as a preoperative functional assessment tool and is a useful adjunct to risk stratification before radical cystectomy [7].

The enhanced recovery pathway implements a series of evidence based interventions that decreases length of stay and complications without compromising patient outcomes [5]. A standard pathway incorporates preoperative education, expectation setting, prehabilitation, nutrition evaluation, carbohydrate loading, venous

© The Editor(s) (if applicable) and The Author(s), under exclusive license to Springer Nature Switzerland AG 2021
S. S. Goonewardene et al., *Management of Muscle Invasive Bladder Cancer*, Management of Urology, https://doi.org/10.1007/978-3-030-57915-9_45

thrombosis prophylaxis, normothermia maintenance, local anaesthesia, no nasogastric tubes or bowel prep, early feeding, and opioid avoidance [5].

Robotics alone is not enough to maximise patient outcome, the benefits of enhanced recovery are also required with robotic cystectomy.

References

1. Xu W, Ahmadi H, Cai J, Miranda G, Shuckman A, Daneshmand S, et al. Post-operative pain management after radical cystectomy: comparing traditional and enhanced recovery after surgery protocol at USC. J Urol. 2015;1:e306.
2. Xu W, Daneshmand S, Bazargani ST, Cai J, Miranda G, Schuckman AK, et al. Postoperative pain management after radical cystectomy: comparing traditional versus enhanced recovery protocol pathway. J Urol. 2015;194(5):1209–13.
3. Goonewardene SS, Rowe E. Radical robotic assisted laparoscopic prostatectomy: a day case procedure. BJU Int. 2014;113:116.
4. Truong H, Nix J, Smith K, Mittal A, Agarwal P. Perioperative management of radical cystectomy patients: a questionnaire survey of the American Urological Association members. J Clin Oncol. 2013;31:316.
5. Kukreja JB, Kiernan M, Schempp B, Hontar A, Ghazi A, Rashid H, et al. Cystectomy enhanced recovery pathway: reduction in length of stay without increased morbidity or readmissions. J Urol. 2015;1:e813–e4.
6. Athanasiadis G, Soares R, Swinn M, Perry M, Jones C, Patil K. Setting up a new robot assisted radical cystectomy service. Eur Urol Suppl. 2014;13(3):31.
7. Hoyland K, Vasdev N, Adshead JM, Thorpe A. Cardiopulmonary exercise testing in patients undergoing radical cystectomy (open, laparoscopic and robotic). J Clin Urol. 2014;7(6):374–9.

MIBC: Quality of Life with Urinary Diversion

46

Filipas et al. [1] compared the quality of life and health in incontinent and continent urinary diversions [1]. Patients with non-tumour disease, a continent reservoir and employment tended to have the highest level of quality of life [1]. The higher the number and severity of psychological symptoms, such as depression and anxiety, the lower the level of global satisfaction with life, health and urinary diversion, and vice versa [1]. This demonstrates the decision for a continent versus an incontinent urinary diversion must consider not only the medical factors of each individual patient, but also the initial diagnosis, psychological condition and employment status.

A questionnaire survey was carried out to assess the quality of life of 60 patients who had undergone cystectomy because of bladder carcinoma [2]. Urinary diversion was by a continent caecal reservoir in 20 patients and by a conduit in 40. The patients' replies showed that cystectomy could cause severe problems in all aspects of life. Diversion with a continent caecal reservoir was associated with fewer stoma-related problems and seemed to allow the patients greater freedom to continue activities such as sport, travel and social life [2]. Sexual problems, disturbed relationships with partners and emotional and mental problems were common and did not differ between the two groups of patients. It is recommended that patients judged to be prone to mental and emotional disturbance after cystectomy should be identified pre-operatively and given extra psychological support.

Protogerou et al., measure the quality-of-life (QoL) outcome and urinary and sexual function and bother after radical cystectomy and different types of urinary tract reconstruction (Bricker vs. modified S-pouch neobladder), also assessing differences between them and a normal population [3]. Sexual function was seriously and similarly affected in groups 1 and 2; the erection rate was 28.9% for group 1, 35.5% for group 2 (p = 0.1) and 83.3% in group 3 (p = 0.003), Women reported equivalent dysfunction in all three groups (15.4%, 20% and 16.6%, p = 0.3). Sexual desire was also equal in all groups (48.2%, 50% and 48.1%). Patients in group 1 expressed more bother, while those in group 2 seemed more satisfied by their sexual

S. S. Goonewardene et al., *Management of Muscle Invasive Bladder Cancer*,
Management of Urology, https://doi.org/10.1007/978-3-030-57915-9_46

life (84.4%, 68% and 68.5%, p = 0.04). Radical cystectomy does not affect QoL whichever urinary reconstruction is used, and this implies a determination by the patients to live and adjust to their new conditions. On the contrary, urinary and sexual function are affected and related to the method used to reconstruct the urinary system.

Bjerre et al., compare the health-related quality of life after bladder substitution with that following ileal conduit diversion [4]. Both day- and night-time urinary leakage occurred more frequently following bladder substitution (18% against 10%, and 21% against 3%) [4]. Nevertheless, urinary leakage affected conduit patients more severely and they scored higher on a leakage distress scale. Furthermore, 58% of the ileal conduit but only 21% of the bladder substitution patients gave urinary leakage as their main concern (p = 0.04) [4]. Ileal conduit patients did not retain their body image as well as those with bladder substitution. The frequency of both sexual and non-sexual physical contacts decreased in the majority of the conduit patients but only in a minority of the bladder substitute patients. Global satisfaction was high and similar in both groups [4]. These results show that the health-related quality of life is retained to a higher degree after bladder substitution and supports the use of this procedure as the standard method of diversion after cystectomy for bladder cancer.

Kitamura et al. compare the QOL in patients with ileal or colon conduits (IC), continent urinary reservoir (CR) and ileal neobladder (NB), a retrospective study was conducted using a questionnaire sent by mail [5]. The IC group frequently complained of changes in bathing habits and loss of using public baths in comparison with the CR and the NB groups [5]. High scores for loss of sexual desire were obtained in the IC, the CR and the NB groups, in this order. Because of the nearly physiological voiding, the NB group desired a voiding condition like pre-operative status as compared with the IC and the CR groups [5]. However, for most of the questionnaire items no difference was seen among the IC, CR and NB groups concerning general condition, reconstruction-related symptoms, psychological status, sexual life, social status, satisfaction with the treatment and global satisfaction with life and health [5]. There was little difference in the QOL score of the questionnaire and satisfaction among the IC, CR and NB groups. It was suggested that almost every patient accepted and adapted to the present status of general quality of life in each group.

Gerharz et al., reassessed the psychological and social aspects of this treatment compared with wet urostomy. There were statistically significant superiority of continent reservoirs regarding all stoma related items, patient global self-assessment of their quality of life (single item, p < 0.005), physical strength, mental capacity, leisure time activities and social competence (p < 0.05) [6]. Continent diversion is clearly advantageous with respect to all items directly related to the stoma. The significant superiority of continent diversion in patient global self-assessment of their quality of life reflects the highly subjective dimension of the concept [6]. Superiority in self-ratings of physical strength, mental capacity, leisure time activities and social competence could be interpreted as indicators of enhanced vitality in those patients, thus, supporting understanding that women and men who actively participate in life have a special benefit from continent reservoirs [6].

Hara compared the health-related quality of life (HRQoL) after radical cystectomy in patients with an ileal conduit or an orthotopic neobladder [7]. Six of the eight scales of HRQoL were favourable in both patients with a neobladder or an ileal conduit, and there was no significant difference between these groups [7]. In addition, the HRQoL of patients with an orthotopic neobladder (except for role-emotional functioning) was unaffected by the segment of the intestine used for neobladder construction [7]. Therefore, patients with both types of urinary diversion were generally satisfied with their overall health and quality of life.

Radical cystectomy remains the gold standard in treatment of muscle invasive bladder cancer [8]. Evolution of pathological guidelines has empowered centres to offer orthotopic substitution (OBS) to patients undergoing radical cystectomy [8]. In a similar age-group population, there was no significant difference in most QoL indices but body image issues persist in ICD patients [8]. OBS patients had significantly better physical function, continuing to have a more active lifestyle [8]. They attained urethral voiding with good continence.

References

1. Filipas D, Egle UT, Budenbender C, et al. Quality of life and health in patients with urinary diversion: a comparison of incontinent versus continent urinary diversion. Eur Urol. 1997;32(1):23–9.
2. Mansson A, Johnson G, Mansson W. Quality of life after cystectomy: comparison between patients with conduit and those with continent caecal reservoir urinary diversion. Br J Urol. 1988;62(3):240–5.
3. Protogerou V, Moschou M, Antoniou N, Varkarakis J, Bamias A, Deliveliotis C. Modified S-pouch neobladder vs ileal conduit and a matched control population: a quality-of-life survey. BJU Int. 2004;94(3):350–4.
4. Bjerre BD, Johansen C, Steven K. "Health-Related Quality of Life after Cystectomy: Bladder Substitution Compared with Ileal Conduit Diversion. A Questionnaire Survey." [In eng]. Br J Urol. 1195;75(2):200–5.
5. Kitamura H, Miyao N, Yanase M, et al. Quality of life in patients having an ileal conduit, continent reservoir or orthotopic neobladder after cystectomy for bladder carcinoma. Int J Urol. 1999;6(8):393–9.
6. Gerharz EW, Weingärtner K, Dopatka T, Köhl UN, Basler HD, Riedmiller HN. Quality of life after cystectomy and urinary diversion: results of a retrospective interdisciplinary study. J Urol. 1997;158(3):778–85.
7. Hara I, Miyake H, Hara S, et al. Health-related quality of life after radical cystectomy for bladder cancer: a comparison of ileal conduit and orthotopic bladder replacement. BJU Int. 2002;89(1):10–3.
8. Philip J, Manikandan R, Venugopal S, Desouza J, Javle MP. "Orthotopic Neobladder Versus Ileal Conduit Urinary Diversion after Cystectomy–a Qualityof-Life Based Comparison." [In eng]. Ann R Coll Surg Engl. 2009;91(2):565–9.

MIBC: Orthotopic vs Ileal Conduit, Which Is Better?

47

Continent urinary diversion has evolved from an investigational method of urinary tract reconstruction to an accepted, and in many instances preferred, option for men and women facing radical cystectomy [1]. At this time, continent diversion should be offered to all appropriate candidates, and these procedures should be considered a part of the standard urologic armamentarium [1].

At most centers with experience in urinary diversion, an orthotopic urinary reservoir is the diversion of choice after radical cystectomy for bladder cancer [2]. The paradigm has shifted in the past 10 years from actively looking for reasons to do an orthotopic diversion to carefully considering why a patient cannot undergo reconstruction to their native urethra [2]. Proper patient selection is the key to success. Notably, chronologic age is not an absolute contraindication to orthotopic diversion [2]. Instead, careful consideration of the patient's comorbid conditions should guide eligibility. In addition, locally advanced disease is not a contraindication to an orthotopic diversion [3].

To have the flexibility to manage whatever situation presents itself intraoperatively, the surgeon performing a urinary diversion after radical cystectomy must be facile with several diversion techniques [3]. At the very least, the surgeon must be comfortable with one type of each major form of urinary diversion, a conduit (incontinent) diversion, a continent cutaneous diversion, and an orthotopic diversion. As a result, radical cystectomy and urinary diversion should be performed at centers with significant experience in all three types of diversions.

Studer et al. reported on 10 years of experience with an ileal low-pressure bladder substitute combined with an afferent tubular segment following cystectomy in 100 consecutive men [4]. The median follow-up period was 30 months (range 3–108 months), with a 2.5-year minimum in survivors. The early complication rate was 11%, including 2 deaths due to postoperative sepsis. In all, 14 patients required reoperation for late complications. For continence: 92% by day (after 1 year) and 80% by night (after 2 years). This demonstrated this technique is straightforward, allows radical cancer surgery, and protects the upper tract. The favorable functional

S. S. Goonewardene et al., *Management of Muscle Invasive Bladder Cancer*, Management of Urology, https://doi.org/10.1007/978-3-030-57915-9_47

results are comparable with those achieved by similar techniques, but meticulous follow-up is essential.

Orthotopic reconstruction following cystectomy has evolved in an attempt to restore anatomy and function to as close as possible to the preoperative state [5]. Lantz et al. [5], reviewed functional outcomes of patients who underwent cystectomy and neobladder reconstruction. This demonstrated orthotopic neobladders have excellent functional outcomes with low rates of incontinence, which improved throughout follow-up [5]. A significant proportion of patients developed hydronephrosis, highlighting the need for close follow-up to prevent reversible renal deterioration [5]. Creatinine increased during follow-up irrespective of the development of hydronephrosis, but the clinical significance is unknown [5].

Mcguire et al. assessed the impact of different forms of urinary diversion on overall quality of life in patients with bladder cancer [6]. Patients with ileal conduits have significantly decreased mental health quality of life whereas patients with continent urinary diversions do not [6]. Therefore, when not medically contraindicated, patients should be offered a continent diversion as the diversion of choice after cystectomy.

Patients frequently complain about changes in their everyday life after radical cystectomy and urinary diversion [7]. Hobisch et al., compared subjective morbidity of ileal neobladder to the urethra versus ileal conduit urinary diversion and to elucidate its influence on quality of life. The results demonstrate patients with an orthotopic neobladder better adapt to the new situation than patients with an ileal conduit [7]. In addition, neobladder to the urethra improves quality of life due to a better self-confidence, better rehabilitation as well as restoration of leisure, professional, traveling, and social activities, and reduced risk of inadvertent loss of urine. The results obtained by this study demonstrate that quality of life is preserved in a higher degree after orthotopic neobladder than after ileal conduit urinary diversion [7].

Health related quality of life after urinary diversion has been increasingly recognized as an important outcome measure [8]. However, few studies have directly compared patients with an ileal conduit with those with a continent orthotopic neobladder and even fewer have used validated quality of life instruments [8]. Dutta et al. compared health related quality of life in patients who underwent neobladder versus ileal conduit creation using validated questionnaires. Patients with an orthotopic neobladder have marginal quality of life advantages over those with an ileal conduit [8, 9]. However, differences in health related quality of life in the two types of urinary diversion are confounded by age since patients who underwent orthotopic diversion were younger and as a result of age would be expected to have a higher health related quality of life score.

References

1. Benson MC, Olsson CA. Continent urinary diversion. Urol Clin N Am. 1999;26(1):125–47.
2. Krupski T, Theodorescu D. Orthotopic neobladder following cystectomy: indications, management, and outcomes. J Wound Ostomy Continence Nurs. 2001;28(1):37–46.

3. Clark PE. Urinary diversion after radical cystectomy. Curr Treat Opt Oncol. 2002;3(5):389–402.
4. Studer UE, Danuser H, Hochreiter W, Springer JP, Turner WH, Zingg EJ. Summary of 10 years' experience with an ileal low-pressure bladder substitute combined with an afferent tubular isoperistaltic segment. World J Urol. 1996;14(1):29–39.
5. Lantz AG, Saltel ME, Cagiannos I. Renal and functional outcomes following cystectomy and neobladder reconstruction. J Can Urol Assoc. 2010;4(5):328–31.
6. McGuire MS, Grimaldi G, Grotas J, Russo P. The type of urinary diversion after radical cystectomy significantly impacts on the patient's quality of life. Ann Surg Oncol. 2000;7(1):4–8.
7. Hobisch A, Tosun K, Kinzl J, et al. Life after cystectomy and orthotopic neobladder, versus, ileal conduit urinary diversion. Semin Urol Oncol. 2001;19(1):18–23.
8. Dutta SC, Chang SS, Coffey CS, Smith JA Jr, Jack G, Cookson MS. Health related quality of life assessment after radical cystectomy: comparison of ileal conduit with continent orthotopic neobladder. J Urol. 2002;168(1):164–7.
9. Philip J, Manikandan R, Venugopal S, Desouza J, Javlé PM. Orthotopic neobladder versus ileal conduit urinary diversion after cystectomy—a quality-of-life based comparison. Ann R Coll Surg Engl. 2009;91(7):565–9.

MIBC: A Systematic Review on Orthotopic Neobladder vs. Ileal Conduit, Which Is Better?

48

A systematic review relating to literature on urinary diversion for muscle invasive bladder cancer was conducted. This was to identify which gave better outcomes. The search strategy aimed to identify all references related to bladder cancer AND urinary diversion. Search terms used were as follows: (Muscle Invasive Bladder cancer) AND (Orthotopic Neobladder) or (Ileal Conduit) The following databases were screened from 1989 to June 2020:

- CINAHL
- MEDLINE (NHS Evidence)
- Cochrane
- AMed
- EMBASE
- PsychINFO
- SCOPUS
- Web of Science

In addition, searches using Medical Subject Headings (MeSH) and keywords were conducted using Cochrane databases. Two UK-based experts in bladder cancer were consulted to identify any additional studies.

Studies were eligible for inclusion if they reported primary research focusing on bladder cancer and screening. Papers were included if published after 1984 and had to be in English. Studies that did not conform to this were excluded. Only primary research was included. The overall aim was to identify the outcomes from Orthotopic neobladder vs. ileal conduit.

Abstracts were independently screened for eligibility by two reviewers and disagreements resolved through discussion or third party opinion. Agreement level was calculated using Cohen's Kappa to test the intercoder reliability of this screening process. Cohens' Kappa allows comparison of inter-rater reliability between papers using relative observed agreement. This also takes account of the comparison

© The Editor(s) (if applicable) and The Author(s), under exclusive license to
Springer Nature Switzerland AG 2021
S. S. Goonewardene et al., *Management of Muscle Invasive Bladder Cancer*,
Management of Urology, https://doi.org/10.1007/978-3-030-57915-9_48

occurring by chance. The first reviewer agreed all 18 papers to be included, the second, agreed on 18.

Data extraction was piloted by the researcher and amended in consultation with the research team (author and two academic supervisors). Data collected included authors, year and country of publication, study aims, setting, intervention aims, number of participants, study design, intervention components and delivery methods, comparison groups and outcome measures, notes and follow-up questions for the authors. Studies were quality assessed using the PRISMA criteria for randomised controlled trials, Mays et al. [1, 2] for the action research and qualitative studies and the Critical Skills Appraisal programme for cohort studies. This was also applied to randomised controlled trials and qualitative studies.

The search identified 49 papers (Fig. 48.1). However, only 18 mapped to the search terms and eligibility criteria. The current systematic reviews were examined to gain further knowledge about the subject. Twenty-one papers were excluded due to not conforming to eligibility criteria or adding to the evidence. Of the 18 papers left, relevant abstracts were identified and the full papers obtained (all of which were in English), to quality assure against criteria. There was considerable heterogeneity of design among the included studies therefore a narrative review of the evidence was undertaken. There was significant heterogeneity within studies, including clinical topic, numbers, outcomes, as a results a narrative review was thought to be best.

48.1   Incidence of Ileal Conduit vs. Orthotopic

Between 2001–2012, approximately 69,049 ICs and 6991 CDs were performed [3]. ICs are conducted at a higher rate than CDs (40–59 years: 79.5% vs. 20.5%; 60–69 years: 88.0% vs. 12.0%; $p < 0.0001$). There was a difference in males vs.

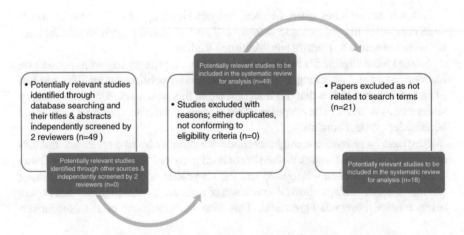

Fig. 48.1 Flow chart of studies identified through the systematic review. (Adapted from PRISMA)

females (10.2% vs. 4.0%; OR 2.36) [3]. Patients are more likely to receive ICs than CDs. Gender, racial, and geographic disparities exist among those receiving CDs.

The utilization rate of neobladder (NB) was 6.9% in 2000 and 9.1% in 2010 (p < 0.001) [4]. Younger, healthier, privately-insured and wealthier male individuals were more likely to receive a NB. High-volume hospitals were more likely to offer NB [4]. In the post-propensity matched cohort, urinary diversion type failed to be significantly associated with the examined endpoints, except for intra- and postoperative complications (IC vs. NB odds ratio [OR]: 1.15, p = 0.04) [4]. Despite comparable morbidity and mortality odds between NB and IC, as of the most contemporary year of the study (2010), IC remains the preferred urinary diversion type. Several sociodemographic factors were associated with NB.

Overall 59% of younger and 26% of older patients received a neobladder (p < 0.001) [5]. There was a significant trend toward ileal conduit urinary diversion. Patients with female gender, advanced age, significant medical comorbidity or locally advanced disease were less likely to undergo neobladder urinary diversion [5]. This trend is partly explained by surgeon preference combined with an aging, more comorbid patient population.

48.2   Health Related Quality of Life

Cerruot examined the health-related quality of life (HR-QoL) outcomes between ileal conduit (IC) and ileal orthotopic neobladder (IONB) with validated self-reported cancer-specific instruments [6]. At univariate analysis IONB was favourable for physical functioning, emotional functioning, cognitive functioning (CF), fatigue, dyspnea, appetite loss, constipation (CO), and abdominal bloating flatulence (AB) [6]. At multivariate analyses, IONB showed better scores for emotional functioning (85 vs. 79, p = 0.023), CF (93 vs. 85, p < 0.001), CO (16 vs. 31, p < 0.001), and AB (12 vs. 25, p < 0.001). A significant worsening of sexual and urinary function was observed for IONB patients in the long-term [6]. IONB provides better results in some aspects of HR-QoL related to bowel function, but a worsening of urinary and sexual functions.

Patients treated with ONR were generally younger and healthier compared with those who underwent ICD (p < 0.01) [7]. Sex, marital status, disease status were similar. Better functional scores in favour of ICD were recorded in the urinary domain (p < 0.01), whereas the corresponding bother scores were roughly identical in both groups [7]. Conversely, although higher functional scores were recorded in the sexual domain of patients with ONR (p < 0.01), the corresponding bother scores in this group were lower compared with their counterparts with ICD (53.2 vs. 65.3; p < 0.05). As patients grew older they were more likely to report on better urinary function and worse sexual function, but were less likely to be bothered by the decline in sexual function.

In the longitudinal analysis of RC patients, functioning and symptoms scores show a similar natural HRQOL course for IC and ONB patients [8]. After 24 months, general HRQOL was significantly higher in the ONB subcohort (60.5 vs. 73.6, p = 0.013). Good general HRQOL was reached by 32.4 (IC) versus 61.1% (ONB; p = 0.019) [8]. In the multivariable analysis, ONB was not an independent predictor of good HRQOL (odds ratio 2.211, 95% confidence interval 0.684–7.150, p = 0.185) [8]. Limitations include the nonbladder specificity of the QLQ-C30 questionnaire and the small sample size.

48.3   Morbidity and Mortality

Kim reported on morbidity and mortality of ileal conduit and neobladder after radical cystectomy [9]. Early and late morbidities were 29.5% (n = 91) and 19.8% (n = 61), and complication-related mortalities were 2.2% and 6.6%, respectively [9]. The type of urinary diversion significantly affected only the late complications (early: neobladder 57 vs. ileal conduit 47, p = 0.096; late: neobladder 67 vs. ileal conduit 37, p < 0.001) [9]. However, after propensity-score matching, no significant differences in early and late morbidities were observed between neobladder and ileal conduit [9].

Abe determined the differences in the type, incidence, and severity of 90-day morbidity after radical cystectomy between two different methods of urinary diversion, ileal conduit and neobladder [10]. There was no significant difference in the overall complication rates between the two groups (ileal conduit: 72% [353/493], neobladder: 74% [129/175], p = 0.5909), whereas the neobladder group had fewer major (grade 3 or more) complications (13% vs. 20%, respectively, p = 0.0271) [10]. The neobladder group had more infectious complications (43% vs. 31%, respectively, p = 0.0037), mainly as a result of urinary tract infection, whereas the ileal conduit group had more wound-related complications (24% vs. 14%, respectively, p = 0.0068), mainly as a result of surgical site infection [10]. The 90-day mortality rates were 1.1% (2/175) in the neobladder group and 1.6% (8/493) in the ileal conduit group (p = 0.6441). There was no significant difference in the overall complication rates between the two methods, and patients with neobladder had fewer major complications. The neobladder group had more infectious complications, whereas the ileal conduit group had more wound-related complications.

48.4   AKI

Ileal conduit and neobladder urinary diversions are frequently performed after radical cystectomy. However, complications after radical cystectomy may be different according to the type of urinary diversion [11]. Acute kidney injury (AKI) is a common complication after surgery and increases costs, morbidity, and mortality of hospitalized patients [11]. The overall incidence of AKI after radical cystectomy was 30.7% (62 out of 202) and the incidences did not significantly differ between the groups (27 [26.7%], ileal conduit group vs. 35 [34.7%], ileal neobladder group, p = 0.268) [11]. Intraoperative data, intensive care unit admission rate, and the duration of hospital stay were not significantly different between the groups [11]. Postoperative AKI did not significantly differ between ileal conduit and neobladder urinary diversions after radical cystectomy [11]. This finding provides additional information useful for appropriate selection of the urinary diversion type in conjunction with radical cystectomy.

48.5 Modified S Pouch Outcomes

There were no differences in the QoL scores among the three groups; group 3 (control) tended to have a better QoL for all domains except emotional functioning [12]. Urinary function was seriously affected in group 1, with more daytime leakage than in groups 2 and 3 (37.8% vs. 10%, p = 0.005, and 9.3%, p = 0.01), night loss of urine (39.5% vs. 28%, p = 0.07, and 3.7%, p = 0.002) and urine odour (58.6% vs. 4%, and 5.5%, both p = 0.001) [12]. Patients in group 2 differed from healthy individuals only in night loss of urine. Consequently, urinary bother was more pronounced in group 1, as fewer were satisfied (68.9% vs. 86% and 83.2%, both p = 0.03). Sexual function was seriously and similarly affected in groups 1 and 2; the erection rate was 28.9% for group 1, 35.5% for group 2 (p = 0.1) and 83.3% in group 3 (p = 0.003), while firm erections were present at 17.7%, 22.2% (p = 0.2) and 83.3% (p = 0.002) [12]. Women reported equivalent dysfunction in all three groups (15.4%, 20% and 16.6%, p = 0.3). Sexual desire was also equal in all groups (48.2%, 50% and 48.1%). Patients in group 1 expressed more bother, while those in group 2 seemed more satisfied by their sexual life (84.4%, 68% and 68.5%, p = 0.04) [12].

Radical cystectomy does not affect QoL whichever urinary reconstruction is used, and this implies a determination by the patients to live and adjust to their new conditions.

48.6 Conversion Factors

Ghodoussipour determined the intraoperative factors result in change in plan from continent orthotopic neobladder to ileal conduit or continent cutaneous diversion at the time of radical cystectomy [13]. Patients who ultimately received a neobladder were significantly more likely to have clinical node-negative disease (p = 0.045), negative soft tissue margins (p = 0.001), lower body mass index (p = 0.045) and higher volume surgeons (p < 0.001). Oncologic reasons for intraoperative conversions were more common than technical reasons (58.3% vs. 35.9%), in both robotic and open surgical techniques [13]. The choice of surgical approach (open vs. robotic) did not influence the rate of intraoperative conversion. The factors influencing intraoperative decision not to perform neobladder are predominantly oncologic rather than technical [13]. A clear understanding of the factors involved in influencing the intraoperative change in the urinary diversion plan may improve shared decision making in patients undergoing radical cystectomy in the future.

48.7   Factors Influencing Selection of Urinary Diversion

Kwan assessed the relative contributions of patient and surgeon factors for predicting selection of ileal conduit (IC), neobladder (NB), or continent pouch (CP) urinary diversions (UD) for patients diagnosed with muscle-invasive/high-risk nonmuscle invasive bladder cancer. The multilevel model with only patient factors showed good fit (area under the curve = 0.93, Hosmer-Lemeshow test p = 0.44), and older age, female sex, estimated glomerular filtration rate <45, 4+ comorbidity index score, and stage III/IV tumors were associated with higher odds of receiving an IC vs. neobladder/continent pouch [14]. However, including surgeon factors (annual cystectomy volume, specialty training, clinical tenure) had no association (p = 0.29).

48.8   Types of Diversion Outcomes

Nieuwenhuijzen examined four different diversions: an ileal conduit according to Bricker (IC; 118 patients), an Indiana pouch (IP; 51 patients), and orthotopic diversions after cystectomy/neobladder (N; 62 patients), or sexuality-preserving cystectomy and neobladder (SPCN; 50 patients) [15]. Forty-four percent developed early complications: IC 48%, IP 43%, N 42%, and SPCN 38%. Late complication rate was 51% with fewer complications in the IC group, IC 39%, IP 63%, N 59%, and SPCN 60% (HR, 0.32; 95% CI: 0.14–0.72), which was explained by fewer uncomplicated urinary tract infections (one third of all late complications) in the IC group [15]. Complete daytime and nighttime continence, respectively, was achieved in 96% and 73% after IP, 90% and 67% after neobladder, and 96% and 67% after SPCN. Cystectomy with any subsequent diversion remains a procedure with considerable morbidity. Orthotopic diversions provide good functional results, but at the cost of more late complications compared with ileal conduits [15].

48.9   Systematic Reviews Relating to Urinary Diversion

Orthotopic neobladder (ONB) and ileal conduit (IC) are the most commonly practiced techniques of urinary diversion (UD) after radical cystectomy (RC) in bladder cancer patients. Data in the literature is still discordant regarding which UD technique offers the best HR-QoL. Ziouziou performed a literature search of PubMed, ScienceDirect, CochraneLibrary and ClinicalTrials.Gov in September 2017 according to the Cochrane Handbook and the Preferred Reporting Items for Systematic Reviews and Meta-Analyzes [16]. The studies were evaluated according to the "Oxford Center for Evidence-Based Medicine" criteria. Four studies met the inclusion criteria. The pooled results demonstrated better UF and UB scores in IC patients: differences were −18.17 (95% CI: −27.49, −8.84, p = 0.0001) and −3.72 (95% CI: −6.66, −0.79, p = 0.01) respectively. There was no significant difference between IC and ONB patients in terms of BF and BB [16]. SF was significantly better in ONB patients: the difference was 12.7 (95% CI, 6.32, 19.08, p < 0.0001). However no significant difference was observed regarding SB. This meta-analysis of non-randomized studies demonstrated a better HR-QoL in urinary outcomes in IC patients compared with ONB patients [16].

References

1. Moher D, Liberati A, Tetzlaff J, Altman DG. "Preferred Reporting Items for Systematic Reviews and Meta-Analyses: The Prisma Statement." [In English]. BMJ (Online) 339, no. 7716 (08 Aug 2009):332–36.
2. Mays N, Pope C, Popay J. "Systematically Reviewing Qualitative and Quantitative Evidence to Inform Management and Policy-Making in the Health Field." [In English]. Journal of Health Services Research and Policy 10, no. SUPPL. 1 (July 2005):6–20.
3. Farber NJ, Faiena I, Dombrovskiy V, Tabakin AL, Shinder B, Patel R, Elsamra SE, Jang TL, Singer EA, Weiss RE. Disparities in the use of continent urinary diversions after radical cystectomy for bladder cancer. Bladder Cancer. 2018;4(1):113–20.
4. Roghmann F, Becker A, Trinh QD, Djahangirian O, Tian Z, Meskawi M, Shariat SF, Graefen M, Karakiewicz P, Noldus J, Sun M. Updated assessment of neobladder utilization and morbidity according to urinary diversion after radical cystectomy: a contemporary US-population-based cohort. Can Urol Assoc J. 2013;7(9–10):E552.
5. Lowrance WT, Rumohr JA, Clark PE, Chang SS, Smith JA Jr, Cookson MS. Urinary diversion trends at a high volume, single American tertiary care center. J Urol. 2009;182(5):2369–74.
6. Cerruto MA, D'Elia C, Siracusano S, Saleh O, Gacci M, Cacciamani G, De Marco V, Porcaro AB, Balzarro M, Niero M, Lonardi C, Iafrate M, Bassi P, Imbimbo C, Racioppi M, Talamini R, Ciciliato S, Serni S, Carini M, Verze P, Artibani W. Health-related quality of life after radical cystectomy: a cross-sectional study with matched-pair analysis on ileal conduit vs ileal orthotopic neobladder diversion. Urology. 2017;108:82–9.
7. Goldberg H, Baniel J, Mano R, Rotlevy G, Kedar D, Yossepowitch O. Orthotopic neobladder vs. ileal conduit urinary diversion: a long-term quality-of-life comparison. Urol Oncol. 2016;34(3):121.e1–7.
8. Kretschmer A, Grimm T, Buchner A, Jokisch F, Ziegelmüller B, Casuscelli J, Schulz G, Stief CG, Karl A. Midterm health-related quality of life after radical cystectomy: a propensity score-matched analysis. Eur Urol Focus. 2020;6:704–10.
9. Kim SH, Yu A, Jung JH, Lee YJ, Lee ES. Incidence and risk factors of 30-day early and 90-day late morbidity and mortality of radical cystectomy during a 13-year follow-up: a comparative propensity-score matched analysis of complications between neobladder and ileal conduit. Jpn J Clin Oncol. 2014;44(7):677–85.
10. Abe T, Takada N, Shinohara N, Matsumoto R, Murai S, Sazawa A, Maruyama S, Tsuchiya K, Kanzaki S, Nonomura K. Comparison of 90-day complications between ileal conduit and neobladder reconstruction after radical cystectomy: a retrospective multi-institutional study in Japan. Int J Urol. 2014;21(6):554–9.
11. Joung KW, Kong YG, Yoon SH, Kim YJ, Hwang JH, Hong B, Kim YK. Comparison of postoperative acute kidney injury between ileal conduit and neobladder urinary diversions after radical cystectomy: a propensity score matching analysis. Medicine (Baltimore). 2016;95(36):e4838.
12. Protogerou V, Moschou M, Antoniou N, Varkarakis J, Bamias A, Deliveliotis C. Modified S-pouch neobladder vs ileal conduit and a matched control population: a quality-of-life survey. BJU Int. 2004;94(3):350–4.
13. Ghodoussipour S, Ahmadi N, Hartman N, Cacciamani G, Miranda G, Cai J, Schuckman A, Djaladat H, Gill I, Daneshmand S, Desai M. Factors influencing intraoperative conversion

from planned orthotopic to non-orthotopic urinary diversion during radical cystectomy. World J Urol. 2019;37:1851–5.

14. Kwan ML, Leo MC, Danforth KN, Weinmann S, Lee VS, Munneke JR, Bulkley JE, Rosetti MO, Yi DK, Banegas MP, Wagner MD, Williams SG, Aaronson DS, Grant M, Krouse RS, Gilbert SM, McMullen CK. Factors that influence selectionof urinary diversion among bladder cancer patients in 3 community-based integrated health care systems. Urology. 2019;125:222–9.

15. Nieuwenhuijzen JA, de Vries RR, Bex A, van der Poel HG, Meinhardt W, Antonini N, Horenblas S. Urinary diversions after cystectomy: the association of clinical factors, complications and functional results of four different diversions. Eur Urol. 2008;53(4):834–42.

16. Ziouziou I, Irani J, Wei JT, Karmouni T, El Khader K, Koutani A, Iben Attya Andaloussi A. Ileal conduit vs orthotopic neobladder: which one offers the best health-related quality of life in patients undergoing radical cystectomy? A systematic review of literature and meta-analysis. Prog Urol. 2018;28(5):241–50.

Urinary Diversion Ileal Conduit vs. Studer vs. Catherisable Stoma

49

49.1 Research Methods

A systematic review relating to muscle invasive bladder cancer, robotic cystectomy and Urinary Diversion was conducted. This was to identify whether outcomes between an ileal conduit, Studer pouch, T Pouch or I Pouch has a role in this cohort. The search strategy aimed to identify all references related to bladder cancer AND muscle invasive disease AND Urinary diversion. Search terms used were as follows: (Bladder cancer) AND (muscle invasive disease) AND (Urinary Diversion). The following databases were screened from 1989 to June 2020:

- CINAHL
- MEDLINE (NHS Evidence)
- Cochrane
- AMed
- EMBASE
- PsychINFO
- SCOPUS
- Web of Science

In addition, searches using Medical Subject Headings (MeSH) and keywords were conducted using Cochrane databases. Two UK-based experts in bladder cancer were consulted to identify any additional studies.

Studies were eligible for inclusion if they reported primary research focusing on muscle invasive bladder cancer and nerve sparing. Papers were included if published after 1984 and had to be in English. Studies that did not conform to this were excluded. Only primary research was included (Fig. 49.1).

Abstracts were independently screened for eligibility by two reviewers and disagreements resolved through discussion or third party opinion. Agreement level was calculated using Cohen's Kappa to test the intercoder reliability of this screening

process. Cohens' Kappa allows comparison of inter-rater reliability between papers using relative observed agreement. This also takes account of the comparison occurring by chance. The first reviewer agreed all 8 papers to be included, the second, agreed on 8.

Data extraction was piloted by the researcher and amended in consultation with the research team (author and two academic supervisors). Data collected included authors, year and country of publication, study aims, setting, intervention aims, number of participants, study design, intervention components and delivery methods, comparison groups and outcome measures, notes and follow-up questions for the authors. Studies were quality assessed using the PRISMA criteria for randomised controlled trials, Mays et al. [1, 2] for the action research and qualitative studies and the Critical Skills Appraisal programme for cohort studies. This was also applied to randomised controlled trials and qualitative studies.

The search identified 56 papers (Fig. 49.1). Eight mapped to the search terms and eligibility criteria. The current systematic reviews were examined to gain further knowledge about the subject. Forty-eight papers were excluded due to not conforming to eligibility criteria or adding to the evidence. Of the 8 papers left, relevant abstracts were identified and the full papers obtained (all of which were in English), to quality assure against search criteria. There was considerable heterogeneity of design among the included studies therefore a narrative review of the evidence was undertaken. There was significant heterogeneity within studies, including clinical topic, numbers, outcomes, as a result a narrative review was thought to be best. There were 7 cohort studies, with a moderate level of evidence, with one RCT with a good level of evidence. These were from a range of countries with minimal loss to follow-up. All participants were identified appropriately.

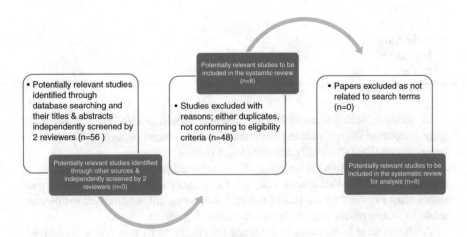

Fig. 49.1 Flow chart of studies identified through the systematic review. (Adapted from PRISMA)

49.2   T-Pouch Neobladder vs. Studer Pouch

Skinner designed the USC-STAR trial to determine whether the T-pouch neobladder that included an antireflux mechanism was superior to the Studer pouch in patients with bladder cancer undergoing radical cystectomy [3]. Between baseline and 3 years the estimated glomerular filtration rate decreased by 6.4 ml/min/1.73 m^2 in the Studer group and 6.6 ml/min/1.73 m^2 in the T-pouch group (p = 0.35) [3]. Multivariable analysis showed that type of ileal orthotopic neobladder was not independently associated with 3-year renal function (p = 0.63) [3]. However, baseline estimated glomerular filtration rate, age and urinary tract obstruction were independently associated with 3-year decline in renal function [3]. Cumulative risk of urinary tract infection and overall late complications were not different between the groups, but the T-pouch was associated with an increased risk of secondary diversion related surgeries [3].

49.3   Studer Pouch vs. I Pouch

Mischinger investigated whether the length of ileum used for ileal orthotopic neobladder (ONB) reconstruction (60 vs. 40 cm) impacts on functional or cancer outcomes [4]. No significant differences were observed for 30-day major- (p = 0.33) and minor (p = 0.96) complication rates between both neobladder types [4]. S-Pouch patients reported higher preoperative stool frequencies (S-pouch: mean 2.7; I-pouch: mean 3.4; p = 0.049) and tended to suffer from urgency (S: mean 2.9; I: mean 3.4; p = 0.059) [4]. No significant differences in postoperative bowel disorders were found between both neobladder types (S-Pouch: 15.9, IQR; I-Pouch: 16.6 IQR; p = 0.84) [4]. No overall-, cancer specific- or recurrence free survival advantage for either of both ONB variants (p = 0.81; 0.65 and 0.78), respectively.

Mischinger investigated whether the ileal length used for the formation of two different orthotopic bladder substitutes [Studer (S)-Pouch vs. I-Pouch; 60 vs. 40 cm] impacts quality of life (QoL) [5]. I-Pouch patients reported better SF-36 physical health status (p = 0.026), QLQ-BLM30 continence scores (p < 0.001) and a more favorable QLQ-C30 total score compared to S-Pouch patients (p = 0.044) [5]. S-Pouch patients reported better QLQ-BLM30 general health status (p = 0.001) [5]. For the TNQ, no significant difference was found between both groups (p = 0.09). S-Pouch patients reported use of condom urinals more frequently (p = 0.026) [5]. I-Pouch patients reported significantly higher micturition volumes (≥300 ml) compared to S-Pouch patients (30/33 vs. 16/23; p = 0.040) [5]. No differences were found with regard to bicarbonate supplementation and recurrent urinary tract infections [5].

49.4   The Studer Neobladder

Studer anastomosed the ileal low-pressure reservoir to the membranous urethra in 22 male patients following radical cystoprostatectomy for bladder cancer [6]. In the following 18 patients, the low-pressure reservoir was anastomosed directly to the membranous urethra [6]. Micturition was good, with no notable residual urine, no bacteriuria and no paroxysmal urinary incontinence [6]. However, a safety pad is used by half of the patients because once or twice a week, mainly at night, a few ml of urine may be lost [6]. No significant changes in serum electrolytes, bicarbonate or creatinine were noted [6]. With the three different antireflux techniques used, no obstructive or inflammatory changes in the upper urinary tracts were found, although no long-term antibiotic prophylaxis was given [6].

Nam analyzed the long-term (>10 years postoperatively) functional outcomes, complications, and urodynamic findings in a single center series of patients who underwent cystectomy and a Studer ileal neobladder substitution [7]. Nam evaluated 19 out of 50 patients who had lived for over 10 years postoperatively [7]. Another 31 patients were not traced: 7 patients died following recurrence, 15 died due to exacerbation of a comorbidity, and 9 patients were lost to follow-up [7]. Concerning complications, 6 patients had an atrophied kidney, 5 patients had moderate hydronephrosis, 5 patients had chronic recurrence of pyelonephritis, and 2 patients had voiding difficulty because of bladder neck stricture due to clean intermittent catheterization [7]. One patient underwent an operation due to intestinal obstruction [7]. Seven patients had incontinence; all 7 patients showed intermittently at night and 2 patients even in waking hours [7].

Atmaca conducted a retrospective comparison of open (n = 42) versus totally intracorporeal (n = 32) robotic-assisted radical cystectomy, bilateral extended pelvic lymph node dissection, and Studer urinary diversion was performed [8]. Positive surgical margin rates were similar between the open (n = 1, 2.4%) and robotic (n = 2, 6.3%) groups (p > 0.05) [8]. Minor and major complication rates were similar between groups (p > 0.05) [8]. Significantly higher percentages were detected in the robotic group regarding bilateral neurovascular bundle-sparing surgery (93.7% vs. 64.3%, p = 0.004) and bilateral extended pelvic lymph node dissection (100% vs. 71.4%, p = 0.001) [8]. The mean lymph node yield was significantly higher in the robotic group (25.4 ± 9.7 vs. 17.2 ± 13.5, p = 0.005) [8]. The number of postoperative readmissions for minor complications was significantly lower in the robotic group (0 vs. 7, p = 0.017) [8]. Better trends were detected in the robotic group concerning daytime continence with no pad use (84.6% vs. 75%, p > 0.05) and severe daytime incontinence (8.3% vs. 16.6%, p > 0.05) [8]. No significant differences were detected regarding postoperative mean International Index of Erectile Function scores between groups (p > 0.05) [8].

Borrell Palanca analysed the outcome, complications and functional results in patients undergoing bladder substitution with the Studer continent urinary pouch [9]. Four patients are free of disease, one died from metastatic disease and one patient with tumour progression and multiple lung metastases at 2 months' follow-up is currently on chemotherapy [9]. The mean operating time was significantly longer for this procedure than for the non-continent Bricker urinary diversion (mean 7.2 vs. 3.5 h, respectively) [9]. The immediate postoperative complications were: ileus (>7 days) in two patients, diarrhoea (>3 days) in two, occlusive ileus due to fecaloma in one, metabolic acidosis in one, wound seroma in one, and wound infection in two patients [9]. The early and late postoperative complications were: incontinence for up to 1 month after removing the urethral catheter in three patients (two of these patients are still incontinent at 2 months' follow-up), wound infection in two and impotence in 6 patients [9].

Saidi analyze the outcome, complications and functional results in patients undergoing bladder substitution with the Studer continent urinary pouch [10]. The transitional cell carcinoma was found to be the most frequent histopathological type [10]. The distribution by grade and pathological stage showed all were high grade infiltrating tumours localized in the bladder [10]. Three patients had neobladder-unrelated complications: one patient with a wound infection and two patients with a prolonged ileus [10].

After radical cystoprostatectomy, an ileal bladder substitute had been performed in 14 male patients à modo Studer [11]. In order to avoid peristalsis with high pressure peaks resulting in incontinence, the antimesenteric border was transsected, and an ileal low-pressure pouch was created [11]. One to two months after operation, the continence for urine was good or excellent [11]. After a follow-up time of 12 months, no metabolic disorders requiring any substitution, nor pyelonephritic changes were observed [11].

49.5   Ileal Conduit vs. Neobladder

Bier reviewed with RARC and intracorporeal diversion using ileal conduit or neobladder [12]. Of the 86 patients, 24 patients (28%) underwent intracorporeal ileal conduit and 62 patients (72%) underwent intracorporeal neobladder formation [12]. A Studer pouch was created in all who underwent intracorporeal neobladder diversion. Minor complications (grade I and II) were reported in 23 patients, while major complications (grade III and above) were reported in 21 patients. The mean nodal yield was 20.3 (range 0–46) [12]. Positive margins were found in in 8% [12]. Continence could be achieved in 88% of patients who received an intracorporeal neobladder [12]. The cancer-specific survival (CSS) and overall survival (OS) were 80% and 70%, respectively [12].

References

1. Moher D, Liberati A, Tetzlaff J, Altman DG. "Preferred Reporting Items for Systematic Reviews and Meta-Analyses: The Prisma Statement." [In English]. BMJ (Online) 339, no. 7716 (08 Aug 2009):332–36.
2. Mays N, Pope C, Popay J. "Systematically Reviewing Qualitative and Quantitative Evidence to Inform Management and Policy-Making in the Health Field." [In English]. Journal of Health Services Research and Policy 10, no. SUPPL. 1 (July 2005):6–20.

3. Skinner EC, Fairey AS, Groshen S, Daneshmand S, Cai J, Miranda G, Skinner DG. Randomized trial of Studer pouch versus T-pouch orthotopic ileal neobladder in patients with bladder cancer. J Urol. 2015;194(2):433–9.

4. Mischinger J, Abdelhafez MF, Rausch S, Todenhöfer T, Neumann E, Aufderklamm S, Stenzl A, Gakis G. Perioperative morbidity, bowel function and oncologic outcome after radical cystectomy and ileal orthotopic neobladder reconstruction: Studer-pouch versus I-pouch. Eur J Surg Oncol. 2018;44(1):178–84.

5. Mischinger J, Abdelhafez MF, Todenhöfer T, Schwentner C, Aufderklamm S, Stenzl A, Gakis G. Quality of life outcomes after radical cystectomy: long-term standardized assessment of Studer pouch versus I-pouch. World J Urol. 2015;33(10):1381–7.

6. Studer UE, Ackermann D, Casanova GA, Zingg EJ. Three years' experience with an ileal low pressure bladder substitute. Br J Urol. 1989;63(1):43–52.

7. Nam JK, Kim TN, Park SW, Lee SD, Chung MK. The Studer orthotopic neobladder: long-term (more than 10 years) functional outcomes, urodynamic features, and complications. Yonsei Med J. 2013;54(3):690–5.

8. Atmaca AF, Canda AE, Gok B, Akbulut Z, Altinova S, Balbay MD. Open versus robotic radical cystectomy with intracorporeal Studer diversion. JSLS. 2015;19(1):e2014.00193.

9. Borrell Palanca A, Chicote Pérez F, Alcalá-Santaella Casanova C, Cisnal Monsalve JM, Pastor Sempere F. [Studer-type orthotopic urinary bladder: our experience]. Arch Esp Urol. 2000;53(10):893–899.

10. Saidi S, Ivanovski O, Petrovski D, Kuzmanoski M, Stavridis S, Banev S, Popov Z. Lower urinary tract reconstruction following a cystectomy: experience and results in 20 patients using the "Studer" orthotopic ileal bladder substitution. Bratisl Lek Listy. 2008;109(8):353–7.

11. Shishkov D. [Orthotopic bladder from the small intestine following radical cystectomy according to Studer's procedure]. Khirurgiia (Sofiia). 2001;57(3–4):41–43.

12. Bier S, Sim A, Balbay D, Todenhöfer T, Aufderklamm S, Halalsheh O, Mischinger J, Böttge J, Rausch S, Stenzl A, Gakis G, Canda E, Schwentner C. [Treatment of invasive bladder cancer: robot-assisted radical cystectomy and intracorporeal urinary diversion]. Urologe A. 2015;54(1):41–46.

Robotic Cystectomy and Intracorporeal Stoma Formation: Robotic Management of Ureteric Strictures

50

Robotic cystectomy to this day, remains the hardest operation a surgeon has to do. Additionally, there is no guarantee, that what is done robotically, this will enable a lack of complications compared to open surgery. Ureteric strictures are incredibly common post robotic radical cystectomy. They are serious complications of urinary diversion, often occurring within a year of surgery. These can also be more common on the left [1].

The question is, what can be done as part of diagnostics and robotics to manage them.

Derangement in renal function is seen in intracoporeal robotic ileal conduit formation. A significant reduction in the ureteric stricture formation is seen with ureteric stents in situ and tension free anatomizing with external stenting [2]. In contrast, one series, over 10 years, demonstrated conservative management may be an option [3]. However, this paper specified, this is only appropriate for a select population. So what can be done for the rest?

The incidence of early uretero-ileal stricture post-cystectomy is 5%, most are symptomatic. The next question, is whether loopograms have a role in diagnostics [1]. The routine 3-month loopograms were not found to change the management of patients significantly [1]. Ureteric strictures post robotic intracorporeal stoma formation can be managed with robot-assisted laparoscopic ureteroileal reimplantation [4]. Robot-assisted ureteral reimplantation for management of post-cystectomy ureteroileal anastomatic stricture is feasible and safe in experienced hands [4].

Complex robotic reconstruction using bowel segments are challenging operative scenarios [4]. This study demonstrates localization and reconstruction of ureteral-ileal anastomotic strictures with the assistance of Indocyanine Green (ICG) using near infrared (NIR) imaging [5]. Intraoperative localization of ureteral-ileal anastomotic strictures involved retrograde and/or antegrade instillation of ICG [5]. The distinction between ureter, bowel and bowel based urinary diversion segments are difficult to demarcate due to distorted anatomy and postoperative adhesions especially in revision surgery. Use of ICG during complex robotic reconstruction allows

S. S. Goonewardene et al., *Management of Muscle Invasive Bladder Cancer*, Management of Urology, https://doi.org/10.1007/978-3-030-57915-9_50

for localization and demarcation of bowel and ureteral segments to improve lysis of adhesions and ureterolysis is one of the methods of dealing with this. This is a safe and feasible option for robotic revision of ureteral-ileal anastomotic strictures.

Post-cystectomy ureteroileal anastomotic strictures that fail percutaneous or endourologic management require operative repair [6]. The longer the stricture, the more challenging the case. Robotic principles apply, dissection of the colonic mesentery, peeling of the ureter off the common iliac vessels, mobilising the ureter appropriately on side of the sigmoid. By addressing these techniques initially, strictures may be prevented [6]. With mean follow up of 16 months no major complications were encountered and all patients remain free of stricture recurrence to date. Robotic ureteroileal anastomotic stricture repair is feasible for both right and left-sided cases [7].

In conclusion, robotics is the way forward for repair of ureteric strictures after robotic radical cystectomy with ileal conduit formation. Additionally, indocyanine green, can be used to guide the surgeon to localise the stricture appropriately and limit the degree of dissection.

References

1. Gan C, Stephenson W, Rottenberg G, Thomas K, Khan MS, O'Brien T. A prospective study of the utility of a routine 'Loopogram' 3 months after surgery for the detection of anastomotic stricture post cystectomy and ileal conduit formation. Eur Urol Suppl. 2015;14(2):e473.
2. Shimpi RK. Renal functional deterioration after urinary diversion a retrospective comparison between ileal conduit and ileal orthotopic neobladder. Eur Urol Suppl. 2014;13(5):153.
3. Baten E, Joniau S, Van Poppel H, Van Der Aa F. When is a conservative management recommended for ureterointestinal strictures following radical cystectomy with ileal conduit? Eur Urol Suppl. 2014;13(1):e284.
4. Carneiro A, Dovirak O, Kaplan J, Chang P, Wagner AA. Robot-assisted ureteroileal reimplantation for post-cystectomy anastomotic stricture. J Urol. 2015;1:e848.
5. Moore BW, Giusto LL, Lee Z, Sterious SN, Mydlo JH, Eun DD. Use of indocyanine green (ICG) for complex robotic reconstruction involving bowel urinary diversions. J Urol. 2014;1:e735.
6. Tobis S, Houman J, Mastrodonato K, Rashid H, Wu G. Robotic repair of post-cystectomy ureteroileal anastomotic strictures: techniques for success. J Laparoendosc Adv Surg Techniq. 2013;23(6):526–9.
7. Tobis S, Houman J, Mastrodonato K, Rashid H, Wu G. Robotic repair of post-cystectomy ureteroileal anastomotic strictures: techniques for success. J Urol. 2013;1:e886.

Management of Ureteric Stricture Disease Post Urinary Diversion in Bladder Cancer

51

A systematic review relating to bladder cancer, ureteric stricture disease and urinary diversion was conducted. This was to identify the bladder cancer, ureteric strictural disease and urinary diversion. The search strategy aimed to identify all references related to bladder cancer, ureteric strictures AND urinary diversion. Search terms used were as follows: (Bladder cancer) AND (ureteric stricture) AND (urinary diversion). The following databases were screened from 1989 to June 2020:

- CINAHL
- MEDLINE (NHS Evidence)
- Cochrane
- AMed
- EMBASE
- PsychINFO
- SCOPUS
- Web of Science

In addition, searches using Medical Subject Headings (MeSH) and keywords were conducted using Cochrane databases. Two UK-based experts in bladder cancer were consulted to identify any additional studies.

Studies were eligible for inclusion if they reported primary research focusing on bladder cancer and screening. Papers were included if published after 1984 and had to be in English. Studies that did not conform to this were excluded. Only primary research was included (Fig. 51.1). The overall aim was to identify bladder cancer risk factors and epidemiology in muscle invasive disease.

Abstracts were independently screened for eligibility by two reviewers and disagreements resolved through discussion or third party opinion. Agreement level was

S. S. Goonewardene et al., *Management of Muscle Invasive Bladder Cancer*, Management of Urology, https://doi.org/10.1007/978-3-030-57915-9_51

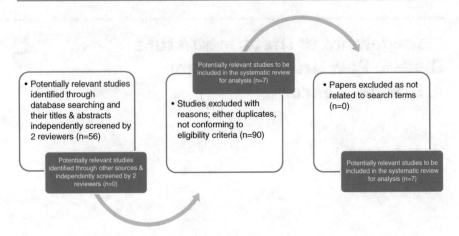

Fig. 51.1 Flow chart of studies identified through the systematic review. (Adapted from PRISMA)

calculated using Cohen's Kappa to test the intercoder reliability of this screening process. Cohens' Kappa allows comparison of inter-rater reliability between papers using relative observed agreement. This also takes account of the comparison occurring by chance. The first reviewer agreed all 7 papers to be included, the second, agreed on 7. Cohens kappa was therefore 1.0.

Data extraction was piloted by the researcher and amended in consultation with the research team (author and two academic supervisors). Data collected included authors, year and country of publication, study aims, setting, intervention aims, number of participants, study design, intervention components and delivery methods, comparison groups and outcome measures, notes and follow-up questions for the authors. Studies were quality assessed using the PRISMA criteria for randomised controlled trials, Mays et al. [1, 2] for the action research and qualitative studies and the Critical Skills Appraisal programme for cohort studies. This was also applied to randomised controlled trials and qualitative studies.

The search identified 56 papers (Fig. 51.1). All 7 mapped to the search terms and eligibility criteria. The current systematic reviews were examined to gain further knowledge about the subject. Three hundred and ninety papers were excluded due to not conforming to eligibility criteria or adding to the evidence. Of the 7 papers left, relevant abstracts were identified and the full papers obtained (all of which were in English), to quality assure against search criteria. There was considerable heterogeneity of design among the included studies therefore a narrative review of the evidence was undertaken. There was significant heterogeneity within studies, including clinical topic, numbers, outcomes, as a result a narrative review was thought to be best. There were 7 cohort studies, with a moderate level of evidence. These were from a range of countries with minimal loss to follow-up. All participants were identified appropriately.

51.1   Systematic Review Results

51.1.1 Ureteric Stricture Rates Post Radical Cystectomy: Ileal Conduit vs. Orthotopic Neobladder

Hosseini reported stricture rates from a single high-volume RARC centre [3]. The median time to stricture formation was 165 days (range 10–495 days) [3]. Twenty-four patients (6.5%) developed strictures [3]. Six of 81 patients (7.4%) in the monofilament group and 18 of 290 (6.2%) in the barbed suture group developed strictures (p = 0.22) [3]. Fifteen patients (63%) had a stricture on the left side, seven (29%) on the right side and two patients (8%) developed bilateral ureteric strictures (p = 0.002) [3]. Strictures occurred in 11 of 131 patients (8.3%) with an orthotopic neobladder and 13 of 240 (5.4%) with an ileal-conduit urinary diversion (p = 0.17) [3].

51.1.2 Rates of Ureteric Strictures: Open vs. Robotic Radical Cystectomy

Goh compared stricture rates of robot-assisted radical cystectomy (RARC) and open radical cystectomy (ORC) using Surveillance, Epidemiology, and End Results-Medicare data [4]. The incidence of ureteroenteric stricture at 6 and 12 months was higher for RARC vs. ORC at 12.1% vs. 7.0% (p < 0.01) and 15.0% vs. 9.5% (p = 0.01), respectively [4]. RARC vs. ORC stricture incidence at 2 years did not differ significantly at 14.6% vs. 11.4% (p = 0.29) [4]. Stricture diagnosis rates were significantly lower following ORC at 6, 12, and 24 months (p < 0.05) [4]. In adjusted analysis, RARC (HR 1.64, 95% CI 1.23–2.19) and preoperative hydronephrosis (HR 1.51, 95% CI 1.17–1.94) were associated with the development of stricture [4]. Higher hospital volume was associated with a lower risk of stricture (HR 0.40, 95% CI 0.26–0.63) [4].

51.1.3 New Techniques in Management of Ureteric Strictures

51.1.3.1   Latero-Lateral Ureteric Re-implantation

Padovani presented a technique of ureteroileal bypass to treat uretero-enteric strictures in urinary diversion, a latero-lateral ureteric re-implantation [5]. All patients had the diagnosis of uretero-enteric anastomotic stricture via computerized tomography and DTPA renal scan [5]. Time between cystectomy and diagnosis of uretero-enteric anastomotic stricture varied from 5 months to 3 years [5]. Mean hospital stay was 3.3 ± 0.62 days (3–4 days) [5]. During follow-up, all patients were asymptomatic and presented improvement in ureterohydronephrosis. Serum creatinine of all patients had been stable [5]. Latero-lateral ureter re-implantation is feasible by open or even robotic surgery with positive results, reasonable operation time, and without complications [5].

51.1.3.2   The Modified Hautmann Neobladder

Elbendary described a simple modification in Hautmann neobladder that involves an elongation of its left chimney to advance it through the pelvic mesocolon in order to reach the left ureter in its original place [6]. This technique was carried out on 27 patients who had Hautmann pouch after radical cystectomy [6]. The modification was applied easily without any perioperative complications that were related to this step in particular [6]. At a mean follow up of 41.3 ± 10.2 months, have not detected any cases of stricture formation or ureteral recurrence at the sites of the ureteroileal anastomosis [6]. There was only one patient who developed acute pyelonephritis (3.7%) as a result of reflux [6].

51.1.4   Ureteric Stricture Rate: Wallace vs. Bricker Anastomosis

Christoph evaluated the outcome and complication rate of the Bricker and Wallace anastomosis [7]. In both groups, the body mass index (BMI) was similar (26.1 kg/m^2 Bricker and 26.4 kg/m^2 Wallace) [7]. the stricture rate after performing the Bricker anastomosis technique was 25.3% (19/75) as compared to 7.7% (5/65) after Wallace anastomosis technique, which was statistically significant ($p = 0.001$) [7]. In the Bricker group, patients with strictures had higher BMI (28.3 vs. 25.7 kg/m^2, $p = 0.05$) [7]. On average it took 8.5 months in the Bricker group and 3 months in the Wallace group ($p = 0.6$) to develop stricture [7].

Kouba evaluated the success and complications of the two most common types of ureteroenteric anastomotic techniques, the Bricker and the Wallace anastomosis [8]. Kouba evaluated the complications of the Bricker and Wallace techniques of ureteroenteric anastomosis in a single surgeon, single institution series [8]. Of the 186 patients 94 underwent a Bricker (51%), 90 underwent a Wallace (48%) and 2 patients underwent both procedures (Wallace on duplicated system on 1 side, Bricker on contralateral side) [8]. Ureteral stricture developed in 5 of 186 (2.6%) patients and the overall stricture rate for all ureters was 7 of 371 (1.9%) [8]. In patients undergoing Bricker anastomosis the total stricture rate for all ureters was 3.7% (7 of 187) [8]. With the Wallace anastomosis the total stricture rate for all ureters was 0% (0 of 184) [8]. This difference in stricture rate in the Bricker vs. Wallace subgroups was significant ($p = 0.015$) [8]. There was no difference in age, gender, creatinine, prior radiation, complications or mode of diversion between the groups [8]. Body mass index was higher in the Bricker vs. the Wallace group (29.0 vs. 25.9 kg/m^2) [8]. Of the 5 patients with strictures 1 underwent successful open repair, 1 had successful interventional radiological repair and 3 were treated with chronic ureteral stents (1 after failed open repair and 2 after failed radiological repair) [8].

51.1.5 Continuous vs. Interrupted Suture Impact on Ureteric Stricture Rate

Large studied the impact of the running vs. the interrupted technique on the uretero-intestinal anastomotic stricture rate [9]. The stricture rate per ureter was 8.5% (25 of 293) and 12.7% (27 of 213) in the interrupted and running groups, respectively (p = 0.14) [9]. Univariate analysis suggested that postoperative urinary tract infection (HR 2.1, 95% CI 1.1–4.1, p = 0.04) and Clavien grade 3 or greater complications (HR 2.6, 95% CI 1.4–4.9, p < 0.01) were associated with ureterointestinal anastomotic stricture [9]. On multivariate analysis postoperative urinary tract infection (HR 2.4, 95% CI 1.2–5.1, p = 0.02) and running technique (HR 1.9, 95% CI 1.0–3.7, p = 0.05) were associated with ureterointestinal anastomotic stricture [9]. Median time to stricture and followup was 289 (IQR 120–352) and 351 days (IQR 132–719) in the running cohort vs. 213 (IQR 123–417) and 497 days (IQR 174–1289) in the interrupted cohort, respectively [9]. Kaplan-Meier analysis controlling for differential followup showed a trend toward higher freedom from stricture for the interrupted ureterointestinal anastomosis (p = 0.06) [9].

51.1.6 Use of Ureteric Stents and Impact on Ureteric Stricture Rates

Mullins determine the impact of stenting ureteroenteric anastomoses on postoperative stricture rate and gastrointestinal recovery in continent and noncontinent urinary diversions (UDs) [10]. Thirty-six percent of patients were stented and 64% were nonstented at the time of UD [10]. Total ureteral stricture rate was 9.9% [10]. There was no statistically significant difference in stricture rate (p = 0.11) or length of hospital stay (p = 0.081) in stented compared to nonstented patients [10]. There was a significantly (p = 0.014) greater rate of ileus in patients who were nonstented in both continent and noncontinent UDs [10].

51.1.7 Impact of Prior Pelvic Irradiation On Ureteric Strictures

Katkoori compared uretero-intestinal anastomotic (UIA) stricture rates after radical cystectomy (RC) with and without previous pelvic radiotherapy (pRT) [11]. In all, 526 patients had RC by one surgical team during the study period; 65 had pRT before RC, 37 for prostate cancer, 23 for bladder cancer and the rest for other pelvic malignancies [11]. All the patients in group 1 had an ileal conduit (IC) diversion [11]. There were 250 IC and 211 neobladder diversions in group 2 [11]. There were 130 (12%) UIAs in group 1, vs. 922 (88%) in group 2 [11]. There was no statistically significant difference between the groups in demographic profile and follow-up [11]. The overall stricture rate for UIA was 1.3%; there were two (1.5%) UIA strictures in group 1 vs. 12 (1.3%) in group 2 [11]. The mean (median, range) time to onset of the stricture was 10 (6, 2–39) months [11]. There was no statistically significant difference in stricture rate between the groups (p > 0.05) [11].

51.1.8 Development of Malignant Ureteric Strictures vs. Benign Strictures

Tsuji designed a proper follow-up for cystectomy and ileal conduit urinary diversion for primary bladder transitional carcinoma and compared the radiographic characteristics of recurrent malignant upper tract lesions with those of benign ureteroileal anastomosis strictures [12]. Five patients (8.2%) developed malignant ureteral obstruction (4 had metachronous upper tract tumors, and 1 patient had retroperitoneal lymph node metastasis which compressed the ureter) [12]. Eleven patients (18.0%) developed benign ureteroileal anastomotic stricture [12]. In all patients with malignant upper tract obstruction, a complete loss of renal function occurred within 10 months after the detection [12]. Conversely, a progressive renal dysfunction was observed in patients with benign ureteroileal anastomotic stricture [12]. All patients were asymptomatic before the detection of lesions on excretory pyelography [12]. These results demonstrated malignant strictures advance rapidly [12].

51.1.9 Risk Factors for Development of Ureteric Strictures

Hautmann evaluated preoperative ureteral obstruction as a risk factor for benign ureteroenteric anastomosis strictures in patients who underwent open radical cystectomy and ileal neobladder diversion [13]. Unilateral or bilateral obstruction developed in 107 of the 953 patients (127 reno-ureteral units, including 63 on the right side and 64 on the left side) [13]. Of the reno-ureteral units 98 had benign and 29 had malignant ureteroenteric anastomosis strictures [13]. The overall stricture rate due to any cause in preoperatively obstructed ureters was 19.3% at 10 years vs. 6.4% in preoperatively undilated ureters [13]. For the refluxing Wallace type technique the 10-year ureteroenteric anastomosis stricture rate was 2.4% for preoperatively undilated and 7.6% for preoperatively obstructed ureters [13]. For the nonrefluxing technique the corresponding rates at 10 years were 14.2% and 35.54%, respectively [13].

51.1.10   Endoureterotomy vs. Open Surgical Revision for Ureteric Strictures

Laven assessed the morbidity or success rate of secondary open anastomotic revision after failed endoureterotomy [14]. One of the 3 patients in whom open revision failed underwent prior pelvic external beam radiation and the other 2 underwent prior endoureterotomies [14]. Overall interventions for right strictures were more successful 85% or 11 of 13 cases than those on the left side (50% or 9 of 18) (p = 0.037) [14]. Average operative time was longer and average estimated blood loss was higher in patients treated with open repair after failed endoureterotomy (p = 0.009 and 0.016, respectively) [14]. No complications developed in patients following endoureterotomy [14].

Kramolowsky evaluated open vs. endourological repair for ureterointestinal anastomotic strictures [15]. The success rate (that is patent ureter and no stent) was 89% for the open revision group and 71% (5 of 7) for the endoscopic group [15]. The endoscopic group had markedly shorter hospitalization, decreased blood loss, diminished patient discomfort and no postoperative complications [15]. While the endoscopic procedure for ureteroileal anastomotic strictures is less successful than open revision, the lower morbidity, decreased cost and shorter hospital stay associated with the endourological approach favor its use over open revision [15]. For elderly patients who fail initial endoscopic revision and for patients with metastatic transitional cell cancer, placement of an indwelling stent is a reasonable alternative [15]. Given these guidelines, less than 30% of the patients who suffer a ureteroileal anastomotic stricture will require open surgical revision [15].

Schöndorf compared the long-term results of minimally invasive endourological intervention and open surgical revision in patients with a nonmalignant ureteroileal stricture [16]. Median followup was 29 months (range 2–177). The overall success rate was 26% (25 of 96 cases) for endourological intervention vs. 91% (32 of 35) for open surgical revision (p < 0.001) [16]. Subgroup analysis showed a significant difference in the success rate of minimally invasive endourological interventions vs. open surgical revision for strictures greater than 1 cm (3 of 52 cases or 6% vs. 19 of 22 or 86%, p < 0.001) [16]. The success rate of endourological and open surgical procedures for strictures 1 cm or less was 50% (22 of 44 cases) and 100% (13 of 13), respectively [16]. After adjusting for multiple preoperative stricture characteristics, only stricture length was strongly and inversely associated with a successful outcome (p < 0.001) [16].

51.1.11   Risk of Ureteric Obstructionwith Antireflux Techniques in Orthotopic Neobladders

Roth attempted to determine the relative risk of ureterointestinal anastomosis using two antireflux techniques of orthotopic bladder substitution, and assessed the degree to which success is determined by surgeon experience [17]. There was a 20.4% rate of nonneoplastic obstructions in the 142 ureters reimplanted with the Le Duc technique (Hautmann group) [17]. The variation in obstruction rates of 16.7%, 18.2% and 25%, respectively, for expert, skilled and learning surgeons was statistically insignificant [17]. Only 3 nonneoplastic obstructions (3.6%) developed in the 83 ureters reimplanted with the Nesbit/Studer technique (Studer group) [17]. The variation in obstruction rates of 5.1%, 0% and 3.6%, respectively, for expert, skilled and learner surgeons was statistically insignificant [17].

51.1.12   Balloon Dilation in Ureterointestinal Anastomotic Stricture

Yagi determined outcomes from a percutaneous antegrade balloon dilation technique in ureterointestinal anastomotic stricture [18]. Additional dilation was necessary in three of ten patients for the recurrent stricture [18]. The balloon dilation was ineffective in two patients with a long stenosis of the ureter or a previous history of radiation therapy for uterine cancer [18]. Eight of 10 patients showed satisfactory outcomes during the mean follow-up period of 47.1 months [18].

References

1. Mays N, Pope C, Popay J. Systematically reviewing qualitative and quantitative evidence to inform management and policy-making in the health field. J Health Serv Res Policy. 2005;10(Suppl. 1):6–20. [in English].
2. Moher D, Liberati A, Tetzlaff J, Altman DG. Preferred reporting items for systematic reviews and meta-analyses: the prisma statement. BMJ (Online). 2009;339(7716):332–6. [in English].
3. Hosseini A, Dey L, Laurin O, Adding C, Hoijer J, Ebbing J, Collins JW. Ureteric stricture rates and management after robot-assisted radical cystectomy: a single-centre observational study. Scand J Urol. 2018;52(4):244–8. [in English].
4. Goh AC, Belarmino A, Patel NA, Sun T, Sedrakyan A, Bochner BH, Hu JC. A population-based study of ureteroenteric strictures after open and robot-assisted radical cystectomy. Urology. 2020;135:57–65. [in English].
5. Padovani GP, Mello MF, Coelho RF, Borges LL, Nesrallah A, Srougi M, Nahas WC. Ureteroileal bypass: a new technic to treat ureteroenteric strictures in urinary diversion. Int Braz J Urol. 2018;44(3):624–8. [in English].
6. Elbendary M, El-Gamal OM, Tawfik AM, Elbahnasy Ael H, El-Mateet MS. Simple modification in Hautmann neobladder to carry out left ureteroileal anastmosis without mobilization of the ureter. Int J Urol. 2014;21(4):413–5. [in English].
7. Christoph F, Herrmann F, Werthemann P, Janik T, Schostak M, Klopf C, Weikert S. Ureteroenteric strictures: a single center experience comparing bricker versus wallace ureteroileal anastomosis in patients after urinary diversion for bladder cancer. BMC Urol. 2019;19(1):100. Published 2019 Oct 24. [in English].
8. Kouba E, Sands M, Lentz A, Wallen E, Pruthi RS. A comparison of the bricker versus wallace ureteroileal anastomosis in patients undergoing urinary diversion for bladder cancer. J Urol. 2007;178(3 Pt 1):945–8; discussion 48–9. [in English].
9. Large MC, Cohn JA, Kiriluk KJ, Dangle P, Richards KA, Smith ND, Steinberg GD. The impact of running versus interrupted anastomosis on ureterointestinal stricture rate after radical cystectomy. J Urol. 2013;190(3):923–7. [in English].
10. Mullins JK, Guzzo TJ, Ball MW, Pierorazio PM, Eifler J, Jarrett TW, Schoenberg MP, Bivalacqua TJ. Ureteral stents placed at the time of urinary diversion decreases postoperative morbidity. Urol Int. 2012;88(1):66–70. [in English].
11. Katkoori D, Samavedi S, Adiyat KT, Soloway MS, Manoharan M. Is the incidence of ureterointestinal anastomotic stricture increased in patients undergoing radical cystectomy with previous pelvic radiation? BJU Int. 2010;105(6):795–8. [in English].
12. Tsuji Y, Nakamura H, Ariyoshi A. Upper urinary tract involvement after cystectomy and ileal conduit diversion for primary bladder carcinoma. Eur Urol. 1996;29(2):216–20. [in English].
13. Hautmann RE, de Petriconi R, Kahlmeyer A, Enders M, Volkmer B. Preoperatively dilated ureters are a specific risk factor for the development of ureteroenteric strictures after open radical cystectomy and ileal neobladder. J Urol. 2017;198(5):1098–106. [in English].

14. Laven BA, O'Connor RC, Gerber GS, Steinberg GD. Long-term results of endoureterotomy and open surgical revision for the management of ureteroenteric strictures after urinary diversion. J Urol. 2003;170(4 Pt 1):1226–30. [in English].
15. Kramolowsky EV, Clayman RV, Weyman PJ. Management of ureterointestinal anastomotic strictures: comparison of open surgical and endourological repair. J Urol. 1988;139(6):1195–8. [in English].
16. Schöndorf D, Meierhans-Ruf S, Kiss B, Giannarini G, Thalmann GN, Studer UE, Roth B. Ureteroileal strictures after urinary diversion with an ileal segment—is there a place for endourological treatment at all? J Urol. 2013;190(2):585–90. [in English].
17. Roth S, van Ahlen H, Semjonow A, Oberpenning F, Hertle L. Does the success of ureterointestinal implantation in orthotopic bladder substitution depend more on surgeon level of experience or choice of technique? J Urol. 1997;157(1):56–60. [in English].
18. Yagi S, Goto T, Kawamoto K, Hayami H, Matsushita S, Nakagawa M. Long-term results of percutaneous balloon dilation for ureterointestinal anastomotic strictures. Int J Urol. 2002;9(5):241–6. [in English].

Neoadjuvant Chemotherapy vs. Radical Cystectomy in Muscle Invasive Bladder Cancer

52

A systematic review relating to muscle invasive bladder cancer and neoadjuvant chemotherapy prior to radical cystectomy was conducted. This was to identify whether neoadjuvant chemotherapy has a role in this cohort. The search strategy aimed to identify all references related to bladder cancer AND muscle invasive disease AND neoadjuvant chemotherapy AND radical cystectomy. Search terms used were as follows: (Bladder cancer) AND (muscle invasive disease) AND (Neoadjuvant chemotherapy) AND (Radical Cystectomy). The following databases were screened from 1979 to June 2020:

- CINAHL
- MEDLINE (NHS Evidence)
- Cochrane
- AMedune
- EMBASE
- PsychINFO
- SCOPUS
- Web of Science

In addition, searches using Medical Subject Headings (MeSH) and keywords were conducted using Cochrane databases. Two UK-based experts in bladder cancer were consulted to identify any additional studies.

Studies were eligible for inclusion if they reported primary research focusing on muscle invasive bladder cancer and palliative cystectomy. Papers were included if published after 1984 and had to be in English. Studies that did not conform to this were excluded. Only primary research was included (Fig. 52.1).

Abstracts were independently screened for eligibility by two reviewers and disagreements resolved through discussion or third-party opinion. Agreement level was calculated using Cohen's Kappa to test the intercoder reliability of this screening process [1]. Cohens' Kappa allows comparison of inter-rater reliability between

S. S. Goonewardene et al., *Management of Muscle Invasive Bladder Cancer*, Management of Urology, https://doi.org/10.1007/978-3-030-57915-9_52

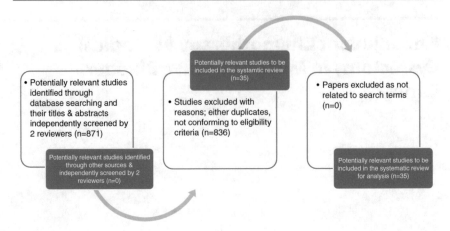

Fig. 52.1 Flow chart of studies identified through the systematic review. (Adapted from PRISMA)

papers using relative observed agreement. This also takes account of the comparison occurring by chance. The first reviewer agreed all 35 papers to be included, the second, agreed on 35.

Data extraction was piloted by the researcher and amended in consultation with the research team (author and two academic supervisors). Data collected included authors, year and country of publication, study aims, setting, intervention aims, number of participants, study design, intervention components and delivery methods, comparison groups and outcome measures, notes and follow-up questions for the authors. Studies were quality assessed using the PRISMA criteria for randomised controlled trials [2, 3] for the action research and qualitative studies and the Critical Skills Appraisal programme for cohort studies. This was also applied to randomised controlled trials and six qualitative studies.

The search identified 871 papers (Fig. 52.1). Thirty-five mapped to the search terms and eligibility criteria. The current systematic reviews were examined to gain further knowledge about the subject. Eight hundred and thirty-six papers were excluded due to not conforming to eligibility criteria or adding to the evidence. Of the 35 papers left, relevant abstracts were identified and the full papers obtained (all of which were in English), to quality assure against search criteria. There was considerable heterogeneity of design among the included studies therefore a narrative review of the evidence was undertaken. There was significant heterogeneity within studies, including clinical topic, numbers, outcomes, as a result a narrative review was thought to be best. There were 28 cohort studies, with a moderate level of evidence and 7 RCTs with a good level of evidence. These were from a range of countries with minimal loss to follow-up. All participants were identified appropriately.

52.1 Systematic Review Results

52.1.1 Neoadjuvant Chemotherapy vs. Radical Cystectomy in Muscle Invasive Bladder Cancer

Osman used a phase III trial to compare outcomes and side effects by neoadjuvant chemotherapy followed by radical cystectomy (arm A), with those treated by radical cystectomy (arm B) in the management of stage II, III urinary bladder cancer [4]. The 3-year OS (overall survival) for arm A, and B were 60% and 50% respectively [4]. The median OS for arm A was 36+ months and that for arm B was 32.5 months [4]. The 3-year progression-free survival (PFS) for arm A, and B were 57% and 43% respectively. The median PFS for arm A was 36+ months and for arm B was 28 months [4]. Both treatment arms were tolerated well with mild toxicities profiles [4].

Grossman et al. [5] evaluated the ability of neoadjuvant chemotherapy to improve the outcome in locally advanced bladder cancer who were treated with radical cystectomy [5]. According to an intention-to-treat analysis, the median survival among patients assigned to surgery alone was 46 months, as compared with 77 months among patients assigned to combination therapy (p = 0.06 by a two-sided stratified log-rank test) [5]. In both groups, improved survival was associated with the absence of residual cancer in the cystectomy specimen. Significantly more patients in the combination-therapy group had no residual disease than patients in the cystectomy group (38% vs. 15%, p < 0.001) [5].

52.1.2 MVAC in Neoadjuvant Chemotherapy in Muscle Invasive Bladder Cancer

Kitamura determined the clinical benefit of neoadjuvant methotrexate, doxorubicin, vinblastine, and cisplatin (MVAC). Patients (N = 130) were randomly assigned to the RC arm (N = 66) and the NAC arm (N = 64) [6]. OS of the NAC arm was better than that of the RC arm, although the difference was not statistically significant [hazard ratio 0.65, multiplicity adjusted 99.99% confidence interval 0.19–2.18, one-sided p = 0.07] [6]. In the NAC arm and the RC arm, 34% and 9% of the patients had pT0, respectively (p < 0.01). In subgroup analyses, OS in almost all subgroups was in favour of NAC [6].

52.1.3 MVAC vs. Gemcitabine and Cisplatin as Neoadjuvant Chemotherapy

MVAC (methotrexate, vinblastine, doxorubicin and cisplatin) has mostly replaced traditional MVAC [7]. Zargar et al. [7] compared pathological response and survival rates in locally advanced bladder cancer who received neoadjuvant chemotherapy with dose dense MVAC vs. gemcitabine and cisplatin [7]. The rate of pT1N0 or less was 30.1% for gemcitabine and cisplatin compared to 41.0% for dose dense MVAC (p = 0.07) [7]. The mean Kaplan-Meier estimates of overall survival in the gemcitabine and cisplatin, and dose dense MVAC groups were 4.2 and 7.0 years, respectively (p = 0.001) [7]. On multivariable cox regression analysis based on preoperative data patients who received gemcitabine and cisplatin were at higher risk for death than patients who received dose dense MVAC (HR 2.07, 95% CI 1.25–3.42, p = 0.003) [7]. Lymph node invasion (HR 1.97, 95% CI 1.15–3.36, p = 0.01) and hydronephrosis (HR 2.18, 95% CI 1.43–3.30, p < 0.001) were also associated with higher risk of death [7].

Kawamura et al. [8] retrospectively evaluated the two chemotherapeutic regimens in the management of muscle-invasive bladder cancer on patients who had had radical cystectomy for clinical stage T2-T4, N and, M0 bladder cancer [8]. Fourteen patients (24.1%) and 44 (75.9%) patients were treated with GC and MVAC therapy, respectively [8]. GC therapy was significantly more effective than MVAC therapy in pathological down-staging (to pT0) rate [8]. On multivariate analysis, the choice of regimen (MVAC) was an independent predictor of the presence of residual cancer after a neoadjuvant chemotherapy [8]. The clinical response to neoadjuvant GC therapy was superior to that to neoadjuvant MVAC therapy [8]. Moreover, GC therapy was associated with less non-hematologic toxicity than MVAC therapy, especially with respect to the occurrence of nausea [8].

Plimack hypothesized that three cycles of neoadjuvant accelerated methotrexate, vinblastine, doxorubicin, and cisplatin (AMVAC) would be safe, shorten the time to surgery, and yield similar pathologic complete response (pT0) rates compared with historical controls [9]. Forty-four patients were accrued; 60% had stage III to IV disease; median age was 64 years. Forty patients were evaluable for response, with 15 (38%; 95% CI 23–53%) showing pT0 at cystectomy, meeting the primary end point of the study [9]. Another six patients (14%) were downstaged to non-muscle invasive disease [9]. Most (82%) experienced only grade 1–2 treatment-related toxicities [9]. There were no grade 3 or 4 renal toxicities and no treatment-related deaths [9]. One patient developed metastases and thus did not undergo cystectomy; all others (n = 43) proceeded to cystectomy within 8 weeks after last chemotherapy administration [9].

52.1.4   Impact of Cisplatin Neoadjuvant Chemotherapy on Muscle Invasive Bladder Cancer Outcomes

The overall direct survival is 37.3% for radical cystectomy and 35.5% for radical cystectomy and cisplatin [10]. The survival rate is 38.2% of the control group and 40.7% for the cisplatin group [10]. Survival rates of patients theoretically rendered free of disease by radical cystectomy (complete response pT0-4a, pN0-2, M0) is 43.7% for 40 control patients and 47.8% for 41 cisplatin treated patients [10]. The time to relapse in complete response patients was significantly longer (p = 0.0298) for those who received cisplatin (arm A 13.1 months versus arm B 30.3 months)

[10]. The time to death (cause specific) did not differ significantly between both groups overall (p = 0.1349) but it was significantly different between controls and responders (p = 0.0501) [10]. The survival of the responders was significantly better than that of nonresponders (p = 0.0142), with specific death rate of 26.3% and 62.5%, respectively.

52.1.5 Gemcitabine and Cisplatin as Neoadjuvant Chemotherapy in Muscle Invasive Bladder Cancer

Okabe et al. [11] evaluated the efficacy of neoadjuvant gemcitabine and cisplatin (GC) therapy for muscle-invasive bladder cancer (MIBC) [11]. Fifty-eight patients receiving neoadjuvant GC therapy and 74 receiving neoadjuvant MVAC were included [11]. The pT0 achieving rates were comparable between the two groups (20.7% vs. 18.9%, p = 0.83) [11]. Neoadjuvant GC was associated with a better 2-year OS rate than neoadjuvant MVAC for clinical T2 disease (95.2% vs. 70.8%, p = 0.036) [11]. In contrast, in patients with clinical T3 or more advanced disease, neoadjuvant MVAC provided more pT0 (20.0% vs. 5.6%, p = 0.07) and better 2-year OS than neoadjuvant GC (71.1% vs. 55.0%, p = 0.142), although the difference did not reach statistical significance [11].

52.1.6 Gemcitabine Plus Carboplatin as Neoadjuvant Chemotherapy in Muscle Invasive Bladder Cancer

Koie conducted a single-arm prospective study to evaluate efficacy and safety of neoadjuvant gemcitabine plus carboplatin (GCarbo) chemotherapy followed by immediate RC in patients with muscle-invasive BC, including cisplatin-unfit patients [12]. The RC specimens of 28 (24.1%) patients showed pT0 [12]. At a median follow-up period of 41 months, the OS and DFS rates were 89.7% and 86.3%, respectively [12]. No patients had grade 3/4 gastrointestinal toxicity or renal impairment [12].

52.1.7 Predictors of Response in Neoadjuvant Chemotherapy for Muscle Invasive Bladder Cancer

Response to neoadjuvant cisplatin treatment in bladder cancer has been linked to expression of Bcl-2 protein by cancer cells [13]. Turker tested Bcl-2 as a predictive marker of neoadjuvant cisplatin chemotherapy response in a patient cohort from randomized cystectomy trials [13]. Bcl-2 expression was positive in 38% and negative in 62% of the 236 evaluable patients [13]. Bcl-2 negative patients receiving neoadjuvant chemotherapy had a significant increase in survival ($p = 0.009$), while Bcl-2 positive patients showed no difference ($p = 0.4$) [13]. When the prognostic value was assessed in the no-chemotherapy group, 5-year overall survival times were significantly better among Bcl-2 positive patients than among Bcl-2 negative patients (42 vs. 33 months, $p = 0.04$), but again Bcl-2 status did not remain independent when other factors were adjusted [13].

When patients with cT3-4aN0 disease in the neoadjuvant chemotherapy group were divided into responders (<pT2) and non-responders (pT2-pT4), responders (<pT2) to neoadjuvant chemotherapy had a better 5-year overall survival rate (83.6%) than non-responders (pT2-pT4; 23.1%; p < 0.05); this was also observed in the non-neoadjuvant chemotherapy group (21.6%; p < 0.05) [14]. On multivariate analysis, the pathological T stage (<pT2 vs. ≥pT2) was a significant predictor of overall survival in the neoadjuvant chemotherapy group [14].

Bhindi evaluated whether survival differed between rUCB at RC after NAC and stage-matched controls who underwent RC alone [15]. The 5-years recurrence-free survival (RFS; 90% vs. 94%; p = 1), cancer-specific survival (CSS; 82% vs. 93%; p = 0.4), and overall survival (OS; 82% vs. 82%; p = 0.5) were not significantly different between the NAC and control groups for patients with ypT0N0/pT0N0 disease (n = 103) [15]. Conversely, among patients with rUCB at RC (n = 401), patients who received NAC had significantly worse 5-years RFS (50% vs. 63%; p = 0.01), CSS (40% vs. 59%; p = 0.003), and OS (33% vs. 48%; p = 0.02) [15]. On multivariable analysis for patients with rUCB, NAC receipt remained independently associated with worse RFS (hazard ratio [HR] 1.84, 95% confidence interval [CI] 1.28–2.66; p = 0.001), CSS (HR 1.81, 95% CI 1.30–2.52; p < 0.001), and OS (HR 1.57, 95% CI 1.18–2.08; p = 0.002) [15].

Parker evaluated pre-treatment clinical factors on the risk of recurrence in patients who were ypT0N0 at RC [16]. A total of 78 patients were identified with ypT0 disease at RC after NAC [16]. Estimated 3-year recurrence-free survival (RFS) of this cohort was 74.8% [16]. In univariate analysis, cT4 disease (HR 3.12; p = 0.04) and time to RC (HR 1.17 for each month increase; p < 0.01) were associated with inferior RFS [16].

Zargar endeavoured to assessed factors predicting adverse pathology in clinically node-negative patients treated with NAC and RC [17]. One hundred and ninety-six patients were included [17]. The clinical stage was cT2 in 115 (61%), cT3 in 62 (33%) and cT4 in 12 (6%) cases. NAC regiments were gemcitabine-cisplatin (GC)-4 cycles 57 (29%), GC-3 cycles 77 (39%), methotrexate, vinblastine, adriamycin, cisplatin (MVAC)-3 cycle 22 (11%) and MVAC-4 cycles 40 (21%). pN+ was seen in 35 (18%) patients [17]. In the logistic regression analysis, cT4 stage (OR 7.50; 95% CI 1.58–33.3) and three compared to four cycles of GC (OR 3.44; 95% CI 1.09–10.9) were significant predictors of pN+ status [17]. Additionally, when controlling for clinical stage, three cycles of GC, compared to four, were significantly associated with higher rates of pT4 disease and lower rates of downstaging to non-muscle-invasive disease [17].

Wang evaluated the spectrum of histologic changes associated with neoadjuvant chemotherapy (NAC) and compared them with those resulting from transurethral resection (TUR) [18]. cases with no/minimal residual disease on RC, it is difficult to attribute the changes to NAC effect only, except if (1) hyalinization of the bladder wall or LN changes are present, or (2) if the preoperative clinical stage was beyond what could be resected by TUR [18].

52.1.8 Gemcitabine, Cisplatin and Lapatinib as Neoadjuvant Chemotherapy

Narayan sought to investigate the safety and efficacy of gemcitabine, cisplatin, and lapatinib (GCL) as neoadjuvant therapy in radical cystectomy [19]. The initial four patients received gemcitabine 1000 mg/m^2 intravenously on days 1 and 8 and cisplatin 70 mg/m^2 intravenously on day 1 of each 21-day treatment cycle [19]. Lapatinib was administered as 1000 mg orally daily starting 1 week prior to the initiation of cycle 1 of gemcitabine and cisplatin (GC) and continuing until the completion of cycle 4 of GC [19]. These initial doses were poorly tolerated, and the final two enrolled patients received a reduced lapatinib dose of 750 mg orally daily [19]. However, reduction of the lapatinib dose did not result in improved tolerance or drug-delivery, and the trial was terminated early due to excessive toxicity [19]. Grade 3/4 toxicities included diarrhea (33%), nausea/vomiting (33%), and thrombocytopenia (33%) [19].

52.1.9 Erlotinib as Neoadjuvant Chemotherapy in Muscle Invasive Bladder Cancer

Pruthi evaluated the clinicopathological efficacy of neoadjuvant erlotinib (an epidermal growth factor receptor, EGFR, inhibitor) for invasive bladder cancer in patients undergoing radical cystectomy (RC) as despite definitive surgical therapy, only half of patients undergoing RC will have long-term disease-free survival, and effective adjunctive therapies, especially using agents with lower toxicity, would be a significant advance in the treatment of invasive bladder cancer [20]. In all, 20 patients with clinical stage T2 disease had neoadjuvant erlotinib therapy followed by RC [20]. On surgical pathology, five patients (25%) were pT0; in addition, seven (35%) were clinically down-staged (≤pT1) and 15 (75%) had organ-confined disease at surgical pathology [20]. At a mean follow-up of 24.8 months, 10 patients remain alive and with no evidence of disease, four with organ-confined disease had progression and nine died, including six from disease and three from other causes [20]. Erlotinib was tolerated in all patients, with drug rash being the most common side-effect, in 15 patients (75%). Interestingly, all pT0 and pTis/T1 patients had a rash [20].

52.1.10 Imaging to Assess Response of Muscle Invasive Bladder Cancer to Neoadjuvant Chemotherapy

Salminen evaluated the accuracy of ^{11}C-acetate Positron Emission Tomography/Magnetic Resonance Imaging (PET/MRI) in bladder cancer (BC) staging and monitoring response to neoadjuvant chemotherapy (NAC) [21]. The sensitivity, specificity and accuracy of ^{11}C-acetate PET/MRI for the detection of muscle invasive BC was 1.00, 0.69 and 0.73 while the area under the receiver operating characteristic curve (95% confidence interval) was 0.85 (0.55–1.0), respectively [21]. All five NAC patients underwent chemotherapy as planned and ^{11}C-acetate PET/MRI correctly staged three patients, overstaged one and understaged one patient compared with RC and ePLND findings [21]. A total of 175 lymph node were removed, median of 35 (range, 27–43) per patient in five patients who had RC and ePLND while 12 (7%) harboured metastases. Sensitivity, specificity, accuracy and AUC for N-staging were 0.20, 0.96, 0.80 and 0.58 on the ePLND template (10 regions) level [21].

52.1.11   Complications from Neoadjuvant Chemotherapy

Michelcompared the peri-operative morbidity in patients treated by NAC then RC and patients having RC alone [22]. Complications rate was 73.9% in the NAC-RC group versus 73.8% in the RC group (p = 1.0) [22]. In multivariate analyses, only the Charlson score was associated with an increased risk of peri-operative complications (p = 0.05) [22]. PT0 tumour rate was significantly higher in the NAC-CR group (50% vs. 7%, p < 0.001) [22].

Iyer et al. [23] assessed the efficacy and tolerability of six cycles of neoadjuvant dose-dense gemcitabine and cisplatin (ddGC) in patients with MIBC [23]. No patient failed to undergo RC as a result of chemotherapy-associated toxicities [23]. The most frequent treatment-related toxicity was anemia (12%; grade 3) [23]. The presence of a presumed deleterious DNA damage response (DDR) gene alteration was associated with chemosensitivity (positive predictive value for <pT2N0 [89%]) [23]. No patient with a deleterious DDR gene alteration has experienced recurrence at a median follow-up of 2 years [23].

Milenkovic compared perioperative and short-term postoperative complication rates between patients receiving radical cystectomy (RC) after neoadjuvant chemotherapy (NAC) and patients undergoing RC alone. Secondary objectives were to compare overall survival (OS) and cancer-specific survival (CSS) [24]. After propensity score covariate adjustment, there was no significant difference in postoperative complications between patients undergoing NAC plus RC and RC alone with an overall complication rate of 69% and 66%, respectively [24]. No significant differences in the 30-day HGC rates (11.76% and 11.83%, respectively) were observed [24]. NAC plus RC patients had worse prognostic factors at baseline; nevertheless, after correction for group differences OS and CSS did not differ from RC only group (5-year OS 61.3% vs. 50.2%, and 5-year CSS 61.8% vs. 57.9% respectively, p > 0.05 for all) [24].

Aldhaam determined the trend of neoadjuvant chemotherapy use for nonmetastatic muscle invasive urothelial bladder cancer and whether it is associated with adverse perioperative morbidity after robot-assisted radical cystectomy [25]. A total of 298 patients (26%) received neoadjuvant chemotherapy [25]. These patients were younger (age 67 vs. 69 years, p = 0.01) and more frequently had an ASA™ (American Society of Anesthesiologists™) score of 3 or greater (62% vs. 55%, p = 0.02) and pathological T3 stage or greater disease (28% vs. 22%, p = 0.04) [25].

The use of neoadjuvant chemotherapy increased significantly from 10% in 2006 to 2007 to 42% in 2016 to 2017 (p < 0.01). On multivariate analysis neoadjuvant chemotherapy was not significantly associated with prolonged operative time, hospital stay, 90-day postoperative complications, reoperation or mortality [25]. Neoadjuvant chemotherapy was associated with 90-day readmissions after robot-assisted radical cystectomy (OR 5.90, 95% CI 3.30–10.90, p < 0.01) [25].

52.1.12 Survival Outcomes in Neoadjuvant Chemotherapy for Muscle Invasive Bladder Cancer

Boeri investigated the prevalence of and factors' association with receiving suboptimal neoadjuvant chemotherapy (NAC) and its impact on survival outcomes in patients with muscle-invasive bladder cancer (MIBC) treated with radical cystectomy (RC) [26]. Before matching, 84/315 (26.6%) patients received a suboptimal NAC regimen [26]. Lower general health status and impaired renal functions were the most significant factors associated with the administration of a suboptimal NAC [26]. After matching, the optimal NAC group achieved higher rates of complete pathological response as compared to the suboptimal group (p = 0.03) [26]. Suboptimal NAC (HR 1.77; p = 0.015) and no NAC (HR 1.52; p = 0.03) were both associated with higher risk of recurrence and OM (HR 1.71; p = 0.02 and HR 1.61; p = 0.02) as compared to optimal NAC [26].

Hanna examined the use of neoadjuvant chemotherapy (NAC) before radical cystectomy [27]. Of 8732 patients who underwent RC, 1619 (19%) received NAC [27]. Following propensity score adjustment, receipt of NAC was not associated with an OS benefit (hazard ratio 0.97; p = 0.591) [27]. On secondary outcome analysis, higher pT0 rates (odds ratio 5.03; p < 0.001) were recorded among patients who received NAC, although rates of pT0 were lower than for patients treated with NAC within the SWOG-8710 trial (13% vs. 38%) [27].

Nitta evaluated the effect of neoadjuvant chemotherapy in patients undergoing radical cystectomy for urothelial bladder cancer [14]. The 5-year overall survival rates were 58.0% and 61.8% in the neoadjuvant chemotherapy and non-neoadjuvant chemotherapy groups, respectively (p = 0.320) [14]. The 5-year overall survival rates for the neoadjuvant chemotherapy and non-neoadjuvant chemotherapy groups were 64.8% and 68.4%, respectively, among cT2N0 patients (p = 0.688) and 38.6% and 21.6%, respectively, among cT3-4aN0 patients (p = 0.290) [14].

Shigyo evaluated the efficacy of neoadjuvant M-VAC (methotrexate, vinblastine, doxorubicin and cisplatin) therapy followed by radical cystectomy [28]. A total of 21 patients with locally invasive bladder cancer received neoadjuvant M-VAC therapy with an average of 2.4 courses (range 2–4) [28]. Of the 21 patients, 4 had stage T2N0M0, 11 had stage T3aN0M0, 5 had stage T3bN0M0 and 1 had stage T4N0M0 at diagnosis [28]. Of the 21 patients, 3 had clinically complete responses (cCR) and 12 had partial responses (cPR), for an overall response rate of 71.4% [28]. The patients who responded to the chemotherapy (cCR + cPR) had a 2-year disease free rate of 80.0% in contrast to 50.0% for the remaining patients who did not respond

[28]. A pathological response (pT0, pT1) was achieved in 6 (28.6%) of the 21 patients [28]. The 5 patients in this group remain free of disease for 15–79 months (mean 58.8 months) [28]. These preliminary results suggest that the patients who achieve either a complete or partial response, in particular those had pathological stage of pT0 or pT1, may have a favorable clinical course [28].

52.1.13   Pathological Impact of Neoadjuvant Chemotherapy in Muscle Invasive Bladder Cancer

Rintala evaluated the benefit of neoadjuvant chemotherapy—given before scheduled low-dose irradiation and cystectomy [29]. The results suggest that a significant downstaging in the group randomized to chemotherapy was found only in T1, grade 3 tumours (56 patients, $p = 0.002$) [29]. The overall survival rate in all 311 patients was significantly higher in the chemotherapy group ($p = 0.03$) and likewise among the 253 patients with T2-T4a tumour ($p = 0.018$) [29]. For the 210 patients who underwent cystectomy for T2-T4a tumour, there was a trend towards longer survival when chemotherapy was given ($p = 0.057$) [29]. Patients with initially muscle-invasive tumour who responded to neoadjuvant treatment survived longer than non-responders ($p = 0.0005$) [29]. The results suggest that neoadjuvant chemotherapy improve the outcome of radical surgery for muscle-invasive bladder cancer, though the effect on long-term survival is inconclusive. Further studies on the effect of neoadjuvant chemotherapy is initiated [29].

Parker et al. [30] evaluated the effect of concomitant clinical carcinoma in situ on cancer specific outcomes after neoadjuvant chemotherapy for muscle invasive bladder cancer [30]. The condition was associated with a significant decrease in the pathological complete response rate (10.7% vs. 26.3%, $p = 0.02$) [30]. This difference was significant on univariate and multivariable analysis (OR 0.34, 95% CI 0.13–0.85, $p = 0.02$ and OR 0.31, 95% CI 0.12–0.81, $p = 0.02$), respectively [30]. Despite the decreased complete response rate clinical carcinoma in situ was not associated with a difference in recurrence-free, cancer specific or overall survival [30]. Additionally, when down-staging to pathological carcinoma in situ only disease was considered a complete response, there was no significant change in recurrence-free, cancer specific or overall survival [30].

Teramukai evaluated the surrogacy of tumor downstaging using data from a follow-up observational study in bladder cancer [31]. The hazard ratios after adjustment for prognostic factors in the intermediate effect patients and the poor effect patients were 1.9 (95% confidence interval, 1.0–3.7) and 5.0 (95% confidence interval, 2.6–9.8), respectively, compared with that in the good effect patients [31]. Neoadjuvant chemotherapy has a statistically significant tumor downstaging effect, [31].

Rosenblattassess the effect of NAC on tumour downstaging and overall survival [32]. Downstaging rates increased significantly in the NAC arm independent of the downstaging threshold [32]. The impact was more prominent in clinical T3 tumours, with a near threefold increase in CD tumours [32]. The combination of CD and

NAC showed an absolute risk reduction of 31.1% in OS at 5 year compared with CD controls [32]. The combination of NAC and CD revealed a hazard ratio of 0.32 compared with 1.0 for the combination of no NAC and no CD [32]. Limitations were the retrospective approach and uncertain clinical TNM staging [32].

Weight evaluated a cohort of patients in a tertiary referral setting [33]. Clinical stage at the time of diagnosis in the NC cohort was T2 in 23 (79%) and T3-4a in 6 (21%) patients [33]. A total of 20 (69%) patients received the combination of gemcitabine and cisplatin (GC), 4 (14%) received MVAC, and 5 (17%) received other regimens [33]. The median interval from the time of diagnosis of muscle-invasive bladder cancer to RC was 208 days (interquartile range, 149–327 days) in the NC cohort [33]. Overall, only 2 patients (7%; 95% confidence interval [95% CI], 0–17 patients) achieved a pathologic complete response, 18 (62%; 95% CI, 43–81 patients) had nonorgan-confined residual cancer, and the overall median progression-free survival was 10.5 months (95% CI, 7–14 months) [33].

52.1.14   Impact of Suboptimal Neoadjuvant Chemotherapy Dosing on Outcomes in Muscle Invasive Bladder Cancer

Hinata evaluated the effect of suboptimal dosing on the outcomes of patients who received neoadjuvant chemotherapy (NAC) and robot-assisted radical cystectomy (RARC) [34]. After propensity-score matching, 69 patients in the cohort received optimal-dose NAC, 41 received suboptimal NAC and 69 did not receive NAC [34]. Complication rates and readmission rates did not differ significantly among the three groups [34]. On multivariable analysis, suboptimal NAC and no NAC were independent predictors of worse RFS (hazard ratio [HR] 2.5, 95% confidence interval [CI] 1.2–5.7, p = 0.01 and HR 2.4, 95% CI 1.28–5.16, p = 0.01) and worse OS (HR 4.5, 95% CI 1.6–15.0, p < 0.01 and HR 4.9, 95% CI 1.9–15.6, p < 0.01) in patients who received NAC and RARC [34]. Failure to achieve pathological complete response (ypT0N0) was also an independent predictor of worse RFS (HR 6.6, 95% CI 1.3–20.9; p = 0.02) and OS (HR 4.9, 95% CI 1.8–15.3; p = 0.02) [34].

52.1.15   Neoadjuvant Chemotherapy in Radical Cystectomy vs. Radiotherapy

Hermans compared complete pathological downstaging (pCD, ≤(y)pT1N0) and overall survival (OS) in patients with cT2 versus cT3-4aN0M0 UC of the bladder undergoing radical cystectomy (RC) with or without neoadjuvant chemo- (NAC) or radiotherapy (NAR) [35]. In cT2 UC, pCD-rate was 25% after upfront RC versus 43% (p < 0.001) and 33% (p = 0.130) after NAC + RC and NAR + RC, respectively [35]. In cT3-4a UC, pCD-rate was 8% after upfront RC versus 37% (p < 0.001) and 16% (p = 0.281) after NAC + RC and NAR + RC, respectively [35]. In cT2 UC, 5-year OS was 57% and 51% for NAC + RC and upfront RC, respectively (p = 0.135), whereas in cT3-4a UC, 5-year OS was 55% for NAC + RC versus 36%

for upfront RC (p < 0.001) [35]. In multivariable analysis for OS, NAC was beneficial in cT3-4a UC (HR: 0.67, 95% CI 0.51–0.89) but not in cT2 UC (HR: 0.91, 95%
CI 0.72–1.15) [35]. NAR did not influence OS [35].

52.1.16 Neoadjuvant Chemotherapy in a Salvage Cystectomy Setting

Malmström conducted a randomized phase III study to assess the possible benefit of
neoadjuvant chemotherapy in patients with bladder cancer undergoing radical cystectomy after short-term radiotherapy [36]. After 5 years the overall survival rate
was 59% in the chemotherapy group and 51% in the control group (p = 0.1) [36].
The corresponding cancer specific survival rate was 64 and 54%, respectively [36].
In regard to treatment, no difference was observed for stages T1 and T2 disease,
while there was a 15% difference in overall survival for patients with stages T3 to
T4a disease (p = 0.03) [36]. In a multivariate analysis only chemotherapy and T
category emerged as independent prognostic factors [36]. The relative death risk for
patients who received chemotherapy was 0.69 (95% confidence interval 0.49–0.98)
compared to the control group after adjustment for the other tested factors [36].

52.1.17 Neoadjuvant Chemotherapy vs. Active Surveillance in Muscle Invasive Bladder Cancer

Mazza et al. [37], reported the outcomes in patients with muscle invasive bladder
cancer from two institutions who experienced a clinically complete response to neoadjuvant platinum based chemotherapy and elected active surveillance [37]. It was
unknown whether conservative treatment could be safely implemented in these
patients [37]. In the 148 patients followed a median of 55 months (range 5–145) the
5-year disease specific, overall, cystectomy-free and recurrence-free survival rates
were 90%, 86%, 76% and 64%, respectively [37]. Of the patients 71 (48%) experienced recurrence in the bladder, including 16 (11%) with muscle invasive disease
and 55 (37%) with noninvasive disease [37]. Salvage radical cystectomy prevented
cancer specific death in 9 of 12 patients (75%) who underwent cystectomy after
muscle invasive relapse and in 13 of 14 (93%) after noninvasive relapse [37].

52.1.18 Systematic Reviews Relating to Neoadjuvant Chemotherapy in Muscle Invasive Bladder Cancer

Lavery analysed the designs, methods and observations of these trials to identify
patient subgroups that appeared most likely to benefit [38]. The greatest apparent
benefit was seen in patients free of cancer at radical cystectomy (pT0) [38]. They
had markedly improved overall and disease specific survival compared to patients
with residual disease [38]. However, improvements occurred regardless of whether

there was down-staging from muscle invasive urothelial bladder cancer to pT0 after transurethral resection alone (controls) or after resection plus neoadjuvant chemotherapy [38]. Thus, the major benefit of chemotherapy appeared to be that more patients achieved pT0 [38].

References

1. Cohen J. Weighted kappa: nominal scale agreement with provision for scaled disagreement or partial credit. Psychol Bull. 1968;70(4):213–20. [in English].
2. Moher D, Liberati A, Tetzlaff J, AltmanDG. "Preferred Reporting Items for Systematic Reviews and Meta-Analyses: The Prisma Statement." [In English]. BMJ (Online) 339, no. 7716 (08 Aug 2009):332–36.
3. Mays N, Pope C, Popay J. "Systematically Reviewing Qualitative and Quantitative Evidence to Inform Management and Policy-Making in the Health Field." [In English]. Journal of Health Services Research and Policy 10, no. SUPPL. 1 (July 2005):6–20.
4. Osman MA, Gabr AM, Elkady MS. Neoadjuvant chemotherapy versus cystectomy in management of stages II, and III urinary bladder cancer. Arch Ital Urol Androl. 2014;86(4):278–83. [in English].
5. Grossman HB, Natale RB, Tangen CM, Speights VO, Vogelzang NJ, Trump DL, deVere White RW, et al. Neoadjuvant chemotherapy plus cystectomy compared with cystectomy alone for locally advanced bladder cancer. N Engl J Med. 2003;349(9):859–66. [in English].
6. Kitamura H, Tsukamoto T, Shibata T, Masumori N, Fujimoto H, Hirao Y, Fujimoto K, et al. Randomised phase III study of neoadjuvant chemotherapy with methotrexate, doxorubicin, vinblastine and cisplatin followed by radical cystectomy compared with radical cystectomy alone for muscle-invasive bladder cancer: Japan Clinical Oncology Group Study JCOG0209. Ann Oncol. 2014;25(6):1192–8. [in English].
7. Zargar H, Shah JB, van Rhijn BW, Daneshmand S, Bivalacqua TJ, Spiess PE, Black PC, Kassouf W. Neoadjuvant dose dense MVAC versus gemcitabine and cisplatin in patients with Ct3-4an0m0 bladder cancer treated with radical cystectomy. J Urol. 2018;199(6):1452–8. [in English].
8. Kawamura N, Matsushita M, Okada T, Ujike T, Nin M, Tsujihata M. [Relative efficacy of neoadjuvant gemcitabine and cisplatin versus methotrexate, vinblastine, adriamycin, and cisplatin in the management for muscle-invasive bladder cancer]. Hinyokika Kiyo. 2013;59(5):277–81. [in Japanese].
9. Plimack ER, Hoffman-Censits JH, Viterbo R, Trabulsi EJ, Ross EA, Greenberg RE, Chen DY, et al. Accelerated methotrexate, vinblastine, doxorubicin, and cisplatin is safe, effective, and efficient neoadjuvant treatment for muscle-invasive bladder cancer: results of a multicenter phase II study with molecular correlates of response and toxicity. J Clin Oncol. 2014;32(18):1895–901. [in English].
10. Martinez-Piñeiro JA, Gonzalez Martin M, Arocena F, Flores N, Roncero CR, Portillo JA, Escudero A, Jimenez Cruz F, Isorna S. Neoadjuvant cisplatin chemotherapy before radical cystectomy in invasive transitional cell carcinoma of the bladder: a prospective randomized phase III study. J Urol. 1995;153(3 Pt 2):964–73. [in English].
11. Okabe K, Shindo T, Maehana T, Nishiyama N, Hashimoto K, Itoh N, Takahashi A, et al. Neoadjuvant chemotherapy with gemcitabine and cisplatin for muscle-invasive bladder cancer: multicenter retrospective study. Jpn J Clin Oncol. 2018;48(10):934–41. [in English].
12. Koie T, Ohyama C, Hashimoto Y, Hatakeyama S, Yamamoto H, Yoneyama T, Kamimura N. Efficacies and safety of neoadjuvant gemcitabine plus carboplatin followed by immediate cystectomy in patients with muscle-invasive bladder cancer, including those unfit for cisplatin: a prospective single-arm study. Int J Clin Oncol. 2013;18(4):724–30. [in English].

13. Turker P, Segersten U, Malmström PU, Hemdan T. Is Bcl-2 a predictive marker of neoadjuvant chemotherapy response in patients with urothelial bladder cancer undergoing radical cystectomy? Scand J Urol. 2019;53(1):45–50. [in English].
14. Nitta M, Kuroda S, Nagao K, Higure T, Zakoji H, Miyakita H, Usui Y, et al. Effect of neoadjuvant chemotherapy in patients undergoing radical cystectomy for muscle-invasive bladder cancer: a retrospective, multi-institutional study. Jpn J Clin Oncol. 2020;50(1):73–9. [in English].
15. Bhindi B, Frank I, Mason RJ, Tarrell RF, Thapa P, Cheville JC, Costello BA, et al. Oncologic outcomes for patients with residual cancer at cystectomy following neoadjuvant chemotherapy: a pathologic stage-matched analysis. Eur Urol. 2017;72(5):660–4. [in English].
16. Parker WP, Ho PL, Boorjian SA, Melquist JJ, Thapa P, Holzbeierlein JM, Frank I, Kamat AM, Lee EK. The importance of clinical stage among patients with a complete pathologic response at radical cystectomy after neoadjuvant chemotherapy. World J Urol. 2016;34(11):1561–6. [in English].
17. Zargar H, Zargar-Shoshtari K, Lotan Y, Shah JB, van Rhijn BW, Daneshmand S, Spiess PE, Black P. Final pathological stage after neoadjuvant chemotherapy and radical cystectomy for bladder cancer-does Pt0 predict better survival than Pta/Tis/T1? J Urol. 2016;195(4 Pt 1):886–93. [in English].
18. Wang HJ, Solanki S, Traboulsi S, Kassouf W, Brimo F. Neoadjuvant chemotherapy-related histologic changes in radical cystectomy: assessment accuracy and prediction of response. Hum Pathol. 2016;53:35–40. [in English].
19. Narayan V, Mamtani R, Keefe S, Guzzo T, Malkowicz SB, Vaughn DJ. Cisplatin, gemcitabine, and lapatinib as neoadjuvant therapy for muscle-invasive bladder cancer. Cancer Res Treat. 2016;48(3):1084–91. [in English].
20. Pruthi RS, Nielsen M, Heathcote S, Wallen EM, Rathmell WK, Godley P, Whang Y, et al. A phase II trial of neoadjuvant erlotinib in patients with muscle-invasive bladder cancer undergoing radical cystectomy: clinical and pathological results. BJU Int. 2010;106(3):349–54. [in English].
21. Salminen A, Jambor I, Merisaari H, Ettala O, Virtanen J, Koskinen I, Veskimae E, et al. (11) C-acetate Pet/Mri in bladder cancer staging and treatment response evaluation to neoadjuvant chemotherapy: a prospective multicenter study (Acebib trial). Cancer Imaging. 2018;18(1):25. [in English].
22. Michel C, Vordos D, Dumont C, Basset V, Meyer F, Gaudez F, Meria P, et al. [Impact of neoadjuvant chemotherapy on the peri-operative morbidity of radical cystectomy for muscle invasive bladder cancer]. Prog Urol. 2018;28(10):495–501. [in French].
23. Iyer G, Balar AV, Milowsky MI, Bochner BH, Dalbagni G, Donat SM, Herr HW, et al. Multicenter prospective phase II trial of neoadjuvant dose-dense gemcitabine plus cisplatin in patients with muscle-invasive bladder cancer. J Clin Oncol. 2018;36(19):1949–56. [in English].
24. Milenkovic U, Akand M, Moris L, Demaegd L, Muilwijk T, Bekhuis Y, Laenen A, et al. Impact of neoadjuvant chemotherapy on short-term complications and survival following radical cystectomy. World J Urol. 2019;37(9):1857–66. [in English].
25. Aldhaam NA, Elsayed AS, Jing Z, Richstone L, Wagner AA, Rha KH, Yuh B, et al. Neoadjuvant chemotherapy is not associated with adverse perioperative outcomes after robot-assisted radical cystectomy: a case for increased use from the IRCC. J Urol. 2020;203(1):57–61. [in English].
26. Boeri L, Soligo M, Frank I, Boorjian SA, Thompson RH, Tollefson M, Tarrel R, et al. Clinical predictors and survival outcome of patients receiving suboptimal neoadjuvant chemotherapy and radical cystectomy for muscle-invasive bladder cancer: a single-center experience. World J Urol. 2019;37(11):2409–18. [in English].
27. Hanna N, Trinh QD, Seisen T, Vetterlein MW, Sammon J, Preston MA, Lipsitz SR, et al. Effectiveness of neoadjuvant chemotherapy for muscle-invasive bladder cancer in the current real world setting in the USA. Eur Urol Oncol. 2018;1(1):83–90. [in English].

28. Shigyo M, Takahashi A, Otani N, Tsukamoto T, Kumamoto Y. [Clinical efficacy of neoadjuvant M-Vac chemotherapy for invasive bladder cancer]. Nihon Hinyokika Gakkai Zasshi. 1995;86(6):1172–6. [in Japanese].
29. Rintala E, Hannisdahl E, Fosså SD, Hellsten S, Sander S. Neoadjuvant chemotherapy in bladder cancer: a randomized study. Nordic Cystectomy Trial I. Scand J Urol Nephrol. 1993;27(3):355–62. [in English].
30. Parker WP, Ho PL, Melquist JJ, Scott K, Holzbeierlein JM, Lopez-Corona E, Kamat AM, Lee EK. The effect of concomitant carcinoma in situ on neoadjuvant chemotherapy for urothelial cell carcinoma of the bladder: inferior pathological outcomes but no effect on survival. J Urol. 2015;193(5):1494–9. [in English].
31. Teramukai S, Nishiyama H, Matsui Y, Ogawa O, Fukushima M. Evaluation for surrogacy of end points by using data from observational studies: tumor downstaging for evaluating neoadjuvant chemotherapy in invasive bladder cancer. Clin Cancer Res. 2006;12(1):139–43. [in English].
32. Rosenblatt R, Sherif A, Rintala E, Wahlqvist R, Ullén A, Nilsson S, Malmström PU. Pathologic downstaging is a surrogate marker for efficacy and increased survival following neoadjuvant chemotherapy and radical cystectomy for muscle-invasive urothelial bladder cancer. Eur Urol. 2012;61(6):1229–38. [in English].
33. Weight CJ, Garcia JA, Hansel DE, Fergany AF, Campbell SC, Gong MC, Jones JS, et al. Lack of pathologic down-staging with neoadjuvant chemotherapy for muscle-invasive urothelial carcinoma of the bladder: a contemporary series. Cancer. 2009;115(4):792–9. [in English].
34. Hinata N, Hussein AA, George S, Trump DL, Levine EG, Omar K, Dasgupta P, et al. Impact of suboptimal neoadjuvant chemotherapy on peri-operative outcomes and survival after robot-assisted radical cystectomy: a multicentre multinational study. BJU Int. 2017;119(4):605–11. [in English].
35. Hermans TJN, Voskuilen CS, Deelen M, Mertens LS, Horenblas S, Meijer RP, Boormans JL, et al. Superior efficacy of neoadjuvant chemotherapy and radical cystectomy in Ct3-4anOmO compared to Ct2nOmO bladder cancer. Int J Cancer. 2019;144(6):1453–9. [in English].
36. Malmström PU, Rintala E, Wahlqvist R, Hellström P, Hellsten S, Hannisdal E. Five-year followup of a prospective trial of radical cystectomy and neoadjuvant chemotherapy: Nordic Cystectomy Trial I. The Nordic Cooperative Bladder Cancer Study Group. J Urol. 1996;155(6):1903–6. [in English].
37. Mazza P, Moran GW, Li G, Robins DJ, Matulay JT, Herr HW, Decastro GJ, McKiernan JM, Anderson CB. Conservative management following complete clinical response to neoadjuvant chemotherapy of muscle invasive bladder cancer: contemporary outcomes of a multi-institutional cohort study. J Urol. 2018;200(5):1005–13. [in English].
38. Lavery HJ, Stensland KD, Niegisch G, Albers P, Droller MJ. Pathological T0 following radical cystectomy with or without neoadjuvant chemotherapy: a useful surrogate. J Urol. 2014;191(4):898–906. [in English].

Radical Cystectomy and Renal Transplant

53

53.1   Research Methods

A systematic review relating to muscle invasive bladder cancer, radical cystectomy and renal transplant was conducted. This was to identify whether outcomes from renal transplant patients in this cohort. The search strategy aimed to identify all references related to radical cystectomy AND renal transplant. Search terms used were as follows: (Radical Cystectomy) AND (Renal Transplant). The following databases were screened from 1989 to June 2020:

- CINAHL
- MEDLINE (NHS Evidence)
- Cochrane
- AMed
- EMBASE
- PsychINFO
- SCOPUS
- Web of Science

In addition, searches using Medical Subject Headings (MeSH) and keywords were conducted using Cochrane databases. Two UK-based experts in bladder cancer were consulted to identify any additional studies.

Studies were eligible for inclusion if they reported primary research focusing on muscle invasive bladder cancer and nerve sparing. Papers were included if published after 1984 and had to be in English. Studies that did not conform to this were excluded. Due to the paucity of studies, all study types were included, including case series and case reports (Fig. 53.1).

Abstracts were independently screened for eligibility by two reviewers and disagreements resolved through discussion or third-party opinion. Agreement level was calculated using Cohen's Kappa to test the intercoder reliability of this

© The Editor(s) (if applicable) and The Author(s), under exclusive license to
Springer Nature Switzerland AG 2021
S. S. Goonewardene et al., *Management of Muscle Invasive Bladder Cancer*,
Management of Urology, https://doi.org/10.1007/978-3-030-57915-9_53

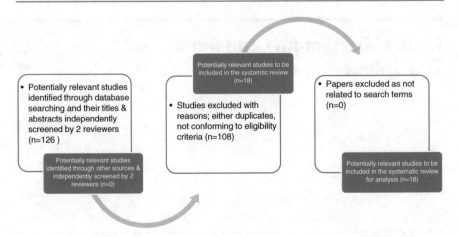

Fig. 53.1 Flow chart of studies identified through the systematic review. (Adapted from PRISMA)

screening process. Cohens' Kappa allows comparison of inter-rater reliability between papers using relative observed agreement. This also takes account of the comparison occurring by chance. The first reviewer agreed all 18 papers to be included, the second, agreed on 18.

Data extraction was piloted by the researcher and amended in consultation with the research team (author and two academic supervisors). Data collected included authors, year and country of publication, study aims, setting, intervention aims, number of participants, study design, intervention components and delivery methods, comparison groups and outcome measures, notes and follow-up questions for the authors. Studies were quality assessed using the PRISMA criteria for randomised controlled trials, Mays et al. [1, 2] for the action research and qualitative studies and the Critical Skills Appraisal programme for cohort studies. This was also applied to randomised controlled trials and qualitative studies.

The search identified 126 papers (Fig. 53.1). Eighteen mapped to the search terms and eligibility criteria. The current systematic reviews were examined to gain further knowledge about the subject. Forty-eight papers were excluded due to not conforming to eligibility criteria or adding to the evidence. Of the 18 papers left, relevant abstracts were identified and the full papers obtained (all of which were in English), to quality assure against search criteria. There was considerable heterogeneity of design among the included studies therefore a narrative review of the evidence was undertaken. There was significant heterogeneity within studies, including clinical topic, numbers, outcomes, as a result a narrative review was thought to be best. There were 18 cohort studies, with a moderate level of evidence. These were from a range of countries with minimal loss to follow-up. All participants were identified appropriately.

53.2   Risk of Bladder Cancer in Renal Transplant Patients

Renal transplant recipients (RTRs) have a two- to seven-fold risk of developing a neoplasm compared to general population [3]. Bladder urothelial neoplasms in this cohort has an incidence of 0.4–2% [3]. Palazzetti et al. [3] described oncologic characteristics of bladder urothelial neoplasms in RTRs and to evaluate its recurrence, progression, and survival rates [3]. A total of 28 de novo bladder transitional cell carcinomas (TCCs) were identified (incidence rate 0.64%) [3]. Cancer-specific survival rates were 100%, 75%, and 70% after 1, 5, and 10 years, respectively [3]. Age at diagnosis superior to 60 years was found to be a statistically significant variable for recurrence risk [3]. Progression rate was 14% [3]. Presence of CIS was significantly associated with progression [3]. All cancer-specific deaths were in the high-risk group and all were progressions from non-muscle invasive to muscle invasive bladder cancer [3].

Huang analyzed the oncologic effect of post-kidney transplantation (KT) immunosuppressive status for end-stage renal disease (ESRD) patients with superficial urothelial carcinoma [4]. Patients with KT were younger [4]. Female predominance was noted in patients with UT-UC and post-KT UB-UC [4]. Pathological stages were distributed similarly in UB-UC and UT-UC groups whether they underwent KT or not [4]. More bladder cancer recurrences within 5 years were found in ESRD patients with KT after TURBT for superficial UB-UC compared with those without KT (77.7% vs. 38%, p = 0.032) [4]. However, systemic disease recurrences were similar in the two groups (11% vs. 1%, p = 0.163) [4].

53.3   Risk and Safety of Radical Cystectomy in the Renal Transplant Patient

Demirdag aimed to evaluate the efficacy and safety of radical cystectomy (RC) and urinary diversion with ileal conduit in renal transplant recipients [5]. Demirdag reviewed 2 patients with prior history of renal transplantation who underwent RC and ileal conduit urinary diversion for bladder cancer [5]. The RC and ileal conduit urinary diversion were performed in the first patient 56 months after renal transplantation and in the second patient 64 months after renal transplantation [5]. Clinical staging was high-grade T2 transitional cell cancer of the bladder for patient 1 and T2 with pure squamous cell cancer of the bladder for patient 2 [5]. No perioperative or postoperative complication and no graft dysfunction occurred in either patient [5].

53.4   Risk According to Type of Urinary Diversion

Zabell identified 4015 patients treated with radical cystectomy for bladder cancer [6]. The outcome of interest was end stage kidney disease stratified by diversion type [6].

End stage kidney disease developed in 7.2% of patients, including 84% with an ileal conduit and 16% with continent urinary diversion [6]. On multivariate analysis no increased risk of end stage kidney disease was associated with continent diversion (HR 1.06, 95% CI 0.78–1.44, p = 0.71) [6]. Overall the estimated risk at 5, 10 and 15 years was 8.3% (95% CI 7.1–9.5), 16.9% (95% 14.6–19.2) and 24.4% (95% CI 20.3–28.5), respectively [6].

53.5 Difficulties Encountered in Renal Transplant Patients

Prabharasuth reviewed management of bladder cancer (BCa) in renal transplantation [7]. Optimal oncologic treatment can be challenging due to the immunosuppressed state and higher comorbidity [7]. Twelve patients were identified with non-muscle invasive (NMI) BCa [7]. Four patients with NMI BCa received intravesical BCG, with no urinary tract infection, fever, or BCG-associated sepsis. Four patients were identified with muscle-invasive bladder cancer (MIBC), and 1 patient had biopsy proven metastatic disease [7]. Five patients underwent radical cystectomy (RC) with diversion, 7 underwent transurethral resection and surveillance, 3 underwent chemotherapy, and 1 received palliative radiation for metastatic disease [7]. Overall, 6 patients were deceased, 4 of whom died of disease at a median of 9.7 months from the time of BCa diagnosis [7].

53.6 A New Technique of Robotic Cystectomy for Renal Transplant Patients

Robotic assisted radical cystectomy (RARC) is an alternative to open radical cystectomy [8]. As experience is gained with the RARC approach the technique is being applied to more complex surgical cases [8]. Caputo describes a new technique for RARC with intracorporeal ileal conduit urinary diversion for a renal transplant recipient [8]. Interestingly his trans-urethral bladder tumour resection specimen surgical technique utilizes 6 trocars, of note a 12-mm assistant trocar is placed 1 cm superior to the pubic symphysis, and this trocar is solely used to pass a laparoscopic stapler to facilitate the excision of the ileal segment and the stapled enteric anastomosis [8]. Surgical steps include: identification of native ureters bilaterally (removed en bloc with the bladder specimen); identification of the transplanted ureter at the right bladder dome; posterior bladder and prostate dissection along Denonvilliers' fascia; development of the space of Retzius; ligation and transection of the bladder and prostate vascular bundles; apical prostate dissection and transection of urethra; left pelvic lymphadenectomy; ilium resection for creation of the ileal conduit; stapled enteric anastomosis; ureteroileal anastomosis; maturation of the ileal conduit stoma [8].

There were no intraoperative complications [8]. Operative time was 443 min (7.4 h) [8]. Estimated blood loss was 250 cc [8]. Length of hospital stay was 5 days

[8]. The patient did not experience any postoperative complications. The patient maintained good renal graft function with no decline in eGFR to date [8].

In the setting of prior renal transplantation, surgical treatment for bladder cancer remains the mainstay but is technically challenging [9]. Moses reported patient outcomes and described a new technique [9]. Four patients were male and one was female, with a median age of 64 years [9]. Gross hematuria was the most common sign at presentation [9]. Clinical staging was T2, T2 with carcinoma in situ (CIS), high-grade (HG) Ta with CIS, T2 with squamous differentiation, and HG T1, and pathologic tumor stage was pTisN1, pT3N0, pTisN0, pT3N0, and pT0N0, respectively [9]. One patient received a Studer-type diversion and four underwent Hautmann diversion [9]. Graft ureteral identification was aided by the use of intravenous dye in all patients [9]. Ipsilateral pelvic lymph node dissection was not possible in any patient [9]. All patients are alive at follow-up, with two experiencing recurrence at 7.2 and 66.8 months. Renal function was maintained.

53.7   Surgical Technique in Renal Transplant Patients

The principles of treatment of de novo bladder tumours in renal transplant patients are comparable to those applied in non-transplant patients [10]. Koutani reports a case of cystectomy with enterocystoplasty for invasive bladder tumour in a renal transplant patient is reported [10]. An invasive urothelial bladder tumour was discovered in a 62-year-old man, 3 months after a second renal transplantation [10]. Treatment consisted of cystectomy with prostatic preservation and nontubulized enterocystoplasty [10]. With a follow-up of 21 months after cystectomy, the patient is alive without recurrence [10]. He is perfectly continent during the day, with normal sexual intercourse and no reflux or residual urine. Renal function is normal [10]. Cystectomy with enterocystoplasty can be an effective treatment for invasive bladder tumour in renal transplant patients [10]. This treatment ensures oncological control and acceptable comfort while preserving the transplant [10].

53.8   BCG vs. MMC in Bladder Cancer

Rodriguez Faba conducted an observational prospective study with a retrospective analysis of 88 patients with BC after RT at 10 European centers [11]. A total of 10,000 RTs were performed [11]. Diagnosis of BC occurred at a median of 73 months after RT [11]. Seventy-one patients (81.6%) had non-muscle invasive bladder cancer, of whom 29 (40.8%) received adjuvant treatment; of these, 6 (20.6%) received bacillus Calmette-Guérin and 20 (68.9%) mitomycin C [11]. At univariate analysis, patients who received bacillus Calmette-Guérin had a significantly lower recurrence rate (p = 0.043) [11]. At multivariate analysis, a switch from immunosuppression to mTOR inhibitors significantly reduced the risk of recurrence (HR 0.24, 95% CI: 0.053–0.997, p = 0.049) while presence of multiple tumors increased it (HR 6.31, 95% CI: 1.78–22.3, p = 0.004) [11]. Globally, 26 patients

(29.88%) underwent cystectomy [11]. No major complications were recorded. Overall mortality (OM) was 32.2% (28 patients); the cancer-specific mortality was 13.8% [11].

53.9 Histological Variants in the Renal Transplant Patient

A rare case of invasive squamous cell carcinoma of the urinary bladder developing 5 years after cadaveric renal transplant is described [12]. The technical precautions to be taken while performing a radical cystectomy in such a situation is highlighted [12]. This patient required chemotherapy in the post-operative period [12].

Moon reported on a 62-year-old woman who developed squamous cell carcinoma of the bladder 16 years after a kidney transplant [13]. She was diagnosed with squamous cell carcinoma of the bladder 16 years later and underwent radical cystectomy with an orthotopic ileal neobladder [13]. The Studer technique was used and the afferent ileal loop was anastomosed to the graft ureter [13]. At the 6-month follow-up visit, the patient showed no evidence of recurrence [13]. Her renal function was stable [13]. The patient was continent during the day and the night [13]. This case shows that the construction of an orthotopic ileal neobladder after cystectomy is safe and feasible in kidney transplant recipients [13].

Davis reviewed the incidence and long-term outcomes of squamous cell carcinoma (SCC) of the bladder in patients after kidney transplantation [14]. Five patients from one center (0.0013%) developed SCC of the bladder after undergoing a deceased donor kidney transplant [14]. Their relevant risk factors included long-term self-intermittent catheterization/indwelling catheter (n = 2), smoking history (n = 2), and a prior history of cyclophosphamide treatment for vasculitis (n = 1) [14]. The latency period between transplantation and bladder SCC was 87 ± 87 (range: 2–228) months, and all five patients were immunosuppressed with tacrolimus, mycophenolate mofetil, and prednisone [14]. Four patients had suspected metastases upon presentation, and one patient presented with organ-confined disease [14]. This patient underwent a radical cystectomy and remains disease free 8 months post-operatively [14]. Despite radical treatment, the remaining four patients died from metastatic disease 7 ± 4.4 (range: 2–11) months after their initial diagnosis [14].

53.10 Presentation and Management of Bladder Cancer in the Renal Transplant Population

Kamal reviewed their experience with bladder cancer among a renal transplant population [15]. There were 7 patients in total [15]. All patients presented with gross haematuria [15]. There was non-muscle-invasive disease in two patients who were treated by transurethral resection and adjuvant intravesical bacille Calmette-Guérin immunotherapy [15]. One patient died 24 months later due to complications of end-stage renal disease [15]. To date the second patient is alive and free of the recurrence

[15]. Five recipients with muscle-invasive disease had a radical cystectomy and orthotopic bladder substitution [15]. The mean (sd) time to the last follow-up or death was 14.6 (3.1) months [15]. Three patients died with stable graft function; two from distant metastasis and one from a cerebrovascular stroke [15]. The remaining two patients are still alive, free of disease and with good graft function [15].

53.11   Orthotopic Neobladders in the Renal Transplant Population

Radical cystectomy and urinary diversion is an effective curative treatment for muscle invasive bladder cancer [16]. The orthotopic ileal neobladder has become a favourable choice of urinary diversion as it offers superior quality of life, cosmetic outcome and the potential for normal voiding [16]. Cooke treated two patients with bladder cancer who previously underwent renal transplant for end-stage renal disease [16]. Radical cystectomy and orthotopic ileal neobladder reconstruction was performed in both patients [16]. One patient had two renal transplants and underwent transplant nephrectomy at the time of cystectomy [16]. In the other patient, the native kidneys were still present and the ureters were anastomosed to the neobladder [16]. There is excellent function of the neobladder [16]. There were no increased complications seen in these patients [16].

Renal transplant recipients with high-risk bladder cancer require cystectomy need a urinary diversion [17]. Manassero et al. [17] described their experience of radical cystectomy and orthotopic ileal neobladder with Studer technique [17]. Manassero et al. [17] performed radical cystectomy and Studer ileal neobladder in four male patients [17]. Pathology revealed pT1HGN+ transitional cell carcinoma in one case, pT1HGN0 in two and pT3aHGN0 in one [17]. Two patients presenting aggressive disease (N+ and pT3a) died of tumour progression after 20 and 14 months, respectively, while the other two are alive after 56 and 36 months of follow-up with no evidence of disease, stable serum creatinine (2.29 and 1.6 mg/dl) and mild metabolic acidosis [17]. Day and night-time urinary continence were satisfactory in all patients [17]. Good functional outcomes have been reported in the 20 cases of ileal orthotopic neobladder with different techniques published so far and the global experience of 24 cases with a median follow-up of 39 months documents a cancer specific survival of 62.5% [17].

Lang analysed the safety and clinical outcome in a single institution experience with orthotopic ileal neobladder reconstruction following radical cystectomy for transitional cell carcinoma in renal transplant recipients [18]. Four renal transplant recipients had bladder cancer a median of 10.5 years after renal transplantation [18]. Two patients died at 11 and 15 months of tumour progression and a pulmonary embolism, respectively, whereas two were alive at a mean follow-up of 90 months with no evidence of disease [18]. No neobladder related reoperations were necessary [18]. Serum creatinine as a marker of renal function was stable in 3 patients. In 1 patient chronic graft rejection led to progressive renal failure and haemodialysis

[18]. Urinary continence was satisfactory during the day and night with spontaneous voiding in all patients and no significant post-void residual urine [18].

53.12 Transplant Post Cystectomy and Urinary Diversion

Fournier reported the long-term survival of transplanted kidneys in patients with a continent urinary diversion [19]. A total of 14 patients presented irreversible dysfunction of the lower urinary tract, and two patients had required radical cystectomy because of bladder cancer [19]. All continent urinary diversions were carried out before the transplantation [19]. There were nine Kock pouches, five Mainz pouches, one Mainz neobladder and one Hautmann neobladder [19]. Two patients died, while six patients lost their transplant and resumed haemodialysis [19]. Nine patients (56.2%) were alive with a functional transplant at the end of follow up [19]. The kidney transplant survival rate was 73.3% after 10 years, and 66.6% after 15 years [19]. Among patients who still had a functional transplant at the time of the study, creatinine clearance was >30 ml/min for seven patients and <30 ml/min for two patients [19].

53.13 Post-operative Complications Post Radical Cystectomy

Cusano reported outcomes of 2 patients who received a single-stage renal transplantation and concomitant urinary-diversion procedure [20]. Two patients underwent a simultaneous renal transplantation-ileal conduit creation to surgically manage their end-stage renal disease [20]. One patient did not have any surgical complications, whereas the other suffered from a postoperative ileus (Clavien grade 3a), atrial fibrillation (Clavien grade 2), hypertension (Clavien grade 2), methicillin-resistant Staphylococcus aureus at the incisional site (Clavien grade 2), and a positive urine culture managed using antibiotics (Clavien grade 2) [20]. No major complications were observed and both have favorable outcomes at 23 and 19 months after surgery, respectively [20].

53.14 Impact of CKD on Oncological Outcomes in MIBC

Hamano evaluated the impact of preoperative chronic kidney disease (CKD) on oncologic outcomes in muscle-invasive bladder cancer patients who underwent radical cystectomy [21]. Of the 581 patients, 215 (37%) were diagnosed with CKD before radical cystectomy [21]. Before the background adjustment, PFS, CSS, and OS after radical cystectomy were significantly lower in the pre-CKD group compared to the non-CKD group [21]. Background-adjusted IPTW analysis showed that preoperative CKD was significantly associated with poor PFS, CSS, and OS after radical cystectomy [21]. The nomogram for predicting 5-year PFS and OS probability showed significant correlation with actual PFS and OS

(c-index $= 0.73$ and 0.77, respectively) [21]. Muscle-invasive bladder cancer patients with preoperative CKD had a significantly lower survival probability than those without CKD [21].

53.15 Reviews Related to Systematic Review

Tillou reviewed the risk and incidence of urological malignancies and the clinical characteristics and outcomes of renal transplant urological malignancies [22]. Comparing to general population, risk of kidney cancer was found to be 7–10 times greater and most of them are incidental low-stage, low-grade tumors with a good prognosis [22]. Papillary carcinomas represented more than 50% of de novo graft carcinomas, which seemed to be low-grade carcinomas with good prognosis [22]. Tillou suggested a three-fold increased risk of developing bladder TCC [22]. Intravesical BCG in superficial bladder cancer and/or CIS is a valid option [22]. For invasive urothelial tumor, radical cystectomy in renal transplant patients remains the best treatment [22]. Oncological outcomes of urological cancers in renal transplant recipients are good and conservative treatment should be preferred each time it is feasible to prevent returning to dialysis following recommendations of urological cancer treatment [22].

References

1. Moher D, Liberati A, Tetzlaff J, Altman DG. "Preferred Reporting Items for Systematic Reviews and Meta-Analyses: The Prisma Statement." [In English]. BMJ (Online) 339, no. 7716 (08 Aug 2009):332–36.
2. Mays N, Pope C, Popay J. "Systematically Reviewing Qualitative and Quantitative Evidence to Inform Management and Policy-Making in the Health Field." [In English]. Journal of Health Services Research and Policy 10, no. SUPPL. 1 (July 2005):6–20.
3. Palazzetti A, Bosio A, Dalmasso E, Destefanis P, Fop F, Pisano F, Segoloni G, Biancone L, Volpe A, Di Domenico A, Terrone C, Iesari S, Famulari A, Todeschini P, Frea B, Gontero P. De novo bladder urothelial neoplasm in renal transplant recipients: a retrospective, multicentered study. Urol Int. 2018;100(2):185–92.
4. Huang GL, Luo HL, Chen YT, Cheng YT. Oncologic outcomes of post-kidney transplantation superficial Urothelial carcinoma. Transplant Proc. 2018;50(4):998–1000.
5. Demirdag C, Citgez S, Talat Z, Onal B. Management of bladder cancer after renal transplantation. Transplant Proc. 2017;49(2):293–6.
6. Zabell JR, Adejoro O, Konety BR, Weight CJ. Risk of end stage kidney disease after radical cystectomy according to urinary diversion type. J Urol. 2015;193(4):1283–7.
7. Prabharasuth D, Moses KA, Bernstein M, Dalbagni G, Herr HW. Management of bladder cancer after renal transplantation. Urology. 2013;81(4):813–9.
8. Caputo PA, Ramirez D, Maurice M, Nelson R, Kara O, Malkoc E, Goldfarb D, Kaouk J. Robotic assisted radical cystoprostatectomy and intracorporeal ileal conduit urinary diversion for a kidney transplant recipient. Int Braz J Urol. 2017;43(6):1192.
9. Moses KA, Bochner BH, Prabharasuth D, Sfakianos JP, Bernstein M, Herr HW, Dalbagni G. Radical cystectomy and orthotopic urinary reconstruction in patients with bladder cancer after renal transplantation: clinical outcomes and description of technique. Transplant Proc. 2013;45(4):1661–6.

10. Koutani A, Lechevallier E, Coulange C. Infiltrating bladder tumor in a renal transplant patient: cystectomy with prostatic conservation and enterocystoplasty. Prog Urol. 1997;7(2):277–80.
11. Rodriguez Faba O, Palou J, Vila Reyes H, Guirado L, Palazzetti A, Gontero P, Vigués F, Garcia-Olaverri J, Fernández Gómez JM, Olsburg J, Terrone C, Figueiredo A, Burgos J, Lledó E, Breda A. Treatment options and predictive factors for recurrence and cancer-specific mortality in bladder cancer after renal transplantation: a multi-institutional analysis. Actas Urol Esp. 2017;41(10):639–45.
12. Srinivas V, Deshmukh R, Shah B, Kapadia A. Radical cystectomy for invasive squamous cell bladder cancer in a renal transplant patient. Urol Int. 1993;51(3):167–70.
13. Moon KC, Soo Ahn H, Min SH, Kim HS, Ku JH. Orthotopic ileal neobladder reconstruction in a woman who developed squamous cell carcinoma of the urinary bladder after kidney transplantation. Tumori. 2011;97(5):20e–3e.
14. Davis NF, McLoughlin LC, Dowling C, Power R, Mohan P, Hickey D, Smyth G, Eng M, Little DM. Incidence and long-term outcomes of squamous cell bladder cancer after deceased donor renal transplantation. Clin Transpl. 2013;27(6):E665–8.
15. Kamal MM, Soliman SM, Shokeir AA, Abol-Enein H, Ghoneim MA. Bladder carcinoma among live-donor renal transplant recipients: a single-centre experience and a review of the literature. BJU Int. 2008;101(1):30–5.
16. Cooke T, Ciancio G, Burke GW, Soloway MS, Manoharan M. Orthotopic ileal neobladder reconstruction after renal transplant. Am J Transplant. 2007;7(11):2630–3.
17. Manassero F, Di Paola G, Mogorovich A, Giannarini G, Boggi U, Selli C. Orthotopic bladder substitute in renal transplant recipients: experience with Studer technique and literature review. Transpl Int. 2011;24(9):943–8.
18. Lang H, de Petriconi R, Wenderoth U, Volkmer BG, Hautmann RE, Gschwend JE. Orthotopic ileal neobladder reconstruction in patients with bladder cancer following renal transplantation. J Urol. 2005;173(3):881–4.
19. Fournier R, Codas-Duarte R, Daily T, Martin X, Badet L, Fassi-Fehri H. Long-term kidney transplant survival in patients with continent urinary diversion. Int J Urol. 2017;24(11):787–92.
20. Cusano A, Meraney AM, Abarzua-Cabezas F, Lally A, Brown M, Shichman S. Single-stage renal transplantation-urinary diversion: a novel surgical approach. Urology. 2014;84(1):232–6.
21. Hamano I, Hatakeyama S, Iwamurau H, Fujita N, Fukushi K, Narita T, Hagiwara K, Kusaka A, Hosogoe S, Yamamoto H, Tobisawa Y, Yoneyama T, Yoneyama T, Hashimoto Y, Koie T, Ito H, Yoshikawa K, Kawaguchi T, Ohyama C. Preoperative chronic kidney disease predicts poor oncological outcomes after radical cystectomy in patients with muscle-invasive bladder cancer. Oncotarget. 2017;8(37):61404–14.
22. Tillou X, Doerfler A. Urological tumors in renal transplantation. Minerva Urol Nefrol. 2014;66(1):57–67.

Radical Cystectomy and Acute Renal Failure

54

A systematic review relating to radical cystectomy and acute renal failure was conducted. The search strategy aimed to identify all references related to Radical Cystectomy AND Acute Renal Failure. Search terms used were as follows: (Radical Cystectomy) AND (Acute Renal Failure). The following databases were screened from 1989 to June 2020:

- CINAHL
- MEDLINE (NHS Evidence)
- Cochrane
- AMed
- EMBASE
- PsychINFO
- SCOPUS
- Web of Science

In addition, searches using Medical Subject Headings (MeSH) and keywords were conducted using Cochrane databases. Two UK-based experts in bladder cancer were consulted to identify any additional studies.

Studies were eligible for inclusion if they reported primary research focusing on bladder cancer and screening. Papers were included if published after 1984 and had to be in English. Studies that did not conform to this were excluded. Only primary research was included (Fig. 54.1).

Abstracts were independently screened for eligibility by two reviewers and disagreements resolved through discussion or third party opinion. Agreement level was calculated using Cohen's Kappa to test the intercoder reliability of this screening process. Cohens' Kappa allows comparison of inter-rater reliability between papers using relative observed agreement. This also takes account of the comparison occurring by chance. The first reviewer agreed all 14 papers to be included, the second, agreed on 14. Cohens kappa was therefore 1.0.

© The Editor(s) (if applicable) and The Author(s), under exclusive license to
Springer Nature Switzerland AG 2021
S. S. Goonewardene et al., *Management of Muscle Invasive Bladder Cancer*,
Management of Urology, https://doi.org/10.1007/978-3-030-57915-9_54

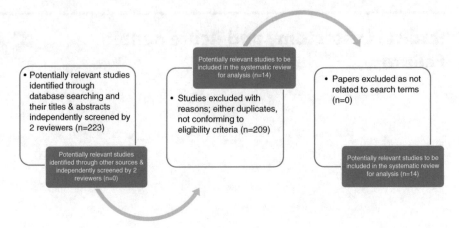

Fig. 54.1 Flow chart of studies identified through the systematic review. (Adapted from PRISMA)

Data extraction was piloted by the researcher and amended in consultation with the research team (author and two academic supervisors). Data collected included authors, year and country of publication, study aims, setting, intervention aims, number of participants, study design, intervention components and delivery methods, comparison groups and outcome measures, notes and follow-up questions for the authors. Studies were quality assessed using the PRISMA criteria for randomised controlled trials, Mays et al. [1, 2] for the action research and qualitative studies and the Critical Skills Appraisal programme for cohort studies. This was also applied to randomised controlled trials and qualitative studies.

The search identified 223 papers (Fig. 54.1). All 14 mapped to the search terms and eligibility criteria. The current systematic reviews were examined to gain further knowledge about the subject. Two hundred and nine papers were excluded due to not conforming to eligibility criteria or adding to the evidence. Of the 14 papers left, relevant abstracts were identified and the full papers obtained (all of which were in English), to quality assure against search criteria. There was considerable heterogeneity of design among the included studies therefore a narrative review of the evidence was undertaken. There was significant heterogeneity within studies, including clinical topic, numbers, outcomes, as a result a narrative review was thought to be best. There were 14 cohort studies, with a moderate level of evidence. These were from a range of countries with minimal loss to follow-up. All participants were identified appropriately.

54.1   AKI Post Major Surgery

Acute kidney injury (AKI) after major surgeries is associated with significant morbidity and mortality [3]. Osman reviewed incidence, predictors and associated comorbidities of AKI after radical cystectomy [3]. Perioperative serum creatinine measurements were used to define AKI according to the RIFLE criteria (as Risk, Injury and Failure) [3]. The predictors of AKI after surgery were determined using univariate and multivariate analyses [3]. Out of 988 evaluable patients, AKI developed in 46 (4.7%) [3]. According to RIFLE criteria; AKI-Risk, AKI-Injury and AKI-Failure occurred in 26 (2.6%), 9 (0.9%) and 11 (1.1%) patients, respectively [3]. AKI is a significant morbidity after radical cystectomy and the term should be included during routine cystectomy morbidity assessment [3].

54.2   Risk Factors for AKI After Radical Cystectomy

Ikehata reviewed the incidence, risk factors and clinical impact of acute kidney injury after radical cystectomy [4]. The incidence of acute kidney injury was evaluated over the first 7 days postoperatively, during which time a ureteral catheter was inserted [4]. Postoperative acute kidney injury was observed in 48 patients (33.1%), with stages 1, 2, and 3 found in 33 (22.7%), 14 (9.6%) and 1 (0.7%), respectively [4]. All patients with stage 1 and 2 acute kidney injury recovered by postoperative day 7, except for one with stage 1. Hypertension (p < 0.001), preoperative estimated glomerular filtration rate <60 ml/min/1.73 m^2 (p = 0.04) and neoadjuvant chemotherapy (p = 0.03) were independent risk factors for postoperative acute kidney injury [4]. Furthermore, postoperative acute kidney injury was an independent risk factor for acute kidney injury after ureteral stent removal [4]. The incidence of acute kidney injury after radical cystectomy is relatively high, although most cases are low grade and can be resolve [4]. The risk for postoperative acute kidney injury is higher in comorbid hypertension, impaired renal function and received naoadjuvant chemotherapy [4].

Furrer identified risk factors for AKI in patients undergoing radical cystectomy and urinary diversion [5]. Early postoperative AKI occurred in 100/912 patients (11%) [5]. An increased risk was seen in patients with surgery lasting >400 min, male and obese patients (>25 kg/m^2) [5]. Independent predictors were duration of surgery (p = 0.020), intraoperative blood loss (p = 0.049), preoperative serum creatinine values (p = 0.004), intraoperative administration of crystalloids (p = 0.032), body mass index (p = 0.031), and fluid balance (p = 0.006) [5]. Patients with AKI had a longer hospitalization time (18 days vs. 17 days, p = 0.040) [5]. An increased risk for AKI was seen in patients with an operative time >400 min [5]. Further independent predictors of postoperative AKI were male sex, obesity, intraoperative blood loss, and a low preoperative plasma creatinine [5].

54.3   Impact of AKI Post Radical Cystectomy on CKD

Kwon investigated the prevalence of acute kidney injury (AKI) after radical cystectomy, and evaluate its impact on chronic kidney disease (CKD) and mortality ([6]. AKI was assessed within 7 days after surgery according to the Acute Kidney Injury Network criteria [6]. The prevalence of AKI after surgery was examined, and the significance of AKI for CKD and mortality was analysed [6]. Of 866 patients, 269 (31.1%) developed AKI in the first week after surgery [6]. Of these, 231 (85.9%) were at stage 1, 32 (11.9%) at stage 2, and 6 (2.2%) at stage 3 [6]. Of 722 patients with a preoperative Modification of Diet in Renal Disease estimated glomerular filtration rate (eGFR) of >60 ml/min/1.73 m^2, CKD developed in 23.0% (118/513) of patients in the non-AKI group and 32.5% (68/209) of patients in the AKI group [6]. Independent factors predicting new-onset CKD were a preoperative eGFR (p < 0.001), age (p = 0.011), urinary tract complication (p < 0.001) and AKI (p = 0.015) [6]. In all, 297 patients died 191 in the non-AKI group and 106 in the AKI group). AKI also correlated significantly with overall survival (p = 0.001) [6].

54.4   Radical Cystectomy with ARF Caused by Rhabdomyolysis

De Gracia-Nieto determined the incidence of acute renal failure secondary to rhabdomyolysis (ARFSR) as a complication of major urological surgery (MUS) [7]. The incidence rates after radical cystectomy were 0.26% (3/1175 cases). No case of rhabdomyolysis was reported among the patients who underwent other major surgical procedures [7]. Two patients required dialysis, and all 4 patients recovered to their baseline renal function at an average of 11 days (7–17) with the appropriate treatment [7]. Male gender, younger age, lower ASA score, prolonged operative time, high body mass index, elevated preoperative serum creatinine and estimated blood loss were possible risk factors for developing ARFSR due to MUS [7].

Pariser studied the epidemiology, risk factors, and outcomes of rhabdomyolysis (RM) after major urologic surgery [8]. This group identified a weighted population of 1,016,074 patients was identified with 870 (0.1%) developing RM, which was significantly more likely for radical or partial nephrectomy and radical cystectomy patients compared with radical prostatectomy patients [8]. On multivariate analysis, independent risk factors for RM included younger age, male sex, diabetes, chronic kidney disease, obesity, and bleeding [8]. Race, minimally invasive technique, and teaching status were not associated with RM when controlling for other factors [8]. Patients with RM experienced increases in mortality, AKI, length of stay, and hospital charges [8].

54.5   Radical Cystectomy, AKI and Association with Uric Acid

Acute kidney injury (AKI) is a common complication after surgery and increases costs, morbidity, and mortality of hospitalized patients [9]. While radical cystectomy associates significantly with an increased risk of serious complications, including AKI, risk factors of AKI after radical cystectomy has not been reported [9]. This study was performed to determine the incidence and independent predictors of AKI after radical cystectomy [9]. Of the 238 patients who met the eligibility criteria, 91 (38.2%) developed AKI [9]. Univariate logistic regression analyses showed that male gender, high serum uric acid level, and long operation time associated with the development of AKI [9]. On multivariate logistic regression analysis, preoperative serum uric acid concentration (odds ratio [OR] = 1.251; 95% confidence interval [CI] = 1.048–1.493; p = 0.013) and operation time (OR = 1.005; 95% CI = 1.002–1.008; p = 0.003) remained as independent predictors of AKI after radical cystectomy [9]. AKI after radical cystectomy was a relatively common complication [9]. Its independent risk factors were high preoperative serum uric acid concentration and long operation [9].

54.6 Radical Cystectomy: Ileal Conduit vs. Neobladder and AKI

Ileal conduit and neobladder urinary diversions are frequently performed after radical cystectomy [10]. Joung reviewed the incidence of postoperative AKI between ileal conduit and neobladder urinary diversions after radical cystectomy [10]. All consecutive patients who underwent radical cystectomy in 2004–2014 in a single tertiary care center were identified [10]. The patients were divided into the ileal conduit and ileal neobladder groups [10]. The overall incidence of AKI after radical cystectomy was 30.7% (62 out of 202) and the incidences did not significantly differ between the groups (27 [26.7%], ileal conduit group vs. 35 [34.7%], ileal neobladder group, p = 0.268) [10]. Intraoperative data, intensive care unit admission rate, and the duration of hospital stay were not significantly different between the groups [10]. Postoperative AKI did not significantly differ between ileal conduit and neobladder urinary diversions after radical cystectomy [10].

54.7 Use of Noradrenaline and Risk of Acute Renal Failure in Radical Cystectomy

Furrer identified risk factors for acute kidney injury (AKI) in patients undergoing cystectomy with urinary diversion and determine whether administration of noradrenaline and intra-operative hydration regimens affect early postoperative renal function (Furrer 2018). A total of 769 consecutive patients scheduled for cystectomy and urinary diversion (Furrer 2018). Postoperative AKI was diagnosed in 86/769 patients (11.1%) (Furrer 2018). Independent predictors for AKI were the amount of crystalloid administered (odds ratio (OR) 0.79 [95% confidence interval (CI), 0.68–0.91], p = 0.002), antihypertensive medication (OR 2.07 [95% CI, 1.25–3.43], p = 0.005), pre-operative haemoglobin value (OR 1.02 [95% CI, 1.01–1.03], p = 0.010), duration of surgery (OR 1.01 [95% CI, 1.00–1.01], p = 0.002), age (OR 1.32 [95% CI, 1.44–1.79], p = 0.002) but not the administration of noradrenaline (OR 1.09 [95% CI, 0.94–1.21], p = 0.097) (Furrer 2018). Postoperative AKI was associated with longer hospital stay (18 [15–22] vs. 16 [15–19] days; p = 0.035) and a higher 90-day major postoperative complication rate (41.9% vs. 27.5%; p = 0.002) (Furrer 2018).

54.8 Radical Cystectomy, Neoadjuvant Chemotherapy and AKI

Chandrasekar evaluated the patterns of impact of neoadjuvant chemotherapy (NAC) on renal function across the initial year following treatment for muscle-invasive bladder cancer (MIBC) with radical cystectomy (RC) [11]. Of the 241 patients who underwent RC for urothelial carcinoma of the bladder, 66 (27%) received NAC and 175 (73%) did not [11]. In multivariable analysis, NAC was significantly associated with a decrease of at least one CKD stage from baseline to post-op (p = 0.009), but not to the 6–12 months follow-up time point ($p = 0.050$) [11]. The loss of GFR in the NAC cohort occurs up-front with chemotherapy, but the peri-operative course is similar to those who underwent cystectomy alone. Of the 15 NAC patients (26.8%) who were Stage 3 CKD prior to chemotherapy, none progressed to a higher stage CKD [11].

References

1. Mays N, Pope C, Popay J. Systematically reviewing qualitative and quantitative evidence to inform management and policy-making in the health field [In English]. J Health Serv Res Pol. 2005;10(SUPPL. 1):6–20.
2. Moher D, Liberati A, Tetzlaff J, Altman DG. Preferred reporting items for systematic reviews and meta-analyses: the prisma statement [In English]. BMJ. 2009;339(7716):332–6.
3. Osman Y, Harraz AM, El-Halwagy S, Laymon M, Mosbah A, Abol-Enein H, Shaaban AA. Acute kidney injury following radical cystectomy and urinary diversion: predictors and associated morbidity [In English]. Int Braz J Urol. 2018;44(4):726–33.
4. Ikehata Y, Tanaka T, Ichihara K, et al. Incidence and risk factors for acute kidney injury after radical cystectomy. Int J Urol. 2016;23(7):558–63.
5. Furrer MA, Schneider MP, Löffel LM, Burkhard FC, Wuethrich PY. Impact of intra-operative fluid and noradrenaline administration on early postoperative renal function after cystectomy and urinary diversion: a retrospective observational cohort study. Eur J Anaesthesiol. 2018;35(9):641–9.
6. Kwon T, Jeong IG, Lee C, You D, Hong B, Hong JH, Ahn H, Kim C-S. Acute kidney injury after radical cystectomy for bladder cancer is associated with chronic kidney disease and mortality [In English]. Ann Surgical Oncol. 2016;23(2):686–93.
7. De Gracia-Nieto AE, Angerri O, Bover J, Salas D, Villamizar JM, Villavicencio H. Acute renal failure secondary to rhabdomyolysis as a complication of major urological surgery: the experience of a high-volume urological center [In English]. Med Princ Pract. 2016;25(4):329–35.
8. Pariser JJ, Pearce SM, Patel SG, et al. Rhabdomyolysis after major urologic surgery: epidemiology, risk factors, and outcomes. Urology. 2015;85(6):1328–32. https://doi.org/10.1016/j.urology.2015.03.018.
9. Joung K-W, Choi S-S, Kong Y-G, Yu J, Lim J, Hwang J-H, Kim Y-K. Incidence and risk factors of acute kidney injury after radical cystectomy: importance of preoperative serum uric acid level [In English]. Int J Med Sci. 2015;12(7):599–604.
10. Joung K-W, Kong Y-G, Yoon S-H, Kim YJ, Hwang J-H, Hong B, Kim Y-K. Comparison of postoperative acute kidney injury between ileal conduit and neobladder urinary diversions after radical cystectomy: a propensity score matching analysis [In English]. Medicine. 2016;95(36):e4838–e38.
11. Chandrasekar T, Pugashetti N, Durbin-Johnson B, et al. Effect of neoadjuvant chemotherapy on renal function following radical cystectomy: is there a meaningful impact? Bladder Cancer. 2016;2(4):441–8.

A Systematic Review on Bladder Cancer, Radical Cystectomy and Complications

55.1 Research Methods

A systematic review relating to muscle invasive bladder cancer, radical cystectomy and complications was conducted. This was to identify whether outcomes from renal transplant patients in this cohort. The search strategy aimed to identify all references related to radical cystectomy AND complications. Search terms used were as follows: (Radical Cystectomy) AND (Complication). The following databases were screened from 1989 to June 2020:

- CINAHL
- MEDLINE (NHS Evidence)
- Cochrane
- AMed
- EMBASE
- PsychINFO
- SCOPUS
- Web of Science

In addition, searches using Medical Subject Headings (MeSH) and keywords were conducted using Cochrane databases. Two UK-based experts in bladder cancer were consulted to identify any additional studies.

Studies were eligible for inclusion if they reported primary research focusing on muscle invasive bladder cancer and nerve sparing. Papers were included if published after 1984 and had to be in English. Studies that did not conform to this were excluded. Due to the paucity of studies, all study types were included, including case series and case reports (Fig. 55.1).

Abstracts were independently screened for eligibility by two reviewers and disagreements resolved through discussion or third party opinion. Agreement level was calculated using Cohen's Kappa to test the intercoder reliability of this screening

© The Editor(s) (if applicable) and The Author(s), under exclusive license to
Springer Nature Switzerland AG 2021
S. S. Goonewardene et al., *Management of Muscle Invasive Bladder Cancer*,
Management of Urology, https://doi.org/10.1007/978-3-030-57915-9_55

process. Cohens' Kappa allows comparison of inter-rater reliability between papers using relative observed agreement. This also takes account of the comparison occurring by chance. The first reviewer agreed all 30 papers to be included, the second, agreed on 30.

Data extraction was piloted by the researcher and amended in consultation with the research team (author and two academic supervisors). Data collected included authors, year and country of publication, study aims, setting, intervention aims, number of participants, study design, intervention components and delivery methods, comparison groups and outcome measures, notes and follow-up questions for the authors. Studies were quality assessed using the PRISMA criteria for randomised controlled trials, Mays et al. [1, 2] for the action research and qualitative studies and the Critical Skills Appraisal programme for cohort studies. This was also applied to randomised controlled trials and qualitative studies.

The search identified 5481 papers (Fig. 55.1). Thirty mapped to the search terms and eligibility criteria. The current systematic reviews were examined to gain further knowledge about the subject. Five thousand four hundred and fifty-one papers were excluded due to not conforming to eligibility criteria or adding to the evidence. Of the 30 papers left, relevant abstracts were identified and the full papers obtained (all of which were in English), to quality assure against search criteria. There was considerable heterogeneity of design among the included studies therefore a narrative review of the evidence was undertaken. There was significant heterogeneity within studies, including clinical topic, numbers, outcomes, as a result a narrative review was thought to be best. There were 30 cohort studies, with a moderate level of evidence. These were from a range of countries with minimal loss to follow-up. All participants were identified appropriately.

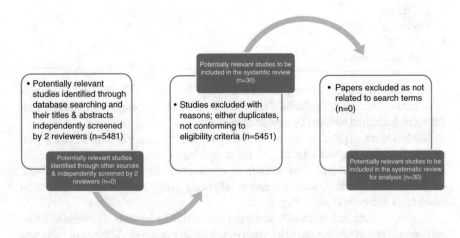

Fig. 55.1 Flow chart of studies identified through the systematic review. (Adapted from PRISMA)

55.2 Impact of Type of Urinary Diversion on Complications

Kim reported on the short and late morbidity and mortality of ileal conduit and neobladder after radical cystectomy with their associated risk factors [3]. During the median follow-up of 46.6 months, early and late morbidities were 29.5% (n = 91) and 19.8% (n = 61), and complication-related mortalities were 2.2% and 6.6%, respectively [3]. The type of urinary diversion significantly affected only the late complications (early: neobladder 57 vs. ileal conduit 47, p = 0.096; late: neobladder 67 vs. ileal conduit 37, p < 0.001) [3]. However, after propensity-score matching, no significant differences in early and late morbidities were observed between neobladder and ileal conduit [3]. For risk factors of morbidity, number of removed lymph node states and hypertension were independently significant for both early and late complications (p < 0.05) [3].

55.3 Perioperative Complications for Robotic Radical Cystectomy and Intracorporeal Urinary Diversion

Tan evaluated the early postoperative morbidity and mortality of patients undergoing iRARC and conduct a critical analysis of complications using standardised reporting criteria as stratified according to urinary diversion [4]. The 90-days all complication rate following ileal conduit and continent diversion was 68% and 82.4%, and major complications were 21.0% and 20.6% respectively [4]. The 90-days mortality was 3% and 2.9% for ileal conduit and continent diversion patients, respectively [4]. On multivariate analysis, the blood transfusion requirement was independently associated with major complications (p = 0.002) and all 30-days (p = 0.002) and 90-days (p = 0.012) major complications [4]. Male patients were associated with 90-days major complications (p = 0.015) [4]. Critical analysis identified that surgical complications were responsible for 39.4% of all 90-days major complications [4]. The incidence of surgical complications did not decline with increasing number of iRARC cases performed (p = 0.742, r = 0.31) [4]. Limitations of this study include its retrospective nature, limited sample size, and limited multivariate analysis due to the low number of major complications events [4].

Pyun analysed the complications after robot-assisted radical cystectomy (RARC) by use of a standardized reporting methodology by a single surgeon [5]. Fifty percent of patients (26 of 52) experienced a complication of any grade <90 days after surgery, and 11 patients (21.2%) experienced a major complication [5]. Complications were grouped in systems-based categories [5]. Fifty complications occurred in 52 patients and hematologic complication (transfusion) was the most common (13 of 52) [5]. Wound dehiscence, anastomotic leakage, urinary tract obstruction, mechanical obstruction, and thromboembolism occurred as major complications [5].

Robot-assisted radical cystectomy (RARC) with totally intracorporeal neoblad-der diversion is a complex procedure that has been reported with good outcomes in small series [6]. Median follow-up of the cohort was 30.3 months (interquartile range: 12.7–35.6) [6]. Tyritzis, recorded negative margins in 69 of 70 patients (98.6%) [6]. Clavien 3–5 complications occurred in 22 of 70 patients (31.4%) at 30 days and 13 of 70 (18.6%) at >30 days [6]. At 90 days, the overall complication rate was 58.5%. Clavien <3 and Clavien ≥3 complications were recorded in 15 of 70 patients (21.4%) and 26 of 70 (37.1%), respectively [6]. Kaplan-Meier estimates for recurrence-free, cancer-specific, and overall survival at 24 months were 80.7%, 88.9%, and 88.9%, respectively [6]. Daytime continence and satisfactory sexual function or potency at 12 months ranged between 70% and 90% in both men and women [6].

Schumacher assessed the surgery-related complications at robot-assisted radical cystectomy with total intracorporeal urinary diversion during the learning curve in treating 45 patients with bladder cancer [7]. Early surgery-related complications were noted in 40% of the patients and late complications in 30% [7]. The early Clavien grade III complications remained significant (27%) and did not decline with time [7]. Overall, fewer complications were observed between the groups over time, with a significant decrease in late versus early complications (p = 0.005 and p = 0.058) [7]. The mean operative times declined from the first group to the second and third groups (p = 0.005) and the hospital stays shortened (p = 0.006) [7]. No significant difference was observed between groups regarding the lymph node yield at cystectomy (p = 0.108), with a mean of 22.5 nodes (range 10–52) removed [7]. More patients received an orthotopic bladder substitute (Studer) in each of the latter two groups than in the first [7].

55.4   Ileal Conduit vs. Orthotopic Neobladder Complication Rate

Abe determined the differences in the type, incidence, and severity of 90-day mor-bidity after radical cystectomy between two different methods of urinary diversion, ileal conduit and neobladder [8]. There was no significant difference in the overall complication rates between the two groups (ileal conduit: 72% [353/493], neoblad-der: 74% [129/175], p = 0.5909), whereas the neobladder group had fewer major (grade 3 or more) complications (13% vs. 20%, respectively, p = 0.0271) [8]. The neobladder group had more infectious complications (43% vs. 31%, respectively, p = 0.0037), mainly as a result of urinary tract infection, whereas the ileal conduit group had more wound-related complications (24% vs. 14%, respectively, p = 0.0068), mainly as a result of surgical site infection [8]. The 90-day mortality rates were 1.1% (2/175) in the neobladder group and 1.6% (8/493) in the ileal con-duit group (p = 0.6441) [8].

55.5 Complications in Ileal Conduit Diversion

Shimko evaluated long-term surgical complications and clinical outcomes in a large group of patients treated with conduit urinary diversion [9]. A total of 844 patients died at a median of 4.1 years (range 0.1–28.1) following cystectomy [9]. There were 643 (60.8%) patients with 1453 complications directly attributable to the urinary diversion performed with a mean of 2.3 complications per patient [9]. Bowel complications were the most common, occurring in 215 patients (20.3%), followed by renal complications in 213 (20.2%), infectious complications in 174 (16.5%), stomal complications in 163 (15.4%) and urolithiasis in 162 (15.3%) [9]. The least common were metabolic abnormalities, which occurred in 135 patients (12.8%), and structural complications, which occurred in 122 (11.5%) [9]. Increasing age at cystectomy (HR 1.21, $p < 0.001$), increasing Eastern Cooperative Oncology Group performance status (HR 1.23, $p = 0.02$) and recent era of surgery (HR 1.68, $p < 0.001$) were significantly associated with a higher incidence of complications [9].

55.6 Risk Factors for Complications Post Radical Cystectomy for Bladder Cancer

Roghmann analysed complications associated with urinary diversion after radical cystectomy (RC) and ileal conduit (IC) for bladder cancer (BCa) [10]. An IC complication (CDC $\geq$I) or a high-grade IC complication (CDC $\geq$III) was experienced by 32.7% and 13.4% of the cohort: 14.8%, 4.3%, 4.6% developed a peristomal hernia, IC stenosis, stenosis of the ureteral anastomosis, respectively [10]. IC revision was required by 10.5% of patients (median follow-up 19.5 months, IQR 7–47 months) [10]. The estimated rate of IC complications at 5 years was 52% (CDC $\geq$I) and 22% (CDC $\geq$III) [10]. The final model of the multivariable analysis showed that patients with a history of previous radiation (HR 4.33), a BMI $\geq$30 (HR 2.24), or longer duration of surgery (HR 1.01; all $p < 0.05$) were at higher risk for IC revision surgery [10]. A BMI $\geq$30 (HR 2.49, $p = 0.011$) was a risk factor for high-grade complications [10]. Previous radiation, obesity, and comorbidities represent risk factors for IC revision surgery [10].

Golan evaluated the accuracy of the American College of Surgeons National Surgical Quality Improvement Programs (ACS-NSQIP) surgical risk calculator in patients undergoing radical cystectomy (RC) with urinary diversion [11]. Of 954 patients undergoing RC, 609 (64%) received ileal conduit and 345 (36%) received ONB [11]. Among patients who received ONB, adequate BS (<0.01) was observed for pneumonia, cardiac complications, and death [11]. A procedure-specific risk calculator is required to better counsel patients in the preoperative setting and generate realistic quality measures.

55.7   Complication by Urinary Diversion Type

Nazmy evaluated perioperative complications stratified by urinary diversion type in patients treated with robot-assisted radical cystectomy [12]. The American Society of Anesthesiologists® (ASA) score was 3 or greater in 80% of patients and continent diversion was performed in 68% [12]. Median followup was 35 months [12]. Within 90 days 77.5% of patients experienced any complication and 32% experienced a major complication [12]. The 90-day mortality rate was 5.3% [12]. Most complications were gastrointestinal, infectious and hematological [12]. On multivariate analysis patients with ileal conduit diversion had a decreased likelihood of complications compared to patients with Indiana pouch and orthotopic bladder substitute diversion despite the selection of a more comorbid population for conduit diversion [12]. Continent diversion was associated with a higher likelihood of urinary tract infection.

Gibert et al. [13] characterized the long-term medical and surgical complications and burden of health care use after urinary diversion [13]. Of the 1565 subjects identified 80% underwent ileal conduit urinary diversion, 7% underwent cutaneous or orthotopic continent diversion and 13% underwent other types of reconstruction [13]. Urinary stone formation, wound complications and fistula complications were more common following continent diversion 5 years after surgery, while ureteral obstruction and renal failure/impairment were more common after ileal conduit diversion [13]. Overall more than 16% of patients experienced renal failure or impairment after urinary diversion [13].

van Hemelrijck, evaluated the risk of different in-hospital complications for patients undergoing a radical cystectomy (RC), as limited nationwide population data on short- and long-term complications after RC is available, despite it being the standard treatment for localised muscle-invasive urinary bladder cancer (UBC) [14]. Urinary tract infection/septicaemia was the most common complication following radical cystectomy, with an incidence of 90.4 per 1000 person years [14]. There was a higher risk of urinary tract infection among patients who had a continent cutaneous reservoir (HR: 1.11 (0.94–1.30)) or orthotopic neobladder (1.21 (1.05–1.39)) than among those with ileal conduit [14]. Similarly, continent cutaneous reservoir and orthotopic neobladder were associated with increased risks for wound and abdominal wall hernias, stones in the urinary tract, hydronephrosis and nephrostomy tube treatment, and kidney failure [14]. In contrast, risk of bowel obstruction was lower among those with orthotopic neobladder than those with ileal conduit (HR: 0.64 (0.50–0.81)) and those with continent cutaneous reservoir (HR: 0.92 (0.73–1.16)) [14].

Smith reported on a multi-institutional, multi-surgeon experience with robotic radical cystectomy with regard to operative and pathologic outcomes and complications to evaluate the feasibility and reproducibility of this technique in a large cohort of patients [15]. One hundred and sixty-eight patients (74%) underwent ileal conduit diversion, 58 (26%) underwent orthotopic ileal neobladder, and 1 patient (<1%) had no diversion (end-stage renal disease) [15]. The urinary diversion was performed extracorporeally in 97% cases, with 7 patients (3%) undergoing an intracorporeal diversion [15]. Sixty-eight patients (30%) experienced complications, with

7% having Clavien grade 3 or higher [15]. A multi-institutional experience with robotic radical cystectomy appears to demonstrate acceptable operative and pathologic outcomes, thus helping to validate the previously reported single-institution case series [15]. Ultimately, oncologic follow-up of these patients will remain as the most important measure of therapeutic success [15].

55.8 Preoperative Anaemia and Impact on Post-operative Complications in Radical Cystectomy

Tan assessed the prevalence of preoperative anemia and the impact of preoperative anemia and blood transfusion requirement on 30- and 90-day complications in a cohort of patients undergoing robot-assisted radical cystectomy with intracorporeal urinary diversion (iRARC) [16]. Preoperative anemia was common (43.4%) and greatest in patients receiving neoadjuvant chemotherapy (48.6%) (p < 0.001) [16]. Patients with preoperative anemia were significantly more likely to have an Ileal conduit (p = 0.033), higher cystectomy stage (≥pT3) (p = 0.028), and a lower lymph node yield (p = 0.031) [16]. Preoperative anemia was not associated with increased perioperative morbidity but was associated with the requirement for blood transfusion (p = 0.001) [16]. Blood transfusion required in 20.4% of patients with intraoperative and postoperative blood transfusion rate was 10.2% and 13.9%, respectively [16]. The 30-day all complication rate and 30-day major complication rate were 55.4% and 15.7%, respectively, while 90-day all complication rate and 90-day major complication rate were 65.7% and 19.3%, respectively [16]. Intraoperative blood transfusion was not associated with increased complications, but postoperative blood transfusion requirement was independently associated with perioperative morbidity: all 30-day complications (p = 0.003), all 90-day complications (p = 0.009), and 90-day major complications (p = 0.004) [16].

55.9 Complications Post Radical Cystectomy Using a Standardised Reporting System

Roghmann examined postoperative complications in a contemporary series of patients after radical cystectomy using a standardized reporting system, and to identify readily available preoperative risk factors [17]. The 90-day rates for overall (Clavien-Dindo classification I–V) and high-grade complications (Clavien-Dindo classification III–V), as well as mortality (Clavien-Dindo classification V), were 56.4%, 18.7% and 3.9%, respectively [17]. Infections (16.4%), bleeding (14.2%) and gastrointestinal complications (10.7%) were the most common adverse outcomes [17]. Independent risk factors for overall complications were body mass index (odds ratio 1.08) and Charlson Comorbidity Index ≥3 (odds ratio 1.93) [17]. Risk factors for high-grade complications were Charlson Comorbidity Index ≥3 (odds ratio 1.86), American Society of Anesthesiologists Score ≥3 (odds ratio 1.92) and body mass index (odds ratio 1.07, all p < 0.03) [17].

55.10 Complications Post Orthotopic Neobladders

Muto presented the long term-results and complications of a large series of stapled ileal orthotopic neobladders [18]. After a median follow-up of 81 months (IQR: 30–144), a total of 147 early (less than 90 days) complications (38 diversion related, 109 diversion unrelated) occurred in 144 patients (24%); 163 late complications (141 diversion related, 22 diversion unrelated) affected 141 patients (23%) [18]. At 60 months, daytime and night-time continence was complete in 96% and 72% of cases, respectively [18].

Torrey evaluated the functional outcomes and complications for patients with bladder cancer undergoing robotic-assisted laparoscopic radical cystectomy with Indiana pouch continent cutaneous urinary diversion [19]. Overall, 175 (123 early and 52 late) complications after surgery were reported in 32 (94%) of 34 patients. Within 90 days of surgery, 31 (91%) of 34 patients experienced ≥ 1 early complication [19]. Of 34 patients, 15 (44%) reported ≥ 1 late complications (>90 days) [19]. Most (85% and 69%, respectively) early and late complications were graded as minor (grade II or less) [19]. Fewer patients with early complications required an additional intervention (grade III) compared with patients with late complications (14% vs. 31%; p = 0.116) [19]. The most common complication in both intervals was infection, reported in 22% and 37% of patients with early and late complications, respectively [19]. The continence data for 31 patients at a mean follow-up of 20.1 months (median 12.0) showed that all but 1 patient (97%) had daytime and nighttime continence [19].

With the purpose to reduce the complications of radical cystectomy and intestinal urinary reconstruction a perioperative protocol based on fast-track surgery principles and technical modifications of the original surgical technique was applied to patient candidates for orthotopic bladder substitution [20]. From 2003 to 2010, 68 consecutive patients participated in the study [20]. Two patients died due to surgical complications (2.9%) [20]. Overall, 24 of 68 patients experienced complications (35.3%) [20]. Surgery was needed under general anaesthesia for seven patients (10.2%) and under local anaesthesia for four (5.9%) [20]. Medical complications were encountered in 13 of 68 patients (19.1%) [20]. According to Clavien grading, complications were grade 5 in two patients, grade 4 in two patients, grade 3b in five patients, grade 3a in four patients, grade 2 in nine patients, and grade 1b in two patients [20].

Hautmann reported the 90-day morbidity of the ileal neobladder in a large, contemporary, homogenous series of patients who underwent radical cystectomy [21]. Of 1013 patients 587 (58%) experienced at least 1 complication within 90 days of surgery [21]. Infectious complications were most common (24%) followed by genitourinary (17%), gastrointestinal (15%) and wound related complications (9%) [21]. The 90-day mortality rate was 2.3%. Of the patients 36% had minor (grade 1–2) and 22% had major (grade 3–5) complications [21]. Radical cystectomy and ileal neobladder formation represent a major surgery with potential relevant early complications even in the most experienced hands. The rate of severe and lethal complications is acceptably low [21].

Porena evaluate the long-term functional results and complications of an orthotopic ileal neobladder, defined as perugia ileal neobladder (PIN), in a group of patients with bladder cancer who underwent radical cystectomy (RC) [22]. The median follow-up was 64 months, and the 5-year overall survival rate was 64% [22]. Early complications were mostly grade I and II; grade III and IV complications were observed in 27 patients [22]. Perioperative mortality rate was 1.6% [22]. The most frequent late complications were neobladder-ureteral reflux, urolithiasis and urethral anastomotic stricture [22]. Daytime and nighttime urinary continence were 93.5% and 83.9%, respectively [22]. All patients were able to completely empty neobladders [22]. Twenty patients were followed up for at least 10 years and presented satisfactory functional results [22].

Jensen reported the complications and function of the Hautmann orthotopic ileal neobladder [23]. There were early complications in 41 patients (61%), and late complications in 32 (48%); 23 (34%) had both early and late complications and 17 (25%) had none [23]. Eighteen of the patients (27%) required a re-operation for complications [23]. At the 4-month follow-up, 90% were continent during the day and 65% during the night; at 1 year after surgery 95% were continent during the day and 73% during the night [23]. The functional bladder capacity and maximum cystometric capacity were close to the natural bladder volume (median 450 and 480 ml, respectively) [23].

55.11   Complications Post Laparoscopic Radical Cystectomy

Huang evaluate operation process and perioperative complications of patients who underwent laparoscopic radical cystectomy (LRC) [24]. For urinary diversion, ileal conduits were constructed in 27 patients (55.1%), ileal neobladders in 16 patients (32.7%), and ureterocutaneostomies in 6 patients (12.2%) [24]. A total of 17 patients (34.7%) developed at least one perioperative complication. Complications of grades 1–2 occurred in 12 patients (24.5%), which included subileus, urinary tract infections, deep venous thrombosis of the lower limbs, pneumonia [24]. Complications of grades 3–5 occurred in 5 patients (10.2%), and one patient died of pulmonary embolism. Ileal neobladders and ileal conduits were similar at the operation time, blood loss, transfusion rates, postoperative hospital stay and morbidity of perioperative complications [24].

55.12   Post-operative Complications of Radical Cystectomy in the Elderly

Ichihara reviewed in 26 patients 75 years old and older who were treated with radical cystectomy including pelvic lymphadenectomy and urinary diversion [25]. Early postoperative complications were found in 9 elderly patients (34%), but there were no deaths in the preoperative and early postoperative periods [25]. There was no significant difference in the rate of early postoperative complications between patients 75 years old and older and those younger than 75 [25]. Preoperative performance status (PS) and the American Society of Anesthesiologists Score (ASA score) were significantly better in elderly patients with the surgery than those without surgery. Therefore, evaluation with PS and the ASA score may allow urologists to appropriately select elderly candidates for radical cystectomy and urinary diversion [25]. Chronological age alone is not a determinant for indicating the surgery [25].

Longo compared peri-operative outcomes and quality of life (QoL) in a series of elderly patients with high comorbidity status who underwent single stoma cutaneous ureterostomy (CU) or ileal conduit (IC) after radical cystectomy (RC) [26]. A total of 70 patients were included in the final comparative analyses [26]. Of these, 35 underwent IC diversion and 35 CU single stoma diversion [26]. Operating times (p < 0.001), estimated blood loss (p < 0.001), need for intensive care unit stay (p = 0.01), time to drain removal (p < 0.001) and length of hospital stay (p < 0.001) were significantly higher in patients undergoing IC diversion [26]. The number of patients with intra- (p = 0.04) and early postoperative (p = 0.02) complications was also significantly higher among those undergoing IC diversion [26]. Interestingly, the mean BCI scores were overlapping in the two groups [26].

Li explored the association of age, gender and urinary diversion category with postoperative complications of radical cystectomy [27]. Among them, 38.8% (145/374) received ileal conduit, 47.9% (179/374) orthotopic ileal neobladder and 13.4% (50/374) orthotopic colonic neobladder [27]. The overall perioperative complication rate was 37.4% (140/374). And 21.4% (80/374) experienced at least one complication within Day 90 postoperation while 16.3% (61/374) had the long-term complications (>day 90) [27]. There was no significant association between patients age (p = 0.15) and perioperative complications or between gender (p = 0.16) and complication [27]. Urinary diversion (OR = 0.26, 95% CI: 0.16–0.43) was the only variable significantly associated with the perioperative urinary complications [27].

55.13 Complications of Radical Cystectomy Post Prior Radiotherapy

Tolhurst assessed the morbidity associated with radical cystectomy in patients who had previously undergone definitive treatment of prostate cancer [28]. An overall complication rate of 76% was seen in this patient cohort, with 47% of patients experiencing a complication that presented later than postoperative day 30 [28]. Radiotherapy was associated with a slightly greater complication rate compared with radical prostatectomy monotherapy (77% versus 71%) [28]. Continent urinary diversion (n = 14) was associated with increased morbidity compared with ileal conduit diversion (n = 21) [28]. However, a greater percentage of the complications occurring in patients undergoing ileal conduit diversion were major (80% versus 67%) [28].

Eisenberg reported early complication rates in patients undergoing cystectomy and urinary diversion after high dose pelvic radiation [29]. Patients received a median of 70 Gy pelvic radiation therapy a median of 2.3 years before surgery [29]. Urinary diversions performed were ileal conduit in 65 patients (43.9%), continent cutaneous pouch in 35 (23.6%) and orthotopic neobladder in 48 (32.4%) [29]. A total of 335 early complications were identified [29]. The highest-grade complication was 0 in 23% of the patients, grade 1 in 12.2%, grade 2 in 32.4%, grade 3 in 18.9%, grade 4 in 7.4% and grade 5 in 6.1% [29]. Age older than 65 years and

American Society of Anesthesiologists score were statistically significant predictors of postoperative complications (p = 0.0264 and p = 0.0252, respectively) [29].

Gschwend determine the risk of post-operative complications in patients receiving high-dose pelvic irradiation before radical cystectomy and urinary diversion [30]. The post-operative course, including the duration of hospital stay, perioperative complications and early functional results, did not differ from a control group of non-irradiated patients, and no patients died [30]. The mean follow-up was 22 months (range 10–37) and revealed satisfactory results in seven of 11 patients [30]. A neovesicoperitoneal fistula developed in one woman 10 months after surgery and was repaired by laparotomy [30]. A neovesicovaginal fistula led to supravesical urinary diversion in the second woman.

55.14   Impact of Metabolic Syndrome on Radical Cystectomy

Cantiello evaluated the effect of (Metabolic syndrome) MetS and its components on the early complications observed in patients treated with RC and urinary diversion [31]. A total of 323 complications occurred in 231 of 346 patients (66.8%) [31]. The rates for low-grade (CCS I-II) and high-grade 19.2% (62 of 323), and 1.7% (6 of 346), respectively [31]. At univariate analysis, MetS patients showed a higher rate of high-grade complications compared with patients without MetS (p < 0.001) [31]. At binary logistic regression analysis, MetS (OR, 1.3; p = 0.010), waist circumference (OR, 1.9; p = 0.022) and, only in single model, urinary diversion (OR, 1.3; p = 0.024) were independent risk factors for high-grade complications [31].

55.15   Mortality Rate and Urinary Diversion

Frazier reviewed 675 patients who underwent radical cystectomy and urinary diversion during two decades [32]. Of the patients 197 were treated from 1969 to 1979 (group 1) and 478 were treated from 1980 until 1990 (group 2) [32]. A total of 215 patients (31.9%) experienced postoperative complications (within 30 days of surgery) [32]. The morbidity rate was nearly identical between the 2 groups (32.0% for group 1 versus 31.8% for group 2, p = 0.962) [32]. Of note, however, there was a decreased incidence of wound infections and wound dehiscence among the patients in group 2 compared to group 1 [32]. Long-term complications occurred in 198 of the 675 patients (29.3%) [32]. At follow-up group 1 had a 35.5% incidence of long-term complications versus 26.8% in group 2 (p = 0.022) [32]. Most notably there was significant improvement in the incidence of ureteroenteric anastomotic strictures when comparing groups 1 (11.2%) and 2 (5.2%) (p = 0.006) [32].

Jarolím made a retrospective analysis of 198 cases [33]. Death during the early postoperative period was recorded in 3 patients (2× ileus and 1× pulmonary embolism) [33]. Other early complications were dehiscence of the intestinal anastomosis (3×), dehiscence of the skin would (3×) and pneumonia (3×) [33]. Clinically relevant late complications were ileus due to adhesions (4×), stenosis of the ureteroenteric anastomosis (21 ureteroenteric units) and urolithiasis (6×) [33]. Metabolic acidosis was recorded frequently (19×) [33]. Complications were more frequent in patients with advanced disease and in a poor biological state [33].

References

1. Moher D, Liberati A, Tetzlaff J, Altman DG. "Preferred Reporting Items for Systematic Reviews and Meta-Analyses: The Prisma Statement." [In English]. BMJ (Online) 339, no. 7716 (08 Aug 2009):332–36.
2. Mays N, Pope C, Popay J. "Systematically Reviewing Qualitative and Quantitative Evidence to Inform Management and Policy-Making in the Health Field." [In English]. Journal of Health Services Research and Policy 10, no. SUPPL. 1 (July 2005):6–20.
3. Kim SH, Yu A, Jung JH, Lee YJ, Lee ES. Incidence and risk factors of 30-day early and 90-day late morbidity and mortality of radical cystectomy during a 13-year follow-up: a comparative propensity-score matched analysis of complications between neobladder and ileal conduit. Jpn J Clin Oncol. 2014;44(7):677–85.
4. Tan WS, Lamb BW, Tan MY, Ahmad I, Sridhar A, Nathan S, Hines J, Shaw G, Briggs TP, Kelly JD. In-depth critical analysis of complications following robot-assisted radical cystectomy with intracorporeal urinary diversion. Eur Urol Focus. 2017;3(2–3):273–9.
5. Pyun JH, Kim HK, Kim JY, Kim SB, Cho S, Kang SG, Ko YH, Cheon J, Lee JG, Kim JJ, Kang SH. Standardized analysis of complications after robot-assisted radical cystectomy: Korea University Hospital experience. Korean J Urol. 2015;56(1):48–55.
6. Tyritzis SI, Hosseini A, Collins J, Nyberg T, Jonsson MN, Laurin O, Khazaeli D, Adding C, Schumacher M, Wiklund NP. Oncologic, functional, and complicationsoutcomes of robot-assisted radical cystectomy with totally intracorporeal neobladder diversion. Eur Urol. 2013;64(5):734–41.
7. Schumacher MC, Jonsson MN, Hosseini A, Nyberg T, Poulakis V, Pardalidis NP, John H, Wiklund PN. Surgery-related complications of robot-assisted radical cystectomy with intracorporeal urinary diversion. Urology. 2011;77(4):871–6.
8. Abe T, Takada N, Shinohara N, Matsumoto R, Murai S, Sazawa A, Maruyama S, Tsuchiya K, Kanzaki S, Nonomura K. Comparison of 90-day complications between ileal conduit and neobladder reconstruction after radical cystectomy: a retrospective multi-institutional study in Japan. Int J Urol. 2014;21(6):554–9.
9. Shimko MS, Tollefson MK, Umbreit EC, Farmer SA, Blute ML, Frank I. Long-term complications of conduit urinary diversion. J Urol. 2011;185(2):562–7.
10. Roghmann F, Gockel M, Schmidt J, Hanske J, von Landenberg N, Löppenberg B, Braun K, von Bodman C, Pastor J, Palisaar J, Noldus J, Brock M. Complications after ileal conduit: urinary diversion-associated complications after radical cystectomy. Urologe A. 2015;54(4):533–41.
11. Golan S, Adamsky MA, Johnson SC, Barashi NS, Smith ZL, Rodriguez MV, Liao C, Smith ND, Steinberg GD, Shalhav AL. National Surgical Quality Improvement Program surgical risk calculator poorly predicts complications in patients undergoing radical cystectomy with urinary diversion. Urol Oncol. 2018;36(2):77.e1–7.
12. Nazmy M, Yuh B, Kawachi MLau CS, Linehan J, Ruel NH, Torrey RR, Yamzon J, Wilson TG, Chan KG. Early and late complications of robot-assisted radical cystectomy: a standardized analysis by urinary diversion type. J Urol. 2014;191(3):681–7.
13. Gilbert SM, Lai J, Saigal CS, Gore JL. Urologic Diseases in America Project. Downstream complications following urinary diversion. J Urol. 2013;190(3):916–22.
14. van Hemelrijck M, Thorstenson A, Smith P, Adolfsson J, Akre O. Risk of in-hospital complications after radical cystectomy for urinary bladder carcinoma: population-based follow-up study of 7608 patients. BJU Int. 2013;112(8):1113–20.
15. Smith AB, Raynor M, Amling CL, Busby JE, Castle E, Davis R, Nielsen M, Thomas R, Wallen EM, Woods M, Pruthi RS. Multi-institutional analysis of robotic radical cystectomy for blad-

der cancer: perioperative outcomes and complications in 227 patients. J Laparoendosc Adv Surg Tech A. 2012;22(1):17–21.

16. Tan WS, Lamb BW, Khetrapal P, Tan MY, Tan ME, Sridhar A, Cervi E, Rodney S, Busuttil G, Nathan S, Hines J, Shaw G, Mohammed A, Baker H, Briggs TP, Klein A, Richards T, Kelly JD. Blood transfusion requirement and not preoperative Anemia are associated with perioperative complications following intracorporeal robot-assisted radical cystectomy. J Endourol. 2017;31(2):141–8.

17. Roghmann F, Trinh QD, Braun K, von Bodman C, Brock M, Noldus J, Palisaar J. Standardized assessment of complications in a contemporary series of European patients undergoing radical cystectomy. Int J Urol. 2014;21(2):143–9.

18. Muto G, Collura D, Simone GMuto GL, Rosso R, Giacobbe A, Castelli E. Stapled orthotopic ileal neobladder after radical cystectomy for bladder cancer: functional results and complications over a 20-year period. Eur J Surg Oncol. 2016;42(3):412–8.

19. Torrey RR, Chan KG, Yip W, Josephson DY, Lau CS, Ruel NH, Wilson TG. Functional outcomes and complications in patients with bladder cancer undergoing rob-assisted radical cystectomy with extracorporeal Indiana pouch continent cutaneous urinary diversion. Urology. 2012;79(5):1073–8.

20. Maffezzini M, Campodonico F, Capponi G, Manuputty E, Gerbi G. Fast-track surgery and technical nuances to reduce complications after radical cystectomy and intestinal urinary diversion with the modified Indiana pouch. Surg Oncol. 2012;21(3):191–5.

21. Hautmann RE, de Petriconi RC, Volkmer BG. Lessons learned from 1,000 neobladders: the 90-day complication rate. J Urol. 2010;184(3):990–4.

22. Porena M, Mearini L, Zucchi A, Zingaro MD, Mearini E, Giannantoni A. Perugia ileal neobladder: functional results and complications. World J Urol. 2012;30(6):747–52.

23. Jensen JB, Lundbeck F, Jensen KM. Complications and neobladder function of the Hautmann orthotopic ileal neobladder. BJU Int. 2006;98(6):1289–94.

24. Huang JL, Qiu M, Ma LL, Huang Y, Hou XF, Tian XJ. [Analysis of perioperative complications of laparoscopic radical cystectomy for bladder cancer]. Beijing Da Xue Xue Bao. 2011;43(4):544–7.

25. Ichihara K, Takahashi A, Hirobe M, Honma I, Fukuta F, Masumori N, Tsukamoto T. Early postoperative complications of radical cystectomy and urinary diversion in elderly patients. Hinyokika Kiyo. 2007;53(8):527–32.

26. Longo N, Imbimbo C, Fusco F, Ficarra V, Mangiapia F, Di Lorenzo G, Creta M, Imperatore V, Mirone V. Complications and quality of life in elderly patients with several comorbidities undergoing cutaneous ureterostomy with single stoma or ileal conduit after radical cystectomy. BJU Int. 2016;118(4):521–6.

27. Li XD, Liu ZW, Zhou FJ, Hou GL, Zhang ZL, Li YH, Dong P, Yao K, Qin ZK, Han H. Effects of age, gender and urinary diversion category on perioperative complications of radical cystectomy. Zhonghua Yi Xue Za Zhi. 2012;92(32):2280–2.

28. Tolhurst SR, Rapp DE, O'Connor RC, Lyon MB, Orvieto MA, Steinberg GD. Complications after cystectomy and urinary diversion in patients previously treated for localized prostate cancer. Urology. 2005;66(4):824–9.

29. Eisenberg MS, Dorin RP, Bartsch G, Cai J, Miranda G, Skinner EC. Early complications of cystectomy after high dose pelvic radiation. J Urol. 2010;184(6):2264–9.

30. Gschwend JE, May F, Paiss T, Gottfried HW, Hautmann RE. High-dose pelvic irradiation followed by ileal neobladder urinary diversion: complications and long-term results. Br J Urol. 1996;77(5):680–3.

31. Cantiello F, Cicione A, Autorino R, De Nunzio C, Salonia A, Briganti A, Aliberti A, Perdonà S, Tubaro A, Damiano R. Metabolic syndrome, obesity, and radical cystectomy complications: a clavien classification system-based analysis. Clin Genitourin Cancer. 2014;12(5):384–93.

32. Frazier HA, Robertson JE, Paulson DF. Complications of radical cystectomy and urinary diversion: a retrospective review of 675 cases in 2 decades. J Urol. 1992;148(5):1401–5.

33. Jarolím L, Babjuk M, Hanus T, Novák K. Complications of urinary diversion after cystectomy in bladder carcinoma. Rozhl Chir. 1997;76(9):425–8.

Part VIII

Patient Fitness, CPEX Testing and Enhanced Recovery

Strategies to improve pre-operative cardiopulmonary fitness could positively impact recovery after surgery. Banerjee, investigated the feasibility of vigorous intensity aerobic interval exercise in bladder cancer patients prior to radical cystectomy (RC) [1]. A total of 60 patients were randomised (1:1) to exercise or control following a cardiopulmonary exercise test (CPET). Improvements in peak values of oxygen pulse (p = 0.001), minute ventilation (p = 0.002) and power output (p < 0.001) were observed at the follow-up CPET in the exercise group versus controls [1]. Although this feasibility study was not powered to detect changes in post-operative recovery outcomes, there were marginal (non-significant) differences in favour of the exercise group in post-operative Clavien-Dindo score and need for high dependency unit inotropic support [1]. Bladder cancer patients responded well to pre-surgical aerobic interval exercise, and the improvements in cardiopulmonary fitness variables are important for post op recovery. These findings provide a strong foundation for an adequately powered randomised controlled trial.

Jensen reviewed feasibility of a short-term physical pre-habilitation program to patients with muscle invasive bladder cancer awaiting surgery [2]. A total of 66% (95% confidence interval (CI) 51; 78) adhered more than 75% of the recommended progressive standardized exercise program [2]. In the intervention group, a significant improvement in muscle power of 18% (p < 0.002) was found at time for surgery. Moreover, muscle power was significantly improved compared to that in the standard group with 0.3 W/kg (95% CI 0.08; 0.5%) (p < 0.006) [2]. Adherence was not associated with pre-operative BMI, nutritional risk, comorbidity, pain, gender, or age [2]. In patients awaiting RC, a short-term exercise-based pre-habilitation intervention is feasible and effective and should be considered in future survivorship strategies [2].

Despite growing evidence of the benefits of exercise in cancer survivors, exercise participation rates are low [3]. Understanding the unique exercise programming and counselling preferences may allow the delivery of optimal exercise programs in these growing populations. The majority of survivors indicated they would be

© The Editor(s) (if applicable) and The Author(s), under exclusive license to
Springer Nature Switzerland AG 2021
S. S. Goonewardene et al., *Management of Muscle Invasive Bladder Cancer*,
Management of Urology, https://doi.org/10.1007/978-3-030-57915-9_56

interested (81.1%) and able (84.3%) to participate in an exercise program designed for bladder cancer survivors [3]. There are strong views for home-based exercise programming (53.7%), walking (81.1%), moderate intensity activity (61.7%) and unsupervised sessions (70.6%). Older survivors were more likely to prefer to exercise at home, do light intensity exercise and want unsupervised exercise sessions. This paper suggests bladder cancer survivors are interested in receiving exercise counseling and prehabilitation.

Radical cystectomy with lymph-node dissection is a complex procedure and often followed by high postoperative morbidity and physical impairments leading to prolonged length of stay (LOS) [4]. Fast-track principles are standard procedure in radical cystectomy. Additional preoperative and postoperative physical exercises and enhanced mobilization may reduce LOS and early complications [4]. Adherence to pre-habilitation, i.e. completion of 75% of the programme, was 59%. Postoperative mobilization was significantly improved by walking distance ($p \leq 0.001$). The ability to perform personal activities of daily living was improved by 1 day ($p \leq 0.05$). Assessment of feasibility and effects of an exercise training programme in patients following cystectomy due to urinary bladder cancer [5]. Eighteen patients (64–78 years), of 89 suitable, cystectomised due to urinary bladder cancer, were randomized after hospital discharge to intervention or control [5].The 12-week exercise programme included group exercise training twice a week and daily walks. Eighteen patients were randomized to intervention or control. Ten patients were evaluated one year postoperatively [5]. The intervention group had continued increasing walking distance, 20 m (19–36), whereas the control group had shortened the distance −15.5 m (−43 to −5) ($p = 0.010$). A 12-week group exercise training programme was not feasible for most cystectomy patients [5]. However, functional capacity and the role-physical domain in HRQoL increased in the short and long term for patients in the intervention group compared with controls.

References

1. Banerjee S, Manley K, Shaw B, Lewis L, Cucato G, Mills R, Rochester M, Clark A, Saxton JM. Vigorous intensity aerobic interval exercise in bladder cancer patients prior to radical cystectomy: a feasibility randomised controlled trial. Support Care Cancer. 2018;26(5):1515–23.
2. Jensen BT, Laustsen S, Jensen JB, Borre M, Petersen AK. Exercise-based pre-habilitation is feasible and effective in radical cystectomy pathways-secondary results from a randomized controlled trial. Support Care Cancer. 2016;24(8):3325–31.
3. Karvinen KH, Courneya KS, Venner P, North S. Exercise programming and counseling preferences in bladder cancer survivors: a population-based study. J Cancer Surviv. 2007;1(1):27–34.
4. Jensen BT, Petersen AK, Jensen JB, Laustsen S, Borre M. Efficacy of a multiprofessional rehabilitation programme in radical cystectomy pathways: a prospective randomized controlled trial. Scand J Urol. 2015;49(2):133–41.
5. Porserud A, Sherif A, Tollbäck A. The effects of a physical exercise programme after radical cystectomy for urinary bladder cancer. A pilot randomized controlled trial. Clin Rehabil. 2014;28(5):451–9.

Exercise Therapy Pre-surgery

57

Assessing the unmet needs of cancer patients can help providers tailor health care services to patients' specific needs [1]. This study examines whether the unmet informational and supportive care needs of the patients with muscle-invasive bladder cancer vary by the patients' age, sex, or individual treatment choices [1].

Participants (N = 30 survivors; 73.3% men) were recruited from the Mount Sinai Medical Center and through advertisements posted on a national Bladder Cancer Advocacy Network [1]. Younger patients (<60 years) were less satisfied with the treatment information received presurgery and more likely to report posttreatment complications, choose a neobladder, and seek and receive professional support regarding sexual function, than were older patients (p < 0.05) [1]. More women than men reported difficulties with self-care and relied on themselves in disease self-management as opposed to relying on spousal support (p < 0.05). Patients with neobladder were more likely to report difficulties with urinary incontinence and deterioration in sexual function, whereas patients with ileal conduit were more likely to require spousal help with self-care. Patients who received chemotherapy were significantly more likely to report changes in everyday life (p < 0.05) [1]. Lastly, regardless of age, sex, or treatment choice, up to 50% of patients reported feeling depressed before or after treatment [1]. Unmet informational and supportive needs of patients with muscle-invasive bladder cancer during survivorship, and vary by age, sex, and treatment choices. Educational and psychological assessments as well as clinical interventions should be tailored to a patient's specific unmet needs, and to specific clinical and demographic characteristics [1].

Reference

1. Jensen BT, Laustsen S, Jensen JB, Borre M, Petersen AK. Exercise-based pre-habilitation is feasible and effective in radical cystectomy pathways-secondary results from a randomized controlled trial. Support Care Cancer. 2016;24(8):3325–31.

S. S. Goonewardene et al., *Management of Muscle Invasive Bladder Cancer*,
Management of Urology, https://doi.org/10.1007/978-3-030-57915-9_57

Patient Fitness for Surgery

58

There have been a number of papers recently, highlighting how supervised exercise training in long-term prostate cancer survivors can increase cardiorespiratory fitness, physical function, muscle strength, and self-reported physical functioning at 6 months [1]. In addition to that, what was also demonstrated, were these effects were maintained with a home based exercise programme. Physical effects are central to addressing care within this cohort of prostate cancer patients.

As part of service evaluation, prostate cancer patients were questioned at a patient conference, regarding physical side effects they were suffering. Sixty-six percent had a lack of energy. In 18% of cases, the needs of their family were not met due to their condition. Side effects of therapy were experienced in 44%. These patients were patients that had been cured with radical prostatectomy, brachytherapy or radiotherapy.

Patient fitness is something which is central to patient care. Whilst this may be taken this into account pre-operatively, by assessing physical fitness, it is not something done post operatively. Modern urological surgery has advanced much, with development of robotic surgery and minimally invasive procedures. However, urological procedures still include major surgery. Precise pre-operative assessment is required, for this often older cohort, with stringent preoperative risks assessment and medical pre-optimisation if required [2].

However, with regards to patients on androgen deprivation therapy, most often, this will be the cohort with locally advanced/metastatic disease. This treatment in itself has significant side effects, especially with regards to cardiovascular events and stroke. Exercise also reduces effects of hormones in creating metabolic syndrome, diabetes and may have anticancer effects regarding recurrence. Yet, this is a cohort that will not be CPEX tested. The same principles apply when considering patients with muscle invasive bladder tumour, pre-cystectomy or pre-neoadjuvant chemotherapy. Whilst they may be CPEX tested pre-cystectomy, if they were to receive neoadjuvant chemotherapy this would not occur prior to receiving chemotherapy.

© The Editor(s) (if applicable) and The Author(s), under exclusive license to Springer Nature Switzerland AG 2021
S. S. Goonewardene et al., *Management of Muscle Invasive Bladder Cancer*, Management of Urology, https://doi.org/10.1007/978-3-030-57915-9_58

So what can be done to help our patients further?

Cardio-pulmonary exercise testing (CPEX) is central to pre-operative assessment as it gives a standardised measure of a patients' function capacity and reserve [3]. This will also serve to add to a patients' physical fitness. CPEX allows assessment of oxygen usage under dynamic stress conditions. This reflects the ability of the patient to meet the physiological challenges of the perioperative period [4]. This also gives us the chance to detect cardiac failure and myocardial ischemia at subclinical levels [5]. The question arises whether all patients, those undergoing major urological surgery and those undergoing medical therapy should be CPEX tested to assess fitness first.

So the question remains, pre-major urological surgery and chemotherapy, how can CPEX be evaluated in this population? Simply, a randomised controlled trial is required, with evaluation of CPEX being central to urological procedures and even pre chemotherapy. The overall motto is 'get fit for surgery, get fit for chemotherapy and get fit for hormones.'

References

1. Galvao DA, Taaffe DR, Spry N, et al. Physical activity and genitourinary cancer survivorship. Recent Results Cancer Res. 2011;186:217–36.
2. Young EL, Karthikesalingam A, Huddart S, et al. A systematic review of the role of cardiopulmonary exercise testing in vascular surgery. Eur J Vasc Endovasc Surg. 2012;44(1):64–71.
3. West M, Jack S, Grocott MPW. Perioperative cardiopulmonary exercise testing in the elderly. Best Pract Res Clin Anaesthesiol. 2011;25(3):427–37.
4. Clayton RA, Bannard-Smith JP, Washington SJ, et al. Cardiopulmonary exercise testing and length of stay in patients undergoing major surgery. Anaesthesia. 2011;66(5):393–4.
5. Gerson MC, Hurst JM, Hertzberg VS, et al. Prediction of cardiac and pulmonary complications related to elective abdominal and noncardiac thoracic surgery in geriatric patients. Am J Med. 1990;88(2):101–7.

59.1 Research Methods

A systematic review relating to muscle invasive bladder cancer, robotic cystectomy and Enhanced Recovery was conducted. This was to identify whether ERAS has a role in this cohort. The search strategy aimed to identify all references related to bladder cancer AND muscle invasive disease AND Robotic Surgery AND enhanced recovery. Search terms used were as follows: (Bladder cancer) AND (muscle invasive disease) AND (Robotic Surgery) AND (Enhanced recovery). The following databases were screened from 1989 to June 2020:

- CINAHL
- MEDLINE (NHS Evidence)
- Cochrane
- AMed
- EMBASE
- PsychINFO
- SCOPUS
- Web of Science

In addition, searches using Medical Subject Headings (MeSH) and keywords were conducted using Cochrane databases. Two UK-based experts in bladder cancer were consulted to identify any additional studies.

Studies were eligible for inclusion if they reported primary research focusing on muscle invasive bladder cancer and nerve sparing. Papers were included if published after 1984 and had to be in English. Studies that did not conform to this were excluded. Only primary research was included (Fig. 59.1).

Abstracts were independently screened for eligibility by two reviewers and disagreements resolved through discussion or third party opinion. Agreement level was calculated using Cohen's Kappa to test the intercoder reliability of this screening

S. S. Goonewardene et al., *Management of Muscle Invasive Bladder Cancer*,
Management of Urology, https://doi.org/10.1007/978-3-030-57915-9_59

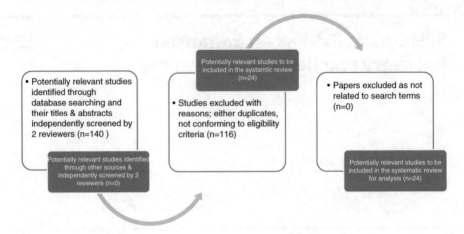

- Potentially relevant studies
  identified through
  database searching and
  their titles & abstracts
  independently screened by
  2 reviewers (n=140)

Potentially relevant studies identified
through other sources &
independently screened by 2
reviewers (n=0)

Potentially relevant studies to be
included in the systamtic review
(n=24)

- Studies excluded with
  reasons; either duplicates,
  not conforming to eligibility
  criteria (n=116)

- Papers excluded as not
  related to search terms
  (n=0)

Potentially relevant studies to be
included in the systematic review
for analysis (n=24)

Fig. 59.1 Flow chart of studies identified through the systematic review. (Adapted from PRISMA)

process. Cohens' Kappa allows comparison of inter-rater reliability between papers using relative observed agreement. This also takes account of the comparison occurring by chance. The first reviewer agreed all 24 papers to be included, the second, agreed on 24.

Data extraction was piloted by the researcher and amended in consultation with the research team (author and two academic supervisors). Data collected included authors, year and country of publication, study aims, setting, intervention aims, number of participants, study design, intervention components and delivery methods, comparison groups and outcome measures, notes and follow-up questions for the authors. Studies were quality assessed using the PRISMA criteria for randomised controlled trials, Mays et al. [1, 2] for the action research and qualitative studies and the Critical Skills Appraisal programme for cohort studies. This was also applied to randomised controlled trials and qualitative studies.

The search identified 140 papers (Fig. 59.1). Twenty-four mapped to the search terms and eligibility criteria. The current systematic reviews were examined to gain further knowledge about the subject. One hundred and forty papers were excluded due to not conforming to eligibility criteria or adding to the evidence. Of the 24 papers left, relevant abstracts were identified and the full papers obtained (all of which were in English), to quality assure against search criteria. There was considerable heterogeneity of design among the included studies therefore a narrative review of the evidence was undertaken. There was significant heterogeneity within studies, including clinical topic, numbers, outcomes, as a result a narrative review was thought to be best. There were 22 cohort studies, with a moderate level of evidence and 2 controlled trials with a good level of evidence. These were from a range of countries with minimal loss to follow-up. All participants were identified appropriately.

59.2   ERAS vs. Standard Care Post Radical Cystectomy

Wei evaluated the application of enhanced recovery after surgery (ERAS) in radical cystectomy (RC) [3]. The times from RC to first water intake, first ambulation, first anal exhaust, first defecation, and pelvic drainage tube removal were significantly shorter and the hospitalization costs were significantly lower in the ERAS than non-ERAS group [3]. The intraoperative blood loss volume, blood transfusion rate, readmission rate, and incidence of postoperative complications were also significantly lower in the ERAS than non-ERAS group [3].

Liu evaluated the safety and efficacy of the ERAS protocol for radical cystectomy for bladder cancer [4]. There was no significant difference in age or gender of patients between the groups [4]. Average length of stay pre-ERAS was 14.25 ± 14.57 days, which is significantly longer than the post-ERAS average of 10.91 ± 8.56 days (p = 0.043) [4]. There was no significant difference in 30-day readmission rate (19.87% pre-ERAS vs. 19.05% post-ERAS; p = 0.873) or complication rate (51.7% pre-ERAS vs. 46.4% post-ERAS; p = 0.425) [4].

59.3   Adherence to ERAS Protocols

Persson assessed the ERAS cystectomy protocol with secondary outcome measures of impact on perioperative complication rate (Clavien-Dindo classification), time to first defecation, postoperative length of stay and hospital readmission rate [5]. There were no significant demographic differences between the two groups, and no differences in complications graded Clavien III or above, or in total length of stay [5]. The ERAS group had statistically significantly shorter mean time to first passage of stool and statistically significantly lower readmission frequency than the pre-ERAS group [5]. The number of patients was small and the study was not randomized; moreover, the use of historical controls inevitably introduced different types of bias [5].

Arumainayagam assessed an enhanced recovery protocol (ERP) for the perioperative management of patients undergoing radical cystectomy (RC) [6]. The median (interquartile range) duration of hospital stay was 17 (15–23) days in the no-ERP group, and 13 (11–17) days in the ERP group (significantly different, p < 0.001, Wilcoxon rank-sum test) [6]. The median duration of recovery after RC was 15 (13–21) days in the no-ERP group and 12 (10–15) days in the ERP group (significantly different, p = 0.001, Wilcoxon rank-sum test) [6].

59.4   Readmission Rates for ERAS

Altobelli evaluated the specific causes of hospital readmissions in RC patients treated before and after adoption of an ERAS protocol [7]. In the post-ERAS time period a total of 56 patients were readmitted, 41 within the first 30 days after surgery (20%) and 15 within the following 60 days (7%) [7]. At 90 days infection accounted for 53% of readmissions [7]. Of all the patients readmitted during the first 90 days after surgery, 32 had positive urine cultures, mostly caused by Enterococcus faecalis isolated in 18 (56%) [7]. Readmission rates did not increase since the introduction of the ERAS protocol, with an incidence of 27% in the post-ERAS group versus 30% in the pre-ERAS group [7].

Baldini estimated the feasibility and the impact of an ERAS program after radical cystectomy for bladder cancer [8]. The ERAS group had statistically significantly shorter median length of stay (D19 versus D14; p: 0.021) [8]. The major complications rate (Clavien ≥3B) were about 23.2% for the control group and 12.1% for the ERAS group [8]. The reinsertion of nasogastric tube were higher in the control group (39.3% vs. 21.9%; P: NS) and the readmission rate was about 7.1% in the control group versus 14.6% in the ERAS group [8].

59.5   Surgical Approach and the Impact of ERUS

Djaladat determined whether surgical approach is a determinant of clinical outcomes following radical cystectomy (RC) and urinary diversion when using an Enhanced Recovery After Surgery (ERAS) protocol [9]. A total of 345 and 143 patients underwent ORC and RARC, respectively [9]. The ORC group had a greater proportion of continent urinary diversion (71.9% vs. 40.6%, p < 0.001), shorter operative time (5.4 vs. 7.3 h, p < 0.001), higher estimated blood loss (500 vs. 200 ml, p < 0.001), and higher intraoperative and postoperative transfusion rates (20.9% vs. 9.1%, p = 0.002 and 20% vs. 11.9%, p = 0.04, respectively) [9]. There was no significant difference between ORC and RARC groups in major complication rates (20% vs. 23.8%, p = 0.51) or readmission rates (32.2% vs. 36.4%, p = 0.4) within 90 days after surgery [9]. Multivariable logistic regression analysis showed that surgical approach was not an independent factor predictive of readmission (p = 0.33) or major complications (p = 0.76) [9].

59.6   Impact of ERAS on Post-operative Recovery

Uña Orejón analysed 124 patients undergoing radical cystectomy [10]. For retrospective analysis, the patients were divided into two groups: Group A (n = 72) included patients whose surgery was performed before the introduction of the ERAS protocol; and Group B (n = 52) included patients who were treated following the items included in the ERAS protocol [10]. Hospital and ICU stay were significantly shorter (p < 0.001) in Group B for patients following the ERAS protocol, which led to reduce seven hospitalization days and 25.7 h of overall ICU stay [10]. Regarding fluid replacement following the ERAS protocol, our study showed a statistically significant reduction in the total amount of fluid administered, both crystalloids and colloids, in Group B (p < 0.001) [10]. The need of blood transfusion was also lower in Group B with a statistically significant difference (p < 0.001) [10]. No statistical differences were observed regarding the incidence of surgical complications [10].

Mukhtar investigated the role of ERP in radical cystectomy [11]. Prospective data were collected from 26 consecutive patients prior to the introduction of the ERP and 51 patients who underwent open radical cystectomy within an ERP [11]. Baseline characteristics for both groups were similar [11]. The median length of hospital stay fell from 11.5 to 10.4 days and the mean ICU stay dropped from 2.4 to 1.0 days (p = 0.01) [11]. Time to removal of nasogastric tube, and time to passage of flatus and faeces were significantly shorter in the ERP group, as was the time to full oral diet [11]. Clavien complication rates and 30-day mortality rates were similar in both groups. There were no readmissions [11].

Collins assessed the effect of introducing an enhanced recovery programme (ERP) to an established robot-assisted radical cystectomy (RARC) service [12]. Following implementation of the ERP, the demographics of the patients (n = 135) changed, with median age increasing from 66 to 70 years (p < 0.01), higher ASA grade (p < 0.001), higher preoperative stage cancer (pT ≥ 2, p < 0.05) and increased likelihood of undergoing an ileal conduit diversion (p < 0.001) [12]. Median LOS before ERP was 9 days [interquartile range (IQR) 8–13 days] and after ERP was 8 days (IQR 6–10 days) (p < 0.001) [12]. ASA grade and neoadjuvant chemotherapy also affected LOS (p < 0.05 and p < 0.01, respectively) [12]. There was no significant difference in 30-day complication rates, readmission rates or 90-day mortality, with 59% experiencing complications before ERP implementation and 57% after implementation [12]. The majority of complications were low grade.

59.7   Patient Nonodifiable Factors Predictive of ERAS Outcomes

Zainfeld identified factors predictive of post-RC outcomes with ERAS protocols [13]. Median LOS was 4 days and 21.1% received intraoperative transfusion [13]. The 30-day complication and readmission rates were 58.8% and 16.6%, respectively [13]. Age >70 ($p = 0.02$), Charlson comorbidity index ≥2 ($p = 0.005$), and intraoperative transfusion ($p = 0.03$) were significantly associated with LOS [13]. Intraoperative transfusion was significantly associated with 30-day complication and readmission ($p = 0.008$, $p = 0.005$, respectively) [13]. No factor was found to be significantly associated with 90-day complication or readmission [13].

59.8   Impact of ERAS on Post-operative Complications

Cerruto described and assessed an enhanced recovery protocol (ERP) in a series of consecutive patients [14]. Thirty-one consecutive patients were recruited to undergo the ERP [14]. No patients died due to surgical complications [14]. Nine of 31 patients experienced complications (29.03%), none requiring surgical intervention [14]. According to Clavien grading, all complications were grade <2 [14].

Dunkman conducted a cohort study of an ERAS pathway for radical cystectomy at a large academic medical center [15]. Implementation of an ERAS pathway for radical cystectomy was associated with reduced hospital length of stay (median

LOS 10 days (IQR = 8–18) vs. 7 days (IQR = 6–11); $p < 0.0001$), reduced time to key recovery milestones, including days to first stool (5.83 vs. 3.99; $p < 0.001$) and days to first solid food (9.68 vs. 3.2; $p < 0.001$), reductions in some complications, and a 26.6% reduction in overall costs ($p < 0.001$) [15].

Djaladat reported 90-day complication rates following radical cystectomy (RC) with enhanced recovery after surgery (ERAS) protocol [16]. One hundred and sixty-nine cases with a median age of 71 years were included in the study [16]. 90-Day major and minor complication rates were 24.3% and 53.9%, respectively [16]. The most common complications were infectious and gastrointestinal [16]. The 90-day ER visit rate was 37.9%, whereas the readmission rate was 29.6% [16]. The most common cause of hospital readmission and ER visits was infections [16].

59.9   Impact of ERAS on Hospital Stay

Thaker evaluated the reasons leading to an extended hospital stay (EHS) in radical cystectomy (RC) with postoperative enhanced recovery after surgery (ERAS) protocol [17]. There were 279/509 (54.8%) patients had an EHS [17]. Univariate analysis demonstrated that age >65 years, CCI >2, increased operative time, anemia requiring transfusion and non-orthotopic diversion were associated with EHS [17]. On multivariate analysis, advanced age, operative time, postop transfusion, CCI >2 as well as surgeon specific preferences was associated with EHS [17]. Within EHS patients, 86% stayed due to an in-house complication; ileus (34.3%), anemia requiring transfusion (9.8%), UTIs (9.4%) and atrial fibrillation (8.5%) [17].

Zhang evaluated the feasibility and effect of implementing enhanced recovery after surgery (ERAS) in patients undergoing radical cystectomy (RC) and urinary diversion [18]. A total of 443 patients were included [18]. The ERAS and non-ERAS groups included 185 and 258 patients, respectively [18]. Compared with the non-ERAS group, there was decreased rates of intraoperative blood loss volumes and transfusion rates in the ERAS group [18]. Patients in the ERAS group also had earlier times to tolerate a clean liquid diet intake, first ambulation and first flatus [18]. The incidences of postoperative pneumonia, urine leakage, intestinal obstruction and deep venous thrombosis were also significantly lower in the ERAS group [18]. The time to pelvic drainage tube removal and the length of stay (LOS) were significantly shorter in the ERAS group than in the non-ERAS group, and the ERAS group also had a significantly lower incidence of 30-day readmission [18].

59.10   Impact of Type of Fluid on ERAS

Bazargani evaluated the association between intraoperative fluid intake and postoperative complications in patients who underwent radical cystectomy (RC) for bladder cancer with an enhanced recovery protocol [19]. One hundred and eighty patients enrolled into the study [19]. Median intraoperative crystalloid and colloid intake were 4000 and 500 cc, respectively [19]. Nineteen percent of patients received blood transfusion [19]. The overall 30- and 90-day complication rates were 59%

and 75%, respectively [19]. Multivariate logistic regressions controlling for a subset of clinically relevant variables showed no significant association between intraoperative fluid intake and complications at 30 or 90 days (p = 0.88 and 0.62, respectively) [19]. A multivariable linear regression similarly showed no association between total intraoperative fluid intake and length of stay (p = 0.099) [19].

59.11   Impact of Multidisciplinary Care on ERAS Outcomes

Patel examined the impact of multidisciplinary care with anesthesiology-related components to an existing ERAS protocol for radical cystectomy [20]. Implementation of a multidisciplinary ERAS protocol was associated with better postsurgical symptom control, as indicated by lower rates of patient-reported nausea (p < 0.05) [20]. Multivariate Poisson regression analysis showed a decrease in estimated intraoperative transfusions (p ≤ 0.001) after adjusting for the effects of potential confounding variables [20]. There were no statistically significant differences noted in length of stay, return of bowel function, 30- and 90-day complications, or readmissions [20].

59.12   Impact of PROMS on ERAS

Kukreja analyzed and compared patient-reported outcomes from those treated with Enhanced Recovery After Surgery (ERAS) methods versus those who received traditional perioperative care [21]. Patients (N = 383) reported dry mouth, disturbed sleep, drowsiness, fatigue, pain, and lack of appetite as the most severe symptoms [21]. Compared with the traditional-care group, the ERAS group had significantly less pain (est. = −0.98, p = 0.005), drowsiness (est. = −0.91, p = 0.009), dry mouth (est. = −1.21, p = 0.002), disturbed sleep (est. = −0.97, p = 0.01), and interference with functioning (est. = −0.70, p = 0.022) (adjusted for age, sex, surgical technique, and neoadjuvant chemotherapy status) [21]. What was highlighted, was the significant reduction in postoperative symptoms burden, with an ERAS pathway.

59.13   Impact of ERAS on Lymphadenectomy

Smith described and assess the evolution of an enhanced recovery programme (ERP) for open radical cystectomy [22]. The overall 90-day mortality was six patients (4.5%) [22]. There were significant differences in ileus rates between the non-ERP, the ERP-1 and the ERP-2 groups: 44.9% (31 patients), 29.7% (11 patients) and 14.8% (four patients), respectively (p = 0.017) [22]. There was a significant difference in the presence of pathological lymphadenopathy in the ERP-2 group: non-ERP group, 10.1%; ERP-1 group, 16.2%; and ERP-2 group, 44.4%; p = 0.002 [22]. There was also a difference in the mean (sd) lymph node yield in ERP-2: non-ERP group, 8.4 (5.4) nodes; ERP-1, 8.2 (6.4) nodes; and ERP-2, 16.7 (5.4) nodes (p < 0.001) [22]. The median (range) LOS was 14 (7–91) days, 10 (6–55) days and 7 (3–99) days in the non-ERP, ERP-1 and ERP-2 groups, respectively (p < 0.001) [22].

59.14 Pain Relief and ERAS After Radical Cystectomy

Xu compared opioid use, pain score and postoperative ileus in consecutive patients on a protocol of enhanced recovery after surgery and those on a traditional protocol after radical cystectomy [23]. Patients on the enhanced recovery after surgery protocol and those on a traditional protocol were similar demographically [23]. When analyzing data up to the median hospital stay on the case group, patients on enhanced recovery used significantly less opioids per day (4.9 vs. 20.67 mg morphine equivalents, $p < 0.001$) and reported more pain (visual analog scale 3.1 vs. 1.14, $p < 0.001$) [23]. They also experienced a significantly lesser incidence of postoperative ileus (7.3% vs. 22.2%, $p = 0.003$) and had a significantly shorter median length of hospital stay (4 vs. 8 days, $p < 0.001$) [23].

59.15 Impact of ERAS on Intracorporeal Urinary Diversion

Tan assessed the cumulative effect of an enhanced recovery after surgery (ERAS) pathway and minimally invasive robot-assisted radical cystectomy with intracorporeal urinary diversion (iRARC) in comparison with open radical cystectomy (ORC) on length of hospital stay (LOS) and peri-operative outcomes [24]. In a propensity score-matched cohort of patients who underwent iRARC, patients who followed the ERAS pathway had significantly lower 90-day readmission rates [24]. Additionally, implementing ERAS in an iRARC cohort resulted in a significantly lower 90-day all ($p < 0.001$) and gastrointestinal-related complications ($p = 0.001$) [24].

59.16 Prognostic Factors for ITU Admission in ERAS

Cheng examined risk factors of ICU admission after Radical Cystectomy (RC) with an Enhanced Recovery After Surgery (ERAS) protocol [25]. A total of 512 patients were identified. ICU admission in index hospitalization was reported in 33 patients (6.4%), 26 with unplanned ICU transfer after initial non-ICU level of care and 7 with planned direct postoperative ICU admission [25]. Higher age and Charlson Comorbidity Index ≥3 were significant risk factors for unplanned ICU admission [25]. Patients who required unplanned ICU transfer had a median length of stay of 11.5 days, compared to a length of stay of 5 days ($p < 0.01$) for non-ICU patients [25]. Ninety-day readmission and mortality rates were higher in the planned ICU cohort when compared to the unplanned ICU cohort [25].

59.17 Grey Matter: ERAS vs. Standard Care
for Radical Cystectomy

Giannarini conducted a systematic review with meta analyses of ERAS vs. standard care [26]. A total of 27 studies were included, namely 3 randomized and 24 non-randomized controlled studies, resulting in 4712 patients, 2690 (57%) participants to some ERAS protocol and 2022 (43%) controls receiving standard of care [26]. A number of primary and secondary outcome measures were assessed in the original studies [26]. Pooled data showed that ERAS protocols were associated with significantly faster recovery of bowel function, faster return to regular diet and shorter hospital stay with no increase in 30-day and 90-day major complication, mortality or readmission rates compared to standard of care [26]. The magnitude of benefit of the various ERAS protocols tested had, however, a non-negligible inter-study variability [26].

References

1. Moher D, Liberati A, Tetzlaff J, Altman DG. "Preferred Reporting Items for Systematic Reviews and Meta-Analyses: The Prisma Statement." [In English]. BMJ (Online) 339, no. 7716 (08 Aug 2009):332–36.
2. Mays N, Pope C, Popay J. "Systematically Reviewing Qualitative and Quantitative Evidence to Inform Management and Policy-Making in the Health Field." [In English]. Journal of Health Services Research and Policy 10, no. SUPPL. 1 (July 2005):6–20.
3. Wei C, Wan F, Zhao H, Ma J, Gao Z, Lin C. Application of enhanced recovery after surgery in patients undergoing radical cystectomy. J Int Med Res. 2018;46(12):5011–8.
4. Liu B, Domes T, Jana K. Evaluation of an enhanced recovery protocol on patients having radical cystectomy for bladder cancer. Can Urol Assoc J. 2018;12:421–6.
5. Persson B, Carringer M, Andrén O, Andersson SO, Carlsson J, Ljungqvist O. Initial experiences with the enhanced recovery after surgery (ERAS) protocol in open radical cystectomy. Scand J Urol. 2015;49(4):302–7.
6. Arumainayagam N, McGrath J, Jefferson KP, Gillatt DA. Introduction of an enhanced recovery protocol for radical cystectomy. BJU Int. 2008;101(6):698–701.
7. Altobelli E, Buscarini M, Gill HS, Skinner C. Readmission rate and causes at 90-day after radical cystectomy in patients on early recovery after surgery protocol. Bladder Cancer. 2017;3(1):51–6.
8. Baldini A, Fassi Fehri H, Cerantola Y, Bayle F, Ravier E, Belot PY, Arnouil N, Colombel M, Badet L. [Do initial experience with an enhanced recovery program after surgery (ERAS) improve postoperative outcomes after cystectomy?]. Prog Urol. 2018;28(6):351–8.
9. Djaladat H, Katebian B, Bazargani ST, Miranda G, Cai J, Schuckman AK, Cystectomy with Enhanced Recovery Protocol: A Prospective Cohort Study." [In eng]. World J Urol. 2017;35(6):907–11.
10. Uña Orejón R, Mateo Torres E, Huercio Martínez I, Jofré Escudero C, Gómez Rivas J, Díez Sebastián J, Ureta Tolsada MP. Application of ERAS (enhanced recovery after surgery) and laparoscopic surgery in the management of patients with bladder cancer. Arch Esp Urol. 2018;71(2):178–86.
11. Mukhtar S, Ayres BE, Issa R, Swinn MJ, Perry MJ. Challenging boundaries: an enhanced recovery programme for radical cystectomy. Ann R Coll Surg Engl. 2013;95(3):200–6.
12. Collins JW, Adding C, Hosseini A, Nyberg T, Pini G, Dey L, Wiklund PN. Introducing an enhanced recovery programme to an established totally intracorporeal robot-assisted radical cystectomy service. Scand J Urol. 2016;50(1):39–46.
13. Zainfeld D, Chen J, Cai J, Miranda G, Schuckman A, Daneshmand S, Djaladat H. The impact of patient-related nonmodifiable factors on perioperative outcomes following radical cystectomy with enhanced recovery protocol. Ther Adv Urol. 2018;10(12):393–401.
14. Cerruto MA, De Marco V, D'Elia C, Bizzotto L, Curti P, Baldassarre R, Artibani W. Introduction of an enhanced recovery protocol to reduce short-term complications following radical cystectomy and intestinal urinary diversion with vescica ileale Padovana neobladder. Urol Int. 2014;92(1):35–40.

15. Dunkman WJ, Manning MW, Whittle J, Hunting J, Rampersaud EN, Inman BA, Thacker JK, Miller TE. Impact of an enhanced recovery pathway on length of stay and complications in elective radical cystectomy: a before and after cohort study. Perioper Med (Lond). 2019;8:9.

16. Djaladat H, Katebian B, Bazargani ST, Miranda G, Cai J, Schuckman AK, Daneshmand S. 90-Day complication rate in patients undergoing radical cystectomy with enhanced recovery protocol: a prospective cohort study. World J Urol. 2017;35(6):907–11.

17. Thaker H, Ghodoussipour S, Saffarian M, Ashrafi A, Miranda G, Cai J, Schuckman AK, Aron M, Desai M, Gill IS, Daneshmand S, Djaladat H. Extended hospital stay after radical cystectomy with enhanced recovery protocol. Can J Urol. 2019;26(1):9654–9.

18. Zhang H, Wang H, Zhu M, Xu Z, Shen Y, Zhu Y, Xu Y, Chen W, Miao C. Implementation of enhanced recovery after surgery in patients undergoing radical cystectomy: a retrospective cohort study. Eur J Surg Oncol. 2020;46:202–8.

19. Bazargani ST, Ghodoussipour S, Tse B, Miranda G, Cai J, Schuckman A, Daneshmand S, Djaladat H. The association between intraoperative fluid intake and postoperative complications in patients undergoing radical cystectomy with an enhanced recovery protocol. World J Urol. 2018;36(3):401–7.

20. Patel SY, Garcia Getting RE, Alford B, Hussein K, Schaible BJ, Boulware D, Lee JK, Gilbert SM, Powsang JM, Sexton WJ, Spiess PE, Poch MA. Improved outcomes of enhanced recovery after surgery (ERAS) protocol for radical cystectomy with addition of a multidisciplinary care process in a US comprehensive cancer care center. World J Surg. 2018;42(9):2701–7.

21. Kukreja JB, Shi Q, Chang CM, Seif MA, Sterling BM, Chen TY, Creel KM, Kamat AM, Dinney CP, Navai N, Shah JB, Wang XS. Patient-reported outcomes are associated with enhanced recovery status in patients with bladder cancer undergoing radical cystectomy. Surg Innov. 2018;25(3):242–50.

22. Smith J, Meng ZW, Lockyer R, Dudderidge T, McGrath J, Hayes M, Birch B. Evolution of the southampton enhanced recovery programme for radical cystectomy and the aggregation of marginal gains. BJU Int. 2014;114(3):375–83.

23. Xu W, Daneshmand S, Bazargani ST, Cai J, Miranda G, Schuckman AK, Djaladat H. Postoperative pain management after radical cystectomy: comparing traditional versus enhanced recovery protocol pathway. J Urol. 2015;194(5):1209–13.

24. Tan WS, Tan MY, Lamb BW, Sridhar A, Mohammed A, Baker H, Nathan S, Briggs T, Tan M, Kelly JD. Intracorporeal robot-assisted radical cystectomy, together with an enhanced recovery programme, improves postoperative outcomes by aggregating marginal gains. BJU Int. 2018;121(4):632–9.

25. Cheng KW, Shah A, Bazargani S, Miranda G, Cai J, Aron M, Schuckman A, Desai M, Gill I, Daneshmand S, Djaladat H. Factors influencing ICU admission and associated outcome in patients undergoing radical cystectomy with enhanced recovery pathway. Urol Oncol. 2019;37(9):572.e13–9.

26. Giannarini G, Crestani A, Inferrera A, Rossanese M, Subba E, Novara G, Ficarra V. Impact of enhanced recovery after surgery protocols versus standard of care on perioperative outcomes of radical cystectomy: a systematic review and meta-analysis of comparative studies. Minerva Urol Nefrol. 2019;71(4):309–23.

Cardio-Pulmonary Exercise Testing and Major Urological Surgery: Risk Stratification and Preoperative Assessment

60

The worldwide increase in elderly is having a significant impact on healthcare systems globally [1]. Between 2009 and 2010, more than 7.4 million individuals aged 60 years and older required some form of hospital in-patient treatment in the UK. This is a rise of 37% since 1999–2000 [1]. Modern urological surgery has advanced much, both technologically and in its delivery; with developments such as robotic surgery and enhanced recovery. However, despite advancement in minimally invasive techniques, major open surgery will always have a role to play. In addition to this even robotic assisted laparoscopic procedures are still considered 'major' procedures or perhaps 'less major than previously'.

Concurrent comorbidities significantly contribute to outcomes. Nevertheless despite increasing challenges of this nature, patient expectation continues to rise unfettered. With surgeon outcomes being in the public domain there is even greater pressure to achieve optimal outcomes.

Rigorous pre-operative assessment is necessary, with stringent preoperative risks assessment and medical pre-optimisation (or 'prehabilitation') [2]. Outcomes after major surgery are dependent in a large part on physiological response to surgery [3]. This worsens with age. Despite the technical ability of the surgeon, the excellent technology at his/her disposal, and the excellent aftercare, outcomes, may still be discouragingly poor. Precise pre-operative assessment, with a dedicated multidisciplinary nursing and speciality based anaesthetic team [4, 5] are central to improving care.

60.1 Cardiopulmonary Exercise Testing

Currently assessment of fitness for surgery, may be crudely based on preoperative comorbidity and mobility status. This is not specific, and if not accurately determined, may lead to suboptimal results. Cardio-pulmonary exercise testing (CPEX) is an accurate means of pre-operative assessment as it gives a standardised measure

S. S. Goonewardene et al., *Management of Muscle Invasive Bladder Cancer*, Management of Urology, https://doi.org/10.1007/978-3-030-57915-9_60

of a patients' function capacity and reserve [1]. It has been used to investigate whether the ability to increase cardiac output and oxygen saturation to compensate for the stress response during surgery is directly related to outcome [6]. It is essentially an exercise test with baseline measurement throughout including ECG, blood pressure and oxygen saturations. This should be central to assessment of a patient, where there is a risk of high operative (or post-operative) mortality. Patient fitness to undergo major surgery can easily be underestimated by the standard pre-assessment questionnaires and pathology tests.

Functional capacity assesses the difference between baseline and greatest function; health status correlates more closely with measures of functional capacity than any resting measurement. CPEX allows measurement of the stress response during surgery, by mimicking it with increasing exercise. This allows assessment of the patient's functional capacity [1]. It also allows monitoring of levels of aerobic work involving the cardiovascular, respiratory and skeletal muscle systems, which form part of the stress response to surgery [7]. Patients who can meet this increased oxygen demand through increased cardiac output, will usually do well after surgery [8]. However, patients who do not have this are unlikely to cope with the operative stress and are more likely to suffer complications [9].

60.2   Other Methods of Assessment

There are others methods of assessing exercise tolerance in these patients. The Duke Activity Status Index allows assessment of physical activity via metabolic equivalents (METs) [10]. Ability to perform levels of exertion are standardised and graded [11]. On the other hand, assessment of patient fitness may be based on mobility. A patient who is unable to climb two flights of stairs has an 89% chance of postoperative cardiorespiratory complications [12].

The Acute Physiology and Chronic Health Evaluation (APACHE) score, allows assessment of physiological components and comorbidities [13]. The Physiological and Operative Severity Score for enumeration of Mortality and morbidity (POSSUM) was designed with surgical patients in mind [14].

60.3   Search Strategy

A systematic review relating to literature on CPEX testing and major surgery was conducted. The search strategy aimed to identify all references related to CPEX testing AND major surgery. The selection criteria specified papers could be related to all levels of research. This was due to paucity of literature available. Search terms used were as follows: (Cardiopulmonary exercise testing) AND (major surgery) OR AND (outcomes). The following databases were screened from 1984 to June 2020: CINAHL and MEDLINE (NHS Evidence), Cochrane, AMed, BNI, EMBASE, Health Business Elite, HMIC, PschINFO. In addition, searches using Medical Subject Headings (MeSH) and keywords were conducted using Cochrane databases.

We examine literature outcomes, including sample sizes and overall conclusions.

60.4 Systematic Review Results

60.4.1 CPEX and Major Surgery: The Research So Far

60.4.1.1 Vascular Surgery

The role of CPEX has been heavily investigated in vascular surgery [2]. The is no conclusive evidence for CPEX to be used as a routine part of pre-operative assessment. This is due to studies having small sample sizes, no randomised control trials with blinding and no standardisation, when reporting results [2]. No large trial has yet been conducted however, between echocardiography, pulmonary function tests and dobutamine stress echocardiography and CPEX.

From the available data, only one small, randomised trial attempted to compare echocardiography, stair climbing and CPEX [15]. The results suggested that stair climbing might be as useful as CPEX in risk stratification of patients.

60.4.1.2 Cardiothoracic Surgery

Low preoperative cardiorespiratory fitness is associated with higher operative and 30-day mortality after CABG [16]. If decreased aerobic fitness is present, this is associated with a higher rate of CABG [16]. Reduced aerobic capacity is also associated with higher operative and 30-day mortality after CABG [16]. A recent meta-analysis by Benzo investigated if VO_2 Max differed between patients who develop postoperative cardiopulmonary complications. Fourteen studies representing a total of 955 men and women were included. They concluded that exercise capacity expressed as VO_2 Max is lower in patients who develop clinically relevant complications after curative lung resection [17].

60.4.1.3 Intraabdominal Surgery

Gerson performed supine exercise ergometry in 177 patients, aged 65 years and over, undergoing elective major abdominal and non-cardiac thoracic surgery [9]. Sixty-nine patients were unable to exercise well with cardiopulmonary complications in 42%, with five deaths [9].

Pre-operative activity of 187 elderly patients undergoing major intra-abdominal surgery was examined by Older et al. [6]. Lower activity levels were associated with increased cardiovascular mortality. If patients' had preoperative ischaemia, the mortality rate rose from 4% to 42% [6]. This was confirmed by Wilson et al. Survival at 90 days was significantly greater in patients with higher activity levels and in patients without ischaemic heart disease [18]. The positive relationship between CPEX and postoperative morbidity after major intra-abdominal surgery was further re-enforced, with a sensitivity (88%) and specificity (79%) in predicting postoperative complications [19]. Consistent with previous reports demonstrating that measures of cardiorespiratory fitness are useful in predicting short-term perioperative outcomes, including extended lengths of hospital stay and 30-day readmission rates, in patients who undergo abdominal aortic aneurysm repair, liver transplantation, bariatric surgery, and other surgical interventions[16].

60.4.2 Future Research: Evaluation of CPEX

So the question remains, prior to major urological surgery, how should we establish or evaluate the role of CPEX testing on patients who are at high risk for surgery? As always the answer is within a trial in which CPEX testing is one of the variables examined in correlation with physiological outcomes. It may also have a role perhaps in selection of patients for other taxing treatments prior to surgery such as neoadjuvant chemotherapy prior to cystectomy. In this setting it may reveal whether patients' fitness for surgery is harmfully impacted on by neoadjuvant treatment erasing any potential advantage to receiving it. This needs to be considered as a serious adjunct to care, whether surgical, or whether patients require chemotherapy—in other words, a trial is required.

References

1. West M, Jack S, Grocott MPW. Perioperative cardiopulmonary exercise testing in the elderly. Best Pract Res Clin Anaesthesiol. 2011;25:427–37.
2. Young EL, Karthikesalingam A, Huddart S, Pearse RM, Hinchliffe RJ, Loftus IM, Thompson MM, Holt PJE. A systematic review of the role of cardiopulmonary exercise testing in vascular surgery. Eur J Vasc Endovasc Surg. 2012;44:64–71.
3. Lee JT, Chaloner EJ, Hollingsworth SJ. The role of cardiopulmonary fitness and its genetic influences on surgical outcomes. Br J Surg. 2006;93:147–57.
4. Patterson BO, Holt PJE, Hinchliffe R, Loftus IM, Thompson MM. Predicting risk in elective abdominal aortic aneurysm repair: a systematic review of current evidence. Eur J Vasc Endovasc Surg. 2008;36:637–45.
5. Tendera M, Aboyans V, Bartelink ML, Baumgartner I, Clment D, Collet JP, Cremonesi A, De Carlo M, Erbel R, Fowkes FGR, Heras M, Kownator S, Minar E, Ostergren J, Poldermans D, Riambau V, Roffi M, Rther J, Sievert H, Van Sambeek M, Zeller TW, Bax J, Auricchio A, Baumgartner H, Ceconi C, Dean V, Deaton C, Fagard R, Funck-Brentano C, Hasdai D, Hoes A, Knuuti J, Kolh P, McDonagh T, Moulin C, Popescu B, Reiner Z, Sechtem U, Sirnes PA, Torbicki A, Vahanian A, Windecker S, Agewall S, Blinc A, Bulvas M, Cosentino F, De Backer T, Gottster A, Gulba D, Guzik TJ, Jnsson B, Ksmrky G, Kitsiou A, Kuczmik W, Larsen ML, Madaric J, Mas JL, McMurray JJV, Micari A, Mosseri M, Mller C, Naylor R, Norrving B, Oto O, Pasierski T, Plouin PF, Ribichini F, Ricco JB, Ruilope L, Schmid JP, Schwehr U, Sol BGM, Sprynger M, Tiefenbacher C, Tsioufis C, Van Damme H. ESC guidelines on the diagnosis and treatment of peripheral artery diseases. Eur Heart J. 2011;32:2851–906.
6. Older P, Hall A, Hader R. Cardiopulmonary exercise testing as a screening test for perioperative management of major surgery in the elderly. Chest. 1999;116:355–62.
7. Clayton RA, Bannard-Smith JP, Washington SJ, Wisely N, Columb M, Rees L. Cardiopulmonary exercise testing and length of stay in patients undergoing major surgery. Anaesthesia. 2011;66:393–4.
8. Shoemaker WC, Appel PL, Kram HB. Role of oxygen debt in the development of organ failure sepsis, and death in high-risk surgical patients. Chest. 1992;102:208–15.

9. Gerson MC, Hurst JM, Hertzberg VS, Baughman R, Rouan GW, Ellis K, Fischer EE, Colthar MS, Burwinkle PM. Prediction of cardiac and pulmonary complications related to elective abdominal and noncardiac thoracic surgery in geriatric patients. Am J Med. 1990;88:101–7.

10. Hlatky MA, Boineau RE, Higginbotham MB, Lee KL, Mark DB, Califf RM, Cobb FR, Pryor DB. A brief self-administered questionnaire to determine functional capacity (the Duke activity status index). Am J Cardiol. 1989;64:651–4.

11. Day JR, Rossiter HB, Coats EM, Skasick A, Whipp BJ. The maximally attainable VO2 during exercise in humans: the peak vs. maximum issue. J Appl Physiol. 2003;95:1901–7.

12. Girish M, Trayner E Jr, Dammann O, Pinto-Plata V, Celli B. Symptom-limited stair climbing as a predictor of postoperative cardiopulmonary complications after high-risk surgery. Chest. 2001;120:1147–51.

13. Berger MM, Marazzi A, Freeman J, Chiolero R. Evaluation of the consistency of acute physiology and chronic health evaluation (APACHE II) scoring in a surgical intensive care unit. Crit Care Med. 1992;20:1681–7.

14. Copeland LA, Elshaikh MA, Jackson J, Penner LA, Underwood W 3rd. Impact of brachytherapy on regional, racial, marital status, and age-related patterns of definitive treatment for clinically localized prostate carcinoma. Cancer. 2005;104:1372–80.

15. Duffty J, Hilditch G. Anaesthesia for urological surgery. Anaesth Inten Care Med. 2009;10:307–12.

16. Smith JL, Verrill TA, Boura JA, Sakwa MP, Shannon FL, Franklin BA. Effect of cardiorespiratory fitness on short-term morbidity and mortality after coronary artery bypass grafting. Am J Cardiol. 2013;112:1104–9.

17. Benzo R, Kelley GA, Recchi L, Hofman A, Sciurba F. Complications of lung resection and exercise capacity: a meta-analysis. Respir Med. 2007;101:1790–7.

18. Wilson RJT, Davies S, Yates D, Redman J, Stone M. Impaired functional capacity is associated with all-cause mortality after major elective intra-abdominal surgery. Br J Anaesth. 2010;105:297–303.

19. Snowden CP, Prentis JM, Anderson HL, Roberts DR, Randles D, Renton M, Manas DM. Submaximal cardiopulmonary exercise testing predicts complications and hospital length of stay in patients undergoing major elective surgery. Ann Surg. 2010;251:535–41.

Robotic Radical Cystectomy and Enhanced Recovery: An Evolving Care Pathway

61

Radical cystectomy with urinary diversion is one of the most complex urologic procedures. Despite improvements in surgical technique, anaesthesia and perioperative care, radical cystectomy is still associated with significant morbidity and prolonged in-patient stay after surgery [1]. Fast-track principles are standard procedure in radical cystectomy, to minimise complications. Robotic surgery has been performed in an effort to reduce surgical stress and decrease perioperative morbidity [2]. Despite the degree of dissection, it remains the gold standard for muscle invasive bladder cancer. The magnitude of the surgical insult is associated with the degree of stress response, particularly in ageing patients with multiple comorbidities. However, there has been a growing trend towards enhanced recovery protocols (ERP).

Enhanced recovery protocols are multimodal perioperative care pathways designed to achieve early recovery after surgical procedures by maintaining preoperative organ function and reducing the stress response following surgery. The key elements of ERP include preoperative counselling, optimization of nutrition, standardized analgesic and anaesthetic regimens and early mobilization. These also have the advantage of not compromising patient outcomes. However, guidelines for perioperative care after open radical cystectomy for bladder cancer were recently published, but these recommendations may differ when considering a robotic approach. Some protocols, have gone as far as incorporating re-operative education, expectation setting, prehabilitation, nutrition evaluation, carbohydrate loading, venous thrombosis prophylaxis, normothermia maintenance, local anesthesia, no nasogastric tubes or bowel prep, early feeding, and opioid avoidance [3]. Part of this involves enhanced mobilization. No single intervention significantly reduces morbidity, but the combination of many interventions at all levels of the pathway is likely to accelerate the patient journey from diagnosis to return to normal function [4]. As a result, both readmission and complications rate are reduced.

S. S. Goonewardene et al., *Management of Muscle Invasive Bladder Cancer*,
Management of Urology, https://doi.org/10.1007/978-3-030-57915-9_61

The enhanced recovery patients have shorter time to GI function and recover more quickly then patients not put through enhanced recovery [5]. This protocol clearly improves clinical outcomes in terms of faster return of bowel function and reduction of readmission within 30 days [6]. These also clearly allow limitation of complications and length of stay [7]. A shorter time to stable health status with no increase of complications.

In contrast, in some cases, enhanced recovery may also have its' readmission rates- incidence of readmission after radical cystectomy still remains relevant, affecting more than 25% of patients, mostly affected by urinary tract infections [8]. Multi-institutional studies would be helpful to externally validate these.

In conclusion, ERP is a safe approach promoting standardization of postoperative care and resulting in decreased length of stay and decreased variability. Incorporating minimal access surgery within an established and continuously evolving care pathway is central to continuously improving care [9]. Early nasogastric tube removal reduced morbidity, bowel recovery time and length of hospital stay [10]. Doppler-guided fluid administration allowed for reduced morbidity [11]. A quicker bowel recovery was observed with a multimodal prevention of ileus, including gum chewing and minimally invasive surgery.

References

1. Preston MA, Lerner SP, Kibel AS. New trends in the surgical management of invasive bladder cancer. Hematol Oncol Clin North Am. 2015;29(2):253–69.
2. Smith J, Pruthi RS, McGrath J. Enhanced recovery programmes for patients undergoing radical cystectomy. Nat Rev Urol. 2014;11(8):437–44.
3. Persson B, Carringer M, Andren O, Andersson SO, Carlsson J, Ljungqvist O. Initial experiences with the enhanced recovery after surgery (ERAS) protocol in open radical cystectomy. Scand J Urol. 2015;49(4):302–7.
4. Porpiglia F, Calza E, Poggio M, Fiori C, Cattaneo G, Morra I, et al. "Enhanced" recovery program in patients undergoing radical cystectomy: our experience. Eur Urol Suppl. 2015;14(2):e434.
5. Adding C, Collins JW, Laurin O, Hosseini A, Wiklund NP. Enhanced recovery protocols (ERP) in robotic cystectomy surgery. Review of current status and trends. Curr Urol Rep. 2015;16(5):32.
6. Kukreja JB, Kiernan M, Schempp B, Hontar A, Ghazi A, Rashid H, et al. Cystectomy enhanced recovery pathway: reduction in length of stay without increased morbidity or readmissions. J Urol. 2015;1:e813–e4.
7. McCombie S, Nack T, Willmott J, Hayne D. The development of a radical cystectomy enhanced recovery pathway at fremantle hospital. BJU Int. 2015;115:98–9.
8. Altobelli E, Buscarini M, Gill H, Skinner E. Readmission rate after radical cystectomy in patients managed following the enhanced recovery after surgery protocols. J Urol. 2015;1:e855–e6.
9. Lim YW, Cheng C, Lee LS. ERAS enhances perioperative outcomes after open radical cystectomy for bladder cancer. BJU Int. 2015;115:23.

10. Campain N, McGrath J, Jackson L, Batchelor N, Daugherty M, Waine E. The robot alone is not enough-how to TO provide a comprehensive enhanced recovery service. Eur Urol Suppl. 2014;13(3):14–5.
11. Cerantola Y, Valerio M, Persson B, Jichlinski P, Ljungqvist O, Hubner M, et al. Guidelines for perioperative care after radical cystectomy for bladder cancer: enhanced recovery after surgery (ERAS) society recommendations. Clin Nutr. 2013;32(6):879–87.

Robotic Radical Cystectomy and Intracorporeal Stoma Formation: A New Technology to Guide Resection

62

Robotic radical cystectomy remains the hardest operation within urology. As surgeons, we consistently look to improve our outcomes. The use of indocyanine green (ICG) fluorescence imaging during robotic assisted laparoscopy has been shown to be helpful in identifying critical structures during cholecystectomies [1]. Additionally, Injection of intavenous ICG highlights pelvic vasculature. This can aid in identifying blood supply to myomas during robotic assisted laparoscopic myomectomy and decrease surgical blood loss [2]. The question then becomes, how can this be used to improve surgical outcomes for robotic radical cystectomy?

There are several steps within cystectomy that can use Firefly fluorescence to guide it further. This technology can assist in localizing a lesion in the bladder. The localization of the disease with this technology is efficient and precise, minimizing the lack of tactile feedback to localize the pathology during robotic assisted surgery [3]. This allows for a much more precise resection. Additionally, by integrating intraoperative near infrared fluorescence imaging into a robotic system, surgeons can identify the vascular anatomy in real-time with the technical advantages of robotics that is useful for meticulous lymphovascular dissection [4]. This technique can allow for precise lymph node dissection within the pelvis and identification of the SMA. This allows for a safe controlled resection.

Indocyanine green (ICG) fluorescence technology has also been used to delineate bowel perfusion. The optimal point of transection can be marked under white (visible) light followed by intravenous injection of 6–8 mg of ICG [5]. The bowel is then visualized via near infrared laparoscopy and the point of transection of the proximal is revised based on optimal bowel perfusion. This demonstrates the feasibility and advantages of the use of fluorescence imaging during creation of anastomosis; the advantages of endoscopic imaging to delineate integrity of the anastomosis as well the technique with regards to creating the anastomosis [6]. This can be used as part of cystectomy, when forming the conduit. To take this one step further, it can also be used, to assess the vasculature of the ileal conduit segment.

© The Editor(s) (if applicable) and The Author(s), under exclusive license to Springer Nature Switzerland AG 2021
S. S. Goonewardene et al., *Management of Muscle Invasive Bladder Cancer*, Management of Urology, https://doi.org/10.1007/978-3-030-57915-9_62

In conclusion, we have another 'pair of eyes' to enable us to conduct a safe controlled resection, with good vascular control, and which also allows us to conduct as safe anastomosis at the most precise location.

References

1. Ma P, Navaran P, Eghbalieh B. Glowing green: case report of indocyanine green uptake in gastrointestinal stromal tumors. Surg Endosc Other Interv Tech. 2015;29:S543.
2. Gutierrez C, Hernansanz S, Rubiales AS, Del Valle ML, Cuadrillero Rodriguez F, Flores LA, et al. Clinical manifestations and care in tumors with pelvic involvement: is there a pelvic syndrome in palliative care? Medicina Paliativa. 2006;13(1):32–6. [Spanish].
3. Rodriguez Morales-Bermudez AR. Fluorescence imaging technology for robotic assisted partial cystectomy and ureteral reconstruction minimizes lack of tactile feedback. Eur Urol Suppl. 2015;14(2):e980.
4. Bae SU, Min BS, Kim NK. Robotic low ligation of the inferior mesenteric artery with real-time identification of the vascular system for rectal cancer using the firefly technique. Surg Endosc Other Interv Tech. 2015;29:S374.
5. Jafari M, Carmichael J, Pigazzi A. Robotic-assisted low anterior resection with transanal extraction: single stapling technique and fluorescence evaluation of bowel perfusion. Dis Colon Rectum. 2015;58(5):e137.
6. Manny T, Hemal A. Novel use of indocyanine green for identification of sentinel lymph nodes and mesenteric angiography to assess bowel vascularity during robotic radical cystectomy with intracorporeal urinary diversion. J Endourol. 2013;27:A95.

A systematic review relating to bladder cancer and obesity was conducted. The search strategy aimed to identify all references related to bladder cancer AND obesity. Search terms used were as follows: (Bladder cancer) AND (obesity). The following databases were screened from 1989 to June 2020:

- CINAHL
- MEDLINE (NHS Evidence)
- Cochrane
- AMed
- EMBASE
- PsychINFO
- SCOPUS
- Web of Science

In addition, searches using Medical Subject Headings (MeSH) and keywords were conducted using Cochrane databases. Two UK-based experts in bladder cancer were consulted to identify any additional studies.

Studies were eligible for inclusion if they reported primary research focusing on bladder cancer and female gender. Papers were included if published after 1984 and had to be in English. Studies that did not conform to this were excluded. Only primary research was included. The overall aim was to identify the impact of obesity on bladder cancer.

Abstracts were independently screened for eligibility by two reviewers and disagreements resolved through discussion or third-party opinion (Fig. 63.1). Agreement level was calculated using Cohen's Kappa to test the intercoder reliability of this screening process. Cohens' Kappa allows comparison of inter-rater reliability between papers using relative observed agreement. This also takes account of the comparison occurring by chance. The first reviewer agreed all 12 papers to be included, the second, agreed on 12 (Fig. 63.1).

S. S. Goonewardene et al., *Management of Muscle Invasive Bladder Cancer*, Management of Urology, https://doi.org/10.1007/978-3-030-57915-9_63

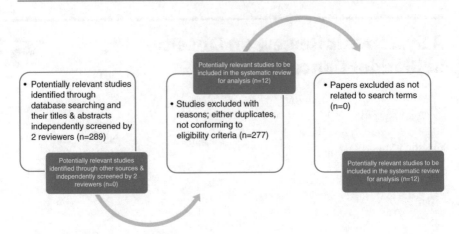

Fig. 63.1 Flow chart of studies identified through the systematic review. (Adapted from PRISMA)

Data extraction was piloted by the researcher and amended in consultation with the research team (author and two academic supervisors). Data collected included authors, year and country of publication, study aims, setting, intervention aims, number of participants, study design, intervention components and delivery methods, comparison groups and outcome measures, notes and follow-up questions for the authors. Studies were quality assessed using the PRISMA criteria for randomised controlled trials, Mays et al. [1, 2] for the action research and qualitative studies and the Critical Skills Appraisal programme for cohort studies. This was also applied to randomised controlled trials and qualitative studies.

63.1   Systematic Review Results on Obesity in Bladder Cancer

63.1.1 Impact of BMI on MIBC and Radical Cystectomy Outcomes

Gierth evaluated the influence of body mass index (BMI) on complications and oncological outcomes in patients undergoing radical cystectomy (RC) [3]. Data of 671 patients were eligible for final analysis. Of these patients, 26% (n = 175) showed obesity. No significant association of obesity on tumour stage, grade, lymph node metastasis, blood loss, type of urinary diversion and 90-day mortality rate was found [3]. According to the American Society of Anesthesiologists score, local lymph node (NT) stage and operative case load patients with higher BMI had significantly higher probabilities of severe complications 30 days after RC (p = 0.037) [3]. The overall survival rate of obese patients was superior to normal weight patients (p = 0.019). There is no evidence of correlation between obesity and worse oncological outcomes after RC [3]. While obesity should not be a parameter to exclude patients from cystectomy, surgical settings need to be aware of higher short-term complication risks and obese patients should be counselled-accordingly.

Dabi to evaluated the association between BMI and oncological outcomes in patients treated with radical cystectomy (RC) for muscle-invasive urothelial carcinoma of the bladder (UCB) [4].

From the 701 patients, 275 (39.2%) had a BMI <25 kg/m², 280 (39.9%) had a BMI between 25 and 29.9 kg/m², and 146 (20.9%) had a BMI ≥30 kg/m² [4]. Within a median follow-up of 45 months (IQR 23–75), 163 patients (23.3%) experienced a disease recurrence and 127 (18.1%) died from the disease. In univariable analyses, BMI ≥30 kg/m² was associated with a higher risk of disease recurrence and cancer-specific mortality (both p values <0.01) [4]. In multivariable analyses that adjusted for the effects of standard clinicopathological features, BMI ≥30 kg/m² was associated with both higher risks of disease recurrence (HR 1.58; 95% CI 1.06–2.34, p = 0.02) and cancer-specific mortality (HR 1.58; 95% CI 1.01–2.48; p = 0.04) [4]. Obesity was independently associated with higher risks of disease recurrence and cancer-specific mortality in patients treated with RC for muscle-invasive UCB. BMI is a modifiable feature that may have significant individual and public health implications in patients with muscle-invasive UCB [4].

Obesity is estimated to account for up to 20% of all cancer deaths. Hafron evaluated the effect of body mass index (BMI) on survival in patients undergoing radical or partial cystectomy for bladder cancer [5]. The BMI distribution was normal weight in 34% of patients, overweight in 41% and obesity in 25%. Mean follow-up was 53.4 months (median 39, range 1–168). BMI was not associated with disease specific survival as a continuous (p = 0.17) or categorical (p = 0.51) variable [5]. Although it was insignificant, unadjusted analysis showed lower disease specific mortality in patients with a BMI of less than 25 mg/kg and organ confined disease (p = 0.08) [5]. There was no significant association between BMI and overall or disease specific survival, although there may be a trend toward better disease specific survival in normal weight (BMI ≤25 kg/m) patients with organ confined disease (p = 0.08) [5].

63.1.2 Impact of BMI on Mortality After Radical Cystectomy

Psutka assessed the impact of obesity, as measured conventionally by body mass index vs. excess adiposity as measured by fat mass index, on mortality after radical cystectomy for bladder cancer, adjusting for the presence of skeletal muscle wasting [6]. Increasing body mass index correlated with improved overall survival (p = 0.03) while fat mass index based obesity did not (p = 0.08). After stratification by sarcopenia, no obesity related 5-year overall survival benefit was observed (68% vs. 51.4%, p = 0.2 obese vs. normal and 40% vs. 37.4%, p = 0.7 sarcopenia vs. sarcopenic/obese) [6]. On multivariable analysis class I obesity according to body mass index (HR 0.79, p = 0.33) or fat mass index criteria (HR 0.85, p = 0.45) was not independently associated with all cause mortality. However, in patients with normal lean muscle mass each 1 kg/m² increase in weight or adipose mass was associated with a 7–14% decrease in all cause mortality [6]. After adjusting for lean muscle wasting, neither measurements of obesity nor adiposity were significantly associated with all cause mortality in patients treated with radical cystectomy, although subanalyses suggest a potential benefit among those with normal lean muscle mass.

63.1.3 Impact of BMI on Recurrence and Progression of Bladder Cancer: High Grade None Muscle Invasive Disease

The body mass index (BMI) may be associated with an increased incidence and aggressiveness of urological cancers [7]. Ferro, evaluated the impact of the BMI on survival in patients with T1G3 non-muscle-invasive bladder cancer (NMIBC) [7]. After re-TURBT, 288 patients (27.53%) showed residual high-grade NMIBC, while 867 (82.89%) were negative. During follow-up, 678 (64.82%) suffered recurrence, and 303 (30%) progression, 150 (14.34%) died of all causes, and 77 (7.36%) died of bladder cancer. Overweight (HR: 4; p < 0.001) and obesity (HR: 5.33; p < 0.001) were significantly associated with an increased risk of recurrence [7]. Overweight (HR: 2.52; p < 0.001) and obesity (HR: 2.521; p < 0.001) were significantly associated with an increased risk of progression. The BMI could have a relevant role in the clinical management of T1G3 NMIBC, if associated with bladder cancer recurrence and progression [7].

Kluth et al. [8] hypothesized that higher body mass index is associated with worse outcomes in patients with clinical primary T1 high grade urothelial carcinoma of the bladder [8]. Of the patients 44.3% were obese and median body mass index was 29.2 kg/m^2 (IQR 8) [8]. On univariable analyses higher body mass index and age were associated with an increased risk of disease recurrence, progression, cancer specific mortality and any cause mortality (all p ≤ 0.001) [8]. On multivariable analyses higher body mass index and age remained independent predictors of disease recurrence, progression, cancer specific mortality and any cause mortality (all p < 0.05) [8]. Patients diagnosed with clinical T1 high grade urothelial carcinoma of the bladder who are obese have worse cancer specific outcomes compared to their nonobese counterparts [8]. Further work is needed to improve our understanding of clinical T1 high grade outcomes in the growing population of obese patients.

63.1.4 BMI and Risk of Recurrence in NMI Bladder Cancer

Xu evaluated the impact of body mass on recurrence and progression in patients with Ta, T1 Urothelial cell carcinoma [9]. Compared with patients with normal weight, overweight and obese counterparts showed significantly shorter recurrence-free or progression-free survival. In multivariate analyses, being overweight was an independent factor for recurrence and obesity was for both recurrence and progression [9]. The presence of diabetes mellitus (DM) was not a strong risk factor for the entire cohort, while it became a significant predictor for both recurrence and progression in the subgroup of overweight and obese patients [9]. Excessive body mass seems to act as independent risk factors for worse oncologic outcomes of Ta, T1 bladder cancer [9].

63.1.5 Obesity and Risk of Bladder Cancer

Increased body size and lack of physical activity are associated with increased risk of several cancers, but the relations of body mass index (BMI) and physical activity to bladder cancer are poorly understood [10]. Koebnick investigated the associations between BMI, physical activity, and bladder cancer in the NIH-AARP Diet and Health Study, a prospective cohort of 471,760 U.S. men and women, followed from 1995 to 2003 [10]. Compared with normal weight, obesity was associated with an up to 28% increased risk for bladder cancer. The multivariate relative risks of bladder cancer for BMI values of 18.5–24.9 (reference), 25.0–29.9, 30.0–34.9, and ≥ 35 kg/m^2 were 1.0, 1.15, 1.22, and 1.28 (95% confidence interval, 1.02–1.61; p trend = 0.028) [10]. The association between BMI and bladder cancer was consistent among subgroups defined by gender, education, smoking status, and other potential effect modifiers [10]. In conclusion, these findings provide support for a modest adverse effect of adiposity on risk for bladder cancer.

Wyszynski identified risk factors that are potentially modifiable to reduce the rate of recurrence are needed [11]. Although being overweight (body mass index >24.9 kg/m^2) at diagnosis was not a strong independent factor (HR = 1.33, 95% CI = 0.94–1.89), among continuing smokers, being overweight more than doubled the risk of recurrence compared to smokers of normal weight (HR = 2.67, 95% CI = 1.14–6.28) [11]. These observational results suggest that adiposity is a risk factor for bladder cancer recurrence, particularly among tobacco users. Future intervention studies are warranted to evaluate whether both smoking cessation and weight reduction strategies reduce bladder tumour recurrences [11].

Cantiello evaluated the pathological characteristics of patients with metabolic syndrome (MetS) undergoing radical cystectomy (RC) for Urothelial cell carcinoma (BCa) [12]. Metabolic syndrome was found in 36.3% of patients. At logistic regression analysis, the presence of MetS did not predict the risk of both higher pathological stage and LVI and LM [12]. Investigating the single components of MetS after adjusting for age, gender, and smoking, the risk of higher pathological stage increased with body mass index [BMI (OR 1.307, 95% CI 1.098–1.555)], waist circumference (OR 1.414, 95% CI 1.364–1.668), and blood hypertension (OR 2.326, 95% CI 1.147–4.717). Higher BMI also predicted the presence of LVI (OR 1.432, 95% CI 1.173–1.748) and LM (OR 1.202, 95% CI 0.951–1.519), whereas HDL cholesterol was inversely associated with the risk of LVI and LM [12]. Metabolic syndrome does not represent an independent risk factor for worse pathological findings in BCa. Conversely, individual components of MetS could increase the risk of higher stage as well as LM.

Anthropometric measures have been related to risk of several cancers. Roswall examined associations between height, weight, waist and hip circumference, waist-hip ratio, waist-height ratio, body mass index (BMI), recalled weight at age 20 and bladder cancer, and investigated effect modification by age, tumor aggressiveness and smoking [13]. Residual analyses on BMI/waist circumference showed a significantly higher disease risk with BMI in men (p = 0.01), but no association with waist circumference [13]. In conclusion, in this large study, height was unrelated to bladder cancer, whereas overweight was associated with a slightly higher bladder cancer risk in men. This association may, however, be distorted by residual confounding by smoking [13].

63.1.6 BMI and Prognosis in MIBC

Kwon investigated the association between body mass index and clinicopathological features of bladder cancer, and to assess the prognostic value of body mass index in patients undergoing radical cystectomy for bladder cancer [14]. Of 714 patients, 304 (42.6%), 184 (25.8%) and 226 (31.7%) had a body mass index of <23 (normal), 23–25 (overweight), and ≥25 (obese) kg/m^2, respectively. Patients with high body mass index had a lower pathological T stage, fewer lymph node metastases and a lower frequency of lymphovascular invasion than those with low body mass index (p < 0.05) [14]. Multivariable analysis showed that obese status was an independent predictor of recurrence-free survival (obese vs. normal: p < 0.001; overweight vs. normal: p = 0.008) and cancer-specific survival (obese vs. normal: p < 0.001; overweight vs. normal: p = 0.019), along with pathological T stage, lymph node metastasis, and lymphovascular invasion [14]. In addition, obesity was significantly associated with recurrence-free survival (p = 0.018) and cancer-specific survival (p = 0.019) in patients with N0M0 status [14]. The present findings suggest that overweight and obesity are associated with favorable pathological features and prognosis in patients with bladder cancer undergoing radical cystectomy.

63.1.7 Reviews on BMI and Bladder Cancer

Urologists are frequently confronted with questions of urinary bladder cancer (UBC) patients about what they can do to improve their prognosis [15]. Unfortunately, it is largely unknown which lifestyle factors can influence prognosis. Westhoff, systematically review the available evidence on the association between body mass index (BMI), diet, dietary supplements, and physical activity and UBC prognosis [15]. In non-muscle invasive bladder cancer (NMIBC) patients, both overweight (3 studies, pooled hazard ratio (HR) 1.29, 95% CI 1.05–1.58, I^2 = 0%) as well as obesity (3 studies, pooled HR 1.82, 95% CI 1.12–2.95, I^2 = 79%) were associated with increased risk of recurrence when compared to normal weight [15]. No association of BMI with risk of progression was found. Results for BMI and prognosis in muscle-invasive or in all stages series were inconsistent. Observational studies on diet and randomized controlled trials with dietary supplements showed inconsistent results [15]. No studies on physical activity and UBC prognosis have been published to date. Evidence for an association of lifestyle factors with UBC prognosis is limited, with some evidence for an association of BMI with risk of recurrence in NMIBC [15]. Well-designed, prospective studies are needed to develop evidence-based guidelines on this topic.

Noguchi evaluated associations of obesity and physical activity with bladder cancer risk by performing a system-wide search of PubMed for cohort and case-control studies focused on obesity, exercise, and bladder cancer [16]. A total of 31 studies were identified that evaluated the associations of obesity and physical activity with bladder cancer risk: Three (100%) of three studies also noted strong positive associations of obesity with bladder cancer progression or recurrence [16]. Ten (91%) of the physical activity studies analysed prevalence or incidence and one (9%) mortality. One (9%) study observed positive, seven (64%) null, and three (27%) negative associations of physical activity with bladder cancer. Obesity is potentially associated with an increased risk of bladder cancer, particularly for progression, recurrence, or death.

Epidemiological studies have reported inconsistent association between obesity and risk of bladder cancer, and the dose-response relationship between them has not been clearly defined [17].

Fifteen cohort studies with 38,072 bladder cancer cases among 14,201,500 participants were included [17]. Compared to normal weight, the pooled relative risks and corresponding 95% confidence intervals of bladder cancer were 1.07 (1.01–1.14) and 1.10 (1.06–1.14) for preobese and obesity, with moderate ($I^2 = 37.6\%$, p = 0.029) and low ($I^2 = 15.5\%$, p = 0.241) heterogeneities between studies, respectively [17]. In a dose-response meta-analysis, body mass index (BMI) was associated with bladder cancer risk in a linear fashion (p(non-linearity) = 0.467) and the risk increased by 4.2% for each 5 kg/m^2 increase. No significant publication bias was found (p = 0.912 for Begg's test, p = 0.712 for Egger's test) [17]. Findings from this dose-response meta-analysis suggest obesity is associated with linear-increased risk of bladder cancer.

References

1. Moher D, Liberati A, Tetzlaff J, Altman DG. "Preferred Reporting Items for Systematic Reviews and Meta-Analyses: The Prisma Statement." [In English]. BMJ (Online) 339, no. 7716 (08 Aug 2009):332–36.
2. Mays N, Pope C, Popay J. "Systematically Reviewing Qualitative and Quantitative Evidence to Inform Management and Policy-Making in the Health Field." [In English]. Journal of Health Services Research and Policy 10, no. SUPPL. 1 (July 2005):6–20.
3. Gierth M, Zeman F, Denzinger S, Vetterlein MW, Fisch M, Bastian PJ, Syring I, Ellinger J, Müller SC, Herrmann E, Gilfrich C, May M, Pycha A, Wagenlehner FM, Vallo S, Bartsch G, Haferkamp A, Grimm MO, Roigas J, Protzel C, Hakenberg OW, Fritsche HM, Burger M, Aziz A, Mayr R. Influence of body mass index on clinical outcome parameters, complication rate and survival after radical cystectomy: evidence from a prospective European multicentre study. Urol Int. 2018;101(1):16–24.
4. Dabi Y, Rouscoff Y, Anract J, Delongchamps NB, Sibony M, Saighi D, Zerbib M, Peyraumore M, Xylinas E. Impact of body mass index on the oncological outcomes of patients treated with radical cystectomy for muscle-invasive bladder cancer. World J Urol. 2017;35(2):229–35.

5. Hafron J, Mitra N, Dalbagni G, Bochner B, Herr H, Donat SM. Does body mass index affect survival of patients undergoing radical or partial cystectomy for bladder cancer? J Urol. 2005;173(5):1513–7.

6. Psutka SP, Boorjian SA, Moynagh MR, Schmit GD, Frank I, Carrasco A, Stewart SB, Tarrell R, Thapa P, Tollefson MK. Mortality after radical cystectomy: impact of obesity versus adiposity after adjusting for skeletal muscle wasting. J Urol. 2015;193(5):1507–13.

7. Ferro M, Vartolomei MD, Russo GI, Cantiello F, Farhan ARA, Terracciano D, Cimmino A, Di Stasi S, Musi G, Hurle R, Serretta V, Busetto GM, De Berardinis E, Cioffi A, Perdonà S, Borghesi M, Schiavina R, Cozzi G, Almeida GL, Bove P, Lima E, Grimaldi G, Matei DV, Crisan N, Muto M, Verze P, Battaglia M, Guazzoni G, Autorino R, Morgia G, Damiano R, de Cobelli O, Shariat S, Mirone V, Lucarelli G. An increased body mass index is associated with a worse prognosis in patients administered BCG immunotherapy for T1 bladder cancer. World J Urol. 2018;37:507–14.

8. Kluth LA, Xylinas E, Crivelli JJ, Passoni N, Comploj E, Pycha A, Chrystal J, Sun M, Karakiewicz PI, Gontero P, Lotan Y, Chun FK, Fisch M, Scherr DS, Shariat SF. Obesity is associated with worse outcomes in patients with T1 high grade urothelial carcinoma of the bladder. J Urol. 2013;190(2):480–6.

9. Xu T, Zhu Z, Wang X, Xia L, Zhang X, Zhong S, Sun F, Zhu Y, Shen Z. Impact of body mass on recurrence and progression in Chinese patients with Ta, T1 urothelial bladder cancer. Int Urol Nephrol. 2015;47(7):1135–41.

10. Koebnick C, Michaud D, Moore SC, Park Y, Hollenbeck A, Ballard-Barbash R, Schatzkin A, Leitzmann MF. Body mass index, physical activity, and bladder cancer in a large prospective study. Cancer Epidemiol Biomark Prev. 2008;17(5):1214–21.

11. Wyszynski A, Tanyos SA, Rees JR, Marsit CJ, Kelsey KT, Schned AR, Pendleton EM, Celaya MO, Zens MS, Karagas MR, Andrew AS. Body mass and smoking are modifiable risk factors for recurrent bladder cancer. Cancer. 2014;120(3):408–14.

12. Cantiello F, Cicione A, Autorino R, Salonia A, Briganti A, Ferro M, De Domenico R, Perdonà S, Damiano R. Visceral obesity predicts adverse pathological features in Urothelial cell carcinomapatients undergoing radical cystectomy: a retrospective cohort study. World J Urol. 2014;32(2):559–64.

13. Roswall N, Freisling H, Bueno-de-Mesquita HB, Ros M, Christensen J, Overvad K, Boutron-Ruault MC, Severi G, Fagherazzi G, Chang-Claude J, Kaaks R, Steffen A, Boeing H, Argüelles M, Agudo A, Sánchez MJ, Chirlaque MD, Barricarte Gurrea A, Amiano P, Wareham N, Khaw KT, Bradbury KE, Trichopoulou A, Papatesta HM, Trichopoulos D, Palli D, Pala V, Tumino R, Sacerdote C, Mattiello A, Peeters PH, Ehrnström R, Brennan P, Ferrari P, Ljungberg B, Norat T, Gunter M, Riboli E, Weiderpass E, Halkjaer J. Anthropometric measures and bladder cancer risk: a prospective study in the EPIC cohort. Int J Cancer. 2014;135(12):2918–29.

14. Kwon T, Jeong IG, You D, Han KS, Hong S, Hong B, Hong JH, Ahn H, Kim CS. Obesity and prognosis in muscle-invasive bladder cancer: the continuing controversy. Int J Urol. 2014;21(11):1106–12.

15. Westhoff E, Witjes JA, Fleshner NE, Lerner SP, Shariat SF, Steineck G, Kampman E, Kiemeney LA, Vrieling A. Body mass index, diet-related factors, and bladder cancer prognosis: a systematic review and meta-analysis. Bladder Cancer. 2018;4(1):91–112.

16. Noguchi JL, Liss MA, Parsons JK. Obesity, physical activity and bladder cancer. Curr Urol Rep. 2015;16(10):74.

17. Sun JW, Zhao LG, Yang Y, Ma X, Wang YY, Xiang YB. Obesity and risk of bladder cancer: a dose-response meta-analysis of 15 cohort studies. PLoS One. 2015;10(3):e0119313.

Part IX

New Techniques in Management of Muscle Invasive Bladder Cancer

A Systematic Review on Immunotherapy in Locally Advanced and Metastatic Bladder Cancer

64

A systematic review relating locally advanced and metastatic bladder and immunotherapy was conducted. This was to identify the bladder cancer, immunotherapy outcomes in locally advanced and metastatic disease. The search strategy aimed to identify all references related to bladder cancer, ureteric strictures AND urinary diversion. Search terms used were as follows: (Bladder cancer) AND (immunotherapy) AND (locally advanced) OR (metastatic). The following databases were screened from 1989 to June 2020:

- CINAHL
- MEDLINE (NHS Evidence)
- Cochrane
- AMed
- EMBASE
- PsychINFO
- SCOPUS
- Web of Science

In addition, searches using Medical Subject Headings (MeSH) and keywords were conducted using Cochrane databases. Two UK-based experts in bladder cancer were consulted to identify any additional studies.

Studies were eligible for inclusion if they reported primary research focusing on bladder cancer and screening. Papers were included if published after 1984 and had to be in English. Studies that did not conform to this were excluded. Only primary research was included (Fig. 64.1). The overall aim was to identify bladder cancer risk factors and epidemiology in muscle invasive disease.

Abstracts were independently screened for eligibility by two reviewers and disagreements resolved through discussion or third-party opinion. Agreement level was calculated using Cohen's Kappa to test the intercoder reliability of this screening

S. S. Goonewardene et al., *Management of Muscle Invasive Bladder Cancer*, Management of Urology, https://doi.org/10.1007/978-3-030-57915-9_64

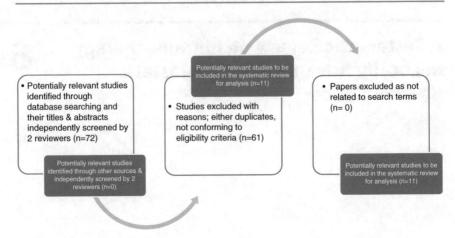

Fig. 64.1 Flow chart of studies identified through the systematic review. (Adapted from PRISMA)

process. Cohens' Kappa allows comparison of inter-rater reliability between papers using relative observed agreement. This also takes account of the comparison occurring by chance. The first reviewer agreed all 11 papers to be included, the second, agreed on 11. Cohens kappa was therefore 1.0.

Data extraction was piloted by the researcher and amended in consultation with the research team (author and two academic supervisors). Data collected included authors, year and country of publication, study aims, setting, intervention aims, number of participants, study design, intervention components and delivery methods, comparison groups and outcome measures, notes and follow-up questions for the authors. Studies were quality assessed using the PRISMA criteria for randomised controlled trials, Mays et al. [1, 2] for the action research and qualitative studies and the Critical Skills Appraisal programme for cohort studies. This was also applied to randomised controlled trials and qualitative studies.

The search identified 72 papers (Fig. 64.1). All 11 mapped to the search terms and eligibility criteria. The current systematic reviews were examined to gain further knowledge about the subject. Sixty-one papers were excluded due to not conforming to eligibility criteria or adding to the evidence. Of the 11 papers left, relevant abstracts were identified and the full papers obtained (all of which were in English), to quality assure against search criteria. There was considerable heterogeneity of design among the included studies therefore a narrative review of the evidence was undertaken. There was significant heterogeneity within studies, including clinical topic, numbers, outcomes, as a result a narrative review was thought to be best. There were 9 cohort studies, with a moderate level of evidence and two RCTs with a good level of evidence. These were from a range of countries with minimal loss to follow-up. All participants were identified appropriately.

64.1 Systematic Review Results

64.1.1 Pembrolizamab and Radiotherapy in Bladder Cancer

Tree conducted the PLUMMB trial (Pembrolizumab in Muscle-invasive/Metastatic Bladder cancer) (NCT02560636) [3]. This was a phase I study—a combination of weekly radiation therapy with pembrolizumab in metastatic or locally advanced urothelial cancer of the bladder [3]. Three patients experienced grade 3 urinary toxicities, 2 of which were attributable to therapy [3]. One patient experienced a grade 4 rectal perforation. In view of these findings, the trial has been paused and the protocol will be amended to reduce radiation therapy dose per fraction [3].

Sundahl conducted a randomized phase 1 trial combining pembrolizumab with either sequential (A) or concomitant (B) stereotactic body radiotherapy (SBRT) in metastatic urothelial carcinoma (mUC) [4]. No dose-limiting toxicity occurred. Treatment-related adverse events (trAEs; Common Terminology Criteria for Adverse Events v4.0) of grade 1–2 occurred in six of nine and all nine patients in arms A and B, respectively [4]. One grade 3 trAE occurred in arm B. No grade 4–5 trAEs occurred [4]. Overall response rates of 0% and 44.4% were noted in arms A and B [4]. The trial was not powered to compare efficacy between arms [4].

64.1.2 Atezolizumab in Locally Advanced or Metastatic Urothelial Carcinoma

Necchi reviewed the impact of atezolizumab in locally advanced or metastatic bladder cancer [5]. Compared with those who discontinued, patients continuing atezolizumab beyond progression were more likely to have had a baseline Eastern Cooperative Oncology Group performance status of 0 (43.1% versus 31.3%), less likely to have had baseline liver metastases (27.0% versus 41.0%), and more likely to have an initial response to atezolizumab (responses in 11.7% versus 1.2%) [5]. Five patients (3.6%) continuing atezolizumab after progression had subsequent responses compared with baseline measurements [5]. Atezolizumab exposure-adjusted adverse event frequencies were generally similar before and following progression [5].

64.1.3 Adjuvant Bestatin Immunotherapy and Radical Radiotherapy in Bladder Cancer

Blomgren examined adjuvant Bestatin immunotherapy after radiotherapy [6]. The results have shown that the disease-free survival of the patients taking Bestatin is significantly improved compared to the controls (p = 0.04) [6]. The beneficial effect of Bestatin seemed to be more marked among men than women [6]. Patients with less advanced disease (T1 and T2) benefitted more from Bestatin treatment than those with more advanced tumours (T3 and T4) [6]. The results of this ongoing trial thus show that patients with bladder cancer benefit from adjuvant Bestatin treatment in terms of disease-free survival [6].

64.1.4 Predictors of Response to Immunotherapy

Raja explored the use of ctDNA to predict survival on durvalumab, an anti-PD-L1 therapy [7]. This was done in 29 patients with urothelial bladder cancer, respectively, to correlate ctDNA changes with clinical outcomes [7]. Somatic variants were detected in 96% of patients [7]. Changes in VAF preceded radiographic responses, and patients with reduction in VAF at 6 weeks had significantly greater reduction in tumor volume, with longer progression-free and overall survival [7]. Early on-treatment reduction in ctDNA VAF may be a useful predictor of long-term benefit from immunotherapy [7].

64.1.5 Markers of Response to Immunotherapy

Tretiakova et al. [8] assessed PD-L1 in relation to primary and metastatic bladder cancer [8]. The antibody panel included three FDA-approved clones (22C3 for pembrolizumab, 28.8 for nivolumab, SP142 for atezolizumab), and a commonly used clone E1L3N [8]. Expression of PD-L1 in tumour cells by ≥ 1 marker was detected in 41/142 (28.9%) primary tumours, 13/77 (16.9%) lymph nodes, and 2/16 (12.5%) distant metastases [8]. In positive cases, high PD-L1 expression (>50% cells) was detected in 34.1% primary and 46.7% metastases [8]. Concordant PD-L1 expression status was present in 71/79 (89.9%) cases of matched primary and metastatic urothelial carcinomas [8].

64.1.6 A Normogram Predicting Survival from Immunotherapy in Locally Advanced and Metastatic Bladder Cancer

Sonpavde developed a nomogram using data from phase 2 trials of historical agents to estimate the 12-month overall survival (OS) for patients to which observed survival of nonrandomized data sets receiving immunotherapies could be compared [9]. Data were available from 340 patients receiving sunitinib, everolimus, docetaxel + vandetanib, docetaxel + placebo, pazopanib, paclitaxel, or docetaxel [9]. Calibration and prognostic ability were acceptable (c index = 0.634; 95% confidence interval [CI], 0.596–0.652) [9]. Observed 12-month survival for patients receiving pemetrexed (n = 127, 23.5%; 95% CI, 16.2–31.7) was similar to nomogram-predicted survival (19%; 95% CI, 16.5–21.5; p > 0.05), while observed results with atezolizumab (n = 403, 39.0%; 95% CI, 34.1–43.9) exceeded predicted results (24.6%; 95% CI, 23.4–25.8; p < 0.001) [9].

64.1.7 Infusion of Autologous T Helper Cells in Metastatic Bladder Cancer

Sherif determined if metinel node detection and subsequent expansion of autologous T-helper cells with subsequent reinfusion was feasible and safe to perform in patients with metastatic UBC [10]. In six patients, it was feasible to administer the treatment [10]. Reinfusion of these T cells was performed without any major adverse effects. In six other patients, technical failures were encountered [10].

64.1.8 Consensus Guidelines on Immunotherapy in Locally Advanced and Metastatic Bladder Cancer

Several immune checkpoint inhibitors have recently been approved for treatment of metastatic disease [11]. The approval of immune checkpoint blockade for patients with platinum-resistant or -ineligible metastatic bladder cancer has led to considerations of expanded use for both advanced and, potentially, localized disease [11]. These NCCN Guidelines also incorporate immunotherapy into second-line therapy for locally advanced or metastatic disease [12].

The SIU (Société Internationale d'Urologie)-ICUD (International Consultation on Urologic Diseases) working group on systemic therapy for metastatic bladder cancer has also highlighted immune checkpoint blockers [13]. This is particularly true in platinum-refractory disease, where supportive randomized data exist [13]. Five checkpoint blockers have been approved in this setting by the FDA: avelumab, atezolizumab, durvalumab, nivolumab, and pembrolizumab. Nivolumab, pembrolizumab, and atezolizumab have been approved in Europe [13].

References

1. Moher D, Liberati A, Tetzlaff J, Altman DG. "Preferred Reporting Items for Systematic Reviews and Meta-Analyses: The Prisma Statement." [In English]. BMJ (Online) 339, no. 7716 (08 Aug 2009):332–36.
2. Mays N, Pope C, Popay J. "Systematically Reviewing Qualitative and Quantitative Evidence to Inform Management and Policy-Making in the Health Field." [In English]. Journal of Health Services Research and Policy 10, no. SUPPL. 1 (July 2005):6–20.
3. Tree AC, Jones K, Hafeez S, et al. Dose-limiting urinary toxicity with pembrolizumab combined with weekly hypofractionated radiation therapy in bladder cancer. Int J Radiat Oncol Biol Phys. 2018;101(5):1168–71.
4. Sundahl N, Vandekerkhove G, Decaestecker K, et al. Randomized phase 1 trial of pembrolizumab with sequential versus concomitant stereotactic body radiotherapy in metastatic urothelial carcinoma. Eur Urol. 2019;75(5):707–11.
5. Necchi A, Joseph RW, Loriot Y, et al. Atezolizumab in platinum-treated locally advanced or metastatic urothelial carcinoma: post-progression outcomes from the phase II IMvigor210 study. Ann Oncol. 2017;28(12):3044–50.

6. Blomgren H, Näslund I, Esposti PL, Johansen L, Aaskoven O. Adjuvant bestatin immunotherapy in patients with transitional cell carcinoma of the bladder. Clinical results of a randomized trial. Cancer Immunol Immunother. 1987;25(1):41–6.

7. Raja R, Kuziora M, Brohawn PZ, et al. Early reduction in ctDNA predicts survival in patients with lung and bladder cancer treated with durvalumab. Clin Cancer Res. 2018;24(24):6212–22.

8. Tretiakova M, Fulton R, Kocherginsky M, et al. Concordance study of PD-L1 expression in primary and metastatic bladder carcinomas: comparison of four commonly used antibodies and RNA expression. Mod Pathol. 2018;31(4):623–32.

9. Sonpavde G, Pond GR, Rosenberg JE, Choueiri TK, Bellmunt J, Regazzi AM, Mullane SA, et al. Nomogram to assess the survival benefit of new salvage agents for metastatic urothelial carcinoma in the era of immunotherapy. Clin Genitourin Cancer. 2018;16(4):e961–e67. [in English].

10. Sherif A, Hasan MN, Marits P, Karlsson M, Winqvist O, Thörn M. Feasibility of T-cell-based adoptive immunotherapy in the first 12 patients with advanced urothelial urinary bladder cancer. Preliminary data on a new immunologic treatment based on the sentinel node concept. Eur Urol. 2010;58(1):105–11.

11. Kamat AM, Bellmunt J, Galsky MD, et al. Society for immunotherapy of cancer consensus statement on immunotherapy for the treatment of bladder carcinoma [published correction appears in J Immunother Cancer. 2017 Sep 28;5(1):80]. J Immunother Cancer. 2017;5(1):68.

12. Clark PE, Spiess PE, Agarwal N, et al. NCCN guidelines insights: bladder cancer, version 2.2016. J Natl Compr Cancer Netw. 2016;14(10):1213–24.

13. Merseburger AS, Apolo AB, Chowdhury S, et al. SIU-ICUD recommendations on bladder cancer: systemic therapy for metastatic bladder cancer. World J Urol. 2019;37(1):95–105.

The Role of Immune Checkpoint Inhibitors in Bladder Cancer

65

A systematic review relating to bladder cancer epidemiology, risk factors and occupational hazards was conducted. This was to identify the bladder cancer epidemiology and risk factors in muscle invasive disease. The search strategy aimed to identify all references related to bladder cancer AND screening. Search terms used were as follows: (Bladder cancer) AND (Immune checkpoint inhibitors). The following databases were screened from 1989 to June 2020:

- CINAHL
- MEDLINE (NHS Evidence)
- Cochrane
- AMed
- EMBASE
- PsychINFO
- SCOPUS
- Web of Science

In addition, searches using Medical Subject Headings (MeSH) and keywords were conducted using Cochrane databases. Two UK-based experts in bladder cancer were consulted to identify any additional studies.

Studies were eligible for inclusion if they reported primary research focusing on bladder cancer and screening. Papers were included if published after 1984 and had to be in English. Studies that did not conform to this were excluded. Only primary research was included (Fig. 65.1). The overall aim was to identify bladder cancer risk factors and epidemiology in muscle invasive disease.

Abstracts were independently screened for eligibility by two reviewers and disagreements resolved through discussion or third party opinion. Agreement level was calculated using Cohen's Kappa to test the intercoder reliability of this screening process. Cohens' Kappa allows comparison of inter-rater reliability between papers

S. S. Goonewardene et al., *Management of Muscle Invasive Bladder Cancer*, Management of Urology, https://doi.org/10.1007/978-3-030-57915-9_65

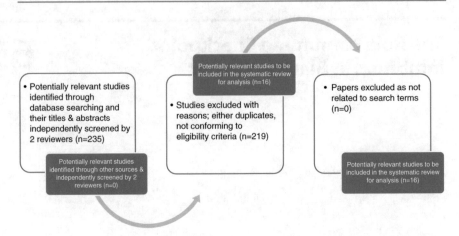

Fig. 65.1 Flow chart of studies identified through the systematic review. (Adapted from PRISMA)

using relative observed agreement. This also takes account of the comparison occurring by chance. The first reviewer agreed all 16 papers to be included, the second, agreed on 16. Cohens kappa was therefore 1.0.

Data extraction was piloted by the researcher and amended in consultation with the research team (author and two academic supervisors). Data collected included authors, year and country of publication, study aims, setting, intervention aims, number of participants, study design, intervention components and delivery methods, comparison groups and outcome measures, notes and follow-up questions for the authors. Studies were quality assessed using the PRISMA criteria for randomised controlled trials, Mays et al. [1, 2] for the action research and qualitative studies and the Critical Skills Appraisal programme for cohort studies. This was also applied to randomised controlled trials and qualitative studies.

The search identified 234 papers (Fig. 65.1). All 16 mapped to the search terms and eligibility criteria. The current systematic reviews were examined to gain further knowledge about the subject. Two hundred and thirty-five papers were excluded due to not conforming to eligibility criteria or adding to the evidence. Of the 16 papers left, relevant abstracts were identified and the full papers obtained (all of which were in English), to quality assure against search criteria. There was considerable heterogeneity of design among the included studies therefore a narrative review of the evidence was undertaken. There was significant heterogeneity within studies, including clinical topic, numbers, outcomes, as a result a narrative review was thought to be best. There were 14 cohort studies, with a moderate level of evidence and two RCTs with a good level of evidence. These were from a range of countries with minimal loss to follow-up. All participants were identified appropriately.

65.1 Systematic Review Results

65.1.1 Pd-L1 Expression in Bladder Cancer

Massard investigated the safety and efficacy of durvalumab, a human monoclonal antibody that binds programmed cell death ligand-1 (PD-L1), and the role of PD-L1 expression on clinical response in patients with advanced urothelial bladder cancer (UBC) [3]. A total of 61 patients (40 PD-L1-positive, 21 PD-L1-negative), 93.4% of whom received one or more prior therapies for advanced disease, were treated (median duration of follow-up, 4.3 months) [3]. The most common treatment-related adverse events (AEs) of any grade were fatigue (13.1%), diarrhea (9.8%), and decreased appetite (8.2%) [3]. Grade 3 treatment-related AEs occurred in three patients (4.9%); there were no treatment-related grade 4 or 5 AEs [3]. One treatment-related AE (acute kidney injury) resulted in treatment discontinuation [3]. The ORR was 31.0% (95% CI, 17.6–47.1) in 42 response-evaluable patients, 46.4% (95% CI, 27.5–66.1) in the PD-L1-positive subgroup, and 0% (95% CI, 0.0–23.2) in the PD-L1-negative subgroup [3]. Responses are ongoing in 12 of 13 responding patients, with median duration of response not yet reached (range, 4.1+ to 49.3+ weeks) [3].

Programmed death-ligand 1 (PD-L1) expression on tumour cells (TC) or tumour-infiltrating immune cells (IC) was examined by Schwamborn [4]. Sections from 30 patients (73.3% cystectomies, 26.7% transurethral resections) were stained by PD-L1 immunohistochemistry using VENTANA SP142, VENTANA SP263, DAKO 22C3, and DAKO 28-8 and scored for PD-L1 expression on IC (% per tumour area) and TC (%). Small, non-significant inter-assay differences were observed for IC [4]. For TC, SP142 showed significantly lower staining percentages [4]. Pairwise comparisons revealed −0.3% to 1.6% differences in adjusted means between assays for IC, and for TC, −10.5% to −7.8% (SP142 versus others) and −1.9% to 2.7% (other comparisons) [4]. Inter-reader and inter-assay agreement was moderate to high for both IC and TC [4]. Allocation to binary cutoffs (1%, 5%, 10%) showed substantial to high Kappa agreement scores (0.440–0.923) for IC and TC between assays for each reader [4]. This first multicenter study, with five independent readers blinded with respect to the assay used, suggests that all four currently clinically relevant assays are analytically similar for evaluation of PD-L1-stained IC and three (SP263, 22C3, and 28-8) for PD-L1-stained TC [4].

Zavalishina assessed the concordance among three validated, commercially available PD-L1 immunohistochemistry assays for patients with urothelial cancer [5]. Tumours from 100 urothelial cancer patients were stained with the antibody clones 22C3 (Agilent), SP142 (Ventana Medical Systems), and SP263 (Ventana Medical Systems), which are used in clinical trials of second-line therapy with checkpoint inhibitors [5]. The percentages of PD-L1 staining in the three assays without using any cutoff were higher in the IC than in the TC (55% versus 24% for 22C3, 45% versus 8% for SP142, and 72% versus 27% for SP263, respectively) [5].

The Pearson correlation coefficients for anti-PD-L1 staining in the IC were 0.5, 0.69, and 0.85 with 22C3/SP142, 22C3/SP263, and SP142/SP263, respectively [5]. The Pearson correlation coefficients for PD-L1 staining in the TC were 0.93, 0.99, and 0.91 for the same pairs [5]. Among the patients who were negative for PD-L1 staining by one test, 91–100% were also negative by the other tests [5]. Among the patients who were positive by one test, 43–100% were also positive by the other tests [5].

Tretiakova characterized PD-L1 expression in 235 urothelial carcinomas including 79 matched pairs of primary and metastatic cancers using a panel of four PD-L1 immunoassays in comparison with RNAscope assay using PD-L1-specific probe (CD274) [6]. The antibody panel included three FDA-approved clones (22C3 for pembrolizumab, 28.8 for nivolumab, SP142 for atezolizumab), and a commonly used clone E1L3N [6]. Expression of PD-L1 in tumour cells by ≥1 marker was detected in 41/142 (28.9%) primary tumours, 13/77 (16.9%) lymph nodes, and 2/16 (12.5%) distant metastases [6]. In positive cases, high PD-L1 expression (>50% cells) was detected in 34.1% primary and 46.7% metastases [6]. Concordant PD-L1 expression status was present in 71/79 (89.9%) cases of matched primary and metastatic urothelial carcinomas [6]. PD-L1 sensitivity ranked from highest to lowest as follows: RNAscope, clone 28.8, 22C3, E1L3N, and SP142 [6]. Despite some heterogeneity in staining, the overall results are highly concordant suggesting diagnostic equivalence of tested assays.

de Jong compared PD-L1 expression in matched transurethral resections of the bladder (TURB), cystectomy specimens and lymph node metastases of urothelial cancer [7]. de Jong performed PD-L1 (SP142) immunohistochemistry on whole tissue slides of 115 urothelial carcinoma patients who had undergone TURB, followed by radical cystectomy and/or pelvic lymph node dissection [7]. The PD-L1 assay was positive if PD-L1 expression in immune cells occupied ≥5% of the tumour area [7]. PD-L1 was positive in 15 of 97 (15.5%) TURB, 17 of 98 (17.3%) cystectomies and nine of 49 (18.4%) lymph node metastases [7]. Urothelial bladder cancer patients showed fair agreement of PD-L1 assay outcome in cystectomies and matched TURB or lymph node specimens [7]. PD-L1 expression was discordant more often after neoadjuvant therapy [7]. Therefore, immune-checkpoint inhibitor studies should take into account specimen type and neoadjuvant therapy in assessing the predictive value of PD-L1 expression [7].

Wang investigated the expression, clinical significance and association of PD-L1 with tumour-infiltrating lymphocytes (TIL) in resectable urothelial cell carcinoma of the bladder (UCB) [8]. Twenty-three percent showed PD-L1 expression in tumour cells and 55% in tumour-infiltrating immune cells. CD8+ TIL, T-bet+ TIL and PD-1+ TIL were distributed throughout the tumour tissues and were more frequently distributed in stromal regions than in intratumoral regions [8]. PD-L1+ tumour cells and PD-L1+ immune cells were positively associated with aggressive clinical features (all p < 0.05). Both PD-L1+ tumour cells and PD-L1+ immune cells were associated with poorer recurrence-free and overall survival (all p < 0.05) [8]. Multivariate analysis showed that PD-L1+ immune cells were an independent prognostic factor for overall (p = 0.001) and recurrence-free survival (p = 0.024) [8]. Notably, high stromal CD8$^+$ TIL and PD-1$^+$ TIL density were associated with poorer overall survival (p = 0.031 and p = 0.001, respectively) [8]. In the stroma, CD8$^+$ TIL density has strong positive association with PD-L1$^+$ immune cells and PD-1$^+$ TIL density (all p < 0.0001) [8].

Burgess sought to characterize PD-L1 expression in primary UC and paired metastatic lesions to gain insight into the potential discordance of tumour PD-L1 expression during the metastatic process [9]. High ($\geq$5%) PD-L1 expression in primary and metastatic biopsies, respectively, was observed in 6.0% and 7.7% of TCs and in 14.5% and 11.5% of ICs [9]. IC PD-L1 expression in primary tumours was not correlated with IC PD-L1 expression in paired metastatic lesions (ρ = 0.05, p = 0.67) and there was poor agreement in high expression rates between primary and metastatic lesions in the IC compartment (κ = 0.086) [9].

Pichler investigated whether compartmentalization of programmed cell death ligand 1 (PD-L1) expression in different locations of RC specimens influences recurrence-free survival (RFS) after RC [10]. PD-L1 ($\geq$1%) was expressed on tumour cells in 33 patients (39.8%) and immune cells in 51 patients (61.4%), respectively. PD-L1 positivity on tumour cells was not associated with RFS (p = 0.455) [10]. In contrast, PD-L1$^+$ expression on immune cells was significantly associated with shorter RFS compared with PD-L1$^-$ expression (p = 0.015) [10].

65.1.2 Anti-PD-L1 and Radiotherapy

Levy assessed preliminary safety and efficacy results of the anti-programmed cell death ligand-1 (anti-PD-L1) durvalumab in combination with radiotherapy (RT) in an expansion cohort of patients included in a phase 1/2 trial [11]. Five patients (50%) reported an irradiation-related adverse event (AE) grade (G) 1 or 2 and one patient had two G2 AEs [11]. The most frequently reported AE (3/6) was G2 mucositis[11]. There was no G3 or more RT-related AEs [11]. All AEs were transient, lasted less than 1 week, and were manageable by standard guidelines [11]. There was no unexpected AE. On 10/15 in-field (IF) evaluable lesions, the objective response (OR) rate was 60% (complete response, 2/10 and partial response, 4/10) and 4/10 stable disease (SD) [11].

65.1.3 Immune Checkpoint Inhibition in Variant Histology in Bladder Cancer

The introduction of immune checkpoint blockade (ICB) therapy has transformed the management of advanced bladder cancer (BC). Reis assessed the potential utility of ICB in patients with histological variants (UCV) [12]. Reis analyzed PD-L1 expression in UCV and compared three commonly used and commercially available PD-L1 antibodies [12]. Full sections from 84 UCV cases were stained with clones SP263, 22C3, and SP142, predictive assays to respond to anti-PD-1/PD-L1 inhibitors durvalumab, pembrolizumab, and atezolizumab, respectively [12]. PD-L1 was expressed in a significant percentage of UCV cases at different cutoff points (cutoff 1% TC: 37–54%, cutoff 5% TC: 23–37%), with the highest expression in UC with squamous differentiation [12]. This is equal to or higher than those for classic/pure UC (4–30%) [12].

Davick immunohistochemical staining of PD-L1 in bladder tumours and its relationship to tumour histologic type, grade, and overall survival has been incompletely analysed [13]. Slides from 165 cystectomy specimens were reviewed for tumour type, grade of urothelial carcinoma, pathologic stage, and overall survival [13]. Squamous cell carcinomas (SCCs) of the bladder demonstrated PD-L1 positivity more frequently than urothelial cell carcinomas (UCCs) [13]. High-grade UCCs were positive for PD-L1 on tumour cells more frequently than low-grade UCCs [13]. There was no difference in survival between PD-L1-positive and PD-L1-negative bladder cancers [13].

65.1.4 Ramucirumab and Docetaxel vs. Placebo in Bladder Cancer

Petrylak assessed the efficacy and safety of treatment with docetaxel plus either ramucirumab-a human IgG1 VEGFR-2 antagonist-or placebo in this patient population [14]. Five hundred and thirty patients were randomly allocated either ramucirumab plus docetaxel (n = 263) or placebo plus docetaxel (n = 267) [14]. Progression-free survival was prolonged significantly in patients allocated ramucirumab plus docetaxel versus placebo plus docetaxel (median 4.07 months [95% CI 2.96–4.47] vs. 2.76 months [2.60–2.96]; hazard ratio [HR] 0.757, 95% CI 0.607–0.943; p = 0.0118) [14]. A blinded independent central analysis was consistent with these results. An objective response was achieved by 53 (24.5%, 95% CI 18.8–30.3) of 216 patients allocated ramucirumab and 31 (14.0%, 9.4–18.6) of 221 assigned placebo [14]. The most frequently reported treatment-emergent adverse events, regardless of causality, in either treatment group (any grade) were fatigue, alopecia, diarrhoea, decreased appetite, and nausea [14]. These events occurred predominantly at grade 1–2 severity [14]. The frequency of grade 3 or worse adverse events was similar for patients allocated ramucirumab and placebo (156 [60%] of 258 vs. 163 [62%] of 265 had an adverse event), with no unexpected toxic effects [14]. Sixty-three (24%) of 258 patients allocated ramucirumab and 54 (20%) of 265 assigned placebo had a serious adverse event that was judged by the investigator to be related to treatment [14]. Thirty-eight (15%) of 258 patients allocated ramucirumab and 43 (16%) of 265 assigned placebo died on treatment or within 30 days of discontinuation, of which eight (3%) and five (2%) deaths were deemed related to treatment by the investigator [14]. Sepsis was the most common adverse event leading to death on treatment (four [2%] vs. none [0%]) [14]. One fatal event of neutropenic sepsis was reported in a patient allocated ramucirumab [14].

65.1.5 T-Cell Immunoglobulin Mucin-3 Expression in Bladder Cancer

Yang investigated Tim-3 expression in BUC and analyze correlations with clinico-pathologic outcomes and postoperative survival [15]. Tim-3 protein was over-expressed in bladder cancer cells, tumour infiltrating lymphocytes and endothelial cells from patients with BUC [15]. The expression levels of Tim-3 were significantly associated with advanced pathological grade and T stage [15]. Multivariate analysis showed that Tim-3 expression, as well as PD-1 expression was both independent predictors of disease-free survival and overall survival in patients with BUC [15].

65.1.6 Inhibition of G9a/DNMT and Immune-Mediated Bladder Cancer Regression

Segovia examined immune checkpoint inhibitors have shown remarkable efficacy but only in a limited fraction of bladder cancer patients [16]. Segovia demonstrated high G9a (EHMT2) expression is associated with poor clinical outcome in bladder cancer and that targeting G9a/DNMT methyltransferase activity with a novel inhibitor (CM-272) induces apoptosis and immunogenic cell death [16]. Segovia demonstrate that CM-272 + cisplatin treatment results in statistically significant regression of established tumours and metastases [16]. The antitumor effect is significantly improved when CM-272 is combined with anti-programmed cell death ligand 1, even in the absence of cisplatin [16]. Increased G9a expression was associated with resistance to programmed cell death protein 1 inhibition in a cohort of patients with bladder cancer [16].

65.1.7 Inhibition of PI3K Pathway Increases Immune Infiltrate in Muscle-Invasive Bladder Cancer

Borcoman found that urothelial bladder cancer from human samples bearing *PIK3CA* gene mutations was significantly associated with lower expression of a defined immune gene signature, compared to unmutated ones [17]. Borcoman identified a reduced 10-gene immune gene signature that discriminates muscle-invasive bladder cancer (MIBC) samples according to immune infiltration and *PIK3CA* mutation [17]. Borcoman observed that BKM120, a pan-PI3K inhibitor, significantly inhibited the growth of a human bladder cancer cell line bearing a *PIK3CA* mutation, associated to increased immune cell infiltration (hCD45+) [17]. This provides a relevant rationale for combination strategies of PI3K inhibitors with immune checkpoint inhibitors to overcome resistance to immune checkpoint inhibitors [17].

65.1.8 Neoantigen-Reactive Tumour-Infiltrating Lymphocytes in Bladder Cancer

Leko examined immune checkpoint inhibitors induce tumour regressions by reactivating a population of endogenous tumour-infiltrating lymphocytes (TILs) that recognize cancer neoantigens [18]. Leko found that CD4$^+$ TILs from one patient recognized mutated C-terminal binding protein 1 in an MHC class II-restricted manner [18]. This finding suggests that neoantigen-reactive TILs reside in bladder cancer, which may help explain the effectiveness of immune checkpoint blockade in this disease and also provides a rationale for the future use of adoptive T cell therapy targeting neoantigens in bladder cancer [18].

65.1.9 Response Rate to Chemotherapy after Immune Checkpoint Inhibition in Metastatic Urothelial Cancer

Immune checkpoint inhibitors (ICIs) are active in metastatic urothelial carcinoma (MUC) [19]. Szabados investigated the activity of chemotherapy (CT) after progression on ICIs. Two cohorts of sequential patients with MUC were described (n = 28) [19]. Cohort A received first-line ICIs followed by CT after progression [19]. Cohort B received CT after failure of first-line platinum-based CT followed by ICIs. Best RR for cohort A was 64% [19]. Two patients experienced clinical progression and died before the first radiographic assessment [19]. RR for cohort B was 21%, which was significantly lower than that for cohort A [19]. Progression of disease occurred in 43% of cohort B patients by the end of CT [19]. These data suggest a lack of cross resistance between CT and ICIs in MUC [19].

References

1. Moher D, Liberati A, Tetzlaff J, Altman DG. "Preferred Reporting Items for Systematic Reviews and Meta-Analyses: The Prisma Statement." [In English]. BMJ (Online) 339, no. 7716 (08 Aug 2009):332–36.
2. Mays N, Pope C, Popay J. "Systematically Reviewing Qualitative and Quantitative Evidence to Inform Management and Policy-Making in the Health Field." [In English]. Journal of Health Services Research and Policy 10, no. SUPPL. 1 (July 2005):6–20.
3. Massard C, Gordon MS, Sharma S, et al. Safety and efficacy of durvalumab (MEDI4736), an anti-programmed cell death ligand-1 immune checkpoint inhibitor, in patients with advanced urothelial bladder Cancer. J Clin Oncol. 2016;34(26):3119–25.
4. Schwamborn K, Ammann JU, Knüchel R, et al. Multicentric analytical comparability study of programmed death-ligand 1 expression on tumor-infiltrating immune cells and tumor cells in urothelial bladder cancer using four clinically developed immunohistochemistry assays. Virchows Arch. 2019;475(5):599–608.
5. Zavalishina L, Tsimafeyeu I, Povilaitite P, et al. RUSSCO-RSP comparative study of immunohistochemistry diagnostic assays for PD-L1 expression in urothelial bladder cancer. Virchows Arch. 2018;473(6):719–24.

6. Tretiakova M, Fulton R, Kocherginsky M, et al. Concordance study of PD-L1 expression in primary and metastatic bladder carcinomas: comparison of four commonly used antibodies and RNA expression. Mod Pathol. 2018;31(4):623–32.

7. de Jong JJ, Stoop H, Nieboer D, Boormans JL, van Leenders GJLH. Concordance of PD-L1 expression in matched urothelial bladder cancer specimens. Histopathology. 2018;73(6):983–9.

8. Wang B, Pan W, Yang M, et al. Programmed death ligand-1 is associated with tumor infiltrating lymphocytes and poorer survival in urothelial cell carcinoma of the bladder. Cancer Sci. 2019;110(2):489–98.

9. Burgess EF, Livasy C, Hartman A, et al. Discordance of high PD-L1 expression in primary and metastatic urothelial carcinoma lesions. Urol Oncol. 2019;37(5):299.e19–25.

10. Pichler R, Fritz J, Lackner F, et al. Prognostic value of testing PD-L1 expression after radical cystectomy in high-risk patients. Clin Genitourin Cancer. 2018;16(5):e1015–24.

11. Levy A, Massard C, Soria JC, Deutsch E. Concurrent irradiation with the anti-programmed cell death ligand-1 immune checkpoint blocker durvalumab: single centre subset analysis from a phase 1/2 trial. Eur J Cancer. 2016;68:156–62.

12. Reis H, Serrette R, Posada J, et al. PD-L1 expression in urothelial carcinoma with predominant or pure variant histology: concordance among 3 commonly used and commercially available antibodies. Am J Surg Pathol. 2019;43(7):920–7.

13. Davick JJ, Frierson HF, Smolkin M, Gru AA. PD-L1 expression in tumor cells and the immunologic milieu of bladder carcinomas: a pathologic review of 165 cases. Hum Pathol. 2018;81:184–91.

14. Petrylak DP, de Wit R, Chi KN, et al. Ramucirumab plus docetaxel versus placebo plus docetaxel in patients with locally advanced or metastatic urothelial carcinoma after platinum-based therapy (RANGE): a randomised, double-blind, phase 3 trial. Lancet. 2017;390(10109):2266–77.

15. Yang M, Yu Q, Liu J, et al. T-cell immunoglobulin mucin-3 expression in bladder urothelial carcinoma: clinicopathologic correlations and association with survival. J Surg Oncol. 2015;112(4):430–5.

16. Segovia C, San José-Enériz E, Munera-Maravilla E, et al. Inhibition of a G9a/DNMT network triggers immune-mediated bladder cancer regression. Nat Med. 2019;25(7):1073–81.

17. Borcoman E, De La Rochere P, Richer W, et al. Inhibition of PI3K pathway increases immune infiltrate in muscle-invasive bladder cancer. Onco Targets Ther. 2019;8(5):e1581556.

18. Leko V, McDuffie LA, Zheng Z, et al. Identification of neoantigen-reactive tumor-infiltrating lymphocytes in primary bladder cancer. J Immunol. 2019;202(12):3458–67.

19. Szabados B, van Dijk N, Tang YZ, et al. Response rate to chemotherapy after immune checkpoint inhibition in metastatic Urothelial Cancer. Eur Urol. 2018;73(2):149–52.

The Role of Chemotherapy in Locally Advanced and Metastatic Bladder Cancer

66

A systematic review relating locally advanced and metastatic bladder and immunotherapy was conducted. This was to identify the bladder cancer, immunotherapy outcomes in locally advanced and metastatic disease. The search strategy aimed to identify all references related to bladder cancer, ureteric strictures AND urinary diversion. Search terms used were as follows: (Bladder cancer) AND (Chemotherapy) AND (locally advanced) OR (metastatic). The following databases were screened from 1989 to June 2020:

- CINAHL
- MEDLINE (NHS Evidence)
- Cochrane
- AMed
- EMBASE
- PsychINFO
- SCOPUS
- Web of Science

In addition, searches using Medical Subject Headings (MeSH) and keywords were conducted using Cochrane databases. Two UK-based experts in bladder cancer were consulted to identify any additional studies.

Studies were eligible for inclusion if they reported primary research focusing on bladder cancer and screening. Papers were included if published after 1984 and had to be in English. Studies that did not conform to this were excluded. Only primary research was included (Fig. 66.1). The overall aim was to identify bladder cancer risk factors and epidemiology in muscle invasive disease.

Abstracts were independently screened for eligibility by two reviewers and disagreements resolved through discussion or third party opinion. Agreement level was calculated using Cohen's Kappa to test the intercoder reliability of this screening

S. S. Goonewardene et al., *Management of Muscle Invasive Bladder Cancer*, Management of Urology, https://doi.org/10.1007/978-3-030-57915-9_66

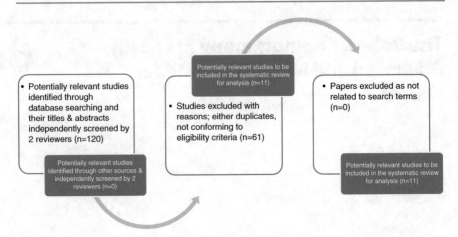

Fig. 66.1 Flow chart of studies identified through the systematic review. (Adapted from PRISMA)

process. Cohens' Kappa allows comparison of inter-rater reliability between papers using relative observed agreement. This also takes account of the comparison occurring by chance. The first reviewer agreed all 11 papers to be included, the second, agreed on 11. Cohens kappa was therefore 1.0.

Data extraction was piloted by the researcher and amended in consultation with the research team (author and two academic supervisors). Data collected included authors, year and country of publication, study aims, setting, intervention aims, number of participants, study design, intervention components and delivery methods, comparison groups and outcome measures, notes and follow-up questions for the authors. Studies were quality assessed using the PRISMA criteria for randomised controlled trials, Mays et al. [1, 2] for the action research and qualitative studies and the Critical Skills Appraisal programme for cohort studies. This was also applied to randomised controlled trials and qualitative studies.

The search identified 72 papers (Fig. 66.1). All 11 mapped to the search terms and eligibility criteria. The current systematic reviews were examined to gain further knowledge about the subject. Sixty-one papers were excluded due to not conforming to eligibility criteria or adding to the evidence. Of the 11 papers left, relevant abstracts were identified and the full papers obtained (all of which were in English), to quality assure against search criteria. There was considerable heterogeneity of design among the included studies therefore a narrative review of the evidence was undertaken. There was significant heterogeneity within studies, including clinical topic, numbers, outcomes, as a result a narrative review was thought to be best. There were 9 cohort studies, with a moderate level of evidence and two RCTs with a good level of evidence. These were from a range of countries with minimal loss to follow-up. All participants were identified appropriately.

66.1   Systematic Review Results

66.1.1 Cis-Diamminedichloroplatinum in Locally Advanced and Metastatic Bladder Cancer

Sixteen patients with locally advanced or metastatic bladder cancer were treated with cis-diamminedichloroplatinum (cis-DDP) alone or in combination with other drugs [3]. Seven patients (44%) had a partial response, 2 a minor response and 4 remained unchanged [3]. Of the 6 patients treated with arterial infusion, 3 achieved a partial response while only 2 of the 8 patients administered intravenously showed a partial response [3]. Eight patients with deeply invasive bladder cancer were treated with cis-DDP alone or in combination with other drugs following radical cystectomy [3]. Cis-DDP was administered every week for 3 courses and every month for 12 courses at a dose of 50 mg and cis-DDP, adriamycin and 5-FU (CAF) were administered at 3 weeks interval for 3 courses and every month for 12 courses [3]. One patient had a recurrence 5 months postoperatively [3].

66.1.2 Gemcitabine in Locally Advanced and Metastatic Bladder Cancer

Moore evaluated the efficacy and toxicity of gemcitabine (2′,2′-difluorodeoxycytidine) in previously untreated patients with advanced transitional cell carcinoma [4]. There were three complete responses and six partial responses seen in 37 assessable patients, for an overall response rate of nine of 37 (24.3%; 95% confidence interval, 12–41) [4]. Four patients remain in remission at 14, 23, 24, and 31 months [4]. The median survival was 8 months with 17% of patients alive at 2 years [4]. Treatment generally was well-tolerated with three patients having ≥grade 3 nonhematologic toxicity, five having grade 3 neutropenia, two having grade 3 thrombocytopenia, and two episodes of febrile neutropenia [4]. Most patients were able to receive the drug as scheduled with the primary reason for dose reduction or dose delay being neutropenia [4].

66.1.3 Gemcitabine and Cisplatin in Locally Advanced and Metastatic Bladder Cancer

De Santis performed a retrospective analysis of patients with stage IV TCC, treated with GC by a standard 4-week or by an alternative 3-week schedule [5]. A total of 212 patients received GC (3-week; n = 151, 4-week; n = 61) [5]. There was no statistical difference in overall survival between the two schedules (hazard ratio 1.15, 95% CI 0.83–1.59), p = 0.40) [5]. Five-year survival rates were 14.9% and 11.8% for the 3- and 4-week schedule, respectively (p = 0.94) [5]. Response rates were 59.7% and 55.6%, respectively (p = 0.61) [5]. Toxicity was less pronounced in the

3-week schedule with regards to neutropenia, thrombocytopenia, and transfusion rates [5]. Hematologic toxicity at day 15 in the 4-week schedule was common, leading to dose omissions in 47% of cycles [5]. Dose intensity for gemcitabine was accordingly lower in the 4 week-schedule [5]. The higher dose intensity of cisplatin in the 3-week schedule, did not lead to increased renal toxicity [5]. In 13 patients with impaired renal function, cisplatin was split into 2 days, which was feasible and efficient [5].

66.1.4 Neoadjuvant Gemcitabine and Cisplatin in Locally Advanced and Metastatic Bladder Cancer

Niedersüss-Beke reported on the efficacy and safety of neoadjuvant GC in patients with locally advanced urothelial cancer [6]. Pathologic complete response (pCR) was achieved in 22.5% and near pCR was seen in 33.7% of the patients [6]. The 1-year PFS rate was 79.5% among those patients achieving ≤pT2 versus 100% among those patients achieving pCR or near pCR (p = 0.041) [6]. Five-year OS was 61.8% (95% CI 67.6 to NA) [6]. GC was well tolerated. Grade 3/4 toxicities occurred in 38% of the patients [6]. There was no grade 3/4 renal toxicity, febrile neutropenia, or death [6].

66.1.5 Gemcitabine and Cisplatin vs. Carboplatin and Gemcitabine in Locally Advanced and Metastatic Bladder Cancer

Dogoiotti conducted a phase 2 randomized study and assessed the efficacy of gemcitabine-cisplatin (GP) and gemcitabine-carboplatin (GC) [7]. No differences between arms were noted in the overall toxicity profiles and any parameter of toxicity [7]. The most frequent grade 3–4 hematologic toxicity was neutropenia in 34.6% of patients for GP and 45.4% for GC [7]. The most frequent grade 3–4 nonhematologic toxicity was nausea and vomiting (GP: 9.1%; GC: 3.6%) [7]. Grade 1–2 nephrotoxicity occurred in 14 GP-treated patients (26.0%) and 9 GC-y patients (16.3%) [7]. Per an intent-to-treat analysis, overall response, evaluated on 80 patients, was 49.1% for GP (CR: 14.5%; PR: 34.5%) and 40.0% for GC (CR: 1.8%; PR: 38.2%) [7].

66.1.6 Paclitaxel, Cisplatin and Gemcitabine vs. Gemcitabine and Cisplatin

The combination of gemcitabine plus cisplatin (GC) is a standard regimen in patients with locally advanced or metastatic urothelial cancer [8]. A phase I/II study suggested that a three-drug regimen that included paclitaxel had greater antitumor activity and might improve survival [8]. From 2001 to 2004, 626 patients were randomly assigned; 312 patients were assigned to PCG, and 314 patients were assigned to GC [8]. OS in the subgroup of all eligible patients was significantly longer on PCG (3.2 months; HR, 0.82; p = 0.03), as was the case in patients with bladder primary tumors. PFS was not significantly longer on PCG (HR, 0.87; p = 0.11) [8]. Overall response rate was 55.5% on PCG and 43.6% on GC (p = 0.0031) [8]. Both treatments were well tolerated, with more thrombocytopenia and bleeding on GC than PCG (11.4% vs. 6.8%, respectively; p = 0.05) and more febrile neutropenia on PCG than GC (13.2% vs. 4.3%, respectively; p < 0.001) [8].

66.1.7   Gemcitabine and Irinotecan in Locally Advanced and Metastatic Bladder Cancer

Chaudhary evaluated the safety and efficacy of gemcitabine and irinotecan (Irinogem) in patients with metastatic bladder cancer [9]. Among the 13 patients evaluable for efficacy, objective radiographic response was documented in 8 patients (2 complete and 6 partial responses), 4 had stable disease, and 1 progressed on therapy [9]. Median progression-free survival was 8.78 months (95% confidence interval, 5.98–15.38) and median overall survival was 13.51 months (95% confidence interval, 8.02–21.93) [9]. Toxicity evaluated in all 16 patients was modest: 2 episodes of febrile neutropenia, grades 3–4 neutropenia in 4 patients, grades 3–4 diarrhea in 2 patients, grades 3–4 fatigue in 1 patient, grades 3–4 nausea/vomiting in 2 patients, grades 3–4 neurological toxicity in 1 patient, and no grades 3–4 thrombocytopenia [9].

66.1.8   Carboplatin Based Chemotherapy for Locally Advanced and Metastatic Bladder Cancer

Waxman examined responses among 72 urothelial cancer patients referred for treatment with MVMJ (methotrexate/vinblastine/mitoxantrone/carboplatin) chemotherapy [10]. Sixty-four evaluable patients, 37 with locally advanced and 27 with metastatic urothelial cancer, were treated [10]. Twenty-nine (45%) of the 64 patients had a complete or partial response, 15 (23%) had stable disease, and 13 (20%) had disease progression [10]. Twelve patients (32%) with locally advanced disease had a complete response to treatment; their median survival has not been reached and ranges up to 1131+ days [10]. Five patients (18%) with metastatic cancer had a complete response to treatment and their median survival was 497 days (range, 184 to 637+) [10]. There were seven deaths within the first treatment month [10].

66.1.9 Gemcitabine vs. Oxaliplatin for Locally Advanced and Metastatic Bladder Cancer

Up to 50% of patients with bladder cancer cannot be treated with cisplatin because they are considered unfit with poor renal function [11]. Gemcitabine and oxaliplatin are active, non-nephrotoxic therapies with non-overlapping toxicity profiles that provide an alternative therapy for this group of patients [11]. Forty-six patients were assessable for response and toxicity [11]. A total of 187 cycles were given with a median of 5 (range 1–6). Haematological toxicity was mild with grade 3–4 peripherical neuropathy occurring in 4% of patients [11]. Overall response rate was 48% (3 complete response, 19 partial response, 7 stable disease and 17 progressive disease). Median time to disease progression was 5 months [11].

Carles, proved the feasibility of a gemcitabine and low-dose cisplatin regimen, delivered every 2 weeks in patients with impaired renal function [11]. Mean creatinine clearance was 47.8 ml/min (range: 37–59 ml/min) [11]. Four patients had previously received chemotherapy with gemcitabine and/or platinum [11]. Median number of cycles per patient was 5 (1–13). No patient developed renal toxicity or worsening of renal function [11]. Main toxicities were (grade 3/4): Anaemia 2/1; leucopenia: 1/2; trombopenia 1/1 [11]. There was one toxic death related to metabolic acidosis, secondary to vomiting [11]. Among 16 patients evaluable for response, we observed one complete response, 7 partial responses (ORR: 53.3%; IC 95%: 28.1–78.5%), 6 stabilizations (37.5%) and 2 progressions (12.5%) [11].

66.1.10 Paclitaxel in Locally Advanced and Metastatic Bladder Cancer

Fourteen patients with previously treated, locally advanced/metastatic transitional cell carcinoma (TCC) of the bladder or ureter received paclitaxel at a dose of 200 mg/m^2 administered as a 3-h infusion every 21 days [12]. The activity of paclitaxel in this group of patients was modest [12]. The response rates were one partial response (PR) (7%) and three stable disease (SD) [12]. There were two early deaths [12].

66.1.11 Neoadjuvant Cisplatin, Methotrexate and Vinblastine in Locally Advanced and Metastatic Bladder Cancer

The International Collaboration of Trialists presents the long-term results of the international multicenter randomized trial that investigated the use of neoadjuvant cisplatin, methotrexate, and vinblastine (CMV) chemotherapy in patients with muscle-invasive urothelial cancer of the bladder treated by cystectomy and/or radiotherapy [13]. Nine hundred seventy-six patients were recruited between 1989 and 1995, and median follow-up is now 8.0 years. This was a randomized phase III trial of either no neoadjuvant chemotherapy or three cycles of CMV [13]. The previously reported possible survival advantage of CMV is now statistically significant at the 5% level [13]. Results show a statistically significant 16% reduction in the risk of death (hazard ratio, 0.84; 95% CI, 0.72–0.99; p = 0.037, corresponding to an increase in 10-year survival from 30% to 36%) after CMV [13].

66.1.12 Larotaxel and Cisplain vs. Gemcitabine and Cisplatin for Locally Advanced or Metastatic Bladder Cancer

Sternberg presents a randomized phase III trial evaluated larotaxel/cisplatin versus gemcitabine/cisplatin as first-line treatment for locally advanced (T4b) or metastatic urothelial tract or bladder cancer [14]. The trial was prematurely closed following the sponsor's decision to stop clinical development of larotaxel (n = 337 randomized) [14]. The larotaxel dose was reduced to 40 mg/m^2 and cisplatin to 60 mg/m^2 following a data monitoring committee safety review of the first 97 patients [14]. At the time of analysis, the median OS was 13.7 months [95% confidence interval (CI) 11.2–17.1] with larotaxel/cisplatin and 14.3 months (95% CI 10.5 to not reached) with gemcitabine/cisplatin [hazard ratio (HR) 1.21; 95% CI 0.83–1.76; p = 0.33] [14]. The median progression-free survival (PFS) was 5.6 months (95% CI 4.1–6.2) with larotaxel/cisplatin and 7.6 months (95% CI 6.6–9.1) with gemcitabine/cisplatin (HR 1.67; 95% CI 1.24–2.25). More myelosuppression was observed with gemcitabine/cisplatin [14].

66.1.13 Mocetinostat in Locally Advanced and Metastatic Bladder Cancer

Grivas evaluated mocetinostat (a class I/IV histone deacetylase inhibitor) in patients with urothelial carcinoma harbouring inactivating mutations or deletions in CREB binding protein [CREBBP] and/or E1A binding protein p300 [EP300] histone acetyltransferase genes in a single-arm, open-label phase 2 study [15]. Genomic testing was feasible in 155 of 175 patients (89%) [15]. Qualifying tumour mutations were CREBBP (15%), EP300 (8%), and both CREBBP and EP300 (1%) [15]. A total of 17 patients were enrolled into stage 1 (the intent-to-treat population); no patients were enrolled in subsequent stages [15]. One partial response was observed (11% [1 of 9 patients; the population that was evaluable for efficacy comprised 9 of the 15 planned patients]); activity was deemed insufficient to progress to stage 2 (null hypothesis: objective response rate of ≤15%) [15]. All patients experienced ≥1 adverse event, most commonly nausea (13 of 17 patients; 77%) and fatigue (12 of 17 patients; 71%) [15]. The median duration of treatment was 46 days; treatment interruptions (14 of 17 patients; 82%) and dose reductions (5 of 17 patients; 29%) were common [15]. Mocetinostat exposure was lower than anticipated (dose-normalized maximum serum concentration [C_{max}] after TIW dosing of 0.2 ng/ml/mg) [15].

66.1.14 Gemcitabine and Cisplatin vs. Methotrexate, Vinblastine, Doxorubicin and Cisplatin for Locally Advanced and Muscle Invasive Bladder Cancer

Gemcitabine plus cisplatin (GC) and methotrexate, vinblastine, doxorubicin, and cisplatin (MVAC) were compared in locally advanced or metastatic transitional-cell carcinoma (TCC) of the urothelium [16]. Overall survival was similar on both arms (hazards ratio [HR], 1.04; 95% confidence interval [CI], 0.82–1.32; p = 0.75), as were time to progressive disease (HR, 1.05; 95% CI, 0.85–1.30), time to treatment failure (HR, 0.89; 95% CI 0.72–1.10), and response rate (GC, 49%; MVAC, 46%) [16]. More GC patients completed six cycles of therapy, with fewer dose adjustments [16]. The toxic death rate was 1% on the GC arm and 3% on the MVAC arm [16]. More GC than MVAC patients had grade 3/4 anaemia (27% vs. 18%, respectively), and thrombocytopenia (57% vs. 21%, respectively) [16]. On both arms, the RBC transfusion rate was 13 of 100 cycles and grade 3/4 haemorrhage or haematuria was 2%; the platelet transfusion rate was four patients per 100 cycles and two patients per 100 cycles on GC and MVAC, respectively [16]. More MVAC patients, compared with GC patients, had grade 3/4 neutropenia (82% vs. 71%, respectively), neutropenic fever (14% vs. 2%, respectively), neutropenic sepsis (12% vs. 1%, respectively), and grade 3/4 mucositis (22% vs. 1%, respectively) and alopecia (55% vs. 11%, respectively) [16]. Quality of life was maintained during treatment on both arms; however, more patients on GC fared better regarding weight, performance status, and fatigue [16].

Adamo evaluated outcomes in a 21-day schedule with GMC and CDDP in patients with advanced/metastatic bladder cancer [17]. Twenty-five patients were valuable for toxic effects, length of survival and tumour response [17]. The overall remission rate (complete response + partial response) was 48% (95% CI 28.4–67.6%) [17]. The median duration of survival for all patients was 13.2 months (range 2–68+), with 1-year and 23-month survival rates of 60% and 20%, respectively [17]. There was no grade 4 toxicity or treatment-related death. Grade 3 anaemia was observed in 4 patients (16%) and grade 3 thrombocytopenia occurred in 6 patients (24%) [17]. No grade 3–4 nausea/vomiting or neutropenia was observed [17].

von der Maase compared long-term survival in patients with locally advanced or metastatic transitional cell carcinoma (TCC) of the urothelium treated with gemcitabine/cisplatin (GC) or methotrexate/vinblastine/doxorubicin/cisplatin (MVAC) [18]. Overall survival was similar in both arms (hazard ratio [HR], 1.09; 95% CI, 0.88–1.34; p = 0.66) with a median survival of 14.0 months for GC and 15.2 months for MVAC [18]. The 5-year overall survival rates were 13.0% and 15.3%, respectively (p = 0.53) [18]. The median progression-free survival was 7.7 months for GC and 8.3 months for MVAC, with an HR of 1.09 [18]. The 5-year progression-free survival rates were 9.8% and 11.3%, respectively (p = 0.63) [18]. Significant prognostic factors favoring overall survival included performance score (>70), TNM staging (M0 vs. M1), low/normal alkaline phosphatase level, number of disease sites (≤3), and the absence of visceral metastases [18]. By adjusting for these prognostic factors, the HR was 0.99 for overall survival and 1.01 for progression-free survival [18]. The 5-year overall survival rates for patients with and without visceral metastases were 6.8% and 20.9%, respectively [18].

Milowsky compare long-term survival in patients with locally advanced or metastatic transitional cell carcinoma (TCC) of the urothelium treated with gemcitabine/cisplatin (GC) or methotrexate/vinblastine/doxorubicin/cisplatin (MVAC) [19]. Overall survival was similar in both arms (hazard ratio [HR], 1.09; 95% CI, 0.88–1.34; p = 0.66) with a median survival of 14.0 months for GC and 15.2 months for MVAC [19]. The 5-year overall survival rates were 13.0% and 15.3%, respectively (p = 0.53) [19]. The median progression-free survival was 7.7 months for GC and 8.3 months for MVAC, with an HR of 1.09 [19]. The 5-year progression-free survival rates were 9.8% and 11.3%, respectively (p = 0.63) [19]. Significant prognostic factors favoring overall survival included performance score (>70), TNM staging (M0 vs. M1), low/normal alkaline phosphatase level, number of disease sites (≤3), and the absence of visceral metastases [19]. By adjusting for these prognostic factors, the HR was 0.99 for overall survival and 1.01 for progression-free survival [19]. The 5-year overall survival rates for patients with and without visceral metastases were 6.8% and 20.9%, respectively [19].

A randomised phase III trial of MVAC (methotrexate, vincristine, doxorubicin, cisplatin) vs. gemcitabine and cisplatin (GC) [20]. A total of 19 patients had glomerular filtration rate <60 ml/min and 19 patients had metastatic disease [20]. Overall response rate was 65.5% on an intention-to-treat analysis (75% [21/28] for assessable patients), with four complete responses (12.5%) and 17 partial responses (53%) [20]. After the median follow-up of 17.2 months (range 13.1–32.4 months), 12 patients remain alive [20]. The overall median survival was 16 months (range 10.1–26.6 months). G plus C every 3 weeks is active and well tolerated in an outpatient setting, even in patients receiving prior platinum-based regimens and with poor renal reserve [20].

66.1.15   Gemcitabine, Cisplatin and Sorafenib vs. Chemotherapy Alone in Locally Advanced and Metastatic Bladder Cancer

Krege evaluate the efficacy and safety of gemcitabine and cisplatin in combination with sorafenib, a tyrosine-kinase inhibitor, compared with chemotherapy alone as first-line treatment in advanced urothelial cancer [21]. The final analysis included 40 patients in the sorafenib and 49 patients in the placebo arm [21]. There were no significant differences between the two arms concerning ORR (sorafenib: complete response [CR] 12.5%, partial response [PR] 40%; placebo: CR 12%, PR 35%), median PFS (sorafenib: 6.3 months, placebo: 6.1 months) or OS (sorafenib: 11.3 months, placebo: 10.6 months) [21]. Toxicity was moderately higher in the sorafenib arm. Diarrrhoea occurred significantly more often in the sorafenib arm and hand-foot syndrome occurred only in the sorafenib arm [21]. The study was closed prematurely because of slow recruitment [21].

66.1.16 Adjuvant Gemcitabine and Cisplatin in Locally Advanced Bladder Cancer

Despite gemcitabine/cisplatin being widely used in metastatic bladder cancer, its role and tolerability in the adjuvant setting, in which renal insufficiency is common, is unclear [22]. Thirty-five patients (90%) completed 4 cycles of chemotherapy [22]. Eleven patients (28%) experienced grade 4 hematologic toxicity, and 14 patients (36%) experienced grade 3 nonhematologic toxicity. The median increase in creatinine was 0.3 mg/dl [22]. Thirteen patients (33%) had recurrent disease, 1 patient at 6 years after completion of therapy [22]. Twelve patients (31%) died, including 11 (28%) with recurrent disease [22].

66.1.17 Gemcitabine and Cisplatin in Renal Dysfunction for Locally Advanced and Metastatic Bladder Cancer

Morales-Barrera et al. [23] evaluated the safety and efficacy of gemcitabine and a split dose administration of cisplatin in renal dysfunction [23]. Thirty-eight patients were treated. Median creatinine clearance was 49 ml/min [23]. There were 15 partial responses (39%) and 12 patients had stable disease (31%) [23]. Grade 3–4 haematological toxicities were: neutropenia 9%, anaemia 6% and thrombocytopenia 16% [23]. No patient developed renal toxicity [23].

66.1.18 Paclitaxel and Gemcitabine in Locally Advanced and Metastatic Bladder Cancer

Fechner evaluated of gemcitabine (Gem) and paclitaxel in transitional cell carcinoma (TCC) [24]. The overall objective response (OR) was 44% (12 of 27) with eight complete remissions (CRs) and four partial remissions [24]. WHO grade III toxicities were seen in schedule A/B as follows: anaemia 3 (23%)/2 (16%) patients, leucopenia 5 (38%)/2 (16%), thrombocytopenia 0/2 (16%) and alopecia 10 (76%)/4 (32%) [24]. The combination of Gem and Pac is an effective second-line regimen in patients with mainly poor prognosis due to PD after cisplatin-based chemotherapy [24]. Except for three SAEs (uncertainly therapy related), both regimens were tolerated well [24].

66.1.19 Paclitaxel, Gemcitabine and Cisplatin in Locally Advanced and Metastatic Bladder Cancer

Ecke evaluated the efficacy of combination chemotherapy with gemcitabine, paclitaxel, and cisplatin in patients with advanced urothelial carcinoma [25]. Forty-eight patients (81%) achieved objective responses to treatment (56% complete responses) [25]. The median survival was 22 months, and the 1-year and 2-year survival rates were 68% and 39%, respectively. After a median follow-up of 17.5 months, 29 patients remained alive and 25 were free of disease progression [25]. The median progression-free survival for the entire group was 10 months [25]. The median survival time for patients with an Eastern Cooperative Oncology Group (ECOG) status of 0, 1, and 2 was 37.5, 17, and 12 months, respectively [25]. Grade 3–4 neutropenia occurred in 39% of the patients [25]. The combination of gemcitabine, paclitaxel, and cisplatin is a highly effective and tolerable regimen for patients with advanced urothelial carcinoma [25].

Sternberg assessed gemcitabine and paclitaxel was adapted for patients with advanced transitional cell carcinoma (TCC) who had received prior cisplatin-based chemotherapy [26]. Response was observed in 24 patients (60%; 95% confidence interval [CI], 45–75%) [26]. Eleven (28%) achieved complete response, and 13 (33%) obtained partial response [26]. Twenty of 25 patients (80%; 95% CI, 64–96%) who had been previously treated in the neoadjuvant or adjuvant setting responded versus 4 of 15 (27%; 95% CI, 5–49%) in patients who received prior methotrexate, vinblastine, doxorubicin, cisplatin (M-VAC) for metastatic disease [26]. The median duration of survival for patients given gemcitabine and paclitaxel after failing neoadjuvant or adjuvant M-VAC was 12 months (range, 2–43+), as compared with only 8 months (range, 2–28) for patients who had been treated after failure of prior therapy for metastatic disease [26]. Thirteen patients (32%) developed World Health Organization Grade 3–4 neutropenia, with febrile neutropenia in 3 (7%) patients [26]. Granulocyte colony-stimulating factor was given to 10 (24%) patients [26]. There was no Grade 3–4 anemia or thrombocytopenia [26].

66.1.20 Paclitaxel, Gemcitabine and Carboplatin in Locally Advanced and Metastatic Bladder Cancer

Hainsworth evaluated the efficacy and toxicity of combination chemotherapy with paclitaxel, carboplatin, and gemcitabine in patients with advanced urothelial carcinoma [27]. Twenty-six patients (43%) had achieved objective responses to treatment (12% complete responses) [27]. The median actuarial survival was 11 months, and the actuarial 1-year and 2-year survival rates were 46% and 27%, respectively [27]. Myelosuppression was the most frequent toxicity, and Grade 3–4 neutropenia (using the National Cancer Institute Common Toxicity Criteria [version 2.0]) occurred in 72% of patients (46% of courses) [27]. Ten patients were hospitalized for the treatment of neutropenia and fever, and 1 patient died of treatment-related causes. Nonhematologic toxicities were relatively uncommon [27].

66.1.21 Paclitaxel in Platin Refractory Locally Advanced and Metastatic Bladder Cancer

Ko assessed efficacy and tolerability of nanoparticle albumin-bound (nab) paclitaxel in platinum-refractory urothelial cancer [28]. Patients received a median of six cycles (range 1–15) [28]. Forty-seven patients were evaluable; one (2.1%) had a CR and 12 (25.5%) had PRs, resulting in an overall response of 27.7% (95% CI 17.3–44.4) [28]. The most frequently recorded adverse events of any grade were fatigue (38 of 48; 79%), pain (37 of 48; 77%), alopecia (34 of 48; 71%), and neuropathy (30 of 48; 77%) [28]. The most frequently recorded adverse events of grade 3 or higher were pain (11 of 48; 23%), fatigue (5 of 48; 23%), hypertension (3 of 48; 6%), neuropathy (3 of 48, 6%), and joint stiffness or pain (2 of 48; 4%) [28].

66.1.22 Docetaxel in Locally Advanced and Metastatic Bladder Cancer

Two patients who achieved CR status remain free of disease at 4 and 3 years respectively [29]. Grade 3–4 granulocytopenia occurred in 27 patients, resulting in five episodes of febrile neutropenia [29]. There was one toxic death in a patient with grade 4 granulocytopenia who developed acute abdomen [29]. Grade 3–4 thrombocytopenia was rare (one patient) [29]. Other grade 3–4 toxicities observed were anaemia (three patients), vomiting (five patients), diarrhoea (four patients), peripheral neuropathy (two patients) and non-neutropenic infections (seven patients) [29].

66.1.23 Docetaxel and Gemcitabine in Locally Advanced and Metastatic Bladder Cancer

Ardavanis investigate the toxicity and efficacy of the combination of gemcitabine and docetaxel in untreated advanced urothelial carcinoma [30]. Toxicity was primarily haematologic, and the most frequent grade 3–4 toxicities were anaemia 11 (6.7%), thrombocytopenia 8 (4.9%), and neutropenia 45 (27.6%), with 10 (6.1%) episodes of febrile neutropenia [30]. No toxic deaths occurred. A number of patients had some cardiovascular morbidity (38.7%) [30]. Non-haematological toxicities except alopecia (29 patients) were mild [30]. Overall response rate was 51.6%, including four complete responses (12.9%) and 12 partial responses (38.7%), while a further five patients had disease stabilisation (s.d. 16.1%) [30]. The median time to progression was 8 months (95% CI 5.1–9.2 months) and the median overall survival was 15 months (95% CI 11.2–18.5 months), with 1-year survival rate of 60% [30].

Gitlitz evaluate the safety and efficacy of gemcitabine plus docetaxel in patients with unresectable (Stage T4 or $\geq$N1) metastatic or locally advanced transitional cell carcinoma (TCC) of the urothelial tract [31]. Neutropenia was the most common adverse event that occurred in patients at the Grade 3 level (in 10 of 27 patients; 37.0%) and the Grade 4 level (in 6 of 27 patients; 22.2%) [31]. There were no other adverse events at the Grade 4 toxicity level [31]. Twenty-five of 27 patients (92.6%) completed more than 1 cycle of combination therapy and were evaluated for antitumor responses [31]. The frequency of objective clinical responses was 33.3% (9 of 27 patients) [31]. Complete responses to therapy were observed in 2 of 27 patients (7.4%), and partial responses were observed in 7 of 27 patients (25.9%) [31]. The median duration of response was 20 weeks (range, 12+ to 152 weeks) [31]. The median survival duration was 52 weeks (range, 12 to 160+ weeks) [31]. Four of 27 patients (14.8%) remained alive at the time of the current data analysis [31].

66.1.24 Cabizataxel vs. Vinflunine in Locally Advanced and Metastatic Bladder Cancer

Bellmunt, using a randomized study compared its efficacy versus vinflunine [32]. Three patients (13%) obtained a partial response on cabazitaxel (95% CI 2.7–32.4) and six patients (30%) in the vinflunine arm (95% CI 11.9–54.3) [32]. Median progression-free survival for cabazitaxel was 1.9 versus 2.9 months for vinflunine (p = 0.039) [32]. The study did not proceed to phase III since the futility analysis showed a lack of efficacy of cabazitaxel [32]. A trend for overall survival benefit was found favouring vinflunine (median 7.6 versus 5.5 months) [32]. Grade 3- to 4-related adverse events were seen in 41% patients with no difference between the two arms [32].

66.1.25 Cisplatin, Epirubicin, Methotrexate in Locally Advanced and Metastatic Bladder Cancer

Forty patients with advanced transitional cell cancer (TCC) of the bladder were treated with cisplatin, epirubicin, methotrexate (PEM, every 3–4 weeks) [33]. The overall response rate was 19/40 (47.5%), 11/23 (48%) for FD and 8/17 (47%) for RD (p = 1.000) (Lelli 1992). 17/40 patients (42.5%) had no-change and 4/40 (10%) had disease progression (Lelli 1992). The median duration of CR and PR was 32 weeks, range 4–82 (22 weeks, range 12–52 for FD; 32 weeks, range 4–82 for RD, cisplatin p = 0.7362) (Lelli 1992). The main side effect was vomiting (35/40 patients, 87.5%, 20/23 = 87% for FD, 15/17 = 90% for RD, p = 1.000) (Lelli 1992). Leukopenia was observed in 12 patients (30%, nadir 3240 range 900–3800, 6/23 = 26% for FD, 6/17 = 35% for RD, p = 0.7285), alopecia in 18 patients (45%, 15/23 = 65% for FD, 3/17 = 18% for RD, p = 0.004). The results of this study show that a dose escalation to 50 mg/m^2 for cisplatin, epirubicin and methotrexate in the PEM regimen results in an increase in overall response (OR) (19/40 = 47.5%) with respect to a historical control using the same drugs at doses of 40 mg/m^2 (12/35 = 34%) (Lelli 1992). In patients with normal renal function the escalated dose was tolerated without a corresponding increase in toxicity (Lelli 1992).

66.1.26 Methotrexate, Carboplatin, Mitoxantrone and Vincristine in Locally Advanced and Metastatic Bladder Cancer

Pectasides examined Chemotherapy with methotrexate, carboplatin, mitoxantrone (Novantrone) and vincristine in locally advanced or metastatic bladder cancer [34]. The overall response rate was 40%, with 15% complete response (CR) [34]. The responses were better for patients with locally advanced disease (CR 25%, partial response, PR, 31.25%, response rate, RR, 56.25%) than for those with metastatic disease (CR 8.3%, PR 20.83%, RR 29.1%) [34]. The differences in these results were probably due to the bad performance status and the presence of visceral metastases in patients with generalized disease [34]. The overall median survival was 14 months, with responders living longer (median survival 28.8 months in patients with locally advanced disease and 22.9 months in patients with metastatic disease) than non-responders (median survival 16 months in patients with locally advanced disease and 8.9 months in patients with metastatic disease) [34]. The difference in survival between responders and non-responders was statistically significant in both groups of patients [34]. Toxicity was moderate, but manageable [34]. The MCNO regimen appears to have a lower efficacy than that obtained with cisplatin-based regimens for the treatment of metastatic disease and rather similar efficacy for the treatment of locally advanced urothelial-cell cancer [34]. Therapy with this regimen, though less toxic, may not be a reliable alternative in elderly patients with visceral metastases and a performance status of ≥ 2 [34].

66.1.27 Methotrexate, Paclitaxel, Epirubicin and Carboplatin in Advanced Bladder Cancer

Tsavaris used a phase II study aimed to define methotrexate, paclitaxel, epirubicin, and carboplatin (M-TEC) in advanced bladder cancer, by substitution of cisplatin by carboplatin, doxorubicin by epirubicin and vinblastine by paclitaxel [35]. Symptomatic improvement was observed in 50% of patients [35]. The median duration of response was 22 (14–32) weeks, median time-to-progression (TTP) 33 (12–44) weeks, and median survival was 56 (20–84) weeks [35]. Toxicity was well accepted and was mainly neutropenia > grade 3: 17%, anemia > grade 3: 16%, thrombocytopenia > grade 2: 6%, nausea and vomiting mainly > grade 2: 31%, according to the administered chemotherapy cycles, whereas fatigue grade 2–3: 19%, neurotoxicity grade 1–2 13% of patients, and alopecia grade 2 [35].

66.1.28 Methotrexate, Carboplatin and Vinblastine in Locally Advanced and Metastatic Bladder Cancer

Bellmunt reviewed a Phase II trial with a new regimen of methotrexate, carboplatin, and vinblastine (M-CAVI) [36]. Among 23 patients assessable for clinical response, the response rate was 48% [36]. The median duration of response for metastatic disease was 7 months [36]. Among nine patients assessable for pathologic response, there were two complete responses and three partial responses. The toxic effects have been moderate [36].

Pronzato assessed 20 outpatients with locally advanced (inoperable) or metastatic transitional cell carcinoma treated with carboplatin, methotrexate, +vinblastine [37]. One patient died of disease progression before completing at least 2 cycles of chemotherapy [37]. Seven patients (35%) obtained a partial response; 8 had disease stabilization (40%) and 4 progressed (20%). Median duration of response was 3 months (range: 3–9), and median overall survival was 12+ months (range: 1–18+) [37]. None of the patients suffered grade IV toxicities, and no nephro-, neuro-, or ototoxicity was observed [37].

66.1.29 Methotrexate, Carboplatin, Vinblastine and Epirubicin in Locally Advanced and Metastatic Bladder Cancer

Skarlos conducted a phase II study in order to assess the efficacy and toxicity of Carbo-MVE (carboplatin, methotrexate, vinblastine, epirubicin) [38]. Toxicity was generally mild and treatment well tolerated [38]. The overall response rate was 54.4%, with 26% complete and 28.3% partial response rates [38]. The median survival was 17.5 months with the complete responders to live significantly longer (64.82 months) than those who had a partial response (20.5 months), stable disease (15 months) or progressive disease (8.5 months) [38]. Survival was also significantly longer in patients with good performance status as well as in patients with locally advanced or locoregional disease [38]. Finally, patients who had cystectomy as definitive treatment survived significantly longer (32 months) than those who had been irradiated (16 months) [38].

66.1.30 Gemcitabine, Cisplatin and Docetxel in Locally Advanced and Metastatic Bladder Cancer

Boukovinas assessed gemcitabine, cisplatin, and docetaxel (GCD) regimen in patients with locally advanced or metastatic urothelial cancer [39]. Sixty patients with an ECOG PS of 0–2 were enrolled. Most (71.7%) patients had stage IV disease [39]. A median number of 4 chemotherapy cycles per patient (range, 1–9) was administered [39]. Eight (13.3%) patients achieved a CR and 16 (26.7%) a partial response (PR) (intention-to-treat: ORR 40%; 95% CI 27.6–52.4%) [39]. Thirteen (21.7%) and 23 (38.3%) patients experienced stable and progressive disease, respectively [39]. Grade 3 and 4 neutropenia occurred in 27 (45%) patients and grade 3 and 4 thrombocytopenia in five (8.3%) [39]. Three (5%) patients developed febrile neutropenia. There were no treatment-related deaths. Severe non-haematological toxicity was infrequent [39].

66.1.31 Everolimus in Locally Advanced and Metastatic Bladder Cancer

Seront, as a phase II study assessed the safety and efficacy of everolimus, an oral mammalian target of rapamycin inhibitor in advanced transitional carcinoma cell (TCC) after failure of platinum-based therapy [40]. Two confirmed PR and eight SD were observed, resulting in a DCR of 27% at 8 weeks [40]. Everolimus was well tolerated [40]. The profile of the plasma angiogenesis-related proteins suggested a role of the everolimus antiangiogenic properties in disease control [40].

66.1.32 Doxorubicin and Gemcitabine Followed by Isofosfamide, Paclitaxel, and Cisplatin in Locally Advanced and Metastatic Bladder Cancer

Milowsky assessed sequential chemotherapy with doxorubicin and gemcitabine (AG) followed by ifosfamide, paclitaxel, and cisplatin (ITP) was previously demonstrated to be well tolerated in patients with advanced transitional cell carcinoma (TCC) [19]. Myelosuppression was seen with 68% of patients who experienced grades 3–4 neutropenia and with 25% who experienced febrile neutropenia [19]. Grade 3 or greater nonhematologic toxicities were infrequent [19]. Forty (73%) of 55 evaluable patients (95% CI, 59–84%) demonstrated a major response (complete, n = 19; partial, n = 21) and had a median response duration of 11.3 months (range, 1.7 to ≥105.6 months) [19]. Twenty-seven (79%) of 34 patients with locally advanced disease (i.e., T4, N0, M0) or with regional lymph node involvement (i.e., T3–4, N1, M0) and 10 (56%) of 18 patients with distant metastases achieved a major response [19].

Dreicer assessed the efficacy and toxicity of vinblastine, ifosfamide, and gallium nitrate (VIG) as first-line chemotherapy in patients with locally advanced or metastatic carcinoma of the urothelium [41]. Twenty of 45 patients (44%; 95% confidence interval, 30–60%) demonstrated an objective response, with 6 patients (13%) achieving a complete clinical response [41]. The median duration of response was 47 weeks and the median survival duration for all patients was 10 months [41]. Hematologic toxicity was significant, with 28 patients and 31 patients experiencing Grade 3 or 4 leukopenia and anemia, respectively [41].

66.1.33 Pemetrexed and Gemcitabine in Locally Advanced and Metastatic Bladder Cancer

von der Maase assessed pemetrexed and gemcitabine have single-agent activity in combination [42]. ORR among 47 patients evaluable for response was 28% (95% CI 16–43%) and ORR for the intention-to-treat population was 20% (95% CI

11–32%) with 3 CR and 10 PR [42]. Median response duration was 11.2 months and median overall survival 10.3 months (95% CI 8.1–14.6 months) [42]. CTC grade 3/4 hematologic toxicities included anemia (19%), thrombocytopenia (9%), neutropenia (38%), febrile neutropenia (17%) and neutropenic sepsis (3%) [42]. Grade 3/4 non-hematologic toxicities included elevated transaminases (12%), dyspnoea (8%), fatigue (8%) and stomatitis (5%). There was one toxic death due to neutropenic sepsis [42].

66.1.34 Paclitaxel and Gemcitabine in Locally Advanced and Metastatic Bladder Cancer

Kaufman evaluated combination gemcitabine and paclitaxel [43]. Of 55 eligible patients, 17 had a partial and 5 had a complete response rate for an overall response rate of 40% (27–54%) [43]. One complete response and one partial response were observed in the 6 previously treated patients [43]. Overall median survival was 11.8 months (11.9 months in the chemonaive cohort) [43]. Grade 3 or 4 myelosuppression occurred in 56%, but only 4 serious infections were observed [43].

66.1.35 Cisplatin, Epirubicin and Docetaxel in Locally Advanced and Metastatic Bladder Cancer

Pectasides evaluated cisplatin (CDDP), epirubicin (EPI) and docetaxel have single agent activity against urothelial transitional cell carcinoma (TCC) [44]. There were 9 (30.0%) complete responses (2, 28.6% in locally advanced and 7, 30.4% in metastatic disease) and 11 (36.7%) partial responses (3, 42.9% in locally advanced and 8, 34.8% in metastatic disease) with an overall response rate (RR) of 66.7% (71.5% in locally advanced, 65.2% in metastatic disease) [44]. Overall median survival was 14.5 months (15 months for locally advanced, 12.5 months for metastatic disease) [44]. The median duration of response in patients with metastatic disease was 8.5 months [44]. 16 (53.3%) patients required one dose reduction and 5 (16.7%) patients required two dose reductions for a nadir AGC $\leq$500/mm^3. Four episodes of febrile neutropenia and sepsis occurred [44]. No patient had a dose reduction or treatment delay for any other grade 3/4 toxicity [44]. There were no treatment delays due to myelotoxicity [44]. Alopecia was universal [44]. Non-haematological toxicity including mucositis, fluid retention, allergy, cutaneous toxicity, diarrhoea and neurotoxicity were mild and infrequent [44]. The combination of EPI, docetaxel and CDDP is an active regimen for urothelial TCC [44]. The response rate and toxicity were comparable with the M-VAC (methotrexate, vinblastine, doxorubicin, cisplastin) regimen [44]. Phase III trials comparing this regimen with M-VAC are warranted [44].

66.1.36 Vinflunine in Locally Advanced and Metastatic Bladder Cancer

Vaughn, evaluated vinflunine in locally advanced or metastatic urothelial carcinoma (UC) [45]. Per the IRRC, 22 patients achieved a partial response, with a response rate of 15% (95% confidence interval, 9–21%) with a median duration of response of 6.0 months [45]. Sixty-four (42%) patients had stable disease [45]. The median progression-free survival was 2.8 months, and the median overall survival was 8.2 months [45]. Myelosuppression was the most frequent adverse event, with grade 3 of 4 (adverse events were evaluated according to the National Cancer Institute Common Toxicity Criteria [version 2.0] guidelines) neutropenia reported in 58% of the patients. Grade 3 of 4 febrile neutropenia occurred in 10 (7%) patients [45]. Nonhematologic treatment-related events (grade 3 of 4) were generally manageable and included constipation (17%), asthenia/fatigue (13%), ileus (5%), and abdominal pain (5%). No cumulative toxicity was observed [45].

66.1.37 Doxorubicin in Locally Advanced and Metastatic Bladder Cancer

Winquist evaluated 34 patients with advanced unresectable or metastatic urothelial carcinoma with doxorubicin as part of a Phase trial [46]. Six of 30 evaluable patients had a partial response to treatment (20%; 95% Confidence Interval (CI), 8–39%) and seven patients had stable disease [46]. Toxicities were primarily non-haematological, but severe palmar-plantar erythrodysesthesia (PPE), lethargy and anorexia were infrequent. Despite a high proportion of patients with poor prognostic features, PLD had clinically significant activity in urothelial cancer in this study [46]. The activity and unique toxicity profile of this drug make it of interest for further study in advanced urothelial cancers in combination with other active agents [46].

Mahjoubi reviewed Doxorubicin in advanced urothelial tumors [47]. Pirarubicin, a new anthracycline, turned out to be equally active and less toxic than its parent compound in preclinical studies [47]. Twenty patients were evaluable for response; there were 2 partial response, 8 stable disease and 10 progressive disease [47]. Hematological toxicity was moderate, however there was one toxic death with grade 4 neutropenia which occurred in a heavily pretreated patient receiving a dose of 25 mg/m^2/day for 3 days [47]. There was no clinical cardiac toxicity [47].

References

1. Moher D, Liberati A, Tetzlaff J, Altman DG. "Preferred Reporting Items for Systematic Reviews and Meta-Analyses: The Prisma Statement." [In English]. BMJ (Online) 339, no. 7716 (08 Aug 2009):332–36.
2. Mays N, Pope C, Popay J. "Systematically Reviewing Qualitative and Quantitative Evidence to Inform Management and Policy-Making in the Health Field." [In English]. Journal of Health Services Research and Policy 10, no. SUPPL. 1 (July 2005):6–20.

3. Uekado Y, Ogawa T, Yoshida T, et al. Hinyokika Kiyo. 1985;31(8):1365–70.
4. Moore MJ, Winquist EW, Murray N, et al. Gemcitabine plus cisplatin, an active regimen in advanced urothelial cancer: a phase II trial of the National Cancer Institute of Canada Clinical Trials Group. J Clin Oncol. 1999;17(9):2876–81.
5. De Santis M, Bachner M, Cerveny M, et al. Combined chemoradiotherapy with gemcitabine in patients with locally advanced inoperable transitional cell carcinoma of the urinary bladder and/or in patients ineligible for surgery: a phase I trial. Ann Oncol. 2014;25(9):1789–94.
6. Niedersüss-Beke D, Puntus T, Kunit T, et al. Neoadjuvant chemotherapy with gemcitabine plus cisplatin in patients with locally advanced bladder cancer. Oncology. 2017;93(1):36–42.
7. Dogliotti L, Carteni G, Siena S, et al. Gemcitabine plus cisplatin versus gemcitabine plus carboplatin as first-line chemotherapy in advanced transitional cell carcinoma of the urothelium: results of a randomized phase 2 trial. Eur Urol. 2007;52(1):134–41.
8. Bellmunt J, von der Maase H, Mead GM, et al. Randomized phase III study comparing paclitaxel/cisplatin/gemcitabine and gemcitabine/cisplatin in patients with locally advanced or metastatic urothelial cancer without prior systemic therapy: EORTC Intergroup Study 30987. J Clin Oncol. 2012;30(10):1107–13.
9. Chaudhary UB, Verma N, Keane T, Gudena V. A phase II study of gemcitabine and irinotecan in patients with locally advanced or metastatic bladder cancer. Am J Clin Oncol. 2014;37(2):188–93.
10. Waxman J, Barton C. Carboplatin-based chemotherapy for bladder cancer. Cancer Treat Rev. 1993;19(Suppl C):21–5.
11. Carles J, Esteban E, Climent M, et al. Gemcitabine and oxaliplatin combination: a multicenter phase II trial in unfit patients with locally advanced or metastatic urothelial cancer. Ann Oncol. 2007;18(8):1359–62.
12. Papamichael D, Gallagher CJ, Oliver RT, Johnson PW, Waxman J. Phase II study of paclitaxel in pretreated patients with locally advanced/metastatic cancer of the bladder and ureter. Br J Cancer. 1997;75(4):606–7.
13. International Collaboration of Trialists, Medical Research Council Advanced Bladder Cancer Working Party (now the National Cancer Research Institute Bladder Cancer Clinical Studies Group), European Organisation for Research and Treatment of Cancer Genito-Urinary Tract Cancer Group. International phase III trial assessing neoadjuvant cisplatin, methotrexate, and vinblastine chemotherapy for muscle-invasive bladder cancer: long-term results of the BA06 30894 trial. J Clin Oncol. 2011;29(16):2171–7.
14. Sternberg CN, Skoneczna IA, Castellano D, et al. Larotaxel with cisplatin in the first-line treatment of locally advanced/metastatic urothelial tract or bladder cancer: a randomized, active-controlled, phase III trial (CILAB). Oncology. 2013;85(4):208–15.
15. Grivas P, Mortazavi A, Picus J, et al. Mocetinostat for patients with previously treated, locally advanced/metastatic urothelial carcinoma and inactivating alterations of acetyltransferase genes. Cancer. 2019;125(4):533–40.
16. von der Maase H, Hansen SW, Roberts JT, et al. Gemcitabine and cisplatin versus methotrexate, vinblastine, doxorubicin, and cisplatin in advanced or metastatic bladder cancer: results of a large, randomized, multinational, multicenter, phase III study. J Clin Oncol. 2000;18(17):3068–77.
17. Adamo V, Magno C, Spitaleri G, et al. Phase II study of gemcitabine and cisplatin in patients with advanced or metastatic bladder cancer: long-term follow-up of a 3-week regimen. Oncology. 2005;69(5):391–8.
18. von der Maase H, Sengelov L, Roberts JT, et al. Long-term survival results of a randomized trial comparing gemcitabine plus cisplatin, with methotrexate, vinblastine, doxorubicin, plus cisplatin in patients with bladder cancer. J Clin Oncol. 2005;23(21):4602–8.
19. Milowsky MI, Nanus DM, Maluf FC, et al. Final results of sequential doxorubicin plus gemcitabine and ifosfamide, paclitaxel, and cisplatin chemotherapy in patients with metastatic or locally advanced transitional cell carcinoma of the urothelium. J Clin Oncol. 2009;27(25):4062–7.

20. Hussain SA, Stocken DD, Riley P, et al. A phase I/II study of gemcitabine and fractionated cisplatin in an outpatient setting using a 21-day schedule in patients with advanced and metastatic bladder cancer. Br J Cancer. 2004;91(5):844–9.
21. Krege S, Rexer H, vom Dorp F, et al. Prospective randomized double-blind multicentre phase II study comparing gemcitabine and cisplatin plus sorafenib chemotherapy with gemcitabine and cisplatin plus placebo in locally advanced and/or metastasized urothelial cancer: SUSE (AUO-AB 31/05). BJU Int. 2014;113(3):429–36.
22. Jin JO, Lehmann J, Taxy J, et al. Phase II trial of adjuvant gemcitabine plus cisplatin-based chemotherapy in patients with locally advanced bladder cancer. Clin Genitourin Cancer. 2006;5(2):150–4.
23. Morales-Barrera R, Bellmunt J, Suárez C, et al. Cisplatin and gemcitabine administered every two weeks in patients with locally advanced or metastatic urothelial carcinoma and impaired renal function. Eur J Cancer. 2012;48(12):1816–21.
24. Fechner G, Siener R, Reimann M, Kobalz L, Albers P, German Association of Urologic Oncology (AUO) Bladder Cancer Study Group. Randomised phase II trial of gemcitabine and paclitaxel second-line chemotherapy in patients with transitional cell carcinoma (AUO Trial AB 20/99). Int J Clin Pract. 2006;60(1):27–31.
25. Ecke TH, Bartel P, Koch S, Ruttloff J, Theissig F. Chemotherapy with gemcitabine, paclitaxel, and cisplatin in the treatment of patients with advanced transitional cell carcinoma of the urothelium. Oncol Rep. 2006;16(6):1381–8.
26. Sternberg CN, Calabrò F, Pizzocaro G, Marini L, Schnetzer S, Sella A. Chemotherapy with an every-2-week regimen of gemcitabine and paclitaxel in patients with transitional cell carcinoma who have received prior cisplatin-based therapy. Cancer. 2001;92(12):2993–8.
27. Hainsworth JD, Meluch AA, Litchy S, et al. Paclitaxel, carboplatin, and gemcitabine in the treatment of patients with advanced transitional cell carcinoma of the urothelium. Cancer. 2005;103(11):2298–303.
28. Ko YJ, Canil CM, Mukherjee SD, et al. Nanoparticle albumin-bound paclitaxel for second-line treatment of metastatic urothelial carcinoma: a single group, multicentre, phase 2 study. Lancet Oncol. 2013;14(8):769–76.
29. Garcia del Muro X, Marcuello E, Gumá J, et al. Phase II multicentre study of docetaxel plus cisplatin in patients with advanced urothelial cancer. Br J Cancer. 2002;86(3):326–30.
30. Ardavanis A, Tryfonopoulos D, Alexopoulos A, Kandylis C, Lainakis G, Rigatos G. Gemcitabine and docetaxel as first-line treatment for advanced urothelial carcinoma: a phase II study. Br J Cancer. 2005;92(4):645–50.
31. Gitlitz BJ, Baker C, Chapman Y, et al. A phase II study of gemcitabine and docetaxel therapy in patients with advanced urothelial carcinoma. Cancer. 2003;98(9):1863–9.
32. Bellmunt J, Kerst JM, Vázquez F, et al. A randomized phase II/III study of cabazitaxel versus vinflunine in metastatic or locally advanced transitional cell carcinoma of the urothelium (SECAVIN). Ann Oncol. 2017;28(7):1517–22.
33. Lelli G, Melotti B, Pannuti F, Rossi AP, Maver P, Mannini D, Corrado G, Severini G, Bercovich E, Beghelli R, et al. Chemotherapy with cisplatin, epirubicin, methotrexate in the treatment of locally advanced or metastatic transitional cell cancer of the bladder (TCC). J Chemother. 1992;4(4):239–43.
34. Pectasides D, Mylonakis A, Antoniou F, et al. Chemotherapy with methotrexate, carboplatin, mitoxantrone (Novantrone) and vincristine (Oncovin) in transitional-cell urothelial cancer. Oncology. 1998;55(2):139–44.
35. Tsavaris N, Kosmas C, Skopelitis H, et al. Methotrexate-paclitaxel-epirubicin-carboplatin (M-TEC) combination chemotherapy in patients with advanced bladder cancer: an open label phase II study [published correction appears in J Chemother. 2005 Oct;17(5): following 573. Kopteridis, P [corrected to Kopterides, P]]. J Chemother. 2005;17(4):441–8.
36. Bellmunt J, Albanell J, Gallego OS, et al. Carboplatin, methotrexate, and vinblastine in patients with bladder cancer who were ineligible for cisplatin-based chemotherapy. Cancer. 1992;70(7):1974–9.

37. Pronzato P, Landucci M, Vaira F, Vigani A, Bertelli G. Carboplatin, methotrexate, and vinblastine in outpatients with advanced transitional cell carcinoma of the bladder. Am J Clin Oncol. 1995;18(3):223–5.
38. Skarlos DV, Aravantinos G, Linardou E, et al. Chemotherapy with methotrexate, vinblastine, epirubicin and carboplatin (Carbo-MVE) in transitional cell urothelial cancer. A Hellenic Co-Operative Oncology Group study. Eur Urol. 1997;31(4):420–7.
39. Boukovinas I, Androulakis N, Kentepozidis N, et al. Chemotherapy with gemcitabine, cisplatin, and docetaxel in the treatment for patients with muscle-invasive bladder cancer: a multicenter phase II study of the Hellenic Oncology Research Group (HORG). Cancer Chemother Pharmacol. 2012;69(2):351–6.
40. Seront E, Rottey S, Sautois B, et al. Phase II study of everolimus in patients with locally advanced or metastatic transitional cell carcinoma of the urothelial tract: clinical activity, molecular response, and biomarkers. Ann Oncol. 2012;23(10):2663–70.
41. Dreicer R, Propert KJ, Roth BJ, Einhorn LH, Loehrer PJ. Vinblastine, ifosfamide, and gallium nitrate—an active new regimen in patients with advanced carcinoma of the urothelium. A phase II trial of the Eastern Cooperative Oncology Group (E5892). Cancer. 1997;79(1):110–4.
42. von der Maase H, Lehmann J, Gravis G, et al. A phase II trial of pemetrexed plus gemcitabine in locally advanced and/or metastatic transitional cell carcinoma of the urothelium. Ann Oncol. 2006;17(10):1533–8.
43. Kaufman DS, Carducci MA, Kuzel TM, et al. A multi-institutional phase II trial of gemcitabine plus paclitaxel in patients with locally advanced or metastatic urothelial cancer. Urol Oncol. 2004;22(5):393–7.
44. Pectasides D, Visvikis A, Aspropotamitis A, et al. Chemotherapy with cisplatin, epirubicin and docetaxel in transitional cell urothelial cancer. Phase II trial. Eur J Cancer. 2000;36(1):74–9.
45. Vaughn DJ, Srinivas S, Stadler WM, et al. Vinflunine in platinum-pretreated patients with locally advanced or metastatic urothelial carcinoma: results of a large phase 2 study. Cancer. 2009;115(18):4110–7.
46. Winquist E, Ernst DS, Jonker D, et al. Phase II trial of pegylated-liposomal doxorubicin in the treatment of locally advanced unresectable or metastatic transitional cell carcinoma of the urothelial tract. Eur J Cancer. 2003;39(13):1866–71.
47. Mahjoubi M, Kattan J, Ghosn M, Droz JP, Philippot I, Herait P. Phase II trial of pirarubicin in the treatment of advanced bladder cancer. Investig New Drugs. 1992;10(4):317–21.

Chemo-radiation in Muscle Invasive Bladder Cancer

67

67.1 Systematic Review Methods

A systematic review relating to muscle invasive bladder cancer and palliative cystectomy was conducted. This was to identify whether radical cystectomy has a role in this cohort. The search strategy aimed to identify all references related to bladder cancer AND muscle invasive disease AND Palliative Cystectomy. Search terms used were as follows: (Bladder cancer) AND (muscle invasive disease) AND (Palliative Cystectomy). The following databases were screened from 1979 to June 2020:

- CINAHL
- MEDLINE (NHS Evidence)
- Cochrane
- AMedune
- EMBASE
- PsychINFO
- SCOPUS
- Web of Science

In addition, searches using Medical Subject Headings (MeSH) and keywords were conducted using Cochrane databases. Two UK-based experts in bladder cancer were consulted to identify any additional studies.

Studies were eligible for inclusion if they reported primary research focusing on muscle invasive bladder cancer and palliative cystectomy. Papers were included if published after 1984 and had to be in English. Studies that did not conform to this were excluded. Only primary research was included (Fig. 67.1).

Abstracts were independently screened for eligibility by two reviewers and disagreements resolved through discussion or third party opinion. Agreement level was calculated using Cohen's Kappa to test the intercoder reliability of this screening

S. S. Goonewardene et al., *Management of Muscle Invasive Bladder Cancer*, Management of Urology, https://doi.org/10.1007/978-3-030-57915-9_67

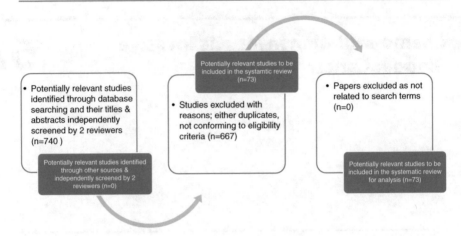

Fig. 67.1   Flow chart of studies identified through the systematic review. (Adapted from PRISMA)

process. Cohens' Kappa allows comparison of inter-rater reliability between papers using relative observed agreement [1]. This also takes account of the comparison occurring by chance. The first reviewer agreed all 73 papers to be included, the second, agreed on 73.

Data extraction was piloted by the researcher and amended in consultation with the research team (author and two academic supervisors). Data collected included authors, year and country of publication, study aims, setting, intervention aims, number of participants, study design, intervention components and delivery methods, comparison groups and outcome measures, notes and follow-up questions for the authors. Studies were quality assessed using the PRISMA criteria for randomised controlled trials, Mays et al. [2, 3] for the action research and qualitative studies and the Critical Skills Appraisal programme for cohort studies. This was also applied to randomised controlled trials and qualitative studies.

The search identified 740 papers (Fig. 67.1). Seventy-three mapped to the search terms and eligibility criteria. The current systematic reviews were examined to gain further knowledge about the subject. Six hundred and sixty-seven papers were excluded due to not conforming to eligibility criteria or adding to the evidence. Of the 73 papers left, relevant abstracts were identified and the full papers obtained (all of which were in English), to quality assure against search criteria. There was considerable heterogeneity of design among the included studies therefore a narrative review of the evidence was undertaken. There was significant heterogeneity within studies, including clinical topic, numbers, outcomes, as a result a narrative review was thought to be best. There were 66 cohort studies, with a moderate level of evidence and 7 RCTs with a good level of evidence. These were from a range of countries with minimal loss to follow-up. All participants were identified appropriately.

67.2 Systematic Review Results

67.2.1 Radical Cystectomy vs. Chemoradiation in Muscle Invasive Bladder Cancer

Haresh et al. [4] compared the two standard treatment approaches in muscle invasive carcinoma of urinary bladder—radical cystectomy and chemo radiation [4]. T2 to T4, N0/N1/N2 and M0 were included with arm A consisted of radical cystectomy [4]. Adjuvant CMV chemotherapy was given for T3/T4 or Node positive disease only [4]. Arm B received two cycles of neoadjuvant CMV chemotherapy followed by concurrent chemo radiation [4]. The actuarial two-year survival rate in surgical arm is 56% while in chemo radiation arm it is 54% [4]. There was no statistically significant difference in disease-free survival also between the two groups [4].

Haque et al. [5] reviewed cystectomy (RC) or concurrent chemoradiation (CRT) [5]. Sixteen thousand nine hundred and sixty patients met the inclusion criteria; 1450 (8.5%) underwent CRT, while 15,510 (91.5%) were treated with RC [5]. CRT was associated with worse median OS (32.8 vs. 36.1 months; $p = 0.0004$) [5]. Older patients are more likely to undergo bladder preservation therapy, while those living farther away from treatment facilities are less likely to under CRT [5].

Kaushik et al. [6] examined whether chemoradiation therapy (CMT) offers overall survival (OS) similar to that of radical cystectomy (RC) in muscle-invasive bladder cancer (MIBC) [6]. Of 484,367 patients with a diagnosis of bladder cancer, 35,856 underwent RC and 4050 received CMT [6]. After applying the exclusion/inclusion criteria, data for 15,854 patients who underwent RC and 2083 who received CMT were available for analysis [6]. Five-year OS was 40.4% in the RC group and 29.4% in the CMT group ($p < 0.001$) [6]. OS was significantly shorter in the CMT group than in the RC group in both multivariate analysis (hazards ratio [HR] 1.15, 95% CI 1.08–1.22; $p < 0.001$) and propensity score-weighted analysis (HR 1.18, 95% CI 1.07–1.30; $p < 0.001$) [6]. Interaction terms indicated better survival after RC in patients younger than 70 years (HR 1.61, 95% CI 1.34–1.93; $p < 0.001$); subgroup analyses identified a survival benefit in patients with N0/N1 disease who underwent RC (HR 1.21, 95% CI 1.09–1.33; $p < 0.001$) [6].

Muscle-invasive bladder cancer (MIBC) may be managed with radical cystectomy (RC) or chemoradiotherapy (CRT) [7]. Of 16,658 patients, 15,208 (91.3%) underwent RC and 1450 (8.7%) CRT [7]. Crude rates of post-treatment mortality at 30 days were 2.7% versus 0.6% ($p < 0.001$) and at 90 days were 7.5% versus 4.5% ($p = 0.017$) for patients treated with RC and CRT, respectively [7].

Ritch et al. [8] compared survival outcome between chemoradiation therapy (CRT) and radical cystectomy (RC) for muscle-invasive bladder cancer (MIBC) [8]. In all, 8379 (6606 RC and 1773 CRT) patients met the inclusion criteria and 1683 patients in each group were propensity matched [8]. On multivariable extended Cox analysis, significant predictors of decreased OS were age, Charlson-Deyo Comorbidity score of 1, Charlson-Deyo Comorbidity score of 2, stage cT3–4, and urothelial histology [8]. CRT was associated with decreased mortality at year 1 (hazard ratio [HR] 0.84, 95% confidence interval [CI] 0.74–0.96; p = 0.01), but at 2 years (HR 1.4, 95% CI 1.2–1.6; p < 0.001) and 3 years onward (HR 1.5, 95% CI 1.2–1.8; p < 0.001) CRT was associated with increased mortality [8]. The 5-year OS was greater for RC than for CRT (38% vs. 30%, p = 0.004) [8].

Gofrit et al. [9] compared outcomes from radical cystectomy vs. chemoradiation [9]. The 2- and 5-year overall survival rates after surgery were 74.4% and 54.8%, respectively, and after chemoradiation were 70.2% and 56.6% (p = 0.8), respectively [9]. The 2- and 5-year disease-free survival rates after surgery were 67.8% and 63.2%, respectively, and after chemoradiation were 63% and 54.3% (p = 0.89), respectively [9]. Side effects were mild in both groups, with grade 3+ toxicity seen in only 2 operated and 4 irradiated patients [9].

Lin et al. [10] tested the hypothesis that bladder preservation therapy consisting of definitive chemoradiotherapy (chemoRT) results in similar overall survival rates to radical cystectomy/chemotherapy when balancing baseline patient characteristics and initial (preoperative) clinical stage [10]. Patients who underwent cystectomy/chemo were significantly younger than ones treated with definitive chemoRT (mean age 63.7 vs. 75.2; p < 0.001) [10]. Patients treated with cystectomy/chemo were younger, healthier with better CDCS, and more likely treated at academic facilities [10]. Before matched pair analyses, OS was significantly better when treated with cystectomy/chemo (3 year 56.4%; 5 year 45.9%) compared to chemoRT (3 year 47.3%; 5 year 33.2%) (p < 0.001); 28.6% of patients undergoing cystectomy were upstaged at the time of surgery [10]. After matched pair analyses matching age, race, sex, CDCS, clinical (presurgical) stage, insurance, and facility type (N = 1750), OS was no longer significantly different between cystectomy/chemo (3 year 52.1% and 5 year 41.0%) vs. chemoRT (3 year 53.3% and 5 year 40.1%) (p = 0.5) [10].

Nagao et al. [11] evaluated the bladder-preservation strategy to Open radical cystectomy [11]. Transurethral resection of the bladder tumor (TURBT) was performed before treatment to confirm pathological stage ≥T2 [11]. Extensive TURBT was performed after chemoradiotherapy to evaluate the pathological response to treatment [11]. The 2- and 5-year progression-free survival, bladder-intact survival, cancer-specific survival, and overall survival (OS) rates after treatment were 70.8% and 63.9%, 64.0% and 49.8%, 86.7% and 71.8%, and 84.3% and 64.8%, respectively [11]. The 2- and 5-year OS rates after CDDP-R were 90.5% and 74.3%, respectively, and those after ORC were 71.8% and 59.9%, respectively, indicating a significant survival advantage conferred by CDDP-R over ORC (p < 0.05, HR 0.45, 95% CI 0.21–0.94) [11].

Radical cystectomy (RC) and radiochemotherapy (RCT) are curative options for muscle-invasive bladder cancer (MIBC), however radical surgery may not be the best option in the elderly [12]. Ninety-two patients underwent RC and 72 patients had RCT [12]. Median OS was 1.99 years (95% CI 1.17–2.76) after RC and 1.97 years (95% CI 1.35–2.64) after RCT (p = 0.73) [12]. Median progression-free survival (PFS) after RC and RCT were 1.25 years (95% CI 0.80–1.75) and 1.52 years (95% CI 1.01–2.04), respectively (p = 0.54) [12]. In multivariate analyses, only disease progression was significantly associated with worse OS (HR = 10.27 (95% CI 6.63–15.91), p < 0.0001) [12]. Treatment modality was not a prognostic factor [12].

Ikeda et al. [13] evaluated the clinical outcomes of radical cystectomy (RC) and concurrent chemoradiotherapy (CRT) with methotrexate, vinblastine, doxorubicin, and cisplatin (MVAC) in patients with locally advanced bladder cancer (BC) [13]. The 3-year progression-free survival (PFS) rates in the RC and CRT groups were 56.2% and 25.6%, respectively (p = −0.015) and the 3-year overall survival (OS) rates were 63.5% and 48.1% (p = 0.272) [13]. Multivariate Cox proportional hazards regression analysis with application of a propensity score indicated that RC was a significant predictor of PFS (p = 0.033) but not of OS (p = 0.291) [13]. Among patients with locally advanced BC, PFS was significantly prolonged in the RC group compared with the CRT group [13]. However, RC was not a significant predictor of OS [13]. Although the sample size in this study was small, the results suggest that patient background and postoperative quality of life should be considered when choosing treatment strategy for locally advanced BC [13].

67.2.2 Predictors of Response to Chemoradiation in Bladder Preservation Therapy

Peyromaure et al. [14] reported outcomes from chemoradiotherapy for clinical Stage T2 bladder cancer [14]. Nine patients underwent early cystectomy for nonresponse, and 2 patients underwent delayed cystectomy [14]. The overall rate of cystectomy was 25.6% [14]. The rate of specific survival at 3 and 5 years was 75% and 60%, respectively [14]. The overall rate of recurrence-free survival at 3 and 5 years was 63% and 33%, respectively [14]. Two factors correlated with patient survival: the presence of carcinoma in situ at first resection (p = 0.01) and the response after the first two cycles (half dose; p = 0.004) [14].

Sanguineti et al. [15] evaluated the predictive role of pretreatment- and treatment-related factors in invasive bladder cancer treated with alternating chemoradiotherapy [15]. Twenty-two patients (76%) developed infiltrative bladder recurrences for an estimated 5-year pelvic control rate of 68 ± 6%; 5-year actuarial survival with intact bladder is 40% ± 6% [15]. Obstructive uropathy at diagnosis, residual disease after TURB, and ARDICT value equal or below the median were independent predictive factors for pelvic failure, with hazard ratios of 2.87 (95% confidence interval [CI], 1.16–7.04), 8.13 (95% CI, 2.74–24.1), and 3.36 (95% CI, 1.29–8.74), respectively [15]. A more detailed model including interactions among these factors showed that the negative prognostic effect of obstructive uropathy at diagnosis was not modified by ARDICT or TURB resection; on the contrary, the risk of local failure for patients with incomplete TURB was markedly affected by different levels of ARDICT [15]. Also, a trend toward a better local outcome was observed for patients with RDIRT above the median [15]. Hydronephrosis and incomplete TURB were also independent predictors of distant metastases and overall survival, but no effect was found for ARDICT on these endpoints [15].

67.2.3 Biochemical Markers of Response to Chemoradiation Therapy in Muscle Invasive Bladder Cancer

Yoshida et al. [16] investigated the effect of C-reactive protein (CRP) level on the prognosis of patients with muscle-invasive bladder cancer treated with chemoradiotherapy (ChRT), as it is increasingly recognized that the presence of a systemic inflammatory response is associated with poor survival in various malignancies [16]. The 5-year cancer-specific survival (CSS) rate was 73% [16]. Ten patients had a high CRP level before ChRT ($\geq$0.5 mg/dl) and their CSS rate was significantly worse than that in the remaining patients (p = 0.003) [16]. Multivariate analysis showed that CRP and cT stage were independent prognostic indicators for CSS, with a hazard ratio of 1.80 (95% confidence interval 1.01–2.97; p = 0.046) [16]. Among 10 patients in those with elevated CRP the CRP levels became normal after ChRT in six, of whom all but one was alive with no evidence of recurrence or metastasis during the follow-up [16]. By contrast, all four with no CRP normalization after ChRT died within 2 years [16].

67.2.3.1 Histological Markers of Response to Chemoradiotherapy

Koga et al. [17] stratified patients with a clinical non-complete response (CR) after induction chemoradiotherapy (CRT) according to their risk of death from cancer, based on pathology of cystectomy specimens [17]. Of 170 patients, 81 (48%) achieved a CR and 62 (36%) met the Partial cystectomy (PC) criteria [17]. After CRT, 122 patients (72%) ultimately underwent PC (n = 44, 26%) or RC (n = 78, 46%) [17]. The 5-year cancer-specific survival (CSS) rate was 96% for the patients with a CR and 50% for patients with non-CR (p < 0.001, median follow-up for survivors: 48 months) [17]. In the 122 patients who underwent cystectomy, pT3–4a (hazard ratio [HR] 8.3 versus pT0-2, p < 0.001) and pN+ (HR 3.0 versus pN0, p = 0.037) were identified as significant and independent risk factors among variables including pT stage, lymph node yield at cystectomy, pN stage, and lymphovascular invasion [17]. A similar result was obtained through analysis of a sub-cohort of 69 patients with non-CR. Patients with non-CR were stratified according to their risk factors into low- (pT0-2pN0, 5-year CSS rate 85%) and high-risk (pT3–4a or pN+, 5-year CSS rate 20%) groups [17].

Weiner et al. [18] determined the association between intravesical tumor location and both adverse pathological outcomes as well as overall survival [18]. Following RC, 822 (24%) patients were pN+ and 1551 (55%) were pT3–4 [18]. Trigonal tumours were most likely to have adverse pathology (31% pN+ and 59% pT3–4), while anterior wall tumours were the least (19% pN+ and 50% pT3–4) [18]. Relative to the anterior wall, trigone (odds ratio [OR] 1.65, 95% confidence interval [CI] 1.12–2.43, p = 0.012) and bladder neck (OR 1.79, 95% CI 1.11–2.90, p = 0.018) tumours were associated with increased odds of pN+ and dome (OR 1.56, 95% CI 1.08–2.24, p = 0.017) with pT3–4 [18]. In those patients treated with primary CRT, trigone involvement was associated with worse survival (HR 1.58, 95% CI 1.17–2.13, p = 0.003) [18].

67.2.3.2 Biomarkers as a Predictor of Response to Chemoradiotherapy

Koga et al. [19] reviewed biomarkers for predicting the clinical outcomes of chemoradiation-based bladder preservation therapy (BPT) [19]. The biomarkers studied were categorized into those related to apoptosis, cell proliferation, receptor tyrosine kinases, DNA damage response genes, hypoxia, molecular subtype, and others [19]. Among these biomarkers, the Ki-67 labeling index (Ki-67 LI) and meiotic recombination 11 may be used for selecting BPT or RC. Ki-67 LI and erythroblastic leukemia viral oncogene homolog 2 (erbB2) may be used for predicting both the chemoradiation response and the prognosis of patients on BPT [19]. Concurrent use of trastuzumab and a combination of carbogen and nicotinamide can overcome chemoradiation resistance conferred by erbB2 overexpression and tumor hypoxia [19].

Tanabe et al. [20] evaluated associations of Ki-67 expression with oncologic outcomes in muscle-invasive bladder cancer (MIBC) patients treated with chemoradiotherapy (CRT)-based bladder-sparing protocol [20]. After induction CRT, 16 (17%) and 53 (56%) patients underwent partial cystectomy and RC, respectively, while the remaining 25 (27%) did not undergo cystectomy [20]. Successful bladder preservation was achieved in 34 patients (36%) [20]. Higher Ki-67 labeling index (LI) independently predicted CRT response clinically and pathologically [20]. Among the clinicopathologic variables available before CRT and cystectomy, high Ki-67 LI ($\geq 20\%$) was independently associated with better cancer-specific survival (CSS) (5-year CSS rate, 78% vs. 46% for low Ki-67 LI; p = 0.019) [20]. The difference in CSS according to Ki-67 expression status was more remarkable in patients with cT3 disease (5-year CSS rate, 72% vs. 29%; p = 0.0098) [20].

Desai et al. [21] wanted to identify potential correlates of response to chemoradiation [21]. Forty-eight patients who had non-metastatic, high-grade UCB and received treatment primarily with chemoradiation were analysed using a next-generation sequencing assay enriched for cancer-related and canonical DNA damage response (DDR) genes [21]. Protein expression of meiotic recombination 11 homolog (MRE11), a previously suggested biomarker, was assessed in 44 patients [21]. Within five pairs of matched primary-recurrent tumours, a median of 92% of somatic mutations were shared [21]. A median 33% of mutations were shared between three matched bladder-metastasis pairs [21]. Of 26 patients (54%) who had DDR gene alterations, 12 (25%) harboured likely deleterious alterations [21]. In multivariable analysis, these patients displayed a trend toward reduced bladder recurrence (hazard ratio, 0.32; p = 0.070) or any recurrence (hazard ratio, 0.37; p = 0.070) [21]. The most common of these alterations, ERCC2 (excision repair cross-complementation group 2) mutations, were associated with significantly lower 2-year metastatic recurrence (0% vs. 43%; log-rank p = 0.044) [21]. No impact of MRE11 protein expression on outcome was detected [21].

67.2.3.3 Immunohistochemistry Response to Chemoradiotherapy

Tanaka et al. [22] evaluated the impact of immunohistochemistry (IHC)-based subtyping in MIBC on prediction of Chemoradiation Therapy (CRT) response

[22]. Patients were classified into urobasal (Uro), genomically unstable (GU), and squamous cell cancer-like (SCCL) subtypes [22]. Clinical complete response (CR) was achieved in 42% of patients overall after CRT, with a significantly higher proportion in GU patients (52%) and SCCL patients (45%) than in Uro patients (15%; p < 0.001 and p = 0.01, respectively) [22]. On multivariate analysis, the GU/SCCL subtype was a significant predictor of clinical CR, as was absence of hydronephrosis or concomitant carcinoma in situ [22]. Analyses for pathologic CR in the cystectomised patients revealed analogous findings [22]. Five-year CSM of Uro, GU, and SCCL patients was 16%, 23%, and 28% overall, respectively, and 19%, 22%, and 23% in cystectomised patients, respectively, with no significant difference among the subtypes [22]. CR status after CRT was significantly and independently correlated with low CSM in both clinical and pathologic evaluations [22].

67.2.3.4   Molecular Pathways Highlighting Response to Chemoradiotherapy in Muscle Invasive Bladder Cancer

Inoue et al. [23] investigated the associations of ERBB 2 overexpression with chemoradiation therapy (CRT) resistance and cancer-specific survival (CSS) in muscle-invasive bladder cancer (MIBC) patients treated with the CRT-based bladder-sparing protocol [23]. CRT resistance was observed clinically in 56% (67 of 119 patients) and pathologically (in cystectomy specimens) in 55% (52 of 95 patients) [23]. ERBB 2 overexpression was observed in 45 patients (38%) [23]. On multivariate analysis, ERBB 2 overexpression was an independent predictor for CRT resistance clinically (odds ratio, 3.6; p = 0.002) and pathologically (odds ratio, 2.9; p = 0.031) [23]. ERBB 2 overexpression was associated with shorter CSS (5-year CSS rates, 56% vs. 87% for the ERBB 2 overexpression group vs. the others; p = 0.001) [23]. ERBB 2 overexpression was also an independent risk factor for bladder cancer death at all time points of our bladder-sparing protocol (pre-CRT, post-CRT, and post-cystectomy) [23].

Shinohara et al. [24] investigated associations between two such polymorphisms, and p53 overexpression, and response to chemoradiotherapy [24]. The study group comprised 96 patients who underwent CRT for transitional cell carcinoma of the bladder [24]. Single nucleotide polymorphisms (SNPs) in TP53 (codon 72, arginine > proline) and MDM2 (SNP309, T > G) were genotyped using PCR-RFLP, and nuclear expression levels of p53 were examined using immunohistochemistry [24]. None of the genotypes or p53 overexpression was significantly associated with response to CRT [24]. However, patients with MDM2 T/G + G/G genotypes had improved cancer-specific survival rates after CRT (p = 0.009) [24]. In multivariate analysis, the MDM2 T/G + G/G genotypes, and more than two of total variant alleles in TP53 and MDM2, were independently associated with improved cancer-specific survival (p = 0.031 and p = 0.015, respectively) [24]. In addition, MDM2 genotypes were significantly associated with cystectomy-free survival (p = 0.030) [24]. These results suggest that the TP53 and MDM2 genotypes might be useful prognostic factors following CRT in bladder cancer, helping patient selection for bladder conservation therapy [24].

Keck et al. [25] studied the prognostic impact of NRP2 and VEGF-C in 247 bladder cancer patients (cN0M0) treated with TURBT and RCT (n = 198) or RT (n = 49) [25]. NRP2 expression emerged as a prognostic factor in overall survival (OS; HR: 3.42; 95% CI: 1.48–7.86; p = 0.004) and was associated with a 3.85-fold increased risk of an early cancer specific death (95% CI: 0.91–16.24; p = 0.066) in multivariate analyses [25]. Cancer specific survival (CSS) dropped from 166 months to 85 months when NRP2 was highly expressed (p = 0.037) [25]. Patients with high VEGF-C expression have a 2.29-fold increased risk of shorter CSS (95% CI: 1.03–5.35; p = 0.043) in univariate analysis [25]. CSS dropped from 170 months to 88 months in the case of high VEGF-C expression (p = 0.041) [25]. Additionally, NRP2 and VEGF-C coexpression is a prognostic marker for OS in multivariate models (HR: 7.54; 95% CI: 1.57–36.23; p = 0.012) [25]. Stratification for muscle invasiveness (T1 vs. T2–T4) confirmed the prognostic role of NRP2 and NRP2/VEGF-C co-expression in patients with T2–T4 but also with high risk T1 disease [25]. In conclusion, immunohistochemistry for NRP2 and VEGF-C has been determined to predict therapy outcome in bladder cancer patients prior to TURBT and RCT [25].

Koga et al. [26], a bladder-sparing alternative strategy using chemoradiation was examined to improve QOL in muscle invasive bladder cancer [26]. Of the 35 patients, 11 (31%) achieved pathological CR, while tumours in the remaining 24 patients (69%) were chemoradiation-resistant [26]. Multivariate analysis identified erbB2 and NFκB overexpression and hydronephrosis as significant and independent risk factors for chemoradiation resistance with respective relative risks of 11.8 (p = 0.014), 15.4 (p = 0.024) and 14.3 (p = 0.038) [26]. The chemoradiation resistance rate was 88.5% for tumours overexpressing erbB2 and/or NFκB, but only 11.1% for those negative for both (p < 0.0001) [26]. The 5-year CSS rate was 74% overall [26]. Through multivariate analysis, overexpression of erbB2 and/or NFκB was identified as an independent risk factor for bladder cancer death with marginal significance (hazard ratio 21.5, p = 0.056) along with chemoradiation resistance (p = 0.003) and hydronephrosis (p = 0.018) [26]. The 5-year CSS rate for the 11 patients achieving pathological CR was 100%, while that for the 24 with chemoradiation-resistant disease was 61% (p = 0.018) [26].

Nicholson et al. [27] examined potential strategies for response to chemoradiation [27]. The MRE11/RAD50/NBS1 (MRN) complex mediates DNA repair pathways, including double-strand breaks induced by radiotherapy [27]. Nicholson et al. [27] identified the mechanism of this downregulation is posttranslational and identify a C-terminally truncated MRE11, which is formed after HDAC inhibition as full-length MRE11 is downregulated [27]. Truncated MRE11 was stabilized by proteasome inhibition, exhibited a decreased half-life after treatment with panobinostat, and therefore represents a newly identified intermediate induced and degraded in response to HDAC inhibition [27]. The E3 ligase cellular inhibitor of apoptosis protein 2 (cIAP2) was upregulated in response to HDAC inhibition and was validated as a new MRE11 binding partner whose upregulation had similar effects to HDAC inhibition [27]. cIAP2 overexpression resulted in downregulation and altered ubiquitination patterns of MRE11 and mediated radiosensitization in response to

HDAC inhibition [27]. These results highlight cIAP2 as a player in the DNA damage response as a posttranscriptional regulator of MRE11 and identify cIAP2 as a potential target for biomarker discovery or chemoradiation strategies in bladder cancer [27].

Abe et al. [28] investigated the long-term results and molecular markers of outcome with selective organ preservation in invasive bladder cancer using chemoradiation therapy [28]. The first assessment after the induction chemoradiotherapy showed that bladder preservation was achieved in 27 patients (84.4%) [28]. The actuarial local control rate with an intact bladder was 56.3% (18 patients) at 3 years [28]. The 1-, 3-, and 5-year cancer-specific survival rate was 90.6%, 84.0%, and 66.9%, respectively [28]. The 5-year cancer-specific survival rate was 75.0%, 67.2%, and 33.3% in T2, T3, and T4, respectively. Bcl-x positivity was significantly associated with a poor cancer-specific survival rate (log-rank test, p = 0.038) [28].

67.2.3.5 Imaging to Predict Response to Chemoradiation

Yoshida et al. [29] investigated whether DW-MRI predicts chemoradiation treatment (CRT) sensitivity of MIBC [29]. Thirteen patients (57%) achieved pathologic complete response (pCR) to CRT [29]. These CRT-sensitive MIBCs showed significantly lower ADC values (median, 0.63×10^{-3} mm^2/s; range, 0.43–0.77) than CRT-resistant (no pCR) MIBCs (median, 0.84×10^{-3} mm^2/s; range, 0.69–1.09; p = 0.0003) [29]. Multivariate analysis identified ADC value as the only significant and independent predictor of CRT sensitivity (p < 0.0001; odds ratio per 0.001×10^{-3} mm^2/s increase, 1.03; 95% confidence interval, 1.01–1.08) [29]. With a cutoff ADC value at 0.74×10^{-3} mm^2/s, sensitivity/specificity/accuracy in predicting CRT sensitivity was 92/90/91%. Ki-67 LI was significantly higher in CRT-sensitive MIBCs (p = 0.0005) and significantly and inversely correlated with ADC values ($\rho = -0.67$, p = 0.0007) [29].

67.2.4 Alternative Regimes in Chemoradiation for Muscle Invasive Bladder Cancer

Fluorouracil plus cisplatin and radiation twice a day (FCT) is an established chemoradiation (CRT) regimen for selective bladder-sparing treatment of muscle-invasive bladder cancer [30]. Gemcitabine and once daily radiation (GD) is an alternative evaluated by [30]. Freedom from distant metastases at 3 years was 78% and 84% for FCT and GD, respectively [30]. Bladder intact distant metastasis free survival was 67% and 72%, respectively [30]. Postinduction CR rates were 88% and 78%, respectively. Of 33 patients in the FCT arm, 21 (64%) experienced treatment-related grade 3 and 4 toxicities during protocol treatment, with 18 (55%), two (6%), and two patients (6%) experiencing grade 3 and 4 hematologic, GI, and genitourinary toxicity, respectively [30]. For the 33 patients in the GD arm, these figures were 18 (55%) overall and 14 (42%), 3 (9%) and 2 patients (6%), respectively [30].

Arias et al. [31] assessed a combination of methotrexate, vinblastine, adriamycin, and cisplatin (M-VAC), followed by radiotherapy and concomitant cisplatin was used [31]. Tumour response was as follows: 34 complete responses (68%), 9 partial responses (18%), and 7 nonresponses (14%) were observed [31]. The 5-year overall survival and local control were 48% and 47%, respectively [31]. For the complete responder patient, 5-year survival and local control were 65% and 70%, respectively [31]. Severe toxicity was uncommon [31]. The most frequent were leucopenia and cystitis [31]. No treatment-related deaths occurred with either treatment protocol [31].

Hussain et al. [32] conducted a phase I/II study investigating synchronous chemoradiotherapy with mitomycin C and infusional 5-fluorouracil (5-FU) in muscle invasive bladder cancer [32]. In all, out of 35 evaluable patients, 25 (71%) had macroscopic complete response at 3-month cystoscopy, and biopsy confirmed in 24 out of 25 [32]. A total of 16 (39%) patients remain alive with a median follow-up of 50.7 (range 23.5–68.8) months, 14 with a functioning bladder with no reported long-term treatment-related bladder or bowel toxicity [32]. Five out of 41 patients have undergone salvage cystectomy: two for persistent CIS, two T1 and one muscle invasive recurrence [32]. Four patients have received intravesical chemotherapy, of whom two remain alive with a functioning bladder [32]. Overall 12-, 24- and 60-month (m) survival rates were 68%, 49% and 36% [32]. Local and distant progression free rates were 82% and 86% at 12-m and 79% and 75% at 24-m [32]. Organ preservation using multimodality therapy is feasible and safe, even in patients with poor renal reserve, and does not compromise salvage therapies [32].

Michaelson et al. [33] treated noncystectomy candidates with daily radiation and weekly paclitaxel for 7 weeks [33]. Patients whose tumours showed her2/neu overexpression were additionally treated with weekly trastuzumab [33]. A total of 20 evaluable patients were treated in group 1 and 46 patients in group 2 [33]. Acute treatment-related adverse events (AEs) were observed in 7 of 20 patients in group 1 (35%) and 14 of 46 patients in group 2 (30.4%) [33]. Protocol therapy was completed by 60% (group 1) and 74% (group 2) of patients [33]. Most incompletions were due to toxicity, and the majority of AEs were gastrointestinal, including 1 grade 5 AE (group 1) [33]. Two other deaths (both in group 2) were unrelated to protocol therapy. No unexpected cardiac, hematologic, or other toxicities were observed [33]. The CR rate at 1 year was 72% for group 1 and 68% for group 2 [33].

The aim of this prospective, phase II trial was to determine the response of muscle-invasive bladder cancer (MIBC) to concurrent chemoradiotherapy of weekly gemcitabine with 4 weeks of radiotherapy (RT; GemX) [34]. All patients completed RT; 46 tolerated all four cycles of gemcitabine [34]. Two patients stopped after two cycles, and two stopped after three cycles, because of bowel toxicity [34]. Forty-seven patients had a post-treatment cystoscopy; 44 (88%) achieved a complete endoscopic response [34]. Fourteen patients died; seven died as a result of metastatic MIBC, five died as a result of intercurrent disease, and two died as a result of treatment-associated deaths [34]. Four patients underwent cystectomy; three because of recurrent disease and one because of toxicity [34]. One patient required a bowel resection for late toxicity [34]. By using Kaplan-Meier analyses, 3-year cancer-specific survival was 82%, and overall survival was 75% [34].

Kageyama et al. [35] investigated chemoradiotherapy with vinblastine [35]. Tolerable toxicity rates were noted. No patient was excluded from the study [35]. The authors report a clinical complete remission rate of 71% at early evaluation of treatment and a 3-year local progression-free survival of 66% (for Group 2 patients) [35]. These results are comparable to those obtained with more aggressive chemoradiation therapy regimens [35]. The authors also noted improved local disease control in patients who received combination therapy in comparison with the 17 patients treated with RT alone [35].

Leng et al. [36] assessed tolerability, efficacy, and toxicity of hypofractionated radiotherapy with capecitabine in muscle invasive bladder cancer [36]. Eleven patients (median age, 80 years) with localized disease (n = 7), locally advanced disease (n = 3), or local-only recurrence after cystectomy (n = 1) were treated [36]. Four patients (35%) had an Eastern Cooperative Oncology Group performance status of 2; median Charlson comorbidity index was 5 [36]. There was 1 acute grade 3 genitourinary event (9%), 6 acute grade 3 hematologic events (55%) of lymphopenia, and no acute grade 4 or higher events or hospitalizations [36]. Ten patients (91%) completed radiotherapy, while 4 patients (36%) temporarily discontinued capecitabine [36]. The complete response rate in the bladder was 64%. Two patients (18%) experienced late grade 1/2 genitourinary toxicities, and 1 (9%) experienced a transient late grade 4 genitourinary toxicity [36]. With a median follow-up of 16.6 months, overall survival, progression-free survival, freedom from local failure, and freedom from distant metastasis at 1 year were 82%, 55%, 100%, and 55%, respectively, and at 2 years were 61%, 41%, 80%, and 55%, respectively [36].

De Santis et al. [37] conducted a phase I trial of gemcitabine (gem) with concurrent radiotherapy in patients with muscle-invasive bladder cancer (BC) ineligible for surgery or cisplatin or refusing organ loss [37]. Thirty-five of 44 patients were assessable for toxicity and thus the primary end point [37]. The 2-year locoregional failure rate was 32% (9/28); 10 of 28 patients (38%) were alive with an intact bladder and no evidence of recurrent disease, 9 patients developed distant metastases and 6 died of their disease [37].

67.2.5 Outcomes from Chemoradiation in Muscle Invasive Bladder Cancer

Matsushita et al. [38] investigated the outcome of selective organ preservation in invasive bladder cancer using chemoradiation therapy [38]. This included transurethral resection of the bladder tumour (TURBT) and 46 Gy radiation (2 Gy/fraction) to the bladder with concurrent cisplatin chemotherapy (20 mg/body/day, 10 days, intravenously) [38]. The first assessment after the chemoradiation therapy showed that the complete remission rate for evaluable cases was 72% (38/53) and bladder preservation was achieved in 56 patients (93%) [38]. The 1-, 3-, and 5-year overall survival rate was 95%, 86%, and 78%, respectively [38]. The 1-, 3-, and 5-year cancer-specific survival rate was 97%, 90%, and 85%, respectively [38]. The 5-year patient survival rate with an intact bladder was 68% [38].

Russell et al. [39] assessed outcomes in chemoradiation. With a median follow-up of 18 months (range 2–45 months), and with 25/34 patients having T3 (16) or T4 (9) tumors, 17 patients are NED, 4 have died of intercurrent deaths, 7 have died with bladder cancer, and 6 are alive with tumour (2 confined to the bladder) [39]. The actuarial cancer-specific survival for the entire group of patients is 64% (±12%) at 45 months, with a freedom from relapse of invasive cancer of 54% (±10%) [39]. Twenty-four of the 34 patients retained intact bladders, with 20/24 reporting entirely normal voiding [39]. Of 18 potential surgical candidates, 13/16 (81%) who underwent pathologic re-staging after 2 cycles of chemoradiotherapy had no histologic evidence of residual cancer [39]. Of these 13 patients, 8 remain NED and 2/13 have locally recurrent non-invasive tumors only [39]. Treatment was well-tolerated, with 28/34 patients having received 100% of the planned 5-FU and 34/34 having received greater than 80% [39].

Pilot study to assess treatment feasibility and results of a 2-drug chemotherapy (CT) regimen administered concurrently with radiotherapy (RT) for muscle-invasive bladder cancer [40]. The feasibility of concurrent CT-RT was excellent: 96% of the patients completed radiotherapy and 100% of them received the two courses of P-FU [40]. The acute toxicity was mild: no haematological toxicity or renal toxicity over grade II, 4 cases of bowel or rectal reversible grade III toxicity and 2 cases of reversible grade III cystitis [40]. A complete response was achieved in 30 out of the 42 evaluable patients (65.2%) [40]. Nine patients received an immediate salvage treatment (3 TUR, 3 additional radiotherapy and 3 cystectomies) [40]. Ten patients had local failure. Projected 3-year locoregional control was 49% for the 46 patients [40]. Projected overall 3-year survival was 53% [40]. Functional results were good for disease-free patients with preserved bladder: 1 grade I, 3 grade II, and no grade III cystitis [40].

Gogna et al. [41] determined the feasibility, toxicity, and clinical effectiveness of concurrent weekly cisplatin chemotherapy as part of a phase 2 study in conjunction with definitive radiation in the treatment of localised muscle invasive bladder cancer [41]. Acute grade 3 urinary toxicity occurred in 23% of the patients [41]. Acute grade 4 pelvic toxicity was not seen [41]. Thirty-eight patients (33%) experienced grade 3 or 4 cisplatin related toxicities with 15 patients (12%) requiring significant dose modification [41]. The reduced dose intensity in Study 99.06 improved tolerability. Incidence of significant late morbidity was low (6%) [41]. Seventy-nine patients (70%) achieved complete remission at the 6 month cystoscopic assessment [41]. Local invasive recurrence was seen in 11 of the 79 patients (14%) [41]. In 18 patients (16%) isolated superficial TCC/CIS were detected (6 months and beyond). The local control rate was 45% with a functional bladder being retained in 69 of the 113 patients (61%) [41]. RFS and DSS at 5 years were 33% and 50%, respectively [41].

Shipley et al. [42] evaluated the outcomes of patients with muscle-invasive Stage T2–4a bladder carcinoma managed by transurethral surgery and concurrent chemoradiation [42]. The 5 and 10-year actuarial overall survival rate was 54% and 36%, respectively (Stage T2, 62% and 41%; Stage T3–T4a, 47% and 31%, respectively) [42]. The 5 and 10-year disease-specific survival rate was 63% and 59% (Stage T2,

74% and 66%; Stage T3–T4a, 53% and 52%), respectively [42]. The 5 and 10-year disease-specific survival rate for patients with an intact bladder was 46% and 45% (Stage T2, 57% and 50%; Stage T3–T4a, 35% and 34%), respectively [42]. The pelvic failure rate was 8.4%. No patient required cystectomy because of bladder morbidity [42].

Lin et al. [43] evaluated a multimodality bladder-preserving therapy in patients with muscle-invasive bladder cancer [43]. Among 30 patients (median, 66 years) enrolled, 17 and 13 patients underwent Protocol A and B, respectively [43]. After induction chemotherapy, 23 patients achieved CR [43]. Five (17%) of 7 patients without CR underwent salvage cystectomy [43]. Overall, 28 patients (93%) completed the protocol treatment [43]. Of 22 patients who completed CCRT, 1 had recurrence with carcinoma in situ and 3 had distant metastases [43]. After a median follow-up of 47 months, overall and progression-free survival rate for all patients were 77% and 54% at 3 years, respectively [43]. Of 19 surviving patients, 15 (79%) retained functioning bladders [43].

Koga et al. [17] evaluated oncological outcomes of muscle-invasive bladder cancer (MIBC) patients who were treated with a selective bladder-sparing protocol consisting of induction low-dose chemoradiotherapy (LCRT) plus partial cystectomy (PC) with pelvic lymph node dissection [17]. Of the 183 patients, 87 (48%) achieved a clinical complete response after LCRT and 65 (36%) met the PC criteria; 46 (25%) patients actually underwent PC, 86 (47%) had RC, and the remaining 51 (28%) had neither PC, nor RC [17]. Histological examination of the 46 PC specimens showed residual muscle-invasive disease in three (7%). Overall, 5-year overall survival and CSS rates were 64% and 71%, respectively (median follow-up for survivors of 45 months) [17]. In the 46 PC patients, neither MIBC, nor pelvic recurrence was observed; 5-year CSS and MRFS rates were both 100% [17]. In 13 non-PC patients who achieved a complete response after LCRT and who met PC criteria but declined PC, 5-year CSS and MRFS rates were 74% and 81%, respectively; CSS and MRFS were significantly better in the PC group than in the non-PC group (p = 0.025 and 0.002, respectively) [17].

Azria et al. [44] presented the long-term results of a phase 1 clinical trial to assess the association of twice-weekly gemcitabine with CDDP and radiation therapy [44]. The overall and disease-specific 5-year survival rates were 62% and 77%, respectively [44]. Among the patients who received the complete treatment, bladder-intact survival was 76% at 5 years, and the median overall survival was 69.6 months [44].

Ishioka et al. [45] evaluated bladder preservation protocol by radical TUR-Bt and subsequent concurrent chemoradiotherapy in muscle invasive bladder cancer [45]. Among 24 evaluable cases, pathological complete response was achieved in 13 cases (50%) and residual tumours were noted in 11 cases (pT1 in 9 and pT2 in 2) [45]. During follow-up period up to 69.8 months, invasive recurrence was observed in 2 cases, superficial recurrence was noted in 5 patients and distant metastasis without evidence of local recurrence was noted in 4 cases [45]. Overall bladder preservation rate was 92%.

Tester et al. [46] evaluated Phase 2 study of a combined chemoradiotherapy program with selective bladder preservation in the management of patients with invasive bladder cancer [46]. Thus, a total of 37 of 91 patients (40%) required cystectomy [46]. The 4-year cumulative risk of invasive local failure (which includes induction failures) was 43% (95% CI, 33–53%) [46]. The 4-year actuarial risk of distant metastasis was 22% (95% CI, 13–31%) [46]. The 4-year actuarial survival rate of the entire group was 62% (95% CI, 52–72%) [46]. The 4-year actuarial rate of survival with bladder intact was 44% (95% CI, 34–54%) [46].

Cervek et al. [47] evaluated the effect and feasibility of bladder-sparing treatment by transurethral resection (TUR) and sequential chemoradiotherapy in patients with biopsy-proven invasive bladder cancer [47]. Complete response after TUR and chemotherapy was achieved in 52% of patients [47]. After a median follow-up of 42 months, 52 of 75 patients (69%) selected for bladder preservation were without evidence of disease in the bladder [47]. Freedom from local failure in complete responders to chemotherapy was 80% [95% confidence interval (CI), 69–91%] at 4 years [47]. The actuarial survival of the entire group was 58% (95% CI, 47–69%), whereas the survival rate with the bladder intact was 45% (95% CI, 34–56%) at 4 years [47]. Survival was significantly better in patients who responded to chemotherapy (79%) than in non-responders (35%, p < 0.0001) [47]. There was no significant difference in survival between non-responders who underwent cystectomy and non-responders who completed treatment with radiotherapy (approximately 30% at 3 years) [47].

67.2.6 Low Dose Chemoradiotherapy Outcomes in Muscle Invasive Bladder Cancer

Koga et al. [48] evaluated the clinical outcomes of patients with muscle-invasive bladder cancer treated with a prospective institutional protocol composed of induction low-dose chemoradiotherapy (LCRT) plus partial or radical cystectomy [48]. LCRT-related toxicity of grade 3 or greater was rare (3%). Of 97 eligible patients, 41 (42%) had a complete response, 29 (30%) a partial response, 24 (25%) had stable disease, and 3 (4%) progressive disease [48]. Of the 97 patients, 19, underwent partial cystectomy, and 58 underwent radical cystectomy, 2 underwent transurethral resection of the bladder tumour, and 18 did not undergo surgery [48]. The 5-year overall survival and cancer-specific survival (CSS) rate was 66% and 74%, respectively [48]. The median follow-up was 43 months (range 3–126). On multivariate analysis, the response to LCRT had the strongest effect on CSS, and CSS was clearly stratified by the response to LCRT (p < 0.0001), with a 5-year CSS rate of 100% for the 41 patients with a complete response [48].

Radiotherapy vs. Chemoradiation in Muscle Invasive Bladder Cancer [35] investigated the feasibility of preoperative low-dose chemoradiotherapy, 50 patients with localized muscle-invasive bladder cancer (T2–T4) were treated with concurrent cisplatin (100 mg/body × 2 courses) and pelvic irradiation (40 Gy) [35]. Among 20 patients (40%) who achieved clinical complete regression, 11 with solitary tumour underwent partial cystectomy because of advanced age, poor condition of the patients, or a reluctance to have radical surgery [35]. Radical cystectomy was carried out in the remaining 39 cases (complete regression 9, partial regression 30) [35]. Pathologic T0 response (no residual tumour) was achieved in 18 (36%) of all the cases. Median follow-up was 19 months (range 2–59 months) [35]. Estimated 3-year disease-free survival was 75% for all patients and 100% for T0 responders [35]. Local recurrence (2 patients) or distant metastasis (6 patients) developed in 8 of 32 patients with pathologic persistent tumour.

As part of a multicenter, phase 3 trial [49] randomly assigned 360 patients with muscle-invasive bladder cancer to undergo radiotherapy with or without synchronous chemotherapy [49]. The regimen consisted of fluorouracil during fractions 1–5 and 16–20 of radiotherapy and mitomycin C on day 1 [49]. Patients were also randomly assigned to undergo either whole-bladder radiotherapy or modified-volume radiotherapy (in which the volume of bladder receiving full-dose radiotherapy was reduced). At 2 years, rates of locoregional disease-free survival were 67% (95% confidence interval [CI], 59–74) in the chemoradiotherapy group and 54% (95% CI, 46–62) in the radiotherapy group [49]. Five-year rates of overall survival were 48% (95% CI, 40–55) in the chemoradiotherapy group and 35% (95% CI, 28–43) in the radiotherapy group (hazard ratio, 0.82; 95% CI, 0.63–1.09; p = 0.16) [49]. Grade 3 or 4 adverse events were slightly more common in the chemoradiotherapy group than in the radiotherapy group during treatment (36.0% vs. 27.5%, p = 0.07) but not during follow-up (8.3% vs. 15.7%, p = 0.07) [49].

Ghate et al. [50] compared outcomes between radiation therapy and chemoradiotherapy [50]. The most common regimens were single-agent Cisplatin (57%, 230/402), single-agent Carboplatin (31%, 125/402) and 5-FU/Mitomycin (4%, 17/402) [50]. Factors associated with CRT include younger age (p < 0.001), lower comorbidity (p = 0.001), and geographic region (range 14–89%, p < 0.001) [50]. Five year CSS and OS among CRT cases were 45% (95% CI 39–51%) and 35% (95% CI 30–40%) [50]. On adjusted analyses CRT was associated with superior survival compared to RT (CSS HR 0.70, 95% CI 0.59–0.84; OS HR 0.74, 95% CI 0.64–0.85); results were consistent on propensity score analysis [50]. There was significant improvement in survival of all RT-treated cases (irrespective or chemotherapy delivery) in 2009–2013 compared to 1999–2003 (CSS HR 0.77, 95% CI 0.61–0.97; OS HR 0.82, 95% CI 0.69–0.98) [50].

Byun et al. [51] evaluated survival rates and prognostic factors related to treatment outcomes after bladder preserving therapy including transurethral resection of bladder tumour, radiotherapy (RT) with or without concurrent chemotherapy in bladder cancer with a curative intent [51]. Thirty patients (60%) showed complete response and 13 (26%) a partial response [51]. All patients could have their own bladder preserved [51]. Five-year overall survival (OS) rate was 37.2%, and the 5-year disease-free survival (DFS) rate was 30.2% [51]. In multivariate analysis, tumor grade and CCRT were statistically significant in OS [51].

The current study was conducted to compare the overall survival (OS) of concurrent chemoradiotherapy (CCRT) versus radiotherapy (RT) alone in elderly patients (those aged ≥80 years) with muscle-invasive bladder cancer (MIBC) [52]. A total of 1369 patients who were treated with RT from 2004 through 2013 met eligibility criteria: 739 patients (54%) received RT alone and 630 patients (46%) received CCRT [52]. When comparing CCRT with RT alone, the 2-year OS rate was 56% versus 42% (p < 0.0001), respectively [52]. Multivariable analysis demonstrated that CCRT (hazard ratio [HR], 0.74; 95% confidence interval [95% CI], 0.65–0.84 [p < 0.0001]) and a higher RT dose (HR, 0.78; 95% CI, 0.67–0.90 [p < 0.001]) were associated with improved OS [52]. T4 disease was associated with worse OS (HR, 1.42; 95% CI, 1.15–1.76 [p = 0.001]). After using 1-to-1 propensity score matching, there remained an OS benefit for the use of CCRT (HR, 0.77; 95% CI, 0.67–0.90 [p < 0.001]) [52].

67.2.7 Chemotherapy vs. Chemoradiotherapy Outcomes in Muscle Invasive Bladder Cancer

Haque et al. [5] evaluated national practice patterns and outcomes of chemotherapy (CT) versus Chemoradiotherapy (CRT) to elucidate the optimal therapy for this patient population. Of 1783 total patients, 1388 (77.8%) underwent CT alone, and 395 (22.2%) CRT [5]. Although patients receiving CRT tended to be of higher socioeconomic status, they were more likely older (p = 0.053), higher T stage, N1 (versus N2) disease, squamous histology, and treated at a non-academic center (p < 0.05) [5]. On Cox multivariate analysis, receipt of CRT was independently associated with improved survival (p < 0.001) [5]. Outcome improvements with CRT persisted on evaluation of propensity-matched populations (p < 0.001) [5].

67.2.8 The Role of Neoadjuvant Chemotherapy Pre Chemoradiation

Jiang et al. [53] examined the role of NAC in fit, cisplatin-eligible patients who opt for bladder preservation warrants further evaluation [53] Most completed planned NAC (95%) [53]. All patients completed external-beam radiotherapy, and 84% completed at least 60% of the planned concurrent weekly cisplatin doses [53]. Two-year OS and disease-specific survival rates were 74% (95% confidence interval, 57.7–84.9) and 88% (95% confidence interval, 78.5–98.1), respectively [53]. Two-year bladder-intact disease-free survival was 64% [53]. Salvage cystectomy was performed in 14% [53]. Distant relapse occurred in 11%, and 9% died of metastatic disease [53]. OS was associated with baseline hydronephrosis and with bladder-intact disease-free survival with residual disease on cystoscopy [53].

Tunio et al. [54] reviewed neoadjuvant chemotherapy prior to concurrent chemo-radiation in muscle-invasive bladder cancer [54]. Out of 43, 32 patients (78.04%) achieved CR at time of cystoscopic evaluation [54]. Six patients who did not achieve CR (14.63%) underwent salvage cystectomies, remaining were not operable [54]. Overall survival was 61% [54]. Local recurrences were seen in 3 patients (10%)

(2pT1, 1pT2), distant metastases were seen in 2 patients (6.6%); 27/41 were alive, of whom 23 (56.1%) were retaining intact diseasefree bladders [54]. The Tumour stage, incomplete TURBT and presence of hydronephrosis were important prognostic factors (log-rank p values 0.0001, 0.0001 and 0.001 respectively) [54].

67.2.9 Neoadjuvant Chemotherapy vs. Concomitant Chemoradiation for Muscle Invasive Bladder Cancer

George et al. [55] described the outcome of patients with muscle-invasive bladder carcinoma treated with neoadjuvant chemotherapy vs. chemoradiotherapy alone [55]. Of the 22 patients who received neoadjuvant chemotherapy, 18 (82%) had received two or more cycles; 51 (85%) of the 60 patients received the concomitant chemotherapy as planned. Radiotherapy was completed in 56 patients [55]. Twenty-eight patients developed relapse either locally (14 did not achieve a complete local response after chemoradiotherapy and 6 had true local relapse during follow-up) or at distant sites [55]. The actuarial 5-year disease-specific survival and freedom from local and distant relapse rate was 54% and 42%, respectively [55]. The actuarial local control rate with an intact bladder was 56% at 5 years [55]. When stratified according to stage and grade, patients with Stage T2–T3, grade 2 tumors had a statistically significantly better chance of remaining relapse free than did the others (p = 0.045) [55]. Salvage cystectomy (n = 11) for isolated local failure in this population achieved limited results [55].

67.2.10 Chemoradiation in the Elderly or Unfit with Muscle Invasive Bladder Cancer

Maebayashi et al. [56] examined whether the feasibility of concurrent use of intra-arterial chemotherapy (IAC) with RT for MIBC in elderly patients [56]. The 2- and 5-year overall survival rates were 80% and 66.7% in the IACRT group [56]. The 1- and 2-year survival rates in the RT-alone group were 50% and 25%, respectively [56]. Regarding late adverse events, only one patient experienced grade 2 genitourinary toxicity [56].

Arias et al. [57] examined a protocol with methotrexate, vinblastine, doxorubicin, and cisplatin (M-VAC regimen) and radiotherapy for these patients [57]. Traditionally, age is an impacting factor, often to the exclusion of the older patients from the oncologic protocols that are considered to be more aggressive [57]. The authors analysed 20 patients (age >70 years) who were treated during this period with the same protocol as the authors' other patients [57]. Tumour response after a dose of 45 Gy included 11 complete responses (55%), 5 partial responses (25%), and 4 nonresponses (20%) [57]. Overall survival was 75%, 34%, and 27% in the second, third, and fifth years of follow-up, respectively [57]. Cause specific survival was 79%, 54%, and 38%, respectively [57]. Survival for patients with complete response was 100%, 60%, and 48%, respectively. Severe toxicity was uncommon, with the most frequent toxicities being leukopenia and cystitis [57]. No treatment-related death occurred with either treatment protocol [57].

Mayadagli et al. [58] observed the outcome of maximal transurethral resection of bladder tumour (TURBT) followed by induction chemotherapy and concurrent chemoradiotherapy in medically inoperable patients with bladder cancer [58]. Radiologically, complete and partial response rates were 60% and 36.7%, while cystoscopically they were 40% and 30%, respectively [58]. Local progression (4 cases) and distant metastasis (11 cases) were noted [58]. Median overall survival and progression free survival were 32 and 21 months, respectively [58]. One -and 2-year overall survival and progression-free survival rates were 97.60% and 83.49%, respectively [58]. Vikram et al. [59] studied rapidly alternating chemotherapy and radiotherapy in patients unfit for cystectomy [59]. There was 1 treatment-related death (5% of patients), but otherwise the acute toxicity was relatively mild [59]. Cystoscopy 1 month after chemoradiotherapy did not reveal invasive cancer in any patient [59]. Subsequent cystoscopies detected recurrent invasive cancer in 3 patients after 30, 44, and 82 months, respectively [59]. The observed survival rate after 5 years was 37%, the cause specific survival rate was 63%, the metastasis free rate was 71%, and the local control rate was 80% [59]. Eighty-four percent of patients had normal bladder function [59].

Demirci et al. [60] determined the efficacy and the toxicity of low dose weekly gemcitabine with radiotherapy, in medically unfit or refused surgery muscle-invasive bladder cancer (BC) patients [60]. A complete response was achieved in 12 patients (80%) [60]. Median progression free survival and overall survival were 15 months (range, 7–23 months) and 18 months (range not calculated), respectively [60]. Local recurrence was found in 3 patients (20%) and distant recurrence was found in 5 patients (33.3%) for the entire group [60]. While salvage surgery was performed on 1 patient, salvage chemotherapy was delivered for 4 patients [60]. Treatment was well tolerated, there was no treatment interruption or instances of toxic death [60]. A serious toxicity (grade 3) cystitis was seen in only 1 patient [60].

Chen et al. [61] investigated the tolerance and efficacy of a modified concurrent chemoradiation (CCRT) protocol for patients with invasive bladder cancer "unfit" for radical cystectomy [61]. Seventy-four percent of patients (17/23) completed the CCRT protocol. Radiation Therapy Oncology Group (RTOG) Grade 3 acute toxicities were observed in 4 patients, which included leucopenia, vomiting, genitourinary (GU) tract infection, and diarrhea [61]. No treatment-related deaths occurred during the CCRT period. RTOG Grade 3 or more late complications were observed in 3 patients; one of them died of radiation cystitis superimposed with GU infection. Of the 18 patients whose response to CCRT was evaluated, a complete tumour response was documented in 16 patients (89%) [61]. With a median follow-up of 3 years, the 3-year overall survival (OS) and disease-free survival (DFS) for all patients was 69% and 65% respectively [61]. Meanwhile, the 3-year overall and DFS rates for patients who completed CCRT vs. those who did not complete CCRT were 82% vs. 33% and 75% vs. 33%, respectively (p = 0.18 for OS and p = 0.04 for DFS) [61].

67.2.11 Female Outcomes with Chemoradiotherapy in Muscle Invasive Bladder Cancer

Kachnic et al. [62] assessed female outcomes with muscle-invading bladder carcinoma treated with chemoradiotherapy [62]. All 21 patients have full urinary continence and no dysuria [62]. Nineteen report unchanged or improved bladder capacity and function [62]. No patient reported loss of bowel continence [62]. Of the five women who were sexually active, two report an increase in intercourse frequency and one noted a decrease [62]. There is no decrease in intercourse satisfaction or orgasm, and no dyspareunia or vaginal bleeding was noted [62]. Eleven patients reported high levels of anxiety related to their bladder cancer before treatment [62]. This was significantly reduced or absent in 9 of 11 after treatment [62]. Actuarial overall survival for all 42 women was 58% at 5 years [62]. Actuarial overall survival with an intact bladder was 47% at 5 years [62].

67.2.12 Patient Reported Outcome Measures in Chemoradiation Therapy

Thompson et al. [63] assessed patient reported outcome measures in concurrent chemoradiation therapy with gemcitabine (GemX) for muscle invasive bladder cancer following neoadjuvant chemotherapy (neoGemX) [63]. The radiation therapy completion rate was 95%, and 96% of patients completed at least 3 cycles of gemcitabine [63]. Bowel toxicity of grade 3 or greater was reported in 7 of 38 patients (18%) in the neoGemX group and 5 of 25 (20%) in the GemX group [63]. Three GemX and two neoGemX patients had grade 3 or greater urinary toxicity [63]. Forty-nine patients completed questionnaires and were included in the analysis. Scores on the late effects in normal tissues-subjective, objective, management, and analytic scales showed an expected peak by week 4 of treatment [63]. There was no statistically significant difference between mean scores at baseline and 12 months after treatment completion or between the neoGemX and GemX groups [63].

Lagrange et al. [64] evaluated bladder preservation and functional quality after concurrent chemoradiotherapy for muscle-invasive cancer in 53 patients included in a Phase II trial [64]. Thirty-two percent of patients had T2a tumors, 46% T2b, 16% T3, and 6% T4 [64]. A visibly complete transurethral resection was possible in 66%. Median follow-up was 8 years. Bladder was preserved in 67% (95% confidence interval, 52–79%) of patients [64]. Overall survival was 36% (95% confidence interval, 23–49%) at 8 years for all patients, and 45% (28–61%) for the 36 patients suitable for surgery [64]. Satisfactory bladder function, according to LENT-SOMA, was reported for 100% of patients with preserved bladder and locally controlled disease 6–36 months after the beginning of treatment [64]. Satisfactory bladder function was reported for 35% of patients before treatment and for 43%, 57%, and 29%, respectively, at 6, 18, and 36 months [64].

Huddart et al. [65] conducted largest randomised trial of bladder-sparing treatment for muscle-invasive bladder cancer, demonstrated improvement of local control and bladder cancer-specific survival from the addition of concomitant 5-fluorouracil and mitomycin C to radiotherapy. The aim was to assess health related quality of life. Data were available for 331 (92%) and 204 (93%) participants at baseline and for 192 (54%) and 114 (52%) at 12 months for the chemotherapy and radiotherapy comparisons, respectively. HRQoL declined at EoT (BLCS -5.06 [99% confidence interval: -6.12 to -4.00, $p < 0.001$]; overall FACT-B TOTAL score -8.22 [-10.76 to -5.68, $p < 0.01$]), recovering to baseline at 6 months and remaining similar to baseline subsequently. There was no significant difference between randomised groups at any time point.

67.2.13 Adjuvant Chemotherapy vs. Chemoradiotherapy for Muscle Invasive Bladder Cancer

Feng et al. [66] investigated bladder preservation therapy with a well-tolerated strategy, 30 patients with bladder cancer underwent concomitant chemoradiotherapy with weekly carboplatin [66]. The 2-year overall survival was 75% for all patients, 43% and 95% for patients without adjuvant chemotherapy or with adjuvant chemotherapy separately [66]. This strategy was well tolerated with 7% of Grade 3/4 late bladder toxicity.

67.2.14 Chemoradiation in Advanced Bladder Cancer

Wu et al. [67] evaluated the feasibility of concurrent chemoradiotherapy (CCRT) in very advanced bladder cancer (stage IV) and further analysed the prognostic factors in these patients [67]. By August 2012, the estimated median progression-free survival (PFS), cancer-specific survival, and overall survival (OS) were 25.7, 64.3 and 35.8 months, respectively; the complete response (CR) rate was 68.8% [67]. Both clinical stage and CR following CCRT, were independent prognostic factors for PFS, cancer-specific survival, and OS [67]. Patients with stage IV disease who achieved CR had significantly better PFS (log-rank $p = 0.01$), cancer-specific survival (log-rank $p = 0.01$), and OS (log-rank $p = 0.01$) than those with stage II/III disease but no CR [67]. The absence of hydronephrosis was the only factor predictive of CR after CCRT (odd ratio, 4.21; $p = 0.04$) [67].

67.2.15 Side Effects of Chemoradiotherapy in Muscle Invasive Bladder Cancer

Gupta et al. [68] assessed outcome of chemoradiotherapy for organ preservation in muscle invasive bladder cancer [68]. Eleven patients have cystitis (5 Gr I, 4 Gr II and 2 Gr III). Five patients have myelosuppression. Ten patients have acute gastrointestinal toxicity (5 Gr-I, 4 Gr-II, 1 Gr-III) [68]. The DFS at 42 months was 54%. Out of 39 patients 3 were lost to follow up (2 in partial bladder group and 1 in whole bladder group) [68]. Out of 36 patients 24 (66.6%) are disease free, 4 (11.1%) patients had recurrence for which 2 underwent salvage cystectomy whereas 2 patients received palliative chemotherapy [68]. Five patients developed distant metastases (4 bone and 1 brain metastasis) [68].

Iwai et al. [69] compared rates of early morbidity after radical cystectomy in patients treated with or without induction chemoradiotherapy (CRT) [69]. Eighty-seven patients underwent radical cystectomy following chemoradiotherapy (chemoradiotherapy group) while the remaining 106 primarily underwent radical cystectomy (no chemoradiotherapy group) [69]. No Grade 4–5 complication was observed [69]. Overall, 118 patients (61%) experienced 36 major and 122 minor complications [69]. There was no significant difference in the incidence of overall complications between the chemoradiotherapy and no chemoradiotherapy groups (67% vs. 57%) [69]. Overall urinary anastomosis-related complications and major gastrointestinal complications, most of which were Grade 3 ileus, were more frequent in the chemoradiotherapy group than the no chemoradiotherapy group (11% vs. 2%, p = 0.007; and 14% vs. 4%, p = 0.02; respectively) [69]. Multivariate analysis identified induction chemoradiotherapy as an independent risk factor for overall urinary anastomosis-related complications (relative risk 6.0, p = 0.01) but not for major gastrointestinal complications [69].

67.2.16 Chemoradiation in Whole Bladder vs. Partial Bladder Treatment

Kang et al. [70] examined experience using definitive chemoradiation via whole bladder (WB) and partial bladder (PB) treatment in muscle-invasive bladder cancer [70]. Freedom from local recurrence was 86% at 2 years (PB 100%, WB 77%) [70]. Overall survival was 80% at 1 year (PB 88%, WB 75%), and 55% at 2 years (PB 70%, WB 48%, p = 0.38) [70]. Failure was predominantly distant [70]. Toxicities were minimal (3 late grade 3 ureteral, 1 acute grade 4 renal), and all resolved [70]. No cystectomies were performed for toxicity [70].

67.2.17 Mortality Outcomes in Chemoradiotherapy for Muscle Invasive Bladder Cancer

Haque et al. [7] assessed short term mortality in radical cystectomy (RC) vs. Chemoradiotherapy (CRT) [7]. Of 16,658 patients, 15,208 (91.3%) underwent RC and 1450 (8.7%) CRT [7]. Crude rates of post-treatment mortality at 30 days were 2.7% versus 0.6% (p < 0.001) and at 90 days were 7.5% versus 4.5% (p = 0.017) for patients treated with RC and CRT, respectively [7]. When stratifying by age, worse 30- and 90-day mortality with RC was observed for patients aged ≥76 years [7].

Kaufman et al. [71] evaluated the safety, tolerance, protocol completion rate, tumour response rate, and patient survival of chemoradiotherapy for patients with muscle-invasive operable bladder cancer [71]. A total of 80 patients met protocol eligibility [71]. TCI resulted in 26% developing grade 3–4 acute toxicity, mainly gastrointestinal (25%) [71]. During consolidation TCI, grade 3–4 acute toxicity, all transient, was reported in 8%. Four cycles of adjuvant chemotherapy were completed per protocol or with minor deviations in 70% of the patients [71]. Adjuvant treatment was associated with grade 3 toxicity in 46% and grade 4 in 26% [71]. One patient had a fatal haemorrhagic stroke [71]. Late bladder radiation toxicity was evaluated in 53 patients with ≥2 years of follow-up. Of these 53 patients, 3 experienced self-limited, late grade 3 bladder toxicity [71]. The postinduction complete response rate was 81% (65/80), 36 of the 80 patients died (22 of bladder cancer) [71]. At a median follow-up of 49.4 months, the actuarial 5-year overall and disease-specific survival rate was 56% and 71%, respectively [71].

Orsatti et al. [72] determined whether chemoradiation in patients with muscle invasive bladder cancer, allowing a better quality of life as part of a phase 2 trial [72]. A clinical complete response was observed in 57 patients (81%), partial response in 7 patients (10%), and a nonresponse in 6 patients (9%) [72]. At a median follow-up of 45 months, 33 patients (47%) were alive and free of tumour [72]. The 6-year overall survival and progression-free survival was 42% and 40%, respectively [72]. Systemic side effects were mild, while a moderate or severe local toxicity was observed in 14 patients and 13 patients (about 20%), respectively [72].

67.2.18 International Reviews and Guidelines on Chemoradiation in Muscle Invasive Bladder Cancer

Leow et al. [73] provided a comprehensive overview and update of the Joint Société Internationale d'Urologie-International Consultation on Urological Diseases (SIU-ICUD) Consultation on Bladder Cancer for muscle-invasive presumably node-negative bladder cancer (MIBC) [73]. Radical cystectomy (RC) is the standard of care for MIBC patients considered to be surgical candidates [73]. While associated with substantial morbidity and mortality, this has been mitigated with improved technique, minimally invasive technology, and better perioperative care pathways (e.g., enhanced recovery after surgery) [73]. Neoadjuvant (NA) cisplatin-based combination chemotherapy improves overall survival and should be offered to eligible ≥cT2N0 patients [73]. Adjuvant (Adj) cisplatin-based combination chemotherapy may be considered, particularly for pT3–4 and/or pN+ disease without prior NA chemotherapy [73]. Trimodal bladder-preserving treatment via maximum transurethral resection of bladder tumour followed by concurrent chemoradiation is safe and, when combined with early salvage RC for recurrence, offers long-term survival rates in selected patients comparable to RC [73]. Immunotherapy is still experimental and is given either alone or in combination with chemotherapy and/or radiation [73].

Milowsky et al. [74] ASCO endorsed the European Association of Urology guideline on muscle-invasive (MIBC) and metastatic bladder cancer [74]. Multidisciplinary care for patients with MIBC and metastatic bladder cancer is critical [74]. Chemoradiotherapy may be offered as an alternative to cystectomy in appropriately selected patients with MIBC and in some patients for whom cystec-tomy is not an option [74]. Metastatic disease should be treated with cisplatin-containing combination chemotherapy or with carboplatin combination chemotherapy or single agents in patients ineligible for cisplatin [74].

References

1. Cohen J. Weighted kappa: nominal scale agreement with provision for scaled disagreement or partial credit. Psychol Bull. 1968;70(4):213–20. [in English].
2. Moher D, Liberati A, Tetzlaff J, Altman DG. "Preferred Reporting Items for Systematic Reviews and Meta-Analyses: The Prisma Statement." [In English]. BMJ (Online) 339, no. 7716 (08 Aug 2009):332–36.
3. Mays N, Pope C, Popay J. "Systematically Reviewing Qualitative and Quantitative Evidence to Inform Management and Policy-Making in the Health Field." [In English]. Journal of Health Services Research and Policy 10, no. SUPPL. 1 (July 2005):6–20.
4. Haresh KP, Julka PK, Sharma DN, Rath GK, Prabhakar R, Seth A. A prospective study eval-uating surgery and chemo radiation in muscle invasive bladder cancer. J Cancer Res Ther. 2007;3(2):81–5. [in English].
5. Haque W, Verma V, Butler EB, Teh BS. Radical cystectomy versus chemoradiation for muscle-invasive bladder cancer: impact of treatment facility and sociodemographics. Anticancer Res. 2017;37(10):5603–8. [in English].
6. Kaushik D, Wang H, Michalek J, Liss MA, Liu Q, Jha RP, Svatek RS, Mansour AM. Chemoradiation vs radical cystectomy for muscle-invasive bladder cancer: a propen-sity score-weighted comparative analysis using the national cancer database. Urology. 2019;133:164–74. [in English].
7. Haque W, Verma V, Aghazadeh M, Darcourt J, Butler EB, Teh BS. Short-term mortality associ-ated with definitive chemoradiotherapy versus radical cystectomy for muscle-invasive bladder cancer. Clin Genitourin Cancer. 2019;17(5):e1069–79. [in English].
8. Ritch CR, Balise R, Prakash NS, Alonzo D, Almengo K, Alameddine M, Venkatramani V, et al. Propensity matched comparative analysis of survival following chemoradiation or radical cystectomy for muscle-invasive bladder cancer. BJU Int. 2018;121(5):745–51. [in English].
9. Gofrit ON, Nof R, Meirovitz A, Pode D, Frank S, Katz R, Shapiro A, et al. Radical cys-tectomy vs. chemoradiation in T2-4an0m0 bladder cancer: a case-control study. Urol Oncol. 2015;33(1):19.e1–5. [in English].
10. Lin HY, Ye H, Kernen KM, Hafron JM, Krauss DJ. National cancer database comparison of radical cystectomy vs chemoradiotherapy for muscle-invasive bladder cancer: implications of using clinical vs pathologic staging. Cancer Med. 2018;7(11):5370–81. [in English].
11. Nagao K, Hara T, Nishijima J, Shimizu K, Fujii N, Kobayashi K, Kawai Y, et al. The efficacy of trimodal chemoradiotherapy with cisplatin as a bladder-preserving strategy for the treat-ment of muscle-invasive bladder cancer. Urol Int. 2017;99(4):446–52. [in English].
12. Boustani J, Bertaut A, Galsky MD, Rosenberg JE, Bellmunt J, Powles T, Recine F, et al. Radical cystectomy or bladder preservation with radiochemotherapy in elderly patients with muscle-invasive bladder cancer: retrospective international study of cancers of the urothelial tract (Risc) investigators. Acta Oncol. 2018;57(4):491–7. [in English].
13. Ikeda M, Matsumoto K, Nishi M, Tabata K, Fujita T, Ishiyama H, Hayakawa K, Iwamura M. Comparison of radical cystectomy and chemoradiotherapy in patients with locally advanced bladder cancer. Asian Pac J Cancer Prev. 2014;15(16):6519–24. [in English].
14. Peyromaure M, Slama J, Beuzeboc P, Ponvert D, Debré B, Zerbib M. Concurrent chemo-radiotherapy for clinical stage T2 bladder cancer: report of a single institution. Urology. 2004;63(1):73–7. [in English].

15. Sanguineti G, Orsatti M, Sormani MP, Canobbio L, Curotto A, Tognoni P, Giudici S, et al. Predictive factors for outcome in invasive bladder cancer treated with alternating chemoradiotherapy. Cancer J Sci Am. 1997;3(4):213–23. [in English].

16. Yoshida S, Koga F, Tatokoro M, Kawakami S, Fujii Y, Kumagai J, Neckers L, Kihara K. Low-dose Hsp90 inhibitors tumor-selectively sensitize bladder cancer cells to chemoradiotherapy. Cell Cycle. 2011;10(24):4291–9. [in English].

17. Koga F, Fujii Y, Masuda H, Numao N, Yokoyama M, Ishioka J, Saito K, Kawakami S, Kihara K. Pathology-based risk stratification of muscle-invasive bladder cancer patients undergoing cystectomy for persistent disease after induction chemoradiotherapy in bladder-sparing approaches. BJU Int. 2012;110(6 Pt B):E203–8. [in English].

18. Weiner AB, Desai AS, Meeks JJ. Tumor location may predict adverse pathology and survival following definitive treatment for bladder cancer: a national cohort study. Eur Urol Oncol. 2019;2(3):304–10. [in English].

19. Koga F, Takemura K, Fukushima H. Biomarkers for predicting clinical outcomes of chemoradiation-based bladder preservation therapy for muscle-invasive bladder cancer. Int J Mol Sci. 2018;19(9):2777. [in English].

20. Tanabe K, Yoshida S, Koga F, Inoue M, Kobayashi S, Ishioka J, Tamura T, et al. High Ki-67 expression predicts favorable survival in muscle-invasive bladder cancer patients treated with chemoradiation-based bladder-sparing protocol. Clin Genitourin Cancer. 2015;13(4):e243–51. [in English].

21. Desai NB, Scott SN, Zabor EC, Cha EK, Hreiki J, Sfakianos JP, Ramirez R, et al. Genomic characterization of response to chemoradiation in urothelial bladder cancer. Cancer. 2016;122(23):3715–23. [in English].

22. Tanaka H, Yoshida S, Koga F, Toda K, Yoshimura R, Nakajima Y, Sugawara E, et al. Impact of immunohistochemistry-based subtypes in muscle-invasive bladder cancer on response to chemoradiation therapy. Int J Radiat Oncol Biol Phys. 2018;102(5):1408–16. [in English].

23. Inoue M, Koga F, Yoshida S, Tamura T, Fujii Y, Ito E, Kihara K. Significance of Erbb2 overexpression in therapeutic resistance and cancer-specific survival in muscle-invasive bladder cancer patients treated with chemoradiation-based selective bladder-sparing approach. Int J Radiat Oncol Biol Phys. 2014;90(2):303–11. [in English].

24. Shinohara A, Sakano S, Hinoda Y, Nishijima J, Kawai Y, Misumi T, Nagao K, Hara T, Matsuyama H. Association of Tp53 and Mdm2 polymorphisms with survival in bladder cancer patients treated with chemoradiotherapy. Cancer Sci. 2009;100(12):2376–82. [in English].

25. Keck B, Wach S, Taubert H, Zeiler S, Ott OJ, Kunath F, Hartmann A, et al. Neuropilin-2 and its ligand Vegf-C predict treatment response after transurethral resection and radiochemotherapy in bladder cancer patients. Int J Cancer. 2015;136(2):443–51. [in English].

26. Koga F, Yoshida S, Tatokoro M, Kawakami S, Fujii Y, Kumagai J, Neckers L, Kihara K. Erbb2 and Nfκb overexpression as predictors of chemoradiation resistance and putative targets to overcome resistance in muscle-invasive bladder cancer. PLoS One. 2011;6(11):e27616. [in English].

27. Nicholson J, Jevons SJ, Groselj B, Ellermann S, Konietzny R, Kerr M, Kessler BM, Kiltie AE. E3 ligase Ciap2 mediates downregulation of Mre11 and radiosensitization in response to hdac inhibition in bladder cancer. Cancer Res. 2017;77(11):3027–39. [in English].

28. Abe T, Yoshioka T, Sato M, Mori N, Sekii K, Itatani H. [Bladder preservation using chemoradiation therapy for locally invasive bladder cancer]. Nihon Hinyokika Gakkai Zasshi. 2011;102(1):14–22. [in Japanese].

29. Yoshida S, Koga F, Kobayashi S, Ishii C, Tanaka H, Tanaka H, Komai Y, et al. Role of diffusion-weighted magnetic resonance imaging in predicting sensitivity to chemoradiotherapy in muscle-invasive bladder cancer. Int J Radiat Oncol Biol Phys. 2012;83(1):e21–7. [in English].

30. Coen JJ, Zhang P, Saylor PJ, Lee CT, Wu CL, Parker W, Lautenschlaeger T, et al. Bladder preservation with twice-a-day radiation plus fluorouracil/cisplatin or once daily radiation plus gemcitabine for muscle-invasive bladder cancer: Nrg/Rtog 0712-a randomized phase II trial. J Clin Oncol. 2019;37(1):44–51. [in English].

31. Arias F, Domínguez MA, Martínez E, Illarramendi JJ, Miquelez S, Pascual I, Marcos M. Chemoradiotherapy for muscle invading bladder carcinoma. Final report of a single institutional organ-sparing program. Int J Radiat Oncol Biol Phys. 2000;47(2):373–8. [in English].

32. Hussain SA, Stocken DD, Peake DR, Glaholm JG, Zarkar A, Wallace DM, James ND. Long-term results of a phase II study of synchronous chemoradiotherapy in advanced muscle invasive bladder cancer. Br J Cancer. 2004;90(11):2106–11. [in English].

33. Michaelson MD, Hu C, Pham HT, Dahl DM, Lee-Wu C, Swanson GP, Vuky J, et al. A phase 1/2 trial of a combination of paclitaxel and trastuzumab with daily irradiation or paclitaxel alone with daily irradiation after transurethral surgery for noncystectomy candidates with muscle-invasive bladder cancer (Trial Nrg Oncology Rtog 0524). Int J Radiat Oncol Biol Phys. 2017;97(5):995–1001. [in English].

34. Choudhury A, Swindell R, Logue JP, Elliott PA, Livsey JE, Wise M, Symonds P, et al. Phase II study of conformal hypofractionated radiotherapy with concurrent gemcitabine in muscle-invasive bladder cancer. J Clin Oncol. 2011;29(6):733–8. [in English].

35. Kageyama Y, Yokoyama M, Sakai Y, Saito K, Koga F, Yano M, Arai G, et al. Favorable outcome of preoperative low dose chemoradiotherapy against muscle-invasive bladder cancer. Am J Clin Oncol. 2003;26(5):504–7. [in English].

36. Leng J, Akthar AS, Szmulewitz RZ, O'Donnell PH, Sweis RF, Pitroda SP, Smith N, Steinberg GD, Liauw SL. Safety and efficacy of hypofractionated radiotherapy with capecitabine in elderly patients with urothelial carcinoma. Clin Genitourin Cancer. 2019;17(1):e12–8. [in English].

37. De Santis M, Bachner M, Cerveny M, Kametriser G, Steininger T, Königsberg R, Schratter-Sehn A, Sedlmayer F, Dittrich C. Combined chemoradiotherapy with gemcitabine in patients with locally advanced inoperable transitional cell carcinoma of the urinary bladder and/or in patients ineligible for surgery: a phase I trial. Ann Oncol. 2014;25(9):1789–94. [in English].

38. Matsushita M, Kitakaze H, Okada K, Minato N, Mori N, Yoshioka T. [Outcome of bladder preservation using low dose chemoradiation therapy in patients with locally invasive bladder cancer]. Nihon Hinyokika Gakkai Zasshi. 2018;109(2):59–67. [in Japanese].

39. Russell KJ, Boileau MA, Higano C, Collins C, Russell AH, Koh W, Cole SB, Chapman WH, Griffin TW. Combined 5-fluorouracil and irradiation for transitional cell carcinoma of the urinary bladder. Int J Radiat Oncol Biol Phys. 1990;19(3):693–9. [in English].

40. Chauvet B, Félix-Faure C, Davin JL, Berger C, Vincent P, Reboul F. [Treatment of infiltrating cancer of the bladder with cisplatin, fluorouracil, and concurrent radiotherapy: results of a pilot study]. Cancer Radiother. 1998;2(Suppl 1):77s–81s. [in French].

41. Gogna NK, Matthews JH, Turner SL, Mameghan H, Duchesne GM, Spry N, Berry MP, Keller J, Tripcony L. Efficacy and tolerability of concurrent weekly low dose cisplatin during radiation treatment of localised muscle invasive bladder transitional cell carcinoma: a report of two sequential phase II studies from the Trans Tasman Radiation Oncology Group. Radiother Oncol. 2006;81(1):9–17. [in English].

42. Shipley WU, Kaufman DS, Zehr E, Heney NM, Lane SC, Thakral HK, Althausen AF, Zietman AL. Selective bladder preservation by combined modality protocol treatment: long-term outcomes of 190 patients with invasive bladder cancer. Urology. 2002;60(1):62–7; discussion 67–8. [in English].

43. Lin CC, Hsu CH, Cheng JC, Huang CY, Tsai YC, Hsu FM, Huang KH, Cheng AL, Pu YS. Induction cisplatin and fluorouracil-based chemotherapy followed by concurrent chemoradiation for muscle-invasive bladder cancer. Int J Radiat Oncol Biol Phys. 2009;75(2):442–8. [in English].

44. Azria D, Riou O, Rebillard X, Thezenas S, Thuret R, Fenoglietto P, Pouessel D, Culine S. Combined chemoradiation therapy with twice-weekly gemcitabine and cisplatin for organ preservation in muscle-invasive bladder cancer: long-term results of a phase 1 trial. Int J Radiat Oncol Biol Phys. 2014;88(4):853–9. [in English].

45. Ishioka J, Kageyama Y, Ichiyanagi N, Saito Y, Nozu S, Nishida K, Fukuda H, Higashi Y. [Bladder preservation by chemoradiotherapy in combination with radical Tur-Bt in muscle invasive bladder cancer]. Nihon Hinyokika Gakkai Zasshi. 2007;98(6):752–6. [in Japanese].

46. Tester W, Caplan R, Heaney J, Venner P, Whittington R, Byhardt R, True L, Shipley W. Neoadjuvant combined modality program with selective organ preservation for invasive bladder cancer: results of radiation therapy oncology group phase II trial 8802. J Clin Oncol. 1996;14(1):119–26. [in English].

47. Cervek J, Cufer T, Zakotnik B, Kragelj B, Borstnar S, Matos T, Zumer-Pregelj M. Invasive bladder cancer: our experience with bladder sparing approach. Int J Radiat Oncol Biol Phys. 1998;41(2):273–8. [in English].

48. Koga F, Yoshida S, Kawakami S, Kageyama Y, Yokoyama M, Saito K, Fujii Y, Kobayashi T, Kihara K. Low-dose chemoradiotherapy followed by partial or radical cystectomy against muscle-invasive bladder cancer: an intent-to-treat survival analysis. Urology. 2008;72(2):384–8. [in English].

49. James ND, Hussain SA, Hall E, Jenkins P, Tremlett J, Rawlings C, Crundwell M, et al. Radiotherapy with or without chemotherapy in muscle-invasive bladder cancer. N Engl J Med. 2012;366(16):1477–88. [in English].

50. Ghate K, Brennan K, Karim S, Siemens DR, Mackillop WJ, Booth CM. Concurrent chemoradiotherapy for bladder cancer: practice patterns and outcomes in the general population. Radiother Oncol. 2018;127(1):136–42. [in English].

51. Byun SJ, Kim JH, Oh YK, Kim BH. Concurrent chemoradiotherapy improves survival outcome in muscle-invasive bladder cancer. Radiat Oncol J. 2015;33(4):294–300. [in English].

52. Korpics MC, Block AM, Martin B, Hentz C, Gaynor ER, Henry E, Harkenrider MM, Solanki AA. Concurrent chemotherapy is associated with improved survival in elderly patients with bladder cancer undergoing radiotherapy. Cancer. 2017;123(18):3524–31. [in English].

53. Jiang DM, Jiang H, Chung PWM, Zlotta AR, Fleshner NE, Bristow RG, Berlin A, et al. Neoadjuvant chemotherapy before bladder-sparing chemoradiotherapy in patients with non-metastatic muscle-invasive bladder cancer. Clin Genitourin Cancer. 2019;17(1):38–45. [in English].

54. Tunio MA, Hashmi A, Rafi M, Qayyum A, Masood R. Bladder preservation by neoadjuvant chemotherapy followed by concurrent chemoradiation for muscle-invasive bladder cancer: experience at Sindh Institute of Urology & Transplantation (Siut). J Pak Med Assoc. 2011;61(1):6–10. [in English].

55. George L, Bladou F, Bardou VJ, Gravis G, Tallet A, Alzieu C, Serment G, Salem N. Clinical outcome in patients with locally advanced bladder carcinoma treated with conservative multimodality therapy. Urology. 2004;64(3):488–93. [in English].

56. Maebayashi T, Ishibashi N, Aizawa T, Sakaguchi M, Sato K, Matsui T, Yamaguchi K, Takahashi S. Radiotherapy for muscle-invasive bladder cancer in very elderly patients. Anticancer Res. 2016;36(9):4763–9. [in English].

57. Arias F, Dueñas M, Martínez E, Domínguez MA, Illarramendi JJ, Villafranca E, Tejedor M, et al. Radical chemoradiotherapy for elderly patients with bladder carcinoma invading muscle. Cancer. 1997;80(1):115–20. [in English].

58. Mayadagli A, Kocak M, Demir O, Karabulut Gul S, Ozkan A, Parlak C, Yaprak G, Gumus M. Elective bladder preservation with multimodality treatment for bladder cancer. J Buon. 2012;17(3):483–9. [in English].

59. Vikram B, Chadha M, Malamud SC, Hecht H, Grabstald H. Rapidly alternating chemotherapy and radiotherapy instead of cystectomy for the treatment of muscle-invasive carcinoma of the urinary bladder: long term results of a pilot study. Cancer. 1998;82(5):918–22. [in English].

60. Demirci U, Dızdar O, Cetindag MF, Altınova S, Ozsavran A, Dede DS, Kızılırmak N, et al. Radiotherapy concurrent with weekly gemcitabine after transurethral tumor resection in muscle invasive bladder cancer. J Cancer Res Ther. 2015;11(4):704–7. [in English].

61. Chen WC, Liaw CC, Chuang CK, Chen MF, Chen CS, Lin PY, Chang PL, et al. Concurrent cisplatin, 5-fluorouracil, leucovorin, and radiotherapy for invasive bladder cancer. Int J Radiat Oncol Biol Phys. 2003;56(3):726–33. [in English].

62. Kachnic LA, Shipley WU, Griffin PP, Zietman AL, Kaufman DS, Althausen AF, Heney NM. Combined modality treatment with selective bladder conservation for invasive bladder

cancer: long-term tolerance in the female patient. Cancer J Sci Am. 1996;2(2):79–84. [in English].

63. Thompson C, Joseph N, Sanderson B, Logue J, Wylie J, Elliott T, Lyons J, Anandadas C, Choudhury A. Tolerability of concurrent chemoradiation therapy with gemcitabine (Gemx), with and without prior neoadjuvant chemotherapy, in muscle invasive bladder cancer. Int J Radiat Oncol Biol Phys. 2017;97(4):732–9. [in English].

64. Lagrange JL, Bascoul-Mollevi C, Geoffrois L, Beckendorf V, Ferrero JM, Joly F, Allouache N, et al. Quality of life assessment after concurrent chemoradiation for invasive bladder cancer: results of a multicenter prospective study (Getug 97-015). Int J Radiat Oncol Biol Phys. 2011;79(1):172–8. [in English].

65. Huddart RA, Hall E, Lewis R, Porta N, Crundwell M, Jenkins PJ, Rawlings C, et al. Patient-reported quality of life outcomes in patients treated for muscle-invasive bladder cancer with radiotherapy ± chemotherapy in the Bc2001 phase III randomised controlled trial. Eur Urol. 2020;77(2):260–8. [in English].

66. Feng YH, Shen KH, Huang KH, Tzeng WS, Li CF, Lin KL. An effective and well tolerated strategy of bladder preservation therapy in cisplatin-ineligible patients with muscle-invasive bladder cancer. Clin Genitourin Cancer. 2016;14(1):e67–74. [in English].

67. Wu CE, Lin YC, Hong JH, Chuang CK, Pang ST, Liaw CC. Prognostic value of complete response in patients with muscle-invasive bladder cancer undergoing concurrent chemoradiotherapy. Anticancer Res. 2013;33(6):2605–10. [in English].

68. Gupta S, De S, Leekha N, Sahay SC, Chaudary P, Srinivasan S, Nandy M. Chemoradiation for organ preservation in the treatment of muscle invasive bladder cancer: our institutional experience. Gulf J Oncol. 2016;1(22):55–60. [in English].

69. Iwai A, Koga F, Fujii Y, Masuda H, Saito K, Numao N, Sakura M, Kawakami S, Kihara K. Perioperative complications of radical cystectomy after induction chemoradiotherapy in bladder-sparing protocol against muscle-invasive bladder cancer: a single institutional retrospective comparative study with primary radical cystectomy. Jpn J Clin Oncol. 2011;41(12):1373–9. [in English].

70. Kang JJ, Steinberg ML, Kupelian P, Alexander S, King CR. Whole versus partial bladder radiation: use of an image-guided hypofractionated IMRT bladder-preservation protocol. Am J Clin Oncol. 2018;41(2):107–14. [in English].

71. Kaufman DS, Winter KA, Shipley WU, Heney NM, Wallace HJ 3rd, Toonkel LM, Zietman AL, Tanguay S, Sandler HM. Phase I-II Rtog Study (99-06) of patients with muscle-invasive bladder cancer undergoing transurethral surgery, paclitaxel, cisplatin, and twice-daily radiotherapy followed by selective bladder preservation or radical cystectomy and adjuvant chemotherapy. Urology. 2009;73(4):833–7. [in English].

72. Orsatti M, Curotto A, Canobbio L, Guarneri D, Scarpati D, Venturini M, Franzone P, et al. Alternating chemo-radiotherapy in bladder cancer: a conservative approach. Int J Radiat Oncol Biol Phys. 1995;33(1):173–8. [in English].

73. Leow JJ, Bedke J, Chamie K, Collins JW, Daneshmand S, Grivas P, Heidenreich A, et al. Siu-Icud consultation on bladder cancer: treatment of muscle-invasive bladder cancer. World J Urol. 2019;37(1):61–83. [in English].

74. Milowsky MI, Rumble RB, Booth CM, Gilligan T, Eapen LJ, Hauke RJ, Boumansour P, Lee CT. Guideline on muscle-invasive and metastatic bladder cancer (European Association of Urology Guideline): American Society of Clinical Oncology clinical practice guideline endorsement. J Clin Oncol. 2016;34(16):1945–52. [in English].

A systematic review relating to trials in bladder cancer was conducted. The search strategy aimed to identify all references related to bladder cancer AND screening. Search terms used were as follows: (Bladder cancer) AND (Trials) AND (Localised). The following databases were screened from 1989 to June 2020:

- CINAHL
- MEDLINE (NHS Evidence)
- Cochrane
- AMed
- EMBASE
- PsychINFO
- SCOPUS
- Web of Science

In addition, searches using Medical Subject Headings (MeSH) and keywords were conducted using Cochrane databases. Two UK-based experts in bladder cancer were consulted to identify any additional studies.

Studies were eligible for inclusion if they reported primary research focusing on bladder cancer and screening. Papers were included if published after 1984 and had to be in English. Studies that did not conform to this were excluded. Only primary research was included (Fig. 68.1). The overall aim was to identify bladder cancer risk factors and epidemiology in muscle invasive disease.

Abstracts were independently screened for eligibility by two reviewers and disagreements resolved through discussion or third party opinion. Agreement level was calculated using Cohen's Kappa to test the intercoder reliability of this screening process. Cohens' Kappa allows comparison of inter-rater reliability between papers using relative observed agreement. This also takes account of the comparison occurring by chance. The first reviewer agreed all 25 papers to be included, the second, agreed on 25. Cohens kappa was therefore 1.0.

© The Editor(s) (if applicable) and The Author(s), under exclusive license to
Springer Nature Switzerland AG 2021
S. S. Goonewardene et al., *Management of Muscle Invasive Bladder Cancer*,
Management of Urology, https://doi.org/10.1007/978-3-030-57915-9_68

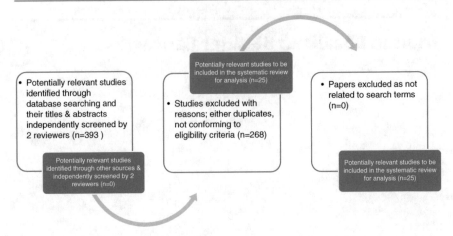

Fig. 68.1 Flow chart of studies identified through the systematic review. (Adapted from PRISMA)

Data extraction was piloted by the researcher and amended in consultation with the research team (author and two academic supervisors). Data collected included authors, year and country of publication, study aims, setting, intervention aims, number of participants, study design, intervention components and delivery methods, comparison groups and outcome measures, notes and follow-up questions for the authors. Studies were quality assessed using the PRISMA criteria for randomised controlled trials, Mays et al. [1, 2] for the action research and qualitative studies and the Critical Skills Appraisal programme for cohort studies. This was also applied to randomised controlled trials and qualitative studies.

The search identified 393 papers (Fig. 68.1). All 25 mapped to the search terms and eligibility criteria. The current systematic reviews were examined to gain further knowledge about the subject. Three hundred and sixty-eight papers were excluded due to not conforming to eligibility criteria or adding to the evidence. Of the 25 papers left, relevant abstracts were identified and the full papers obtained (all of which were in English), to quality assure against search criteria. There was considerable heterogeneity of design among the included studies therefore a narrative review of the evidence was undertaken. There was significant heterogeneity within studies, including clinical topic, numbers, outcomes, as a result a narrative review was thought to be best. There were 25 Trials, with a good level of evidence. These were from a range of countries with minimal loss to follow-up. All participants were identified appropriately.

68.1 Systematic Review Results

68.1.1 Bladder Preservation Therapy

Coen evaluated fluorouracil plus cisplatin and radiation twice a day (FCT) is an established chemoradiation (CRT) regimen for selective bladder-sparing treatment of muscle-invasive bladder cancer [3]. Gemcitabine and once daily radiation (GD) is a well-supported alternative [3]. Patients with cT2-4a muscle-invasive bladder cancer were randomly assigned to FCT or GD [3]. Patients underwent transurethral resection and induction CRT to 40 Gy [3]. Patients who achieved a complete response (CR) received consolidation CRT to 64 Gy and others underwent cystectomy [3]. Adjuvant gemcitabine/cisplatin chemotherapy was given [3]. DMF3 was 78% and 84% for FCT and GD, respectively [3]. BI-DMFS3 was 67% and 72%, respectively [3]. Postinduction CR rates were 88% and 78%, respectively [3]. Of 33 patients in the FCT arm, 21 (64%) experienced treatment-related grade 3 and 4 toxicities during protocol treatment, with 18 (55%), 2 (6%), and 2 patients (6%) experiencing grade 3 and 4 hematologic, GI, and genitourinary toxicity, respectively [3]. For the 33 patients in the GD arm, these figures were 18 (55%) overall and 14 (42%), 3 (9%) and 2 patients (6%), respectively [3].

Mitin investigated muscle-invasive bladder cancer treated with induction chemoradiation and then completed bladder-preserving therapy with chemoradiation therapy (chemo-RT) [4]. Thirty-six of 101 T0 patients (36%) versus 5 of 18 Ta or Tis patients (28%) experienced bladder recurrence (p = 0.52) [4]. Thirteen patients among complete responders eventually required late salvage cystectomy for tumour recurrence, compared with 1 patient among near-complete responders (p = 0.63) [4]. Disease-specific, bladder-intact, and overall survivals were not significantly different between T0 and Ta/Tis cases [4].

Royce et al. [5] compare the effectiveness of trimodality therapy vs. radical cystectomy [5]. For all patients with MIBC, although the model showed identical survival, TMT was the most effective strategy with an incremental gain of 0.59 QALYs over RC (7.83 vs. 7.24 QALYs, respectively) [5]. When limiting the model to favourable, contemporary cohorts in both the TMT and RC strategies, TMT remained more effective with an incremental gain of 1.61 QALYs (9.37 vs. 7.76 QALYs, respectively) [5]. One-way sensitivity analyses demonstrated the model was sensitive to the quality of life parameters (i.e., the utilities) for RC and TMT [5]. When testing the 95% confidence interval of the RC utility parameter the model demonstrated an incremental gain with TMT from −0.54 to 4.23 QALYs [5]. Probabilistic sensitivity analysis demonstrated that TMT was more effective than RC for 63% of model iterations [5].

68.1.2 Pre-operative Fitness

Banerjee investigated the feasibility of vigorous intensity aerobic interval exercise in bladder cancer patients prior to radical cystectomy (RC) [6]. Over half of the 112 eligible patients approached in the clinic were recruited to the study (53.5%), with recruited patients attending a median of 8 (range 1–10) exercise sessions over a pre-operative period of 3–6 weeks. Improvements in peak values of oxygen pulse (p = 0.001), minute ventilation (p = 0.002) and power output (p < 0.001) were observed at the follow-up CPET in the exercise group versus controls and there were no adverse events [6]. Although this feasibility study was not powered to detect changes in post-operative recovery outcomes, there were marginal (nonsignificant) differences in favour of the exercise group in post-operative Clavien-Dindo score and need for high dependency unit inotropic support [6].

Moeen compared the results of urethral anastomosis to a buttonhole and to the lowest part of the anterior suture line during orthotopic neobladder substitution [7]. Early postoperative complications occurred in 9 patients (5 in group I and 4 in group II, p = 0.484) [7]. Prolonged urinary leakage persisted for 11 and 14 days in 2 patients in group I and 10 and 16 days in 2 patients in group II [7]. Delayed postoperative complications occurred in 11 patients (5 [12.5%] in group I and 6 [15.6%] in group II) (p = 0.711) [7]. Three patients developed urethro-enteric strictures (2 in group I and 1 in group II) (p = 0.571) [7].

Furrer aimed to identify risk factors for AKI in patients undergoing RC and UD [8]. Early postoperative AKI occurred in 100/912 patients (11%). An increased risk was seen in patients with surgery lasting >400 min, male and obese patients (>25 kg/ m^2) [8]. Independent predictors were duration of surgery (p = 0.020), intraoperative blood loss (p = 0.049), preoperative serum creatinine values (p = 0.004), intraoperative administration of crystalloids (p = 0.032), body mass index (p = 0.031), and fluid balance (p = 0.006) [8]. Patients with AKI had a longer hospitalization time (18 vs. 17 days, p = 0.040) [8].

68.1.3 Partial Cystectomy

Ebbing evaluated the oncological results, associated complications, and postoperative health-related quality of life (HR-QoL) in patients treated with partial cystectomy (PC) for muscle-invasive bladder cancer (MIBC) [9]. Final pathological tumour stages in PC specimen were: pT0: 18.5%, non-MIBC: 3.7%, MIBC: 74.1%, pCIS: 14.8% [9]. Estimated 5-year overall- and progression-free survival rates were 53.7% and 62.1%. Five (18.5%) patients experienced local recurrence with MIBC [9]. Overall, the salvage cystectomy rate was 18.5%. The 90-day mortality rate was 0% [9]. Significant risk factors for progression-free survival were vascular invasion (HR 5.33) and tumour multilocularity (HR 4.5) in the PC specimen, and a ureteric reimplantation during PC (HR 4.53) [9]. The rates of intraoperative complications, 30- and 90-day major complications were 7.4%, respectively and 14.8% for overall long-term complications [9]. Postoperatively, median (IQR) global health status and QoL in our PC cohort was 79.2 (52.1–97.9) [9].

68.1.4 Open vs. Robotic Radical Cystectomy

Khan compared the outcomes of patients undergoing open radical cystectomy (ORC), RARC, and LRC [10]. The 30-day complication rates (classified by the Clavien-Dindo system) varied significantly between the three arms (ORC: 70%; RARC: 55%; LRC: 26%; p = 0.024) [10]. ORC complication rates were significantly higher than LRC (p < 0.01) [10]. The 90-day complication rates did not differ significantly between the three arms (ORC: 70%; RARC: 55%; LRC: 32%;

p = 0.068) [10]. ORC resulted in a slower return to oral solids than RARC or LRC [10].

The RAZOR (Randomized Open versus Robotic Cystectomy) trial revealed non-inferior 2-year progression-free survival for robotic radical cystectomy [11]. Venkatramani reported 3-year overall survival and sought to identify factors predicting recurrence, and progression-free and overall survival [11]. Estimated progression-free survival at 36 months was 68.4% (95% CI 60.1–75.3) and 65.4% (95% CI 56.8–72.7) in the robotic and open groups, respectively (p = 0.600) [11]. At 36 months overall survival was 73.9% (95% CI 65.5–80.5) and 68.5% (95% CI 59.8–75.7) in the robotic and open groups, respectively (p = 0.334) [11]. There was no significant difference in the cumulative incidence rates of recurrence (p = 0.802) [11].

Parekh compare progression-free survival in patients with bladder cancer treated with open cystectomy and robot-assisted cystectomy [12]. The RAZOR study is a randomised, open-label, non-inferiority, phase 3 trial done in 15 medical centres in the USA [12]. Eligible participants (aged ≥18 years) had biopsy-proven clinical stage T1–T4, N0–N1, M0 bladder cancer or refractory carcinoma in situ [12]. Three hundred and fifty participants were randomly assigned to treatment [12]. Three hundred and two patients (150 in the robotic cystectomy group and 152 in the open cystectomy group) were included in the per-protocol analysis set. Two-year progression-free survival was 72.3% (95% CI 64.3–78.8) in the robotic cystectomy group and 71.6% (95% CI 63.6–78.2) in the open cystectomy group (difference 0.7%, 95% CI −9.6% to 10.9%; $p_{non-inferiority}$ = 0.001), indicating non-inferiority of robotic cystectomy [12]. Adverse events occurred in 101 (67%) of 150 patients in the robotic cystectomy group and 105 (69%) of 152 patients in the open cystectomy group [12]. The most common adverse events were urinary tract infection (53 [35%] in the robotic cystectomy group vs. 39 [26%] in the open cystectomy group) and postoperative ileus (33 [22%] in the robotic cystectomy group vs. 31 [20%] in the open cystectomy group) [12].

Bochner compare cancer outcomes in BCa patients managed with ORC or robotic-assisted radical cystectomy (RARC) [13]. No differences were observed in recurrence (hazard ratio [HR]: 1.27; 95% confidence interval [CI]: 0.69–2.36; p = 0.4) or cancer-specific survival (p = 0.4) [13]. No difference in overall survival was observed (p = 0.8) [13]. However, the pattern of first recurrence demonstrated a nonstatistically significant increase in metastatic sites for those undergoing ORC (sub-HR [sHR]: 2.21; 95% CI: 0.96–5.12; p = 0.064) and a greater number of local/abdominal sites in the RARC-treated patients (sHR: 0.34; 95% CI: 0.12–0.93; p = 0.035) [13].

Bochner compared perioperative complications between robot-assisted radical cystectomy (RARC) and ORC techniques (Bochner 2015). The trial enrolled 124 patients, of whom 118 were randomized and underwent RC/PLND (Bochner 2015). Sixty were randomized to RARC and 58 to ORC (Bochner 2015). At 90 days, grade 2–5 complications were observed in 62% and 66% of RARC and ORC patients, respectively (95% confidence interval for difference, −21% to −13%; p = 0.7)

(Bochner 2015). The similar rates of grade 2–5 complications at our mandated interim analysis met futility criteria; thus, early closure of the trial occurred (Bochner 2015). The RARC group had lower mean intraoperative blood loss (p = 0.027) but significantly longer operative time than the ORC group (p < 0.001) (Bochner 2015). Pathologic variables including positive surgical margins and lymph node yields were similar (Bochner 2015). Mean hospital stay was 8 days in both arms (standard deviation, 3 and 5 days, respectively; p = 0.5) (Bochner 2015).

68.1.5 Neoadjuvant Chemotherapy in Muscle Invasive Bladder Cancer

Iyer assessed the efficacy and tolerability of six cycles of neoadjuvant dose-dense gemcitabine and cisplatin (ddGC) in patients with MIBC [14]. Patients and Methods In this prospective, multicenter phase II study, patients received ddGC (gemcitabine 2500 mg/m^2 on day 1 and cisplatin 35 mg/m^2 on days 1 and 2) every 2 weeks for 6 cycles followed by RC [14]. Fifty-seven percent of 46 evaluable patients downstaged to <pT2N0 [14]. Pathologic response correlated with improved recurrence-free survival and overall survival [14]. Nineteen patients (39%) required toxicity-related dose modifications [14]. No patient failed to undergo RC as a result of chemotherapy-associated toxicities [14]. The most frequent treatment-related toxicity was anemia (12%; grade 3) [14]. The presence of a presumed deleterious DNA damage response (DDR) gene alteration was associated with chemosensitivity (positive predictive value for <pT2N0 [89%]) [14].

Kim investigated trends in perioperative chemotherapy use, and determined factors associated with neoadjuvant chemotherapy (NAC) and adjuvant chemotherapy (AC) use in Korean patients with muscle-invasive bladder cancer (MIBC) [15]. Complete remission was defined as histologically confirmed T0N0M0 after RC [15]. NAC and AC were administered to 7.3% and 18.1% of the patients, respectively [15]. The median time interval between completing NAC and undergoing RC was 32 days and the mean number of cycles was 3.2 [15]. Gemcitabine and cisplatin were most frequently used in combination for NAC (49.0%) and AC (74.9%) [15]. NAC use increased significantly from 4.6% between 2003 and 2005 to 8.4% between 2010 and 2013 (p < 0.05), but AC use did not increase [15]. Only 1.9% of patients received NAC and AC. Complete remission after NAC was achieved in 12 patients (12.5%) [15].

Necchi examined sorafenib with gemcitabine and cisplatin chemotherapy (SGC) in an open-label, single-arm, phase 2 trial [16]. Pathologic T0 response was obtained in 20 patients (43.5%, 95% CI: 28.9–58.9); pT ≤ 1 in 25 (54.3%, 95% CI: 39.0–69.1) [16]. After a median follow-up of 35 months, the median progression-free survival was not reached (NR, interquartile range: 23.6-NR), nor was median overall survival (interquartile range: 30.3-NR) [16]. Hematologic and extrahematologic grade 3 to 4 adverse events occurred in 45.6% and 26.1% of patients, respectively [16]. In 29 samples from responders (pT ≤ 1) and nonresponders, different distribution of missense mutations involved DNA-repair genes, RAS-RAF pathway genes, chromatin-remodeling genes, and HER-family genes [16].

68.1.6 Extended vs. Limited Lymph Node Dissection in Radical Cystectomy

Gschwend evaluated whether extended versus limited LND prolongs recurrence-free survival (RFS) [17]. Prospective, multicenter, phase-III trial patients with locally resectable T1G3 or muscle-invasive urothelial BCa (T2–T4aM0) [17]. In total, 401 patients were randomized from February 2006 to August 2010 (203 limited, 198 extended) [17]. The median number of dissected nodes was 19 in the limited and 31 in the extended arm [17]. Extended LND failed to show superiority over limited LND with regard to RFS (5-year RFS 65% vs. 59%; hazard ratio [HR] = 0.84 [95% confidence interval 0.58–1.22]; p = 0.36), CSS (5-year CSS 76% vs. 65%; HR = 0.70; p = 0.10), and OS (5-year OS 59% vs. 50%; HR = 0.78; p = 0.12) [17]. Clavien grade ≥3 lymphoceles were more frequently reported in the extended LND group within 90 days after surgery. Inclusion of T1G3 tumors may have contributed to the negative study result [17].

68.1.7 Sentinel Node Detection in Muscle Invasive Bladder Cancer

Rosenblatt determined whether sentinel node detection (SNd) in muscle-invasive urothelial bladder cancer (MIBC) can be performed in patients undergoing neoadjuvant chemotherapy (NAC) and determine whether SNd is feasible in all pT stages, including pT0 [18]. Totally 1063 lymph nodes were removed (total SNs; 222–227) [18]. NAC patients with pT0 (n = 24) displayed a true positive detection in 91.7% by either SNdef, with a median of 3.0 SNs. NACpT >0 patients had a true positive detection in 87% (SNdef1) and 91.3% (SNdef2) [18]. In a univariate analysis, patient group neither NAC nor tumor downstaging influenced detection rates, regardless of SN definition [18]. In total eight patients, 4/22 metastatic nodes were SNs while 18/22 were non-SNs [18].

68.1.8 Urinary Diversion Post Radical Cystectomy

Skinner determined whether the T-pouch neobladder that included an antireflux mechanism was superior to the Studer pouch in patients with bladder cancer undergoing radical cystectomy [19]. Multivariable analysis showed that type of ileal orthotopic neobladder was not independently associated with 3-year renal function (p = 0.63) [19]. However, baseline estimated glomerular filtration rate, age and urinary tract obstruction were independently associated with 3-year decline in renal function [19]. Cumulative risk of urinary tract infection and overall late complications were not different between the groups, but the T-pouch was associated with an increased risk of secondary diversion related surgeries [19].

68.1.9 ERAS in Radical Cystectomy

Lin evaluated ERAS compared with the conventional recovery after surgery (CRAS) for RC-IUD [20]. There were 144 ERAS and 145 CRAS patients [20]. Postoperative complications occurred in 25.7% and 30.3% of the ERAS and CRAS patients with 55 complications in each group, respectively (p = 0.40) [20]. There was no significant difference between groups in major complications (p = 0.82), or type of complications (p = 0.99) [20]. The ERAS group had faster recovery of bowel movements (median 88 versus 100 h, p = 0.01), fluid diet tolerance (68 versus 96 h, p < 0.001), regular diet tolerance (125 versus 168 h, p = 0.004), and ambulation (64 versus 72 h, p = 0.047) than the CRAS group, but similar time to flatus and LOS [20].

68.1.10 Radiotherapy in Muscle Invasive Bladder Cancer

Whalley described the feasibility of image guided intensity modulated radiotherapy (IG-IMRT) using daily soft tissue matching in the treatment of bladder cancer [21]. Three patients ceased chemotherapy early due to toxicity. Six patients (21%) had acute Grade ≥2 genitourinary (GU) toxicity and six (21%) had acute Grade ≥2 gastrointestinal (GI) toxicity [21]. Five patients (18%) developed Grade ≥2 late GU toxicity and no ≥2 late GI toxicity was observed [21]. Nineteen patients underwent cystoscopy following radiation, with complete response (CR) in 16 cases (86%), including all patients treated with chemoradiotherapy [21]. Eight patients relapsed, four of which were local relapses [21]. Of the patients with local recurrence, one underwent salvage cystectomy [21]. For patients treated with definitive intent, freedom from locoregional recurrence (FFLR) and overall survival (OS) was 90%/100% for chemoradiotherapy versus 86/69% for radiotherapy alone [21].

68.1.11 Chemoradiotherapy in Muscle Invasive Bladder Cancer

Michaelson treated noncystectomy candidates with daily radiation and weekly paclitaxel for 7 weeks. Patients whose tumors showed her2/neu overexpression were additionally treated with weekly trastuzumab [22]. A total of 20 evaluable patients were treated in group 1 and 46 patients in group 2 [22]. Acute treatment-related adverse events (AEs) were observed in 7 of 20 patients in group 1 (35%) and 14 of 46 patients in group 2 (30.4%) [22]. Protocol therapy was completed by 60% (group 1) and 74% (group 2) of patients [22]. Most incompletions were due to toxicity, and the majority of AEs were gastrointestinal, including 1 grade 5 AE (group 1) [22]. Two other deaths (both in group 2) were unrelated to protocol therapy [22]. No unexpected cardiac, hematologic, or other toxicities were observed. The CR rate at 1 year was 72% for group 1 and 68% for group 2 [22].

Thompson assessed the tolerability of concurrent chemoradiation therapy with gemcitabine (GemX) in muscle invasive bladder cancer following neoadjuvant chemotherapy (neoGemX) by use of patient- and provider-reported outcomes [23].

Bowel toxicity of grade 3 or greater was reported in 7 of 38 patients (18%) in the neoGemX group and 5 of 25 (20%) in the GemX group [23]. Three GemX and two neoGemX patients had grade 3 or greater urinary toxicity [23]. Forty-nine patients completed questionnaires and were included in the analysis [23]. Scores on the late effects in normal tissues-subjective, objective, management, and analytic scales showed an expected peak by week 4 of treatment [23]. There was no statistically significant difference between mean scores at baseline and 12 months after treatment completion or between the neoGemX and GemX groups [23].

Datta evaluated the outcomes of loco-regional hyperthermia (HT) with radiotherapy (RT) and/or chemotherapy (CT) in elderly patients with muscle-invasive bladder cancers (MIBC) [24]. HTRT patients received a mean RT dose of 51.0 Gy compared to 57.1 Gy with HTCTRT (p < 0.001) in a shorter overall treatment time (OTT) (30.8 ± 6.9 versus 43.9 ± 4.0 days, p < 0.001) [24]. All HTRT patients had long-term local disease control, while 41.6% of HTCTRT recurred during follow-up [24]. None of the HTRT patients experienced grade III/IV acute and late toxicities, while these were evident in two and one HTCTRT patients respectively [24]. Taken together, the 3-year bladder preservation, local disease-free survival, cause-specific survival and overall survival were 86.6%, 60.7%, 55% and 39.5% respectively [24]. Even though the mean biological effective dose (BED) for both groups was similar (57.8 Gy15), the thermo-radiobiological BED estimated from HT-induced reduction of α/β was significantly higher for HTRT patients (91 ± 4.4 versus 85.8 ± 4.3 Gy3, p = 0.018) [24].

68.1.12 Brachytherapy in Muscle Invasive Bladder Cancer

van der Steen-Banasik reported experience and early results of laparoscopic implantation for interstitial brachytherapy (BT) of solitary bladder tumors and the feasibility of a high-dose-rate (HDR) schedule [25]. These modifications resulted in an average postoperative hospitalization of 6 days, minimal blood loss, and no wound healing problems [25]. Two patients had severe acute toxicity: 1 pulmonary embolism grade 4 and 1 cardiac death [25]. Late toxicity was mild (n = 2 urogenital grade 3 toxicity). The median follow-up was 2 years [25]. Using cumulative incidence competing risk analysis, the 2-year overall, disease-free, and disease-specific survival and local control rates were 59%, 71%, 87%, and 82%, respectively [25].

References

1. Moher D, Liberati A, Tetzlaff J, Altman DG. "Preferred Reporting Items for Systematic Reviews and Meta-Analyses: The Prisma Statement." [In English]. BMJ (Online) 339, no. 7716 (08 Aug 2009):332–36.
2. Mays N, Pope C, Popay J. "Systematically Reviewing Qualitative and Quantitative Evidence to Inform Management and Policy-Making in the Health Field." [In English]. Journal of Health Services Research and Policy 10, no. SUPPL. 1 (July 2005):6–20.

3. Coen JJ, Zhang P, Saylor PJ, et al. Bladder preservation with twice-a-day radiation plus fluorouracil/cisplatin or once daily radiation plus gemcitabine for muscle-invasive bladder cancer: NRG/RTOG 0712—a randomized phase II trial. J Clin Oncol. 2019;37(1):44–51.

4. Mitin T, George A, Zietman AL, et al. Long-term outcomes among patients who achieve complete or near-complete responses after the induction phase of bladder-preserving combined-modality therapy for muscle-invasive bladder cancer: a pooled analysis of NRG oncology/RTOG 9906 and 0233. Int J Radiat Oncol Biol Phys. 2016;94(1):67–74.

5. Royce TJ, Feldman AS, Mossanen M, et al. Comparative effectiveness of bladder-preserving tri-modality therapy versus radical cystectomy for muscle-invasive bladder cancer. Clin Genitourin Cancer. 2019;17(1):23–31.e3.

6. Banerjee S, Manley K, Shaw B, et al. Vigorous intensity aerobic interval exercise in bladder cancer patients prior to radical cystectomy: a feasibility randomised controlled trial. Support Care Cancer. 2018;26(5):1515–23.

7. Moeen AM, Safwat AS, Gadelmoula MM, et al. Does the site of the orthotopic neobladder outlet matter? A prospective randomized comparative study. Eur J Surg Oncol. 2018;44(6):847–52.

8. Furrer MA, Schneider MP, Burkhard FC, Wuethrich PY. Incidence and perioperative risk factors for early acute kidney injury after radical cystectomy and urinary diversion. Urol Oncol. 2018;36(6):306.e17–23.

9. Ebbing J, Heckmann RC, Collins JW, et al. Oncological outcomes, quality of life outcomes and complications of partial cystectomy for selected cases of muscle-invasive bladder cancer. Sci Rep. 2018;8(1):8360.

10. Khan MS, Gan C, Ahmed K, et al. A single-centre early phase randomised controlled three-arm trial of open, robotic, and laparoscopic radical cystectomy (CORAL). Eur Urol. 2016;69(4):613–21.

11. Venkatramani V, Reis IM, Castle EP, et al. Predictors of recurrence, and progression-free and overall survival following open versus robotic radical cystectomy: analysis from the RAZOR trial with a 3-year followup. J Urol. 2020;203(3):522–9.

12. Parekh DJ, Reis IM, Castle EP, et al. Robot-assisted radical cystectomy versus open radical cystectomy in patients with bladder cancer (RAZOR): an open-label, randomised, phase 3, non-inferiority trial. Lancet. 2018;391(10139):2525–36.

13. Bochner BH, Dalbagni G, Marzouk KH, et al. Randomized trial comparing open radical cystectomy and robot-assisted laparoscopic radical cystectomy: oncologic outcomes. Eur Urol. 2018;74(4):465–71.

14. Iyer G, Balar AV, Milowsky MI, et al. Multicenter prospective phase II trial of neoadjuvant dose-dense gemcitabine plus cisplatin in patients with muscle-invasive bladder cancer. J Clin Oncol. 2018;36(19):1949–56.

15. Kim SH, Seo HK, Shin HC, et al. Trends in the use of chemotherapy before and after radical cystectomy in patients with muscle-invasive bladder cancer in Korea. J Korean Med Sci. 2015;30(8):1150–6.

16. Necchi A, Lo Vullo S, Raggi D, et al. Neoadjuvant sorafenib, gemcitabine, and cisplatin administration preceding cystectomy in patients with muscle-invasive urothelial bladder carcinoma: an open-label, single-arm, single-center, phase 2 study. Urol Oncol. 2018;36(1):8.e1–8.

17. Gschwend JE, Heck MM, Lehmann J, et al. Extended versus limited lymph node dissection in bladder cancer patients undergoing radical cystectomy: survival results from a prospective, randomized trial. Eur Urol. 2019;75(4):604–11.

18. Rosenblatt R, Johansson M, Alamdari F, et al. Sentinel node detection in muscle-invasive urothelial bladder cancer is feasible after neoadjuvant chemotherapy in all pT stages, a prospective multicenter report. World J Urol. 2017;35(6):921–7.

19. Skinner EC, Fairey AS, Groshen S, et al. Randomized trial of studer pouch versus T-pouch orthotopic ileal neobladder in patients with bladder cancer. J Urol. 2015;194(2):433–9.

20. Lin T, Li K, Liu H, et al. Enhanced recovery after surgery for radical cystectomy with ileal urinary diversion: a multi-institutional, randomized, controlled trial from the Chinese bladder cancer consortium. World J Urol. 2018;36(1):41–50.

21. Whalley D, Caine H, McCloud P, Guo L, Kneebone A, Eade T. Promising results with image guided intensity modulated radiotherapy for muscle invasive bladder cancer. Radiat Oncol. 2015;10:205.
22. Michaelson MD, Hu C, Pham HT, et al. A phase 1/2 trial of a combination of paclitaxel and trastuzumab with daily irradiation or paclitaxel alone with daily irradiation after transurethral surgery for noncystectomy candidates with muscle-invasive bladder cancer (Trial NRG Oncology RTOG 0524). Int J Radiat Oncol Biol Phys. 2017;97(5):995–1001.
23. Thompson C, Joseph N, Sanderson B, et al. Tolerability of concurrent chemoradiation therapy with gemcitabine (GemX), with and without prior neoadjuvant chemotherapy, in muscle invasive bladder cancer. Int J Radiat Oncol Biol Phys. 2017;97(4):732–9.
24. Datta NR, Eberle B, Puric E, et al. Is hyperthermia combined with radiotherapy adequate in elderly patients with muscle-invasive bladder cancers? Thermo-radiobiological implications from an audit of initial results. Int J Hyperth. 2016;32(4):390–7.
25. van der Steen-Banasik EM, GAHJ S, Oosterveld BJ, Janssen T, Visser AG. The Curie-Da Vinci connection: 5-years' experience with laparoscopic (robot-assisted) implantation for high-dose-rate brachytherapy of solitary T2 bladder tumors. Int J Radiat Oncol Biol Phys. 2016;95(5):1439–42.

Trials in Locally Advanced and Metastatic Bladder Cancer

69

A systematic review relating to trials in locally advanced and metastatic bladder cancer was conducted. Search terms used were as follows: (Bladder cancer) AND (Trials) AND (Locally Advanced) OR (Metastatic). The following databases were screened from 1989 to June 2020:

- CINAHL
- MEDLINE (NHS Evidence)
- Cochrane
- AMed
- EMBASE
- PsychINFO
- SCOPUS
- Web of Science

In addition, searches using Medical Subject Headings (MeSH) and keywords were conducted using Cochrane databases. Two UK-based experts in bladder cancer were consulted to identify any additional studies.

Studies were eligible for inclusion if they reported primary research focusing on bladder cancer and screening. Papers were included if published after 1984 and had to be in English. Studies that did not conform to this were excluded. Only primary research was included (Fig. 69.1). The overall aim was to identify bladder cancer risk factors and epidemiology in muscle invasive disease.

Abstracts were independently screened for eligibility by two reviewers and disagreements resolved through discussion or third-party opinion. Agreement level was calculated using Cohen's Kappa to test the intercoder reliability of this screening process. Cohens' Kappa allows comparison of inter-rater reliability between papers using relative observed agreement. This also takes account of the comparison occurring by chance. The first reviewer agreed all 22 papers to be included, the second, agreed on 22. Cohens kappa was therefore 1.0.

© The Editor(s) (if applicable) and The Author(s), under exclusive license to
Springer Nature Switzerland AG 2021
S. S. Goonewardene et al., *Management of Muscle Invasive Bladder Cancer*,
Management of Urology, https://doi.org/10.1007/978-3-030-57915-9_69

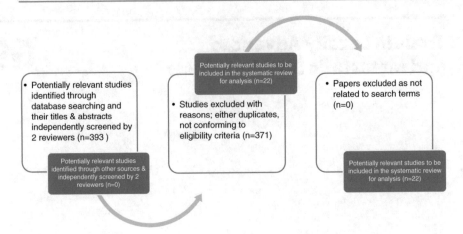

Fig. 69.1 Flow chart of studies identified through the systematic review. (Adapted from PRISMA)

Data extraction was piloted by the researcher and amended in consultation with the research team (author and two academic supervisors). Data collected included authors, year and country of publication, study aims, setting, intervention aims, number of participants, study design, intervention components and delivery methods, comparison groups and outcome 1 measures, notes and follow-up questions for the authors. Studies were quality assessed using the PRISMA criteria for randomised controlled trials, Mays et al. [1, 2] for the action research and qualitative studies and the Critical Skills Appraisal programme for cohort studies. This was also applied to randomised controlled trials and qualitative studies.

The search identified 393 papers (Fig. 69.1). All 22 mapped to the search terms and eligibility criteria. The current systematic reviews were examined to gain further knowledge about the subject. Three hundred and seventy-one papers were excluded due to not conforming to eligibility criteria or adding to the evidence. Of the 22 papers left, relevant abstracts were identified and the full papers obtained (all of which were in English), to quality assure against search criteria. There was considerable heterogeneity of design among the included studies therefore a narrative review of the evidence was undertaken. There was significant heterogeneity within studies, including clinical topic, numbers, outcomes, as a result a narrative review was thought to be best. There were 22 Trials, with a good level of evidence. These were from a range of countries with minimal loss to follow-up. All participants were identified appropriately.

69.1 Systematic Review Results

69.1.1 Adjuvant Chemoradiation vs. Chemotherapy Alone in Locally Advanced Bladder Cancer

Zaghloul investigated if adjuvant sequential RT plus chemotherapy can improve locoregional recurrence-free survival (LRFS) compared with adjuvant chemotherapy alone [3]. The chemotherapy plus RT arm accrued 75 patients, and the chemotherapy-alone arm accrued 45 patients, with a weighted randomization to speed accrual [3]. Fifty-three percent (64 of 120) had urothelial carcinoma, and 46.7% (56 of 120) had squamous cell carcinoma or other [3]. The arms were balanced except for age (median, 52 vs. 55 years; p = 0.04) and tumor size (mean, 4.9 vs. 5.8 cm; p < 0.01), both favoring chemotherapy plus RT [3]. Two-year outcomes and overall adjusted hazard ratios (HRs) for chemotherapy plus RT vs. chemotherapy alone were 96% vs. 69% (HR, 0.08; 95% CI, 0.02–0.39; p < 0.01) for LRFS, 68% vs. 56% (HR, 0.53; 95% CI, 0.27–1.06; p = 0.07) for disease-free survival, and 71% vs. 60% (HR, 0.61; 95% CI, 0.33–1.11; p = 0.11) for overall survival (OS) [3]. Five patients (7%) had RT-associated late grade 3 gastrointestinal tract adverse effects in the chemotherapy plus RT arm [3].

69.1.2 Neaoadjuvant Chemotherapy in Locally Advanced Bladder Cancer

Neoadjuvant chemotherapy with methotrexate-vinblastine-doxorubicin-cisplatin (MVAC) is the standard of care for muscle-invasive urothelial bladder cancer [4]. Niedersüss-Beke et al. [4] reported on the efficacy and safety of neoadjuvant GC in patients with locally advanced urothelial cancer [4]. In all, 83 patients finished chemotherapy; 80 patients were evaluable for the primary endpoint [4]. Pathologic complete response (pCR) was achieved in 22.5% and near pCR was seen in 33.7% of the patients [4]. The 1-year PFS rate was 79.5% among those patients achieving ≤pT2 versus 100% among those patients achieving pCR or near pCR (p = 0.041). Five-year OS was 61.8% (95% CI 67.6 to NA) [4]. GC was well tolerated. Grade 3/4 toxicities occurred in 38% of the patients [4]. There was no grade 3/4 renal toxicity, febrile neutropenia, or death.

69.1.3 Chemotherapy in Locally Advanced and Metastatic Bladder Cancer

Bellmunt conducted a randomized study was conducted to compare cabizataxel versus vinflunine in locally advanced bladder cancer [5]. Seventy patients were included in the phase II across 19 institutions in Europe [5]. Baseline characteristics were well balanced between the two arms [5]. Three patients (13%) obtained a partial response on cabazitaxel (95% CI 2.7–32.4) and six patients (30%) in the vinflunine arm (95% CI 11.9–54.3) [5]. Median progression-free survival for cabazitaxel was 1.9 versus 2.9 months for vinflunine (p = 0.039) [5]. The study did not proceed to phase III since the futility analysis showed a lack of efficacy of cabazitaxel [5]. A trend for overall survival benefit was found favouring vinflunine (median 7.6 versus 5.5 months) [5]. Grade 3- to 4-related adverse events were seen in 41% patients with no difference between the two arms [5].

Pulido assessed the efficacy of temsirolimus in a homogenous cohort of patients with recurrent or metastatic bladder cancer following first-line chemotherapy [6]. A total of 22 (48.9%) non-progressions were observed at 2 months with 3 partial responses and 19 stable diseases [6]. Remarkably, 4 patients were treated for more than 30 weeks [6]. Fifty patients experienced at least a related grade 1/2 (94%) and 28 patients (52.8%) a related grade 3/4 adverse event [6]. Eleven patients had to stop treatment for toxicity [6]. This led to recruitment being halted by an independent data monitoring committee with regard to the risk-benefit balance and the fact that the primary objective was already met [6].

Powles established whether maintenance lapatinib after first-line chemotherapy is beneficial in human epidermal growth factor receptor (HER) 1/HER2-positive metastatic urothelial bladder cancer (UBC) [7]. The overall survival for lapatinib and placebo was 12.6 (95% CI, 9.0–16.2) and 12.0 (95% CI, 10.5–14.9) months, respectively (hazard ratio, 0.96; 95% CI, 0.70–1.31; p = 0.80). Discontinuation due to adverse events were similar in both arms (6% lapatinib and 5% placebo) [7]. The rate of grade 3–4 adverse events for lapatinib and placebo was 8.6% versus 8.1% (p = 0.82) [7]. Preplanned subset analysis of patients strongly positive for HER1/HER2 (3+ on immunohistochemistry; n = 111), patients positive for only HER1 (n = 102), and patients positive for only HER2 (n = 42) showed no significant benefit with lapatinib in terms of PFS and overall survival (p > 0.05 for each) [7].

Cao compared the chemotherapeutic regimens of gemcitabine plus cisplatin (GC) vs. pemetrexed plus cisplatin (PC) in bladder cancer (BC) with vascular invasion and/or distant metastasis [8]. The median overall survival (OS) and the median progression-free survival (PFS) in the GC group were significantly higher than that in the PC group (OS: p = 0.033 and PFS: p = 0.039, respectively) [8]. Besides, the response rates and disease control were obviously higher in the GC group (68% and 86%, respectively) compared to the PC group (44% and 56%, respectively), although without statistical significance [8]. Regarding toxicity, higher rates of neutropenia and nausea in the PC group were noted, while thrombocytopenia was more frequent in the GC group [8].

Petrylak did a randomised, double-blind, phase 3 trial in patients with advanced or metastatic urothelial carcinoma who progressed during or after platinum-based chemotherapy [9]. Five hundred and thirty patients were randomly allocated either ramucirumab plus docetaxel (n = 263) or placebo plus docetaxel (n = 267) [9]. Progression-free survival was prolonged significantly in patients allocated ramucirumab plus docetaxel versus placebo plus docetaxel (median 4.07 months [95% CI 2.96–4.47] vs. 2.76 months [2.60–2.96]; hazard ratio [HR] 0.757, 95% CI 0.607–0.943; p = 0.0118) [9]. An objective response was achieved by 53 (24.5%, 95% CI 18.8–30.3) of 216 patients allocated ramucirumab and 31 (14.0%, 9.4–18.6) of 221 assigned placebo [9]. The most frequently reported treatment-emergent adverse events, regardless of causality, in either treatment group (any grade) were fatigue, alopecia, diarrhoea, decreased appetite, and nausea [9]. These events occurred predominantly at grade 1–2 severity [9]. The frequency of grade 3 or worse adverse events was similar for patients allocated ramucirumab and placebo (156 [60%] of 258 vs. 163 [62%] of 265 had an adverse event), with no unexpected toxic effects. 63 (24%) of 258 patients allocated ramucirumab and 54 (20%) of 265 assigned placebo had a serious adverse event [9]. Thirty-eight (15%) of 258 patients allocated ramucirumab and 43 (16%) of 265 assigned placebo died on treatment or within 30 days of discontinuation, of which 8 (3%) and 5 (2%) deaths were deemed related to treatment by the investigator [9]. Sepsis was the most common adverse event leading to death on treatment (four [2%] vs. none [0%]) [9]. One fatal event of neutropenic sepsis was reported in a patient allocated ramucirumab [9].

Cerbone determined the maximum tolerated dose (MTD) of lapatinib in combination with GC for metastatic bladder cancer [10]. No dose-limiting toxicities (DLTs) were observed in cohort 1 or 2 (3 patients each); in cohort 3 (2 × 3 patients), 1 of the 6 patients presented DLTs (grade 4, treatment-related febrile neutropenia and renal failure) [10]. Twelve patients received 6 cycles [10]. Lapatinib at 750–1250 mg combined with GC appears safe and tolerable [10]. The MTD of lapatinib combined with GC in bladder cancer was 1250 mg [10].

McConkey explore clinical outcomes for patients treated with dose-dense (DD) methotrexate, vinblastine, doxorubicin, and cisplatin (MVAC) and bevacizumab (B) and the impact of UC subtype [11]. Sixty patients enrolled in a neoadjuvant trial of four cycles of DDMVAC + B between 2007 and 2010 [11]. Chemotherapy was active, with pT0N0 and ≤pT1N0 downstaging rates of 38% and 53%, respectively, and 5-year overall survival (OS) of 63% [11]. Bevacizumab had no appreciable impact on outcomes. Basal tumors had improved survival compared to luminal and p53-like tumors (5-year OS 91%, 73%, and 36%, log-rank p = 0.015), with similar findings on multivariate analysis [11]. Bone metastases within 2 years were exclusively associated with the p53-like subtype (p53-like 100%, luminal 0%, basal 0%; p ≤ 0.001) [11]. Tumors enriched with the p53-like subtype at cystectomy suggested chemoresistance for this subtype [11]. A separate cohort treated with perioperative MVAC confirmed the UC subtype survival benefit (5-year OS 77% for basal, 56% for luminal, and 56% for p53-like; p = 0.021) [11]. Limitations include the small number of pretreatment specimens with sufficient tissue for GEP [11].

Petrioli determined the activity and safety of carboplatin, methotrexate, vinblastine, and epirubicin (the M-VECa regimen) in patients with advanced bladder cancer after failure of at least one chemotherapy line [12]. Treatment consisted of carboplatin 250 mg/m on day 1, methotrexate 30 mg/m on days 1 and 22, vinblastine 3 mg/m on days 2 and 22, and epirubicin 50 mg/m on day 2 every 28 days until disease progression or death. Response rate was the main endpoint [12]. Twenty-five patients were enrolled: the median age was 67 years (range 42–83) and there were 14 patients aged at least 70 years (56%) [12]. Fourteen patients had previously received vinflunine as a second-line treatment [12]. Complete remission occurred in one patient (4%), partial remission in five patients (20%), and stable disease in eight patients (32%) [12]. The overall response rate was 24% [95% confidence interval (CI), 9.3–45.1%] and the overall disease control rate was 56% (95% CI, 34.9–75.5%) [12]. The median progression-free survival was 5.1 months (95% CI, 3.9–6.4) and the median overall survival was 9.5 months (95% CI, 7.1–11.2) [12]. Treatment was well tolerated: grade 3 neutropenia was documented in five patients and grade 3 nausea and vomiting in two patients [12].

Izumi assessed gemcitabine/cisplatin (GC) split or gemcitabine/carboplatin (GCarbo) in renal dysfunction [13]. Patients with normal renal function treated with GC were also reviewed as a reference group [13]. A total of 41 patients, including 10 treated with GCsplit, 16 treated with GCarbo, and 15 treated with GC, were analysed [13]. The median overall and progression-free survival in GCsplit and GCarbo groups were 18.1 and 12.5 months (p = 0.0454) and 9.9 and 6.4 months (p = 0.0404), respectively [13]. Neutropenia was relatively more severe in the GCsplit group than the GCarbo group (p = 0.0103) [13].

De Santis assessed the efficacy and tolerability profile of two vinflunine-based cytotoxic regimens in this setting [14]. Sixty-nine patients were enrolled (34 VG, 35 VC). Less G3/4 haematological adverse events (AEs) were reported with VG: neutropaenia was seen in 38% (versus 68% with VC) and febrile neutropaenia in 3% (versus 14% with VC) of patients [14]. No major differences were observed for non-haematological AEs. DCR was 77% in both groups; overall response rate (ORR) was 44.1% versus 28.6%, with a median progression-free survival of 5.9 versus 6.1 months and median OS of 14.0 versus 12.8 months with VG and VC, respectively [14].

Miyata examined the anticancer effects, changes in the quality of life (QoL), and safety of combined therapy of low-dose gemcitabine, paclitaxel, and sorafenib (LD-GPS) in patients with CDDP-resistant UC [15]. Twenty patients were treated with gemcitabine (700 mg/m^2 on day 1), paclitaxel (70 mg/m^2 on day 1), and sorafenib (400 mg/day on days 8–22) [15]. QoL and pain relief were evaluated using the short-form survey (SF)-36 for bodily pain and the visual analog scale (VAS). VAS scores were significantly decreased by both the second- and third-line therapies (p = 0.012 and 0.028, respectively) [15]. The bodily pain score from the SF-36 survey was also significantly (p = 0.012) decreased [15]. Complete responses, partial responses, and stable disease were found in 0 (0.0%), 1 (5.0%), and 13 patients (65%), respectively [15]. Three patients (15.0%) stopped therapy because of grade 3 fatigue and hand-foot reactions [15]. LD-GPS therapy was well tolerated by patients with CDDP-resistant UC [15].

Vinflunine is recommended in the European guideline for the treatment of advanced or metastatic urothelial cell carcinoma (UCC) after failure of platinum-based therapy [16]. Seventy-seven platinum-pretreated patients were recruited [16]. Vinflunine was predominantly administered as second-line (66%) therapy or in subsequent treatment lines (21%) [16]. One third of the patients received at least six cycles of vinflunine and the average number was 4.7 cycles [16]. A vinflunine starting dose of 320 mg/m^2 was chosen in 48% of patients and 280 mg/m^2 in 39% [16]. Grade 3/4 toxicities were leucopenia 16.9%, anemia 6.5%, elevated liver enzymes 6.5% and constipation 5.2%. ORR was 23.4% and OS was 7.7 (CI 4.1–10.4) months

[16]. Patients with zero, one, two or ≥three risk factors displayed a median OS of 18.2, 9.5, 4.1 and 2.8 months, respectively (p = 0.0005; HR = 1.82) [16].

69.1.4 Immunotherapy in Locally Advanced and Metastatic Bladder Cancer

Massard investigated the safety and efficacy of durvalumab, a human monoclonal antibody that binds programmed cell death ligand-1 (PD-L1), and the role of PD-L1 expression on clinical response in patients with advanced urothelial bladder cancer (UBC) [17]. A total of 61 patients (40 PD-L1-positive, 21 PD-L1-negative), 93.4% of whom received one or more prior therapies for advanced disease, were treated (median duration of follow-up, 4.3 months) [17]. The most common treatment-related adverse events (AEs) of any grade were fatigue (13.1%), diarrhea (9.8%), and decreased appetite (8.2%) [17]. Grade 3 treatment-related AEs occurred in three patients (4.9%); there were no treatment-related grade 4 or 5 AEs [17]. One treatment-related AE (acute kidney injury) resulted in treatment discontinuation [17]. The ORR was 31.0% (95% CI, 17.6–47.1) in 42 response-evaluable patients, 46.4% (95% CI, 27.5–66.1) in the PD-L1-positive subgroup, and 0% (95% CI, 0.0–23.2) in the PD-L1-negative subgroup [17]. Responses are ongoing in 12 of 13 responding patients, with median duration of response not yet reached (range, 4.1+ to 49.3+ weeks) [17].

Necchi assessed efficacy and safety of atezolizumab, a programmed death-ligand 1-directed antibody, in patients with platinum-treated locally advanced or metastatic urothelial carcinoma [18]. In total, 220 patients who experienced progression from the overall cohort (n = 310) were analyzed: 137 continued atezolizumab for ≥1 dose after progression, 19 received other systemic therapy, and 64 received no further systemic therapy [18]. Compared with those who discontinued, patients continuing atezolizumab beyond progression were more likely to have had a baseline Eastern Cooperative Oncology Group performance status of 0 (43.1% versus 31.3%), less likely to have had baseline liver metastases (27.0% versus 41.0%), and more likely to have had an initial response to atezolizumab (responses in 11.7% versus 1.2%) [18]. Five patients (3.6%) continuing atezolizumab after progression had subsequent responses compared with baseline measurements [18]. Median post-progression overall survival was 8.6 months in patients continuing atezolizumab, 6.8 months in those receiving another treatment, and 1.2 months in those receiving no further treatment [18]. Atezolizumab exposure-adjusted adverse event frequencies were generally similar before and following progression [18].

Atezolizumab (anti-programmed death ligand 1) has demonstrated safety and activity in advanced and metastatic urothelial carcinoma, but its long-term clinical profile remains unknown [19]. Petrylak et al. [19] reported long-term clinical outcomes with atezolizumab therapy for patients with metastatic urothelial carcinoma [19]. Atezolizumab was given intravenously every 3 weeks until unacceptable toxic effects, protocol nonadherence, or loss of clinical benefit [19]. Ninety-five patients were evaluable (72 [76%] male; median age, 66 years [range, 36–89 years]) [19].

Forty-five (47%) received atezolizumab as third-line therapy or greater [19]. Nine patients (9%) had a grade 3–4 treatment-related adverse event, mostly within the first treatment year; no serious related adverse events were observed thereafter [19]. One patient (1%) discontinued treatment due to a related event [19]. No treatment-related deaths occurred [19]. Responses occurred in 26% (95% CI, 18–36%) of patients [19]. Median overall survival was 10.1 months (95% CI, 7.3–17.0 months); 3-year OS rate was 27% (95% CI, 17–36%) [19]. Response occurred in 40% (95% CI, 26–55%; n = 40) and 11% (95% CI, 4–25%; n = 44) of patients with programmed death ligand 1 expression of at least 5% tumor-infiltrating immune cells (IC2/3) or less than 5% (IC0/1), respectively [19].

Plimack aimed to assess the safety and activity of an anti-PD-1 antibody pembrolizumab in patients with locally advanced or metastatic urothelial cancer [20]. Sixty-one (53%) patients were PD-L1 positive, of whom 33 were enrolled in this study [20]. The most common treatment-related adverse events were fatigue (six [18%] of 33 patients) and peripheral oedema (4 [12%]) [20]. Five (15%) patients had 11 grade 3 treatment-related adverse events; no single event occurred in more than one patient [20]. Three (9%) patients experienced five serious treatment-related adverse events [20]. After median follow-up of 13 months (range 1–26, IQR 5–23), an overall response was achieved in seven (26% [95% CI 11–46]) of 27 assessable patients, with three (11% [2–29]) complete and four (15% [4–34]) partial responses [20]. Of the four deaths that occurred during the study (cardiac arrest, pneumonia, sepsis, and subarachnoid haemorrhage), none were deemed treatment related [20].

Levy assessed preliminary safety and efficacy results of the anti-programmed cell death ligand-1 (anti-PD-L1) durvalumab in combination with radiotherapy (RT) in an expansion cohort of patients included in a phase 1/2 trial [21]. Five patients (50%) reported an irradiation-related adverse event (AE) grade (G) 1 or 2 and one patient had two G2 AEs [21]. The most frequently reported AE (3/6) was G2 mucositis [21]. There was no G3 or more RT-related AEs [21]. All AEs were transient, lasted less than one week, and were manageable by standard guidelines [21]. There was no unexpected AE [21]. On 10/15 in-field (IF) evaluable lesions, the objective response (OR) rate was 60% (complete response, 2/10 and partial response, 4/10) and 4/10 stable disease (SD) [21]. All evaluated IF lesions had a TGR decrease resulting in a significant decrease in the TGR between the two periods (before versus after RT; p < 0.01) [21]. Outfields disease evaluation retrieved 10/14 SD and 4/14 progressive disease (PD). There was no out-field OR, no abscopal effect and no out-field difference between the two periods according to TGR (p = 0.09) [21].

Alisertib is an orally available, selective inhibitor of the aurora kinase A [22]. From 10/2014 to 04/2015, 22 patients were enrolled (20 evaluable for response), 8 (36.4%) in second-line and 14 (63.6%) beyond the second-line [22]. Eight (36.4%) had an ECOG-performance status 1–2 [22]. Two partial responses (PR, ORR: 9.1%), 7 stable disease (SD) and 11 PD were obtained [22]. Median follow-up was 8.3 months (IQR: 7–10.3), 6-month progression-free survival (PFS) was 13.6% (95%CI: 4.8–39.0) [22]. Two SD are still receiving treatment after 11.5 and 6.3 months [22]. Hb <10 g/dl was significantly associated with shorter PFS and OS multivariably (p = 0.031 and p = 0.033) [22]. Tissue of the case with 11.5 month SD harbored a missense mutation of mTOR (E1813D), the nonsense mutation Q527STOP of TSC1, HER3 and TAF1L missense mutations [22]. Grade 3–4 adverse events (AE) were: 40.9% mucositis, 36.4% fatigue, 18.2% neutropenia (13.6% febrile neutropenia) [22]. There were 2 treatment-related deaths.

69.1.5 Immunotherapy and Radiotherapy in Metastatic Bladder Cancer

Tree examined The PLUMMB trial (Pembrolizumab in Muscle-invasive/Metastatic Bladder cancer), a phase I study to test the tolerability of a combination of weekly radiation therapy with pembrolizumab in patients with metastatic or locally advanced urothelial cancer of the bladder [23]. In the first dose-cohort, patients received pembrolizumab 100 mg 3-weekly, starting 2 weeks before commencing weekly adaptive bladder radiation therapy to a dose of 36 Gy in 6 fractions [23]. The first dose-cohort was stopped after 5 patients, having met the predefined definition of dose-limiting toxicity [23]. Three patients experienced grade 3 urinary toxicities, 2 of which were attributable to therapy [23]. One patient experienced a grade 4 rectal perforation [23]. In view of these findings, the trial has been paused and the protocol will be amended to reduce radiation therapy dose per fraction [23].

69.1.6 Chemoradiotherapy in the Elderly

Christodoulou evaluated the efficacy and tolerability of concurrent radical radiotherapy with gemcitabine radiosensitisation (GemX) in elderly patients with MIBC and compared outcomes to those from the bladder carbogen and nicotinamide (BCON) phase III trial [24]. Out of 167 patients who received GemX, 61 were elderly (36.5%) with a median age of 78 years [24]. Elderly patients had worse performance status (p = 0.020) and co-morbidities (p = 0.030) [24]. A similar proportion of patients received planned dose radiotherapy in both groups (p = 0.260), although fewer elderly patients received all four cycles of concurrent chemotherapy (p = 0.017) due to toxicity [24]. For OS, age had some prognostic power; HR 1.04 (95% CI 1.00–1.08; p = 0.068) [24]. Overall survival and LPFS in elderly patients were comparable between CON and GemX (HR 1.13, 95% CI 0.69–1.85; p = 0.616 and HR 0.85, 95% CI 0.41–1.74; p = 0.659 respectively) [24].

References

1. Moher D, Liberati A, Tetzlaff J, Altman DG. "Preferred Reporting Items for Systematic Reviews and Meta-Analyses: The Prisma Statement." [In English]. BMJ (Online) 339, no. 7716 (08 Aug 2009):332–36.

2. Mays N, Pope C, Popay J. "Systematically Reviewing Qualitative and Quantitative Evidence to Inform Management and Policy-Making in the Health Field." [In English]. Journal of Health Services Research and Policy 10, no. SUPPL. 1 (July 2005):6–20.

3. Zaghloul MS, Christodouleas JP, Smith A, et al. Adjuvant sandwich chemotherapy plus radiotherapy vs adjuvant chemotherapy alone for locally advanced bladder cancer after radical cystectomy: a randomized phase 2 trial. JAMA Surg. 2018;153(1):e174591.

4. Niedersüss-Beke D, Puntus T, Kunit T, et al. Neoadjuvant chemotherapy with gemcitabine plus cisplatin in patients with locally advanced bladder cancer. Oncology. 2017;93(1):36–42.

5. Bellmunt J, Kerst JM, Vázquez F, et al. A randomized phase II/III study of cabazitaxel versus vinflunine in metastatic or locally advanced transitional cell carcinoma of the urothelium (SECAVIN). Ann Oncol. 2017;28(7):1517–22.

6. Pulido M, Roubaud G, Cazeau AL, et al. Safety and efficacy of temsirolimus as second line treatment for patients with recurrent bladder cancer. BMC Cancer. 2018;18(1):194.

7. Powles T, Huddart RA, Elliott T, et al. Phase III, double-blind, randomized trial that compared maintenance lapatinib versus placebo after first-line chemotherapy in patients with human epidermal growth factor receptor 1/2-positive metastatic bladder cancer. J Clin Oncol. 2017;35(1):48–55.

8. Cao Y, He Y, Chen H, et al. Phase I study of gemcitabine-cisplatin versus pemetrexed cisplatin for patients with advanced or metastatic bladder cancer. J BUON. 2018;23(2):475–81.

9. Petrylak DP, de Wit R, Chi KN, et al. Ramucirumab plus docetaxel versus placebo plus docetaxel in patients with locally advanced or metastatic urothelial carcinoma after platinum-based therapy (RANGE): a randomised, double-blind, phase 3 trial. Lancet. 2017;390(10109):2266–77.

10. Cerbone L, Sternberg CN, Sengeløv L, et al. Results from a phase I study of lapatinib with gemcitabine and cisplatin in advanced or metastatic bladder cancer: EORTC Trial 30061. Oncology. 2016;90(1):21–8.

11. McConkey DJ, Choi W, Shen Y, et al. A prognostic gene expression signature in the molecular classification of chemotherapy-naïve urothelial cancer is predictive of clinical outcomes from neoadjuvant chemotherapy: a phase 2 trial of dose-dense methotrexate, vinblastine, doxorubicin, and cisplatin with bevacizumab in urothelial cancer. Eur Urol. 2016;69(5):855–62.

12. Petrioli R, Roviello G, Fiaschi AI, et al. Carboplatin, methotrexate, vinblastine, and epirubicin (M-VECa) as salvage treatment in patients with advanced bladder cancer: a phase II study. Anti-Cancer Drugs. 2015;26(8):878–83.

13. Izumi K, Iwamoto H, Yaegashi H, et al. Gemcitabine plus cisplatin split *versus* gemcitabine plus carboplatin for advanced urothelial cancer with cisplatin-unfit renal function. In Vivo. 2019;33(1):167–72.

14. De Santis M, Wiechno PJ, Bellmunt J, et al. Vinflunine-gemcitabine versus vinflunine-carboplatin as first-line chemotherapy in cisplatin-unfit patients with advanced urothelial carcinoma: results of an international randomized phase II trial (JASINT1). Ann Oncol. 2016;27(3):449–54.

15. Miyata Y, Asai A, Mitsunari K, Matsuo T, Ohba K, Sakai H. Safety and efficacy of combination therapy with low-dose gemcitabine, paclitaxel, and sorafenib in patients with cisplatin-resistant urothelial cancer. Med Oncol. 2015;32(10):235.

16. Retz M, de Geeter P, Goebell PJ, Matz U, de Schultz W, Hegele A. Vinflunine in routine clinical practice for the treatment of advanced or metastatic urothelial cell carcinoma—data from a prospective, multicenter experience. BMC Cancer. 2015;15:455.

17. Massard C, Gordon MS, Sharma S, et al. Safety and efficacy of durvalumab (MEDI4736), an anti-programmed cell death ligand-1 immune checkpoint inhibitor, in patients with advanced urothelial bladder cancer. J Clin Oncol. 2016;34(26):3119–25.

18. Necchi A, Joseph RW, Loriot Y, et al. Atezolizumab in platinum-treated locally advanced or metastatic urothelial carcinoma: post-progression outcomes from the phase II IMvigor210 study. Ann Oncol. 2017;28(12):3044–50.

19. Petrylak DP, Powles T, Bellmunt J, et al. Atezolizumab (MPDL3280A) monotherapy for patients with metastatic urothelial cancer: long-term outcomes from a phase 1 study. JAMA Oncol. 2018;4(4):537–44.

20. Plimack ER, Bellmunt J, Gupta S, et al. Safety and activity of pembrolizumab in patients with locally advanced or metastatic urothelial cancer (KEYNOTE-012): a non-randomised, open-label, phase 1b study. Lancet Oncol. 2017;18(2):212–20.

21. Levy A, Massard C, Soria JC, Deutsch E. Concurrent irradiation with the anti-programmed cell death ligand-1 immune checkpoint blocker durvalumab: single centre subset analysis from a phase 1/2 trial. Eur J Cancer. 2016;68:156–62.

22. Necchi A, Lo Vullo S, Mariani L, et al. An open-label, single-arm, phase 2 study of the Aurora kinase A inhibitor alisertib in patients with advanced urothelial cancer. Investig New Drugs. 2016;34(2):236–42.

23. Tree AC, Jones K, Hafeez S, et al. Dose-limiting urinary toxicity with pembrolizumab combined with weekly hypofractionated radiation therapy in bladder cancer. Int J Radiat Oncol Biol Phys. 2018;101(5):1168–71.

24. Christodoulou M, Reeves KJ, Hodgson C, et al. Outcomes of radiosensitisation in elderly patients with advanced bladder cancer. Radiother Oncol. 2018;129(3):499–506.

Part X

Salvage Therapy

A Systematic Review on Salvage Cystectomy

70.1   Research Methods

A systematic review relating to muscle invasive bladder cancer and salvage cystectomy was conducted. This was to identify whether salvage radical cystectomy has a role in this cohort. The search strategy aimed to identify all references related to bladder cancer AND muscle invasive disease AND salvage cystectomy. Search terms used were as follows: (Bladder cancer) AND (muscle invasive disease) AND (Salvage Cystectomy). The following databases were screened from 1979 to June 2020:

- CINAHL
- MEDLINE (NHS Evidence)
- Cochrane
- AMed
- EMBASE
- PsychINFO
- SCOPUS
- Web of Science

In addition, searches using Medical Subject Headings (MeSH) and keywords were conducted using Cochrane databases. Two UK-based experts in bladder cancer were consulted to identify any additional studies.

Studies were eligible for inclusion if they reported primary research focusing on muscle invasive bladder cancer and nerve sparing. Papers were included if published after 1984 and had to be in English. Studies that did not conform to this were excluded. Only primary research was included (Fig. 70.1).

Abstracts were independently screened for eligibility by two reviewers and disagreements resolved through discussion or third-party opinion. Agreement level was calculated using Cohen's Kappa to test the intercoder reliability of this

© The Editor(s) (if applicable) and The Author(s), under exclusive license to
Springer Nature Switzerland AG 2021
S. S. Goonewardene et al., *Management of Muscle Invasive Bladder Cancer*,
Management of Urology, https://doi.org/10.1007/978-3-030-57915-9_70

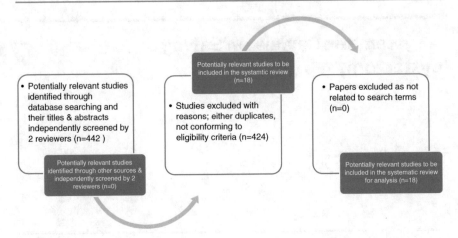

Fig. 70.1 Flow chart of studies identified through the systematic review. (Adapted from PRISMA)

screening process. Cohens' Kappa allows comparison of inter-rater reliability between papers using relative observed agreement. This also takes account of the comparison occurring by chance. The first reviewer agreed all 18 papers to be included, the second, agreed on 18.

Data extraction was piloted by the researcher and amended in consultation with the research team (author and two academic supervisors). Data collected included authors, year and country of publication, study aims, setting, intervention aims, number of participants, study design, intervention components and delivery methods, comparison groups and outcome measures, notes and follow-up questions for the authors. Studies were quality assessed using the PRISMA criteria for randomised controlled trials, Mays et al. [1, 2] for the action research and qualitative studies and the Critical Skills Appraisal programme for cohort studies. This was also applied to randomised controlled trials and qualitative studies.

The search identified 442 papers (Fig. 70.1). Eighteen mapped to the search terms and eligibility criteria. The current systematic reviews were examined to gain further knowledge about the subject. Four hundred and twenty-four papers were excluded due to not conforming to eligibility criteria or adding to the evidence. Of the 18 papers left, relevant abstracts were identified and the full papers obtained (all of which were in English), to quality assure against search criteria. There was considerable heterogeneity of design among the included studies therefore a narrative review of the evidence was undertaken. There was significant heterogeneity within studies, including clinical topic, numbers, outcomes, as a result a narrative review was thought to be best. There were 16 cohort studies, with a moderate level of evidence and 2 controlled trials with a good level of evidence. These were from a range of countries with minimal loss to follow-up. All participants were identified appropriately.

70.2   Is Salvage Cystectomy Required?

Treatment of a series of 194 patients with T3 (B2/C) tumors by radical radiotherapy, 5000–5500 rad in 4 weeks, produced a 5-year survival of 40% [3]. Patients whose tumor completely disappeared after treatment (N = 97) had a 5-year survival of 69% [3]. These results raise doubts about the necessity of performing elective cystectomy in patients who achieve complete response after radiotherapy, though the significantly better survival of partial responders who underwent salvage cystectomy emphasizes the need for an active policy of cystectomy once failure to respond completely to radiotherapy has been established and a need for techniques to give early indication of nonresponse to radiotherapy [3].

Seven hundred and four patients with bladder cancer treated by radiotherapy at the London Hospital between 1965 and 1974 have been followed for a minimum period of 5 years [4]. Invasive tumours were usually treated by radical radiotherapy [4]. Cystectomy was reserved for patients whose tumours did not respond to radiation, recurred later on, or who developed complications from radiotherapy [4]. The crude 5-year survival rate for T3 tumours in this series was 38%—similar to that obtained in other centres using pre-operative radiation followed by cystectomy, but this overall figure conceals the important difference between two distinct tumour populations [4]. Nearly half of these tumours appear to be radiosensitive, giving a 56% crude 5-year survival rate for T3 tumours [4]. The remainder are radioinsensitive, with only a 17% crude 5-year survival rate for T3 tumours. When there is a good initial response to radiotherapy there would seem to be no necessity to insist upon cystectomy [4].

Nineteen salvage cystectomies were performed during a period of 17 years, either on patients who failed definitive radiation therapy of bladder carcinoma or on those with massive bleeding or incapacitating irritative bladder symptoms after irradiation [5]. In 16 cases a single-stage and in 3 a two-stage procedure was used. The postoperative hospital mortality rate was 11% [5]. Early complications developed in 63%, late complications in 47% of the patients [5]. The 5-year survival rate was 5%. In 11 cases, widespread transitional cell carcinoma was the cause of death [5]. With more accurate preoperative tumor staging and subsequent patient selection, better results can be obtained by this procedure [5]. A proposal for the treatment of patients with T3 bladder cancer is made [5].

70.3   Survival Outcomes in Salvage Cystectomy

Abratt studied 46 patients who underwent salvage cystectomy [6]. The overall 5-year survival rate was 43% [6]. There was a higher 5-year survival rate in patients with an incomplete response compared with those with a complete response to their prior irradiation (50% and 36%), in patients with grades 1 or 2 compared with grade 3 histology (75% and 28%), and in patients with T1 or T2 tumours compared with T3 tumours (59% and 32%) [6]. A worsening of tumour grade and category was found in some patients when comparing the findings at cystectomy with those prior to irradiation [6]. This was consistently higher in patients with a prior complete response than in those with an incomplete response [6]. There were 3 deaths and 12 non-fatal major complications due to the prior irradiation or surgery, with a mortality rate of 7% and an overall 5-year complications rate of 35% [6].

Recent clinical studies have revealed the superiority of planned preoperative irradiation therapy followed by cystectomy compared to either treatment modality alone [7]. Crawford examined 37 consecutive patients who failed definitive irradiation therapy and had salvage cystectomy [7]. The mortality rate for this group was 8.1% and the early complication rate was 24% [7]. However, none of the patients who underwent a 2-stage procedure or who had an early perineal approach died. In addition, only 1 (7%) of the staged patients had an early complication [7]. The overall survival for the entire group of 37 patients was 38% [7]. However, those patients with pathological stage O or A disease had a 63% survival compared to a dismal 19% for those with stage B or greater disease.

Cooke established the long-term outcome for muscle-invasive transitional cell carcinoma of the bladder treated by radiotherapy with or without neoadjuvant cisplatin [8]. Minimum follow-up was 9 (median 11) years, at which time 29 patients (18%) remain alive [8]. Median survival was 24 months with no difference between the treatment groups (chi(2) = 0.08, p = 0.77) [8]. Overall cystectomy rate was 24% (radiotherapy alone 20%, combined therapy 28%; p = 0.24) [8]. Median time to cystectomy from primary treatment was 12 months; range 56 days to 10 years [8]. The risk of cystectomy was 11%, 10% and 7% for the first, second and third years after radiotherapy respectively, and 8% in total after the third year [8]. The proportion of patients alive in each successive year who had required a cystectomy was between 20% and 30% for 5 of the first 8 years after treatment [8].

The results of salvage cystectomy for persistent or recurrent tumour following definite radiotherapy in 47 patients are reviewed [9]. The calculated 5-year survival rate was 25% for all stages, with a significantly better survival for the low pathological stages [9]. Operative mortality was 12.8% [9]. It was concluded that salvage cystectomy is a suitable supplement in the treatment of bladder cancer in spite of the considerable operative mortality and complication rate [9].

70.4   Salvage Cystectomy After EBRT

Nieuwenhuijzen evaluated the long-term results of salvage cystectomy after interstitial radiotherapy (IRT) and external beam radiotherapy (EBRT) [10]. Salvage cystectomy was used after failure of IRT in 14 or EBRT in 13 patients, with a 3- and 5-year survival probability of 46% (95% confidence interval 26–65) and 33 (11–54)% [10]. The 5-year overall survival after cystectomy was 54% after IRT and 14% after EBRT (p = 0.12) [10]. Tumour category, response to radiation, American Society of Anesthesiology score, and complete tumour resection had a significant influence on survival [10]. Five of seven patients with incomplete resection died because of local disease, with a median survival of 5 months [10]. There was clinical understaging after radiotherapy in 41% of patients [10]. Nine patients had an orthotopic neobladder, with complete day- and night-time continence in eight and four, respectively [10].

Sixty-two patients with carcinoma of the bladder who had received external radiation as definitive therapy underwent radical cystectomy for persistent or recurrent tumor [11]. A preoperative clinical assessment correctly predicted whether the tumor was superficial or advanced in 74% of patients, which correlated with prognosis [11]. Overall 5-year survival rate after cystectomy was 43%, while 5-year survival rates for patients with clinically staged superficial and advanced tumors were 64% and 25%, respectively [11]. There have been no postoperative deaths, and morbidity was not greater than that of patients undergoing cystectomy after planned preoperative radiation therapy [11].

Between 1976 and 1983, 70 patients who underwent cystectomy for transitional cell carcinoma (TCC) of the bladder were retrospectively divided into two groups: 39 patients were treated by a protocol using 2000 rad of radiation over a period of 5 days followed by immediate cystectomy (group 1); 31 patients who failed to be cured by definitive radiotherapy of 6000 rad were treated by salvage cystectomy (group 2) [12]. The 5-year disease-specific survival rate was not significantly different in the two groups of patients (64.5% and 65.5%) [12]. The postoperative early complication rates were similar as well (36.8% in group 1 and 35.5% in group 2) [12]. One patient of the group treated with 2000 rad died 19 days after surgery, giving an operative mortality of 1.4% [12].

Sell examined 183 patients with transitiocellular carcinoma of the urinary bladder, category T2–T4a, entered a randomized study [13]. The treatment plan was followed by 66 patients (75%) in the planned cystectomy group and by 88 (92%) in the radical radiotherapy group of which 27 (28%) were treated with salvage cystectomy [13]. The results showed a trend to a higher survival rate following the combined treatment with preoperative irradiation and cystectomy compared to radical irradiation followed by salvage cystectomy in case of residual tumor, but a statistical significant difference could not be demonstrated [13]. The lack of difference also applied according to the actually given treatment. There was no difference in surgical complications between planned and salvage cystectomy and there were no postoperative deaths among the cystectomized patients.

70.5   Prognostic Factors in Salvage Cystectomy

Bruins reported the clinical outcomes and prognostic factors in patients undergoing salvage radical cystectomy (sRC) for recurrent urothelial carcinoma (UC) of the bladder following partial cystectomy (PC) [14]. Peri-operative mortality was 2.8% [14]. After sRC, 44 patients (61.2%) had pathologically organ-confined disease, 14 patients (19.4%) extravesical disease and 14 patients (19.4%) lymph node positive disease [14]. Five-year recurrence-free survival and overall survival following sRC were 56% and 41%, respectively [14]. On multivariate analysis, the presence of pathological tumor stage $\geq$pT3a (hazard ratio 6.86, p < 0.001) and the presence of lymph node metastases (hazard ratio 8.78, p < 0.001) were associated with increased risk of recurrence after sRC [14].

Droller conducted a retrospective review of patients who underwent salvage cystectomy, patients with muscle-invasive cancers who had initially presented with tumors that were pathologically TA or T1 appeared to have a better prognosis than those who had muscle-invasive (T2 or T3) cancers on initial clinical presentation [15]. Prognosis in each group appeared to correlate with the stage of tumor at initial clinical presentation rather than with stage of tumor at recurrence after radiation therapy [15]. Prognosis also appeared to correlate with architectural configuration of the presenting tumor as well as the type of invasion [15]. Thus, papillary lesions with muscle invasion by a broad front of histologically cohesive blocks of cells appeared to have a better prognosis than did solid or nodular lesions that appeared to invade the muscle wall in a tentacular fashion with finger like tumor cell extensions that seemed to percolate through the bladder wall [15]. Taken together, the results of treatment in these patients may have represented the intrinsic nature of their particular tumors [15].

Analysis of 86 patients who underwent salvage cystectomy following a radical course of radiotherapy for bladder cancer and 37 patients who underwent primary cystectomy has shown a greater survival for women than men [16]. The following factors were associated with a significant deterioration in survival: (1) Age at time of cystectomy: post-operative mortality and tumour recurrence are greater over the age of 70. (2) Non-function of one kidney on IVU. (3) Grade 3 tumour on cystectomy specimen. (4) pT3 or pT4 tumour on cystectomy specimen [16].

70.6   Post Operative Complications for Salvage Cystectomy

Eswara characterized complications associated with salvage cystectomy [17]. Complications of any grade within 90 days occurred in 69% (63 of 91) of patients and 16% (15 of 91) experienced major complications within 90 days [17]. Of the patients 21% (19 of 91) required hospital readmission within 90 days [17]. The 90-day mortality rate was 2.2% (2 of 91) [17]. Significant cardiovascular/hematological complications (pulmonary embolism, myocardial infarction, deep vein thrombosis, transfusion) within 90 days were more common in the immediate than in the delayed cystectomy group (37% vs. 15%, p = 0.02) [17]. Tissue healing complications (fascial dehiscence, wound infection, ureteral stricture, anastomotic stricture, stoma/loop revisions) were more common in the delayed than in the immediate cystectomy group (35% vs. 12%, p = 0.05) [17].

Jenkins examined salvage cystectomy was reserved for patients whose tumours either did not respond completely to radiation or recurred later, provided they were fit for surgery and had not developed distant metastases [18]. The overall corrected 5-year survival rate was 40%; 75 patients responded to radiation and did not relapse during the period of follow-up; 20 patients had an initial response to radiation but subsequently relapsed, with a 5-year survival rate following relapse of 20% [18]. Of these, 11 patients had a cystectomy with a 5-year survival following relapse of 36%, whereas all 9 patients who did not have a cystectomy died within 3 years; 87 patients who did not respond to radiation had a 5-year survival rate of 18% [18]. Of these, 22 patients underwent salvage cystectomy with a 5-year survival of 47%, whereas the 65 patients who did not have a cystectomy had a 5-year survival of 3% [18]. These results justify a policy of radical radiotherapy and salvage cystectomy rather than elective cystectomy in the treatment of invasive bladder cancer [18].

Twenty patients with bladder carcinoma underwent total cystectomy and one-stage urinary diversion after a definitive external radiotherapy [19]. The indication for surgery was a persistent or locally recurrent tumor and/or intractable voiding symptoms [19]. There was no operative mortality [19]. Early or late complications occurred in 14 patients (70%) and in 7 of these cases a reoperation was necessary [19]. The overall 5-year survival rate after the operation was 61%[19]. The prognosis of the patients was dependent on the pathological stage of the tumor in cystectomy specimens [19].

70.7 Salvage Cystectomy and Orthotopic Neobladder

Bochner described their salvage surgery and orthotopic bladder substitution following failed radical radiation therapy [20]. Operative characteristics, postoperative outcomes and postoperative complications related or unrelated to urinary reconstruction were similar between irradiated and nonirradiated patients [20]. Good day and night continence following surgery was reported by 67 and 56% of irradiated patients, respectively [20]. Patients with poor postoperative continence were successfully treated with the placement of an artificial urinary sphincter [20].

References

1. Moher D, Liberati A, Tetzlaff J, Altman DG. "Preferred Reporting Items for Systematic Reviews and Meta-Analyses: The Prisma Statement." [In English]. BMJ (Online) 339, no. 7716 (08 Aug 2009):332–36.
2. Mays N, Pope C, Popay J. "Systematically Reviewing Qualitative and Quantitative Evidence to Inform Management and Policy-Making in the Health Field." [In English]. Journal of Health Services Research and Policy 10, no. SUPPL. 1 (July 2005):6–20.
3. Hope-Stone HF, Oliver RT, England HR, Blandy JP. T3 bladder cancer: salvage rather than elective cystectomy after radiotherapy. Urology. 1984;24(4):315–20.
4. Blandy JP, England HR, Evans SJ, Hope-Stone HF, Mair GM, Mantell BS, Oliver RT, Paris AM, Risdon RA. T3 bladder cancer—the case for salvage cystectomy. Br J Urol. 1980;52(6):506–10.
5. Lindell O. Salvage cystectomy. Review of 19 cases. Eur Urol. 1987;13(1–2):17–21.
6. Abratt RP, Wilson JA, Pontin AR, Barnes RD. Salvage cystectomy after radical irradiation for bladder cancer-prognostic factors and complications. Br J Urol. 1993;72(5 Pt 2):756–60.
7. Crawford ED, Skinner DG. Salvage cystectomy after irradiation failure. J Urol. 1980;123(1):32–4.
8. Cooke PW, Dunn JA, Latief T, Bathers S, James ND, Wallace DM. Long-term risk of salvage cystectomy after radiotherapy for muscle-invasive bladder cancer. Eur Urol. 2000;38(3):279–86.

9. Rasmussen RB, Knudsen JB, Sørensen BL, Walbom-Jørgensen S. Radical cystectomy for residual of recurrent tumour after definitive radiotherapy (salvage cystectomy). Dan Med Bull. 1988;35(1):98–100.

10. Nieuwenhuijzen JA, Horenblas S, Meinhardt W, van Tinteren H, Moonen LM. Salvage cystectomy after failure of interstitial radiotherapy and external beam radiotherapy for bladder cancer. BJU Int. 2004;94(6):793–7.

11. Swanson DA, von Eschenbach AC, Bracken RB, Johnson DE. Salvage cystectomy for bladder carcinoma. Cancer. 1981;47(9):2275–9.

12. Nissenkorn I, Baniel J, Slucker D, Servadio C, Winkler H. Comparison between short-course high-dose preoperative irradiation with immediate radical cystectomy and salvage cystectomy after full-dose irradiation. Eur Urol. 1990;18(1):23–6.

13. Sell A, Jakobsen A, Nerstrøm B, Sørensen BL, Steven K, Barlebo H. Treatment of advanced bladder cancer category T2 T3 and T4a. A randomized multicenter study of preoperative irradiation and cystectomy versus radical irradiation and early salvage cystectomy for residual tumor. DAVECA protocol 8201. Danish Vesical Cancer Group. Scand J Urol Nephrol Suppl. 1991;138:193–201.

14. Bruins HM, Wopat R, Mitra AP, Cai J, Miranda G, Skinner EC, Daneshmand S. Long-term outcomes of salvage radical cystectomy for recurrent urothelial carcinoma of the bladder following partial cystectomy. BJU Int. 2013;111(3 Pt B):E37–42.

15. Droller MJ, Walsh PC. Therapeutic efficacy of salvage cystectomy. Do results reflect natural history of bladder cancer? Urology. 1983;22(2):118–22.

16. Osborn DE, Honan RP, Palmer MK, Barnard RJ, McIntyre D, Pointon RS. Factors influencing salvage cystectomy results. Br J Urol. 1982;54(2):122–5.

17. Eswara JR, Efstathiou JA, Heney NM, Paly J, Kaufman DS, McDougal WS, McGovern F, Shipley WU. Complications and long-term results of salvage cystectomy after failed bladder sparing therapy for muscle invasive bladder cancer. J Urol. 2012;187(2):463–8.

18. Jenkins BJ, Caulfield MJ, Fowler CG, Badenoch DF, Tiptaft RC, Paris AM, Hope-Stone HF, Oliver RT, Blandy JP. Reappraisal of the role of radical radiotherapy and salvage cystectomy in the treatment of invasive (T2/T3) bladder cancer. Br J Urol. 1988;62(4):343–6.

19. Nurmi M, Valavaara R, Puntala P, Ekfors T. Single-stage salvage cystectomy: results and complications in 20 patients. Eur Urol. 1989;16(2):89–91.

20. Bochner BH, Figueroa AJ, Skinner EC, Lieskovsky G, Petrovich Z, Boyd SD, Skinner DG. Salvage radical cystoprostatectomy and orthotopic urinary diversion following radiation failure. J Urol. 1998;160(1):29–33.

A systematic review relating to bladder cancer and survivorship was conducted. This was to identify the bladder cancer and Survivorship. The search strategy aimed to identify all references related to bladder cancer AND Survivorship. Search terms used were as follows: (Bladder cancer) AND (Survivorship). The following databases were screened from 1989 to June 2020:

- CINAHL
- MEDLINE (NHS Evidence)
- Cochrane
- AMed
- EMBASE
- PsychINFO
- SCOPUS
- Web of Science

In addition, searches using Medical Subject Headings (MeSH) and keywords were conducted using Cochrane databases. Two UK-based experts in bladder cancer were consulted to identify any additional studies.

Studies were eligible for inclusion if they reported primary research focusing on bladder cancer and screening. Papers were included if published after 1984 and had to be in English. Studies that did not conform to this were excluded. Only primary research was included (Fig. 71.1). The overall aim was to identify the role and components of bladder cancer screening.

Abstracts were independently screened for eligibility by two reviewers and disagreements resolved through discussion or third-party opinion. Agreement level was calculated using Cohen's Kappa to test the intercoder reliability of this screening process. Cohens' Kappa allows comparison of inter-rater reliability

S. S. Goonewardene et al., *Management of Muscle Invasive Bladder Cancer*, Management of Urology, https://doi.org/10.1007/978-3-030-57915-9_71

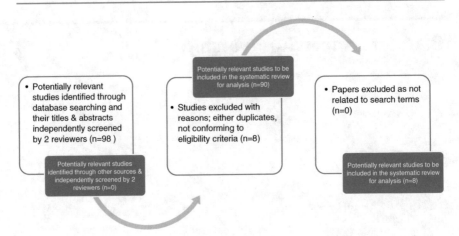

Fig. 71.1 Flow chart of studies identified through the systematic review. (Adapted from PRISMA)

between papers using relative observed agreement. This also takes account of the comparison occurring by chance. The first reviewer agreed all 8 papers to be included, the second, agreed on 8.

Data extraction was piloted by the researcher and amended in consultation with the research team (author and two academic supervisors). Data collected included authors, year and country of publication, study aims, setting, intervention aims, number of participants, study design, intervention components and delivery methods, comparison groups and outcome measures, notes and follow-up questions for the authors. Studies were quality assessed using the PRISMA criteria for randomised controlled trials, Mays et al. [1, 2] for the action research and qualitative studies and the Critical Skills Appraisal programme for cohort studies. This was also applied to randomised controlled trials and qualitative studies.

The search identified 8 papers (Fig. 71.1). All 20 mapped to the search terms and eligibility criteria. The current systematic reviews were examined to gain further knowledge about the subject. Ninety papers were excluded due to not conforming to eligibility criteria or adding to the evidence for bladder cancer screening. Of the 8 papers left, relevant abstracts were identified and the full papers obtained (all of which were in English), to quality assure against search criteria. There was considerable heterogeneity of design among the included studies therefore a narrative review of the evidence was undertaken. There was significant heterogeneity within studies, including clinical topic, numbers, outcomes, as a result a narrative review was thought to be best. There were 8 cohort studies, with a moderate level of evidence. These were from a range of countries with minimal loss to follow-up. All participants were identified appropriately.

71.1 Systematic Review

71.1.1 Survivorship Differences in Demographic Factors

Seo examine survivorship disparities in demographic factors and risk status for non-muscle-invasive bladder cancer (NMIBC), which accounts for more than 75% of all urinary bladder cancers, but is highly curable with early identification and treatment [3]. Among all urinary bladder cancer patients, the majority of NMIBCs were in male (74.1%), non-Latino white (86.7%), married (67.8%), and low-risk (37.6%) to intermediate-risk (44.8%) patients [3]. Survivorship (in median life years) was highest for non-Latino white (5.4 years), married (5.4 years), and low-risk (5.7 years) patients (K-M analysis, p < 0.001) [3]. There was significantly lower survivorship for elderly, male (female hazard ratio [HR], 0.96), Latino (HR, 1.20), and unmarried (married HR, 0.93) patients [3].

71.1.2 Health Related Quality of Life

Physical activity has been shown to significantly improve health-related quality of life (HRQOL) and survivorship in a variety of patients with cancer [4]. Gopalakrishna et al. [4] described self-reported physical activity patterns and HRQOL and examine the association between these measures in a large cohort of bladder cancer survivors [4]. A total of 472 subjects (49% response rate) completed the survey [4]. The mean age was 74 years; 81% were male and 87% were white [4]. Similarly, subjects reporting "high" physical activity had a 2.2-fold increased odds of reporting higher global HRQOL compared with subjects reporting "low" physical activity [4].

Chung assessed the quality of life (QoL), informational needs, and supportive care needs (SCN) in a large sample of muscle invasive (MIBC) and non-muscle invasive (NMIBC) bladder cancer survivors across the treatment trajectory (newly diagnosed and undergoing treatment, post-treatment follow-up, and treatment for advanced/recurrent disease) [5]. Of the 1126 surveys distributed, 586 were completed (response = 52%) [5]. Eighty-eight percent (95% CI 85–91%) of respondents reported at least one SCN, with a median of 12 [5]. Over half of the participants (54%, 95% CI 49–59%) had at least one unmet need and 15% had ≥10 unmet needs. Newly diagnosed participants had the highest number of unmet needs [5].

Mohamed examined unmet patient needs along the illness trajectory [6]. At diagnosis unmet informational needs were predominant, consisting of insufficient discussion of certain topics, including urinary diversion options and their side effects, self-care, the recovery process and medical insurance trajectory [6]. Unmet psychological needs related to depression, and worries about changes in body image and sexual function were reported trajectory [6]. Postoperative unmet needs revolved around medical needs (e.g. pain and bowel dysfunction) and instrumental needs (e.g. need of support for stomal appliances, catheters and incontinence) trajectory

[6]. During survivorship (i.e. 6–72 months postoperatively) unmet needs centered around psychological support (i.e. depression, poor body image and sexual dysfunction) and instrumental support (e.g. difficulty adjusting to changes in daily living) trajectory [6].

71.1.3 Unmet Informational Needs in Bladder Cancer Survivorship

Mohamed examined whether the unmet informational and supportive care needs of the patients with muscle-invasive bladder cancer vary by the patients' age, sex, or individual treatment choices [7]. Younger patients (<60 years) were less satisfied with the treatment information received presurgery and more likely to report post-treatment complications, choose a neobladder, and seek and receive professional support regarding sexual function, than were older patients ($p < 0.05$) [7]. More women than men reported difficulties with self-care and relied on themselves in disease self-management as opposed to relying on spousal support ($p < 0.05$) [7]. Patients with neobladder were more likely to report difficulties with urinary incontinence and deterioration in sexual function, whereas patients with ileal conduit were more likely to require spousal help with self-care [7]. Patients who received chemotherapy were significantly more likely to report changes in everyday life ($p < 0.05$) [7]. Lastly, regardless of age, sex, or treatment choice, up to 50% of patients reported feeling depressed before or after treatment [7].

71.1.4 Exercise Programming and Counselling in Bladder Cancer Survivorship

Karvinen exercise programming and counseling preferences of different cancer survivor groups may facilitate the delivery of optimal exercise programs in these growing populations [8]. The majority of survivors indicated they would be interested (81.1%) and able (84.3%) to participate in an exercise program designed for bladder cancer survivors [8]. Strong preferences for home-based exercise programming (53.7%), walking (81.1%), moderate intensity activity (61.7%) and unsupervised sessions (70.6%) were also noted [8]. Logistic regression analyses showed that older survivors were more likely to prefer to exercise at home (77% vs. 68%; OR = 4.21, 95% CI = 0.188–0.962, $p = 0.040$), do light intensity exercise (33% vs. 16%; OR = 4.50, 95% CI = 0.208–0.940, $p = 0.034$) and want unsupervised exercise sessions (75% vs. 62%; OR = 4.60, 95% CI = 1.07–4.08, $p = 0.032$) [8].

71.1.5 Health Behaviours in Bladder Cancer Survivorship

Chung examine health behaviours in bladder cancer survivors including physical activity (PA), body mass index, diet quality, smoking and alcohol consumption, and to explore their relationship with health-related quality of life (HRQoL) [9]. A total of 586 participants completed the questionnaire (52% response rate) [9]. In all, 60.9% (n = 357) were overweight/obese, and the vast majority met alcohol recommendations (n = 521, 92.5%) and were current non-smokers (n = 535, 91.0%) [9]. Health behaviours did not differ between MIBC and NMIBC, and cancer treatment stages [9]. Sufficient PA, healthy diet, and non-smoking were significantly associated with HRQoL, and the number of health behaviours participants engaged in was positively associated with HRQoL (p < 0.001) [9].

71.1.6 Survivorship Care Plans

Linscott determine the prevalence of SCP receipt for survivors of genitourinary (GU) malignancy including kidney, prostate, and bladder cancer and evaluate whether receipt was associated with a measurable health benefit [10]. SCP distribution increased from 27.5% in 2012 to 39.5% in 2017 [10]. Patients with low income, less formal education, and extremes of age were less likely to receive an SCP [10]. Those receiving an SCP were less likely to report poor physical health (OR 0.70; CI 0.52–0.96; p = 0.026) [10]. Sub-analysis showed a similar result for physical health of prostate patients (OR 0.68; CI 0.48–0.96; p = 0.030) and general health of kidney patients (OR 0.37; CI 0.19–0.75; p = 0.006) [10].

71.1.7 Physical Prehabilitation Prior to Cystectomy

Jensen investigate the feasibility, the adherence, and the efficacy of a short-term physical pre-habilitation program to patients with invasive bladder cancer awaiting radical cystectomy (RC) [11]. A total of 66% (95% confidence interval (CI) 51; 78) adhered more than 75% of the recommended progressive standardized exercise program [11]. In the intervention group, a significant improvement in muscle power of 18% (p < 0.002) was found at time for surgery [11]. Moreover, muscle power was significantly improved compared to that in the standard group with 0.3 W/kg (95% CI 0.08; 0.5%) (p < 0.006) [11]. Adherence was not associated with pre-operative BMI, nutritional risk, comorbidity, pain, gender, or age [11].

References

1. Moher D, Liberati A, Tetzlaff J, Altman DG. "Preferred Reporting Items for Systematic Reviews and Meta-Analyses: The Prisma Statement." [In English]. BMJ (Online) 339, no. 7716 (08 Aug 2009):332–36.
2. Mays N, Pope C, Popay J. "Systematically Reviewing Qualitative and Quantitative Evidence to Inform Management and Policy-Making in the Health Field." [In English]. Journal of Health Services Research and Policy 10, no. SUPPL. 1 (July 2005):6–20.
3. Seo M, Langabeer JR II. Demographic and survivorship disparities in non-muscle-invasive bladder cancer in the United States. J Prev Med Public Health. 2018;51(5):242–7.

4. Gopalakrishna A, Longo TA, Fantony JJ, Harrison MR, Inman BA. Physical activity patterns and associations with health-related quality of life in bladder cancer survivors. Urol Oncol. 2017;35(9):540.e1–6.
5. Chung J, Kulkarni GS, Morash R, et al. Assessment of quality of life, information, and supportive care needs in patients with muscle and non-muscle invasive bladder cancer across the illness trajectory. Support Care Cancer. 2019;27(10):3877–85.
6. Mohamed NE, Chaoprang Herrera P, Hudson S, et al. Muscle invasive bladder cancer: examining survivor burden and unmet needs. J Urol. 2014;191(1):48–53.
7. Mohamed NE, Pisipati S, Lee CT, et al. Unmet informational and supportive care needs of patients following cystectomy for bladder cancer based on age, sex, and treatment choices. Urol Oncol. 2016;34(12):531.e7–531.e14.
8. Karvinen KH, Courneya KS, Venner P, North S. Exercise programming and counseling preferences in bladder cancer survivors: a population-based study. J Cancer Surviv. 2007;1(1):27–34.
9. Chung J, Kulkarni GS, Bender J, et al. Modifiable lifestyle behaviours impact the health-related quality of life of bladder cancer survivors. BJU Int. 2020; https://doi.org/10.1111/bju.15007.
10. Linscott JA, Rutan MC, Han PKJ, et al. Receipt of survivorship care plans and self-reported health status among patients with genitourinary malignancy. J Urol. 2020;204:564–9.
11. Jensen BT, Laustsen S, Jensen JB, Borre M, Petersen AK. Exercise-based pre-habilitation is feasible and effective in radical cystectomy pathways-secondary results from a randomized controlled trial. Support Care Cancer. 2016;24(8):3325–31.

Cancer affects both patients and their caregivers. Caregiver burden may change during different stages of the patients' cancer trajectory [1]. Limited research has focused on the impact of being a caregiver, assessed by the caregiver's mental health and quality of life (QOL) during the curative and the palliative phases of the patient's disease [1].

Girgis et al. [2], began to test the psychometric properties of a measure designed to capture the multi-dimensional supportive care needs of cancer caregivers: the Supportive Care Needs Survey-Partners and Caregivers (SCNS-P&C) [2]. Draft SCNS-P&C items were developed with reference to the literature and existing instruments and reviewed for face and content validity [2]. The final SCNS-P&C was then completed by 547 cancer caregivers. Psychometric analyses conducted included principal factor analysis, internal consistency, and construct validity through the known-group approach [2]. Across all domains, individuals with anxiety or depression were more likely to report at least one unmet moderate or high need in comparison to non-anxious or non-depressed participants [2]. A greater proportion of younger participants experienced at least one unmet moderate or high need within the Psychological and Emotional Needs and Work and Social Needs domains. Proportion of reported unmet needs varied across cancer types for the Health Care Service Needs and Information Needs domains [2]. The SCNS-P&C has the potential to comprehensively assess the range of caregivers' supportive care needs, across the illness trajectory [2]. The SCNS-P&C can be used by researchers and clinicians to determine caregivers' unmet needs, prioritize health-care resources, and tailor supportive cancer care services accordingly.

Scherbring identified the level of lay caregiver burden and perception of preparedness that exists for the oncology population prior to and just after hospital discharge [3]. Caregivers completed Robinson's Caregiver Strain Index and Archbold's Preparedness Scale questionnaires immediately prior to discharge, 7–10 days postdischarge, and 28–30 days postdischarge [3]. Preparedness levels ranged from "somewhat" to "pretty well" prepared and were consistent over time [3].

S. S. Goonewardene et al., *Management of Muscle Invasive Bladder Cancer*,
Management of Urology, https://doi.org/10.1007/978-3-030-57915-9_72

Burden levels were moderate and also consistent over time. Increased levels of preparedness were associated with decreased levels of burden, and that relationship was consistent over time [3]. Caregivers' levels of preparedness can be enhanced, although no significant differences were reported in the period from prehospital discharge to 1 month following discharge [3]. Burden experiences of caregivers are real and not affected by the transition from hospital to home. Burden experiences can be influenced by perceptions of preparedness [3]. Efforts to enhance the preparedness of lay caregivers can influence their burden experience.

Cancer affects not only the quality of life (QOL) of individuals with the disease but also that of their family members and close friends [4]. The impact on various aspects of the family caregivers' QOL is significant throughout the trajectory of the illness. Kim and Given reviewed literature on the QOL of family caregivers at the acute and middle- to long-term survivorship phases as well as the bereavement phase [4]. The findings suggested that the QOL of family caregivers of individuals with cancer varies along the illness trajectory [4]. This highlights were importance of assessing the ongoing adjustment of the caregivers over time. However, there were few theory-driven studies, and significant gaps remain in the current understanding of the effects of family caregiving beyond the time of diagnosis and treatment [4]. Accumulating evidence has supported the concept that cancer affects not only the patients/survivors but also their family members. However, theoretically and methodologically rigorous research on various aspects of the family's QOL, including not only the psychological but also the physical, spiritual, and behavioral adjustment to cancer in the family, remains sparse [4]. Family-based interventions across the trajectory of the illness also are needed.

Although cancer has been considered as a chronic disease for those diagnosed, the long-term impact of cancer on the family caregivers' quality of life (QOL) remains unknown [5]. Thus, the current study aimed: (a) to characterize family caregivers of cancer survivors, (b) to describe the multidimensional aspects of QOL of family caregivers of cancer survivors, and (c) to identify demographic and caregiving experience factors that may play significant roles in the caregivers' QOL around 5 years after the relative's initial diagnosis [5]. The findings help to increase evidence-based awareness of the long-term impact of cancer on the family caregivers' QOL [5]. Findings also have implications for developing programs, whereby family caregivers in the various phases of caregivership will benefit by improving their QOL.

This study describes the concordance between advanced cancer patients' self-report of quality of life and their caregivers' perception of the patients' quality of life at two time points. It is often necessary for health professionals to rely on information about the patients' quality of life that is provided by family caregivers (proxy), even though information from the patients is considered 'the gold standard' [6]. Therefore, it is important to establish how reliable this proxy information is. Data were collected 4–6 weeks following diagnosis of recurrent or progressive disease, and again 12 weeks later [6]. Fifty-one patients and their caregivers completed the European Organization for Research and Treatment of Cancer (EORTC) Quality of Life Questionnaire (QLQ-C30), version 2.0 at both time points [6]. In general, most caregivers were able to accurately rate the global quality of life, the level of functioning and the degree of symptom distress experienced by the person they were caring for, when compared with the patients' self-rating [6]. Caregiver ratings for physical domains tended to be more in agreement with those of patients as compared with ratings of the psychosocial domains [6]. This study suggests information from proxy raters is reliable when the proxy is a family caregiver, and this remains true over time.

When a patient is diagnosed with cancer, family members often assume responsibility for providing care. They are typically involved not only with the diagnostic and treatment phases of care but also across the care trajectory and into survivorship [7]. These caregivers are a primary source of support to individuals with cancer. The purpose of this article is to present an overview of the challenges, needs, and roles of family caregivers over the course of the cancer treatment trajectory and to discuss what support the professionals can provide [7]. Caregivers require support, coordination, and communication with health care providers if they are to be successful in carrying out tasks of care [7]. Concern for caregivers as partners in patient care and caregiver outcomes deserves attention from health care professionals. Considering the caregivers' value to the health care team, this role should not be underestimated.

Grov and Valeberg [1] compared caregivers of cancer patients during the curative and a palliative phases with respect to their mental health and health-related QOL [1]. This descriptive, cross-sectional study combines data from two studies. The first group consists of caregivers of patients with cancer in the late palliative phase and the second group consists of caregivers of outpatients with cancer who suffer from pain and/or use analgesics [1]. Based on this material, no significant differences in mental health and health-related QOL were revealed for caregivers of cancer patients in the palliative and the curative phases, respectively [1]. Neither education level in the caregivers, nor the patients' functional status influenced caregivers' mental health or QOL. Younger caregivers seem to have better physical QOL [1]. Being caregivers of cancer patients seems to have a similar pattern of impact on caregivers' mental health and quality of life regardless of the patient's disease stage [1].

To understand family caregivers' needs for better preparation and care, this state-of-the-science review examines the effect of caregiving on the health and well-being of caregivers, the efficacy of research-tested interventions on patient and caregiver outcomes, implications of the research on policy and practice, and recommendations for practice and future research [8]. Research findings indicate that caregiver stress can lead to psychological and sleep disturbances and changes in caregivers' physical health, immune function, and financial well-being [8]. Research-tested interventions delivered to caregivers of patients with cancer or other chronic illnesses can reduce many of these negative effects and improve caregivers' coping skills, knowledge, and quality of life [8]. Although these interventions also decrease patients' symptoms, reduce mortality (non-dementia patients), and improve patients' physical and mental health, they are seldom implemented in practice [8]. Recommendations for practice include development of standardized guidelines that address caregiver assessment, education, and resources; identification of "caregiver champions" in practice settings; provision of referrals to established support organizations for caregivers (e.g., Cancer Support Community, Cancer Care); and collaboration among caregiving, professional, and cancer-related organizations to advocate policy and practice changes for family caregivers.

References

1. Grov EK, Valeberg BT. Does the cancer patient's disease stage matter? A comparative study of caregivers' mental health and health related quality of life. Palliat Support Care. 2012;10(3):189–96.
2. Girgis A, Lambert S, Lecathelinais C. The supportive care needs survey for partners and caregivers of cancer survivors: development and psychometric evaluation. Psychooncology. 2011;20(4):387–93.
3. Scherbring M. Effect of caregiver perception of preparedness on burden in an oncology population. Oncol Nurs Forum. 2002;29(6):E70–6.
4. Kim Y, Given BA. Quality of life of family caregivers of cancer survivors: across the trajectory of the illness. Cancer. 2008;112(11 Suppl):2556–68.
5. Kim Y, Spillers RL, Hall DL. Quality of life of family caregivers 5 years after a relative's cancer diagnosis: follow-up of the national quality of life survey for caregivers. Psychooncology. 2012;21(3):273–81.
6. Milne DJ, Mulder LL, Beelen HC, Schofield P, Kempen GI, Aranda S. Patients' self-report and family caregivers' perception of quality of life in patients with advanced cancer: how do they compare? Eur J Cancer Care (Engl). 2006;15(2):125–32.
7. Given BA, Given CW, Sherwood PR. Family and caregiver needs over the course of the cancer trajectory. J Support Oncol. 2012;10(2):57–64.
8. Northouse L, Williams AL, Given B, McCorkle R. Psychosocial care for family caregivers of patients with cancer. J Clin Oncol. 2012;30(11):1227–34.

Muscle Invasive Bladder Cancer: What is the Impact of Radical Cystectomy on Patient Reported Outcome Measures?

73

73.1 Definition of Bladder Cancer Survivorship

The definition of cancer survivorship is varied. Survivorship is defined by Macmillan Cancer Support [1], as 'someone who has completed initial cancer management with no evidence of apparent disease'. According to the National Cancer Institute in the USA, cancer survivorship encompasses the "physical, psychosocial, and economic issues of cancer from diagnosis until the end of life." *The National Coalition of Cancer Survivors defines being a survivor as 'from diagnosis of cancer onwards'.* This has been extended to include 'the experience of living with, through and beyond a diagnosis'.

Bladder cancer (BC) is a common with variable treatments and variable outcomes as a result. Despite the disease's high prevalence, little is known of the experience of patients [2]. National patient experience surveys suggest that those with BC have poorer experiences than those with other common cancers. The aim of this review is to identify first-hand accounts of the lived experiences of diagnosis through to survivorship.

73.2 Bladder Cancer Survivorship and Patient Reported Outcome Measures: Code 1 Erectile Dysfunction

Post TURBT, 7 patients were involved. Comments made were as followed:

Code 1: Erectile dysfunction	Comments made were as followed
Age related disease	'ED does apply to elderly.'
No requirement for treatment	'Op does not affect erectile problem.'

S. S. Goonewardene et al., *Management of Muscle Invasive Bladder Cancer*, Management of Urology, https://doi.org/10.1007/978-3-030-57915-9_73

Code 1: Erectile dysfunction	Comments made were as followed
Side effects of surgery and requirement for a pathway	'ED afterwards—1 month-age dependant—would initially try to see if it resolved, then seek CNS help—an opt in pathway would help.'

This clearly indicates, that ED is an age-related problem, which would be of more concern to younger patients. There clearly needs to be a pathway in place to support this.

Post MMC instillation, 5 patients were involved there were no side effects experienced.

Post cystectomy, there were 10 patients involved. Comments made were as follows:

Code 1: Erectile dysfunction	Comments made as follows
Side effects of treatment	Problems getting erections, prolonged time to get prescription, have to order in caverject.
Psychological impact	Biggest psychological effect from lack of erections.
Requirement for pathway	Specialised pathway would make a difference, with CNS, and counsellor, but needs to start 6 months after cystectomy.
Requirement for pathway	Lack of support in a timely manner.
Age related disease	ED present, age related as to whether it is treated.
Requirement for pathway	No erections—not prepared—pathway few months after.

73.3 Bladder Cancer Survivorship and Patient Reported Outcome Measures: Code 2 Age Related disease

Post TURBT, 7 patients were involved. Comments made were as followed:

Code 2: Age related disease	Comments made were as followed
Age related disease	'ED does apply to elderly.'
Age related disease	'ED afterwards—1 month-age dependant—would initially try to see if it resolved, then seek CNS help—an opt in pathway would help.'
Side effects of surgery	

Post BCG/MMC there were 7 patients involved, there were no age related effects experienced.

Post radical cystectomy, there were 10 patients involved, the comments made were as follows:

Code 2: Age related disease	Comments made were as followed
Age related disease	Operation went well, not ready for prolonged healing process. Not prepared for hernia.
Age related disease	Not prepared for length of rehabilitation.
Side effects of surgery	Nutritionist needed. Taken erections away, but age related.

This demonstrates, there is a clear requirement for a pathway, and to specific indivisualised age related focus for treatment.

73.4   Bladder Cancer Survivorship and Patient Reported Outcome Measures: Code 3 Side Effects Post Operatively

Post TURBT, 7 patients were involved. Comments made were as followed:

Code 3: Side effects post operatively	Comments made were as followed
Age related disease	No side effects.
Age related disease	Op does not affect erectile problem.
Side effects of surgery	Recurrent problems with chest and UTI-managed medically-really happy.

Post BCG/MMC there were 7 patients involved, there were no age related effects experienced.

Code 3: Side effects post surgery	Comments made were as followed
Side effects post surgery	Prepared for side effects.
Education pre op	Shock at diagnosis but well supported.
Side effects of surgery	No side effects experienced.

Post radical cystectomy, there were 10 patients involved, the comments made were as follows:

Code 3: Side effects post surgery	Comments made were as followed
Side effects post surgery	Operation went well, not ready for prolonged healing process. Not prepared for hernia.
Requirement for pathway	Specialised pathway would make a difference, with CNS, and counsellor, but needs to start 6 months after cystectomy.
Side effects of surgery	Minor infection post op-wound infection. Not fully prepared for operation or side effects. Not prepared for length of rehabilitation.
Side effects of surgery	Lymphoedema-currently present. Pathway needed with CNS, but difficult to get a time as to when to start-pt dependant.

This demonstrates, there is a clear requirement for a pathway, more so to address side effects of surgery and age related diseases.

73.5   Bladder Cancer Survivorship and Patient Reported Outcome Measures: Code 4 Psychological Impact

There were no psychological issues experienced in either the TURBT/MMC/BCG groups.

There were 10 patients who underwent radical cystectomy. Comments made were as follows:

Code 4: Psychological impact from ED	Comments made were as followed
Impact of operation	Biggest psychological effect from lack of erections.
Impact of operation	Operation went well, not ready for prolonged healing process.
Impact of operation	Not fully prepared for operation or side effects.

All of these issues could be dealt with by a bladder cancer survivorship pathway.

73.6   Bladder Cancer Survivorship and Patient Reported Outcome Measures: Code 5 Impact of Operation on General Health

There were 7 patients involved with TURBTs.

Code 5: Impact of operation on general health	Comments made were as followed
Impact of operation	No side effects
Impact of operation	ED afterwards—1 month-age dependant—would initially try to see if it resolved, then seek CNS help—an opt in pathway would help
Impact of operation	Recurrent problems with chest and UTI-managed medically-really happy

There was no impact of procedure experience for BCG/MMC patients.

There were 10 patients who underwent radical cystectomy. Comments made were as follows:

Code 5: Impact of operation on general health	Comments made were as followed
Requirement for pathway	Peer support group with CNS beforehand would have helped.
Nutritionist requirement	Nutritionist needed. Taken erections away, but age related. Lymphoedema-currently present. Pathway needed with CNS, but difficult to get a time as to when to start-pt dependant.

Code 5: Impact of operation on general health	Comments made were as followed
Impact of operation	Problem post op-hernia post op.

References

1. Maher EJ. Managing the consequences of cancer treatment and the English National Cancer Survivorship Initiative. Acta Oncol. 2013;52(2):225–32.
2. Rowland JH, Hewitt M, Ganz PA. Cancer survivorship: a new challenge in delivering quality cancer care. J Clin Oncol. 2006;24:5101–4.

Survivorship Issues in Muscle Invasive Bladder Cancer

Bladder cancer is the fifth most commonly diagnosed cancer and the most expensive adult cancer in average healthcare costs incurred per patient in the USA [1]. However, little is known about factors influencing patients' treatment decisions, quality of life, and responses to treatment impairments. MIBC may be treated with curative intent by either external beam radiation therapy (with or without chemotherapy) or radical cystectomy, with or without perioperative chemotherapy. Radical cystectomy necessitates urinary diversion using one of three major methods: incontinent cutaneous (e.g., the ileal conduit), continent cutaneous, or orthotopic (e.g., the neobladder) diversion.

The Functional Assessment of Cancer Therapy (FACT-BL) instrument was used to evaluate QOL in a population-based sample of bladder cancer patients [2]. QOL scores were compared between those undergoing radical cystectomy (RC) or those with an intact bladder (BI) and between continent and conduit urinary diversion groups [2]. There were no differences in general QOL scores between RC and BI groups and between the two urinary diversion groups, but patients undergoing RC had worse sexual function scores. QOL scores for BI patients tended to decrease with increasing age (p = 0.01). Presence of comorbid conditions lowered QOL (p < 0.05). This demonstrates general QOL does not vary among long-term bladder cancer survivors regardless of treatment, but sexual functioning can be adversely affected in those undergoing cystectomy. Long-term QOL declines even in those with intact bladders, particularly in those with comorbidities.

Physical exercises offer a variety of health benefits to cancer survivors during and post-treatment. Jensen et al., investigated the feasibility, the adherence, and the efficacy of a short-term physical pre-habilitation program to patients with invasive bladder cancer awaiting radical cystectomy (RC) [3]. A prospective randomized controlled clinical trial investigated efficacy of a multidisciplinary rehabilitation program on length of stay following RC. A total of 107 patients were included in the intension-to-treat population revealing 50 patients in the intervention group and 57 patients in the standard group. A total of 66% (95% confidence interval (CI) 51; 78)

S. S. Goonewardene et al., *Management of Muscle Invasive Bladder Cancer*, Management of Urology, https://doi.org/10.1007/978-3-030-57915-9_74

adhered more than 75% of the recommended progressive standardized exercise program. In the intervention group, a significant improvement in muscle power of 18% ($p < 0.002$) was found at time for surgery. Moreover, muscle power was significantly improved compared to that in the standard group with 0.3 W/kg (95% CI 0.08; 0.5%) ($p < 0.006$). Adherence was not associated with pre-operative BMI, nutritional risk, comorbidity, pain, gender, or age. This demonstrates in patients awaiting RC, a short-term exercise-based pre-habilitation intervention is feasible and effective and should be considered in future survivorship strategies [3].

Kulaksizoglu et al., reviewed the time it takes cystectomized patients' to adapt to their new health status. The mean follow-up of the study group was 27.7 ± 7.3 months (range 12–46 months). At the 12th-month and thereafter the symptom scores of the patients decreased significantly in comparison to both the pre-operative and the post-operative 3–6 months (23.4 ± 13.7 and 21.8 ± 18.5, respectively; $p < 0.01$ for all) [4]. There was a 23% pre-operative depression rate, which comes down to 16% at the 12th-month control. The peak depression scores suggesting depression are observed at the third-month controls. There is a gradual decrease in depression score starting from the sixth-month controls and all reach minimum scores after 12 months [4]. This demonstrates both psychological and health-related quality of life measures come to baseline values and stabilize after the 12th-month period, suggesting that the time frame for the adaptation of patients is 12 months in patients undergoing radical cystectomy surgery.

Several unmet needs emerged about 6 months after surgery, when patients and their families are transitioning into the survivorship phase [1]. Many patients reported that they were unable to resume some of the usual physical or social activities because of treatment sequelae. Changes in sexual function (43.33%) were reported by both men (36.36%) and women (62.50%) [1]. Changes in sexual function reported by men included erectile dysfunction and low libido. Women reported difficulties related to vaginal dryness, pain during sexual intercourse, and lost desire for sex because of changes in body image and having a stoma [1]. About 36% of these patients (25% women, 40.91% men) were bothered by these changes and only 16.67% (12.50% women, 18.18% men) received professional advice concerning sexual dysfunction However, when asked whether they would have made a different treatment decision if they [1] had known what they knew now, many patients indicated they would not have changed their decision. One-fifth of the sample (20%; 25% women and 36.36% men) reported difficulties in adjusting to a changed body image.

In the USA radical surgery remains the golden standard for invasive bladder cancer [5]. Yet in most other areas of surgical oncology the trend of the 1990s has been towards organ conservation with chemoradiation with or without limited local surgery. Five and 8-year survival rates for clinically staged patients treated by transurethral resection and chemoradiation (trimodality therapy) in several modern, large and mature series show survival rates comparable to those reported in contemporary radical cystectomy series [5]. Eighty percent of those alive 5 years after chemoradiation still retain their native bladder. Although NMI relapse occurs in 20% of cases, it remains responsive to BCG (Bacilles bilie de Calmette-Guerin) in the manner of de novo NMI disease [5]. Quality-of-life studies show that the retained bladder functions well.

References

1. Mohamed NE, Diefenbach MA, Goltz HH, Lee CT, Latini D, Kowalkowski M, Philips C, Hassan W, Hall SJ. Muscle invasive bladder cancer: from diagnosis to survivorship. Adv Urol. 2012;2012:142135.
2. Allareddy V, Kennedy J, West MM, Konety BR. Quality of life in long-term survivors of bladder cancer. Cancer. 2006;106:2355–62.
3. Jensen BT, Laustsen S, Jensen JB, Borre M, Petersen AK. Exercise-based pre-habilitation is feasible and effective in radical cystectomy pathways-secondary results from a randomized controlled trial. Support Care Cancer. 2016;24(8):3325–31.
4. Kulaksizoglu H, Toktas G, Kulaksizoglu IB, Aglamis E, Unluer E. When should quality of life be measured after radical cystectomy? Eur Urol. 2002;42(4):350–5.
5. Zietman AL, Shipley WU, Kaufman DS. Organ-conserving approaches to muscle-invasive bladder cancer: future alternatives to radical cystectomy. Ann Med. 2000;32(1):34–42.

Survivors of muscle invasive bladder cancer (MIBC) experience physical and psychosocial side effects of cancer diagnosis and treatment [1]. These negative side effects have a crucial impact on their health-related quality of life (HRQoL). To date, there is evidence that rehabilitation interventions such as physical activity and psychosocial support have a positive effect on the HRQoL of cancer survivors [1].

Health-related quality of life (HRQOL) in patients with bladder cancer is important, because radical cystectomy and urinary diversion significantly affect urinary and sexual function, and lead to associated sex-specific morbidity [2]. This study found HRQOL is achieved with a particular type of urinary diversion after cystectomy for bladder cancer. Patients should be counseled on all reconstructive alternatives and a diversion chosen on the basis of patient preference, patient anatomy and tumor status, rather than on a potential difference in HRQOL [2]. Prospective studies with appropriate adjustment for confounding factors, which use validated and disease-specific questionnaires, are needed for HRQOL research on bladder cancer.

Patient-reported outcomes (PRO), including health-related quality of life (HRQOL) measures, represent important means for evaluating patients' health outcomes and for guiding health care decisions made by patients, practitioners, investigators, and policy makers [3]. Establishing a useful model of perceived general health or specific symptoms is the first and most important step in developing the responsive bladder cancer HRQOL measures necessitated by clinical settings [4].

Okada et al., assessed whether CUR enhanced postoperative QOL, we surveyed patients with CUR and ileal conduit (IC) using a questionnaire sent by mail [5]. Basic physical conditions were similar in the two groups, except for sleeping habits. Regarding social life, however, the CUR group showed better scores in bathing habits and frequency of overnight travel. Parastomal dermatitis was more frequent in the IC group and the patients were more hesitant to show their stoma to others. On the other hand, about half of the patients in the CUR group complained of troublesomeness in self-catheterization, especially at night. Overall, 74% and 41% of the patients in the CUR and IC group were satisfied with their urinary diversion [5].

S. S. Goonewardene et al., *Management of Muscle Invasive Bladder Cancer*, Management of Urology, https://doi.org/10.1007/978-3-030-57915-9_75

When the Kock pouch and Indiana pouch were compared, no statistically significant differences were found in average capacity, maximum capacity, or frequency of self-catheterization. This study demonstrates, CUR recipients have enhanced QOL regarding the stoma, travel and sleeping habits as compared to ileal conduit [5]. However, troublesomeness of night time self-catheterization was noted in the CUR group. Individualized selection of the type of urinary diversion with informed consent is essential.

Hardt et al., examined the changes in the quality of life (QoL) of 44 patients observed prospectively from pre-surgery to 1 year post-surgery. Two kinds of surgeries were compared: continent and incontinent urinary diversion [6]. In most areas the QoL returned to the prior level within 1 year after surgery. However, patients were restricted in their physical activity, sexual activity, and emotional well-being. Using individual weights for different aspects of life, QoL was higher than when using an unweighted measurement (Short Form 36, MOS). Two trends for the different developments in the QoL were established: general life satisfaction and social functioning tended to improve after a continent diversion but decreased after an incontinent diversion [6]. The perceived global satisfaction with both kinds of diversion was high—75% of the patients would choose the same kind of diversion again.

Not much is generally known regarding the burden imposed by bladder cancer upon patient health-related quality of life (HRQL) [7]. The role of HRQL in affecting patient preferences and utility assessment and, ultimately, the selection of therapeutic regimen, or patient satisfaction with that selection, is considered increasingly important by the medical community [7]. Most studies have identified urinary and sexual HRQL domains as being of greatest concern to patients. Increased awareness and use of the HRQL instruments such as the FACT-BL as well as the EORTC-QLQ-BLS24 and the EORTC-QLQ-BLM30 (when they are validated for SBC and IBC, respectively), should increase our understanding of the impact of this disease and its management options on patient HRQL [7].

References

1. Rammant E, Bultijnck R, Sundahl N, Ost P, Pauwels NS, Deforche B, Pieters R, Decaestecker K, Fonteyne V. Rehabilitation interventions to improve patient-reported outcomes and physical fitness in survivors of muscleinvasive bladder cancer: a systematic review protocol. BMJ Open. 2017;7(5):e016054.
2. Wright JL, Porter MP. Quality-of-life assessment in patients with bladder cancer. Nat Clin Pract Urol. 2007;4:147–54.
3. Mohamed NE, Gilbert F, Lee CT, et al. Pursuing quality in the application of bladder cancer quality of life research. Bladder Cancer. 2016;2:139–49.
4. Mohamed NE, Pisipati S, Lee CT, Goltz HH, Latini DM, Gilbert FS, Wittmann D, Knauer CJ, Mehrazin R, Sfakianos JP, McWilliams GW, Quale DZ, Hall SJ. Unmet informational and supportive care needs of patients following cystectomy for bladder cancer based on age, sex, and treatment choices. Urol Oncol. 2016;34(12):531.e7–531.e14.

5. Okada Y, Oishi K, Shichiri Y, et al. Quality of life survey of urinary diversion patients: comparison of continent urinary diversion versus ileal conduit. Int J Urol. 1997;4(1):26–31.
6. Hardt J, Filipas D, Hohenfellner R, Egle UT. Quality of life in patients with bladder carcinoma after cystectomy: first results of a prospective study. Qual Life Res. 2000;9:1):1–12.
7. Botteman MF, Pashos CL, Hauser RS, Laskin BL, Redaelli A. Quality of life aspects of bladder cancer: a review of the literature. Qual Life Res. 2003;12(6):675–88.

Body Image in Bladder Cancer

Although improvements in perioperative care have decreased surgical morbidity after radical cystectomy for muscle invasive bladder cancer, treatment side effects still have a negative impact on patient quality of life. At diagnosis unmet informational needs were predominant, consisting of insufficient discussion of certain topics, including urinary diversion options and their side effects, self-care, the recovery process and medical insurance. Unmet psychological needs related to depression, and worries about changes in body image and sexual function were reported [1]. Postoperative unmet needs revolved around medical needs (e.g. pain and bowel dysfunction) and instrumental needs (e.g. need of support for stomal appliances, catheters and incontinence) [1]. During survivorship unmet needs centered around psychological support (i.e. depression, poor body image and sexual dysfunction) and instrumental support (e.g. difficulty adjusting to changes in daily living).

Cancer diagnosis is often perceived as a traumatic event that changes an individual's basic assumptions about the self as effective and powerful, and the world as benevolent, controllable, and predictable. This event is even more devastating when cancer patients undergo extensive surgeries that severely debilitate their body image and their psychological and social well-being [2]. The 5-year CSM-free survival rate was 63.9% at RC, and increased to 71.0%, 77.5%, 81.7%, 85.9% and 86.3% in patients who survived ≥1, 2, 3, 4 and 5 years, respectively [3]. Patients with pT2–4 disease benefitted from the highest increase in survivorship 2 years after RC. The same findings were recorded according to patients' nodal status [3].

Somani et al. examined whether health and body image are important determinants of quality of life (QoL) for patients undergoing urinary diversion (UD) [4]. Patients with advanced bladder cancer who undergo cystectomy and UD face potential serious morbidity (25–40%) and a small risk of mortality (0–4%) [4]. The systematic review compares QoL and body image for different types of diversions. One researcher trained in using schedule for evaluation of individual quality of life-direct weighting interviewed 32 consecutive patients undergoing radical cystectomy. The European Organization for Research and Treatment of Cancer QLQ-C30 and the

S. S. Goonewardene et al., *Management of Muscle Invasive Bladder Cancer*, Management of Urology, https://doi.org/10.1007/978-3-030-57915-9_76

Satisfaction With Life Scale questionnaire were also administered before cystectomy and 9–12 months postcystectomy [4]. Family, relationships, health, and
finance were the most important determinants of QoL, whereas body image was not
mentioned by anyone. On using European Organization for Research and Treatment
of Cancer QLQ-C30 and Satisfaction With Life Scale, it was found that there was
no difference in QoL of patients pre- and postcystectomy. In our review of published data, 40 studies were identified reporting on 3645 patients. Only two studies
reported a better QoL in favor of neobladders, whereas two other studies suggest a
better body image perception in patients with neobladder. This prospective cohort
study suggests that health and body image may not always be important to patients
for their QoL. Our systematic review suggests an overall good QoL in most studies
irrespective of the type of UD, with no significant differences among the different
diversion types.

Patients being treated for bladder cancer share issues in common with other cancer patients, but also experience issues that are unique to their surgical treatment [5].
This study used a descriptive qualitative approach to explore the experiences of
patients who had undergone radical cystectomy for bladder cancer. Participants
described the shock of their diagnosis, their lack of information about bladder cancer, the importance of clear communication with care providers, and the types of
adjustments they had to make following surgery [5]. Specifically, changes in bodily
function, body image, sexual relationships, and intimacy presented challenges for
these participants. Although there was a sense of acceptance about the treatment-
related events, there were still significant adjustments required by individuals following their surgery [5]. Information, open communication, and support from
family and friends and medical team were seen as important factors in helping
patients adjust after surgery.

There has been a recent marked increase in interest in continent urinary diversions [6]. While considerable time has been spent on the technical aspects of these
diversions the psychological impact has not yet been fully explored. Boyd et al. [6],
studied this in detail. The results revealed that all patients surveyed generally were
satisfied with the diversions and they had adapted reasonably socially, physically
and psychologically [6]. The key to adaptation seemed to be a detailed, realistic
preoperative education about the type of diversion used [6]. Patients with ileal conduit diversions had the lowest expectations of the form of diversion as defined by
the preoperative awareness of the need to wear an external ostomy appliance with
its associated inconveniences and change in the external body image [6].
Postoperatively, ileal conduit patients also had the poorest self-images as defined by
a decrease in sexual desire and in all forms of physical contact (sexual and nonsex-
ual) [6]. The subset of patients who underwent conversion from conduit diversions
to Kock pouches, however, were statistically the most satisfied, and they were the
most physically and sexually active [6].

Patients undergoing radical cystectomy with neobladder for bladder cancer are
hypothesized to tolerate worse urinary function than ileal conduit patients because
of improved body image [7]. Hedgepeth et al. to compared body image and quality
of life between the two diversion types after surgery. Radical cystectomy has a

significant impact on body image that improves slowly over time. No difference in body image scores between ileal conduit and neobladder patients exists after surgery.

Nowadays, psychological and social aspects of treatment of urinary diversion after cystectomy, have become of utmost importance [8]. Body image, potency, continence, emotional distress and dissatisfaction, functional and social activities are majors factors to improve quality of life after surgery. Conde Redondo [8], compare health-related quality of life after bladder substitution with ileal conduit diversion. Patients with ileal consuit presented higher body image dissatisfaction than those who underwent bladder substitution Nowadays, psychological and social aspects of treatment of urinary diversion after cystectomy, have become of utmost importance [8]. When urine leakage occurred it caused more distress to the conduit patients, indicating urinary leakage as their main problem. Bladder substitution patients did not consider continence problems as very important, they had not interrupted social activities such as travelling or seeing friends. Hundred percent of of bladder substitution patients would not mind to undergo this operation again, while only 66% of ileal conduit patients would. Health-related quality of life is higher after bladder substitution.

DeFrank explored medical and psychosocial factors associated with body image dissatisfaction in male and female cancer survivors [9]. One hundred and sixty-five male and 234 female cancer survivors of six cancer types (bladder, female breast, colorectal, endometrial, prostate, and melanoma) who were 2, 5, and 10 years beyond diagnosis [9]. Results of multiple regression analysis indicated that male survivors of prostate cancer were more likely to express positive body images than men who had other types of cancer [9]. A composite variable that included a history of cancer recurrence, multiple cancers, or metastatic cancer was the strongest predictor of body image dissatisfaction for female survivors. Body image was not associated with age, length of time since diagnosis, or general treatment type for either gender [9]. Body image was associated with various medical and psychosocial factors, and the factors differed for male and female cancer survivors.

References

1. Mohamed NE, Chaoprang Herrera P, Hudson S, Revenson TA, Lee CT, Quale DZ, Zarcadoolas C, Hall SJ, Diefenbach MA. Muscle invasive bladder cancer: examining survivor burden and unmet needs. J Urol. 2014;191(1):48–53.
2. Mohamed NE, Diefenbach MA, Goltz HH, Lee CT, Latini D, Kowalkowski M, Philips C, Hassan W, Hall SJ. Muscle invasive bladder cancer: from diagnosis to survivorship. Adv Urol. 2012;2012:142135.
3. Sun M, Abdollah F, Bianchi M, Trinh QD, Shariat SF, Jeldres C, Tian Z, et al. "Conditional Survival of Patients with Urothelial Carcinoma of the Urinary Bladder Treated with Radical Cystectomy." [In eng]. Eur J Cancer. 2012;48(10):1503–11.
4. Somani BK, Gimlin D, Fayers P, N'Dow J. Quality of life and body image for bladder cancer patients undergoing radical cystectomy and urinary diversion—a prospective cohort study with a systematic review of literature. Urology. 2009;74(5):1138–43.

5. Fitch MI, Miller D, Sharir S, McAndrew A. Radical cystectomy for bladder cancer: a qualitative study of patient experiences and implications for practice. Can Oncol Nurs J. 2010;20(4):177–87.
6. Boyd SD, Feinberg SM, Skinner DG, Lieskovsky G, Baron D, Richardson J. Quality of life survey of urinary diversion patients: comparison of ileal conduits versus continent Kock ileal reservoirs. J Urol. 1987;138(6):1386–9.
7. Hedgepeth RC, Gilbert SM, He C, Lee CT, Wood DP. Body image and bladder cancer specific quality of life in patients with ileal conduit and neobladder urinary diversions. Urology. 2010;76(3):671–5.
8. Conde Redondo C, Estebanez Zarranz J, Rodriguez Tovez A, Amon Sesmero J, Alonso Fernandez D, Martinez Sagarra JM. "[Quality of Life in Patients Treated with Orthotopic Bladder Substitution Versus Cutaneous Ileostomy]." [In spa]. Actas Urol Esp. 2001;25(6):435–44.
9. DeFrank JT, Mehta CC, Stein KD, Baker F. Body image dissatisfaction in cancer survivors. Oncol Nurs Forum. 2007;34(3):E36–41.

Psychological Impact in Bladder Cancer

A systematic review relating to bladder cancer and psychological impact was conducted. This was to identify the bladder cancer epidemiology and risk factors in muscle invasive disease. The search strategy aimed to identify all references related to bladder cancer AND screening. Search terms used were as follows: (Bladder cancer) AND (psychological impact). The following databases were screened from 1989 to June 2020:

- CINAHL
- MEDLINE (NHS Evidence)
- Cochrane
- AMed
- EMBASE
- PsychINFO
- SCOPUS
- Web of Science

In addition, searches using Medical Subject Headings (MeSH) and keywords were conducted using Cochrane databases. Two UK-based experts in bladder cancer were consulted to identify any additional studies.

Studies were eligible for inclusion if they reported primary research focusing on bladder cancer and screening. Papers were included if published after 1984 and had to be in English. Studies that did not conform to this were excluded. Only primary research was included (Fig. 77.1). The overall aim was to identify bladder cancer risk factors and epidemiology in muscle invasive disease.

Abstracts were independently screened for eligibility by two reviewers and disagreements resolved through discussion or third-party opinion. Agreement level was calculated using Cohen's Kappa to test the intercoder reliability of this screening process. Cohens' Kappa allows comparison of inter-rater reliability between papers

S. S. Goonewardene et al., *Management of Muscle Invasive Bladder Cancer*, Management of Urology, https://doi.org/10.1007/978-3-030-57915-9_77

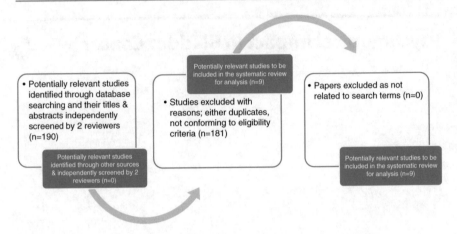

Fig. 77.1   Flow chart of studies identified through the systematic review. (Adapted from PRISMA)

using relative observed agreement. This also takes account of the comparison occurring by chance. The first reviewer agreed all 9 papers to be included, the second, agreed on 9. Cohens kappa was therefore 1.0.

Data extraction was piloted by the researcher and amended in consultation with the research team (author and two academic supervisors). Data collected included authors, year and country of publication, study aims, setting, intervention aims, number of participants, study design, intervention components and delivery methods, comparison groups and outcome measures, notes and follow-up questions for the authors. Studies were quality assessed using the PRISMA criteria for randomised controlled trials, Mays et al. [1, 2] for the action research and qualitative studies and the Critical Skills Appraisal programme for cohort studies. This was also applied to randomised controlled trials and qualitative studies.

The search identified 397 papers (Fig. 77.1). All 9 mapped to the search terms and eligibility criteria. The current systematic reviews were examined to gain further knowledge about the subject. One hundred and ninety-one papers were excluded due to not conforming to eligibility criteria or adding to the evidence. Of the 9 papers left, relevant abstracts were identified and the full papers obtained (all of which were in English), to quality assure against search criteria. There was considerable heterogeneity of design among the included studies therefore a narrative review of the evidence was undertaken. There was significant heterogeneity within studies, including clinical topic, numbers, outcomes, as a result a narrative review was thought to be best. There were 9 cohort studies, with a moderate level of evidence. These were from a range of countries with minimal loss to follow-up. All participants were identified appropriately.

77.1 Systematic Review Results

77.1.1 Psychological Impairment in Patients Referred for Bladder Cancer Investigations

Smith assessed the influence of trait emotional intelligence (trait EI) and perceived social support on psychological impairment in a sample of patients urgently referred for bladder cancer investigations [3]. Thirty-one percent of patients were considered to be suffering from clinical levels of state anxiety [3]. Trait EI was a significant predictor of state anxiety, worry regarding the appointment, worry regarding the outcome of the appointment and perceived social support [3]. In contrast, perceived social support was not predictive of psychological impairment on any measure and did not moderate the relationship between trait EI and psychological impairment [3].

Tan determined patient experience and perception following a diagnosis of non-muscle-invasive bladder cancer (NMIBC) [4]. A total of 213 patients completed the Brief-IPQ [4]. Patients felt that they had minimal symptoms (median [interquartile range, IQR] score 2 [0–5]) and were not particularly affected emotionally (median [IQR] score 3 [1–6]) with a minimal effect to their daily life (median [IQR] score 2 [0–5]) [4]. However, they remained concerned about their cancer diagnosis (median [IQR] score 5 [3–8]) and felt that they had no personal control over the cancer (median [IQR] score 2 [2–5]) and believed that their illness would affect them for some time (median [IQR] score 6 [3–10]) [4]. A significant association with a lower personal control of the disease ($p < 0.05$) and a poorer understanding of the management of NMIBC ($p < 0.05$) was seen in patients aged >70 years [4]. Many patients were uncertain about the cause of bladder cancer [4]. Qualitative analysis found that at initial presentation of haematuria, most patients were not aware of the risk of bladder cancer [4]. Patients were most anxious and psychologically affected between the interval of cystoscopy diagnosis and transurethral resection of bladder tumour (TURBT) [4]. Following TURBT, most patients were positive about their cancer prognosis [4].

77.1.2 Psychological Distress and Radical Cystectomy

Palapattu determined the prevalence of psychological distress in patients with bladder cancer prior to and following radical cystectomy [5]. The preoperative prevalence of psychological distress in patients diagnosed with bladder cancer was 45% and it remained somewhat increased at 34% approximately 4 weeks after cystectomy [5]. In the entire study group there was a statistically significant decrease in general distress ($p = 0.028$), depression ($p = 0.034$) and anxiety ($p = 0.0004$) from the preoperative to the postoperative assessments [5]. Pathological stage was significantly associated with post-cystectomy anxiety ($p = 0.040$) and general distress ($p = 0.042$) [5].

Månsson investigated (1) if early psychosocial intervention after cystectomy for bladder cancer can assist psychosocial rehabilitation; (2) if the outcome of such intervention correlates with the patient's psychological defensive strategies as revealed with the meta-contrast technique (MCT); and (3) if the patient's general philosophical outlook is important in this context [6]. There was no significant difference in the results of the SIP between the intervention and the non-intervention group, as a whole or in its psychosocial dimension [6]. However, intervention benefited patients with continent cutaneous diversion, whose scores on the psychosocial SIP dimension were lower than in the groups with ileal conduit diversion or orthotopic bladder replacement ($p < 0.05$) [6]. The MCT analysis of defensive strategies identified three clusters of patients characterized mainly by isolation and repression, repression and stereotypy or sensitivity and stereotypy [6]. Analysis for cluster identification showed no significant SIP score differences between intervention and non-intervention groups [6]. In an analysis of single defensive strategies, stereotypy was associated with higher total SIP score, but not significantly [6]. Three clusters of philosophical outlook were identified; in one cluster, characterized by a belief in a supernatural power and philosophical interest, the psychosocial SIP scores were lower in the patients who obtained emotional support and the reverse in a cluster with contrary attitudes, although neither differences were significant [6].

77.1.3 Psychological Distress in Smokers with Bladder Cancer

Kowalkowski identified actionable targets for educational intervention to increase adherence to cystoscopic monitoring for disease recurrence or progression [7]. Compared to non-smokers, current smokers reported increased fear of recurrence and psychological distress ($p < 0.05$) [7]. In regression analyses, non-adherence was associated with smoking (OR = 33.91, $p < 0.01$), providing a behavioral marker to describe a survivor group with unmet needs that may contribute to low cystoscopic adherence [7].

77.1.4 Psychological Impact of Type of Urinary Diversion

Månsson assessed if there is relationship between: (1) preoperative psychological defensive strategies, mood and type of lower urinary tract reconstruction, and (2) psychosocial adaptation after radical cystectomy for bladder cancer [8]. The remembered difficulties during the first month after discharge from hospital differed between the 'risk' and 'no risk' groups after 1 and 5 years [8]. On a visual analogue scale (VAS) the 'risk' patients had very low scores (less difficulty) or very high, while the 'no risk' patients had intermediate scores [8]. VAS score were also higher, although not significantly so, in patients using primitive defence strategies [8]. The psychosocial situation did not differ between the groups in the first year, but at 5 years there were differences in self-esteem and interpersonal contact-seeking [8]. High depression scores before surgery were associated with high VAS scores at

3 months when recalling the first month after discharge, but the anxiety score was not predictive [8]. Men with orthotopic bladder replacement adapted less well throughout the 5 year follow-up [8]. Elderly patients with stereotypy (the commonest defensive strategy at these ages) adapted relatively well to ileal conduit diversion [8]. About 20% of patients had difficulty in accepting the postoperative situation, regardless of urinary diversion modes [8].

Kitamura compared the QOL in patients with ileal or colon conduits (IC), continent urinary reservoir (CR) and ileal neobladder (NB), a retrospective study was conducted using a questionnaire sent by mail [9]. The IC group frequently complained of changes in bathing habits and loss of using public baths in comparison with the CR and the NB groups [9]. High scores for loss of sexual desire were obtained in the IC, the CR and the NB groups, in this order [9]. Because of the nearly physiological voiding, the NB group desired a voiding condition like preoperative status as compared with the IC and the CR groups [9]. However, for most of the questionnaire items no difference was seen among the IC, CR and NB groups concerning general condition, reconstruction-related symptoms, psychological status, sexual life, social status, satisfaction with the treatment and global satisfaction with life and health [9].

77.1.5 Quality of Life During Chemotherapy or Immunotherapy in Bladder Cancer

Taarnhøj reported correlations between selected PROs and QoL and thus to present symptoms that influence QoL [10]. Identification of these symptoms during treatment can lead to earlier symptom management and thus secure improvements in QoL [10]. In this study, 78 BC patients reported 724 questionnaires. Spearman's analysis showed significant correlations between almost all PRO-CTCAE items and the expected domain of QoL [10]. The PRO-CTCAE items with the strongest correlations with QoL were anxiety (F, frequency item) and emotional function ($r_s = -0.603$, $p < 0.0001$), concentration (S, severity item) and cognitive function ($r_s = -0.704$, $p < 0.0001$), discouraged (F) and emotional function ($r_s = -0.659$, $p < 0.0001$), fatigue (S) and role function ($r_s = -0.659$, $p < 0.0001$) and sad (F) and emotional function ($r_s = -0.711$, $p < 0.0001$) [10]. The weakest correlations were found for the PRO-CTCAE items urinary frequency, incontinence and urge, all with variations in the direction and significance of the correlations [10].

77.1.6 Psychological Issues in Metastatic Bladder Cancer

Sengeløv described self-reported functional and psychological status of patients using The European Organization for Research and Treatment of Cancer Quality of Life Questionnaire (QLQ-C30) and relates this to the prognosis [11]. There was a significant relation between functional, emotional, and social status and survival [11]. The self-assessment of functional status was a better prognostic factor for survival than performance status evaluated by the clinician [11]. The value of the global quality of life scale did not relate to survival after recurrence [11]. Functional, emotional, and quality of life scales declined during the progression of the disease [11]. The study suggests that evaluation with self-reporting questionnaires may provide the physician with useful information, and it may aid in making treatment decisions in patients with metastatic bladder cancer [11].

References

1. Moher D, Liberati A, Tetzlaff J, Altman DG. "Preferred Reporting Items for Systematic Reviews and Meta-Analyses: The Prisma Statement." [In English]. BMJ (Online) 339, no. 7716 (08 Aug 2009):332–36.
2. Mays N, Pope C, Popay J. "Systematically Reviewing Qualitative and Quantitative Evidence to Inform Management and Policy-Making in the Health Field." [In English]. Journal of Health Services Research and Policy 10, no. SUPPL. 1 (July 2005):6–20.
3. Smith SG, Turner B, Pati J, Petrides KV, Sevdalis N, Green JS. Psychological impairment in patients urgently referred for prostate and bladder cancer investigations: the role of trait emotional intelligence and perceived social support. Support Care Cancer. 2012;20(4):699–704.
4. Tan WS, Teo CH, Chan D, et al. Exploring patients' experience and perception of being diagnosed with bladder cancer: a mixed-methods approach. BJU Int. 2020;125:669–78. https://doi.org/10.1111/bju.15008. [Published online ahead of print, 2020 Jan 23].
5. Palapattu GS, Haisfield-Wolfe ME, Walker JM, et al. Assessment of perioperative psychological distress in patients undergoing radical cystectomy for bladder cancer. J Urol. 2004;172(5 Pt 1):1814–7.
6. Månsson A, Colleen S, Hermerén G, Johnson G. Which patients will benefit from psychosocial intervention after cystectomy for bladder cancer? Br J Urol. 1997;80(1):50–7.
7. Kowalkowski MA, Goltz HH, Petersen NJ, Amiel GE, Lerner SP, Latini DM. Educational opportunities in bladder cancer: increasing cystoscopic adherence and the availability of smoking-cessation programs. J Cancer Educ. 2014;29(4):739–45.
8. Månsson A, Christensson P, Johnson G, Colleen S. Can preoperative psychological defensive strategies, mood and type of lower urinary tract reconstruction predict psychosocial adjustment after cystectomy in patients with bladder cancer? Br J Urol. 1998;82(3):348–56.
9. Kitamura H, Miyao N, Yanase M, et al. Quality of life in patients having an ileal conduit, continent reservoir or orthotopic neobladder after cystectomy for bladder carcinoma. Int J Urol. 1999;6(8):393–9.
10. Taarnhøj GA, Johansen C, Lindberg H, Basch E, Dueck A, Pappot H. Patient reported symptoms associated with quality of life during chemo- or immunotherapy for bladder cancer patients with advanced disease. Cancer Med. 2020;9:3078–87. https://doi.org/10.1002/cam4.2958.
11. Sengeløv L, Frølich S, Kamby C, Jensen NH, Steven K. The functional and psychosocial status of patients with disseminated bladder cancer. Urol Oncol. 2000;5(1):20–4.

Part XII

Palliative Therapy in Muscle Invasive Bladder Cancer

The Role of Palliative Cystectomy in Bladder Cancer

78

78.1 Research Methods

A systematic review relating to muscle invasive bladder cancer and palliative cystectomy was conducted. This was to identify whether radical cystectomy has a role in this cohort. The search strategy aimed to identify all references related to bladder cancer AND muscle invasive disease AND Palliative Cystectomy. Search terms used were as follows: (Bladder cancer) AND (muscle invasive disease) AND (Palliative Cystectomy). The following databases were screened from 1979 to June 2020:

- CINAHL
- MEDLINE (NHS Evidence)
- Cochrane
- AMedune
- EMBASE
- PsychINFO
- SCOPUS
- Web of Science

In addition, searches using Medical Subject Headings (MeSH) and keywords were conducted using Cochrane databases. Two UK-based experts in bladder cancer were consulted to identify any additional studies.

Studies were eligible for inclusion if they reported primary research focusing on muscle invasive bladder cancer and palliative cystectomy. Papers were included if published after 1984 and had to be in English. Studies that did not conform to this were excluded. Only primary research was included (Fig. 78.1).

Abstracts were independently screened for eligibility by two reviewers and disagreements resolved through discussion or third-party opinion. Agreement level

S. S. Goonewardene et al., *Management of Muscle Invasive Bladder Cancer*, Management of Urology, https://doi.org/10.1007/978-3-030-57915-9_78

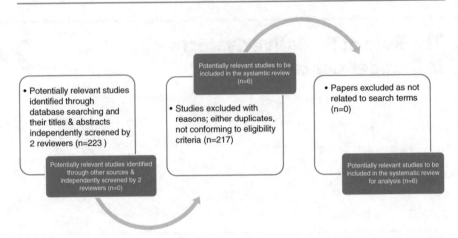

Fig. 78.1   Flow chart of studies identified through the systematic review. (Adapted from PRISMA)

was calculated using Cohen's Kappa to test the intercoder reliability of this screening process. Cohens' Kappa allows comparison of inter-rater reliability between papers using relative observed agreement. This also takes account of the comparison occurring by chance. The first reviewer agreed all 18 papers to be included, the second, agreed on 18.

Data extraction was piloted by the researcher and amended in consultation with the research team (author and two academic supervisors). Data collected included authors, year and country of publication, study aims, setting, intervention aims, number of participants, study design, intervention components and delivery methods, comparison groups and outcome measures, notes and follow-up questions for the authors. Studies were quality assessed using the PRISMA criteria for randomised controlled trials, Mays et al. [1, 2] for the action research and qualitative studies and the Critical Skills Appraisal programme for cohort studies. This was also applied to randomised controlled trials and qualitative studies.

The search identified 223 papers (Fig. 78.1). Six mapped to the search terms and eligibility criteria. The current systematic reviews were examined to gain further knowledge about the subject. Two hundred and seventeen papers were excluded due to not conforming to eligibility criteria or adding to the evidence. Of the 6 papers left, relevant abstracts were identified and the full papers obtained (all of which were in English), to quality assure against search criteria. There was considerable heterogeneity of design among the included studies therefore a narrative review of the evidence was undertaken. There was significant heterogeneity within studies, including clinical topic, numbers, outcomes, as a result a narrative review was thought to be best. There were 6 cohort studies, with a moderate level of evidence. These were from a range of countries with minimal loss to follow-up. All participants were identified appropriately.

78.2   Systematic Review Results

78.2.1   Lymph Node Positive Bladder Cancer and Outcomes with Cystectomy

Bae examined the treatment strategy for lymph node-positive bladder cancer [3] and compared the treatment outcomes of chemotherapy, surgery, and combination therapy [3]. Patients with bladder cancer presenting local lymph node metastasis at the time of diagnosis were treated with a single treatment strategy [3]. Treatment outcomes were retrospectively analyzed on the basis of clinical indices and survival time [3]. Out of 230 patients with bladder cancer, 44 (19.1%) were treated with palliative chemotherapy, 30 (13.0%) with neoadjuvant chemotherapy followed by cystectomy, 129 (56.1%) with cystectomy followed by adjuvant chemotherapy, and 27 (11.7%) with cystectomy alone [3]. Median survival among all groups was 30.4 months. For each group, median overall survival was 19.3, 49.1, 42.6, and 11.2 months, respectively [3].

Stanik evaluated oncological results in bladder cancer patients with clinically regional and supraregional lymph-adenopathy treated with induction chemotherapy (IC) and consolidative cystectomy [4]. Twenty-five patients with clinically node-positive bladder cancer (including pelvic and retroperitoneal nodes) were treated with 2–4 cycles of IC followed by consolidative cystectomy [4]. Pathologic complete response (pCR) was defined as no residual tumor in the final specimen (ypT0N0) [4]. The 3-year cancer-specific (CSS) and recurrence-free survival (RFS) for the whole cohort were 52% and 39%, respectively [4]. The 3-year RFS differed according to volume of nodal metastases, the rates were 56% for minimal nodal disease (cN1) versus 33% for cN2-3 and 0% for cM1 disease (p < 0.001) [4]. pCR was seen in 7 (28%) patients; 50% in cN1 versus 13% in cN3-M1 [4]. pCR associated with 3-year CSS of 80% versus 45% in patients with persistent disease after IC [4].

Guru evaluated the lymph node yield (LNY) during robot-assisted radical cystectomy (RC), as it has been questioned as to whether robot assistance allows adequate pelvic LN dissection (LND), especially during the initial experience [5]. Six underwent palliative cystectomy) and the remainder were divided into five groups [5]. The mean operative duration for the robot-assisted pelvic LND was 44 (19–85) min. There was one postoperative complication that required exploration for vascular injury [5]. The mean number of LNs retrieved was 18 (6–43). The mean LNY for each of the five groups was 13, 16, 21, 19 and 23, respectively, and neither BMI nor previous major abdominal surgery affected LNY [5]. Robot-assisted RC with pelvic LND was performed safely. LNY was oncologically acceptable and increased with experience [5].

Patients with clinically node-positive bladder cancer were historically considered to have uniformly poor prognosis and were frequently treated with palliative chemotherapy (CHT) only [6]. Stanik compared the efficacy of different treatment modalities [6]. The 5-year OS for CHT alone, RC alone, and RC + CHT were 21.7% (95% confidence interval [CI], 15.4–28.0%), 12.1% (95% CI, 7.4–16.7%), and 25.4% (95% CI, 18.9–31.9%), respectively (p < 0.001) [6]. The median survivals were 17, 10, and 23 months, respectively. In multivariate analysis, age >60 years (hazard ratio, 1.29; 95% CI, 1.06–1.56; p = 0.011) and clinical stage cT3–4 (hazard ratio, 1.39; 95% CI, 1.12–1.71; p = 0.002) were negative predictors of survival [6]. When compared with CHT, RC + CHT reduced the risk of overall mortality by 21% (p = 0.044) [6].

78.2.2 Outcomes from Palliative Cystectomy

Zebic evaluated the morbidity and mortality of radical cystectomy in a group of unselected patients aged ≥75 years who were treated with curative and palliative intent [7]. Forty-six were treated with curative intent (Group A), seven with palliative intent (group B). The indications for cystectomy in group A were recurrent and otherwise therapy-resistant bladder cancer, the indications in group B were advanced pelvic malignancy [7]. Complications and mortality before, during and after surgery, and the duration of hospital stay and clinical outcome, were assessed [7]. The early mortality rate in group A was 4% (2/46); in group B two patients died after prolonged complications [7]. The median (range) hospital stay was 28 (6–56) days, and was significantly longer in patients with complications, at a median (range) of 36 (6–70) days [7]. The complication rates early and late after surgery in group A were 22% and 11%, respectively, and in group B, five of seven (early) [7].

78.2.3 Outcomes from Palliative Robotic Cystectomy

Bianchi assessed surgical and functional outcomes of 17 consecutive patients undergoing robot-assisted radical cystectomy (RARC) with palliative intent in a monocentric single surgeon series [8]. Median age at surgery was 78 years, with median Charlson Comorbidity Index (CCI) and age-adjusted CCI of 3 and 7, respectively [8]. Clinical stage was T2, T3 or T4 in 7, 8 and 2 patients respectively, with 52.9% and 29.4% with cN+ and cM+ disease [8]. Median estimated blood loss was 200 ml, with 1 patient requiring intra-operative blood transfusion [8]. Median hospital stay was 7 days. A total of 3 and 2 patients were re-hospitalized during the first 30 and 30-90 post-operative days, respectively [8]. One major Clavien grade complication was recorded [8]. At median follow-up of 8 months, 9 and 2 patients succumbed due to tumor progression and other causes [8]. Pre-operative and post-operative FACT-BL scores improved significantly in each domain [8].

Flamm presented 19 patients with inoperable urinary bladder carcinoma in which urinary diversion was performed by ileal conduit without cystectomy [9]. The post-operative mortality rate was 10.5% and the incidence of complications was 16%. The average time of survival was 5.1 months and varied from between 1 and 23 months [9]. This paper highlighted palliative ileal conduit should not be considered a suitable method for urinary diversion in patients with advanced carcinoma of the urinary bladder [9].

A retrospective study is presented of 19 patients with inoperable urinary bladder carcinoma in which urinary diversion was performed by ileal conduit without cystectomy [10]. The postoperative mortality rate was 10.5% and the incidence of complications was 16% [10]. The average time of survival was 5.1 months and varied from between 1 and 23 months [10]. This paper highlighted palliative ileal conduit should not be considered a suitable method for urinary diversion in patients with advanced carcinoma of the urinary bladder [10].

78.2.4 Systematic Reviews Relating to Palliative Cystectomy

Palliative surgery is performed in order to relieve symptoms as well as to increase survival in selected tumour entities [11]. For urothelial cancer, its role is limited and clinical data are limited, too [11]. For patients with low metastatic load, or if the tumour is restricted to lymph nodes inside and outside the pelvis, as well as for singular pulmonary metastasis, there seems to be a survival benefit in select cases [11]. Calculation of risks and benefits is difficult and, for now, should be reconsidered for every individual patient [11].

Neuzillet was to review situations where surgical resection of the bladder tumor and/or metastatic urothelial carcinoma has been reported and analyze its results [12]. Synchronous or metachronous urothelial carcinoma metastases were diagnosed in 4% and 50% of the cases, respectively [12]. The surgical treatment of metastatic urothelial carcinoma of the bladder has been proposed to achieve oncologic resection of all detectable lesions after a first-line chemotherapy or to treat symptoms, which were refractory to other treatment modalities [12]. In achieving complete resection of the primary tumor and metastases after MVAC chemotherapies, the 5 years overall survival was 28% [12].

References

1. Moher D, Liberati A, Tetzlaff J, Altman DG. "Preferred Reporting Items for Systematic Reviews and Meta-Analyses: The Prisma Statement." [In English]. BMJ (Online) 339, no. 7716 (08 Aug 2009):332–36.
2. Mays N, Pope C, Popay J. "Systematically Reviewing Qualitative and Quantitative Evidence to Inform Management and Policy-Making in the Health Field." [In English]. Journal of Health Services Research and Policy 10, no. SUPPL. 1 (July 2005):6–20.
3. Bae WK, Lee HJ, Park SH, et al. Comparative effectiveness of palliative chemotherapy versus neoadjuvant chemotherapy followed by radical cystectomy versus cystectomy followed by adjuvant chemotherapy versus cystectomy for regional node-positive bladder cancer: a retrospective analysis: KCSG GU 17-03. Cancer Med. 2019;8(12):5431–7.
4. Stanik M, Poprach A, Macik D, et al. Clinically node-positive bladder cancer: oncological results of induction chemotherapy and consolidation surgery. Neoplasma. 2018;65(2):287–91.
5. Guru KA, Sternberg K, Wilding GE, et al. The lymph node yield during robot-assisted radical cystectomy. BJU Int. 2008;102(2):231–4.

6. Stanik M, Poprach A, Zapletalová M, et al. Comparison of different treatment modalities outcomes in clinically node-positive bladder cancer: analysis of a population-based cancer registry. Clin Genitourin Cancer. 2019;17(4):e759–67.
7. Zebic N, Weinknecht S, Kroepfl D. Radical cystectomy in patients aged > or = 75 years: an updated review of patients treated with curative and palliative intent. BJU Int. 2005;95(9):1211–4.
8. Bianchi FM, Romagnoli D, D'Agostino D, et al. Is robotic approach useful to palliate advanced bladder cancer? A monocentric single surgeon experience. Cent Eur J Urol. 2019;72(2):113–20.
9. Flamm J, Kiesswetter H. Das palliative Ilealconduit beim inoperablen Harnblasenkarzinom [Palliative ileal conduit in inoperable cancer of the urinary bladder]. Wien Klin Wochenschr. 1987;99(2):58–9.
10. Li Z, Zhang S, Qi F. Zhonghua Wai Ke Za Zhi. Nontransitional cell tumor of the bladder. 1999;37(1):29–31.
11. Hübner N, Shariat SF. Palliative Chirurgie beim metastasierten Urothelkarzinom [Palliative surgery for metastatic urothelial cancer]. Aktuelle Urol. 2018;49(5):412–6.
12. Neuzillet Y, Larré S, Comperat E, et al. Traitement chirurgical du carcinome urothélial de vessie métastatique: revue du Comité de cancérologie de l'Association française d'urologie [Surgical treatment of metastatic urothelial carcinoma of the bladder: review of the Cancer Committee of the French Association of Urology]. Prog Urol. 2013;23(12):951–7.

Palliative Care in Bladder Cancer

A systematic review relating to muscle invasive bladder cancer and palliative cystectomy was conducted. This was to identify whether radical cystectomy has a role in this cohort. The search strategy aimed to identify all references related to bladder cancer AND muscle invasive disease AND Palliative Care. Search terms used were as follows: (Bladder cancer) AND (muscle invasive disease) AND (Palliative). The following databases were screened from 1979 to June 2020:

- CINAHL
- MEDLINE (NHS Evidence)
- Cochrane
- AMedune
- EMBASE
- PsychINFO
- SCOPUS
- Web of Science

In addition, searches using Medical Subject Headings (MeSH) and keywords were conducted using Cochrane databases. Two UK-based experts in bladder cancer were consulted to identify any additional studies.

Studies were eligible for inclusion if they reported primary research focusing on muscle invasive bladder cancer and palliative cystectomy. Papers were included if published after 1984 and had to be in English. Studies that did not conform to this were excluded. Only primary research was included (Fig. 79.1).

Abstracts were independently screened for eligibility by two reviewers and disagreements resolved through discussion or third-party opinion. Agreement level was calculated using Cohen's Kappa to test the intercoder reliability of this screening process. Cohens' Kappa allows comparison of inter-rater reliability

S. S. Goonewardene et al., *Management of Muscle Invasive Bladder Cancer*,
Management of Urology, https://doi.org/10.1007/978-3-030-57915-9_79

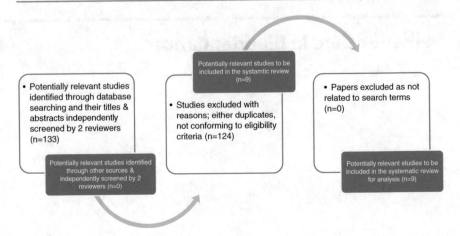

Fig. 79.1 Flow chart of studies identified through the systematic review. (Adapted from PRISMA)

between papers using relative observed agreement. This also takes account of the comparison occurring by chance. The first reviewer agreed all 9 papers to be included, the second, agreed on 9.

Data extraction was piloted by the researcher and amended in consultation with the research team (author and two academic supervisors). Data collected included authors, year and country of publication, study aims, setting, intervention aims, number of participants, study design, intervention components and delivery methods, comparison groups and outcome measures, notes and follow-up questions for the authors. Studies were quality assessed using the PRISMA criteria for randomised controlled trials, Mays et al. [1, 2] for the action research and qualitative studies and the Critical Skills Appraisal programme for cohort studies. This was also applied to randomised controlled trials and qualitative studies.

The search identified 133 papers (Fig. 79.1). Nine mapped to the search terms and eligibility criteria. The current systematic reviews were examined to gain further knowledge about the subject. One hundred and twenty-four papers were excluded due to not conforming to eligibility criteria or adding to the evidence. Of the 9 papers left, relevant abstracts were identified and the full papers obtained (all of which were in English), to quality assure against search criteria. There was considerable heterogeneity of design among the included studies therefore a narrative review of the evidence was undertaken. There was significant heterogeneity within studies, including clinical topic, numbers, outcomes, as a result a narrative review was thought to be best. There were 9 cohort studies, with a moderate level of evidence. These were from a range of countries with minimal loss to follow-up. All participants were identified appropriately.

79.1 Systematic Review Results

79.1.1 Surgery in Palliation

Bianchi assessed surgical and functional outcomes of 17 consecutive patients undergoing robot-assisted radical cystectomy (RARC) with palliative intent in a monocentric single surgeon series [3]. Clinical stage was T2, T3 or T4 in 7, 8 and 2 patients respectively, with 52.9% and 29.4% with cN+ and cM+ disease [3]. One major Clavien grade complication was recorded [3]. At median follow-up of 8 months, 9 and 2 patients succumbed due to tumor progression and other causes [3]. Pre-operative and post-operative FACT-BL scores improved significantly in each domain [3].

79.1.2 Patient Selection in Palliative Radiotherapy

Ali investigated the effectiveness of palliative pelvic radiation therapy (PRT) in patients with bladder cancer and identify factors associated with treatment outcome [4]. Two hundred forty-one patients were identified as receiving PRT [4]. At first follow-up at about 6 weeks after the last fraction of radiation therapy, symptoms were reported in 150 of 200 (75%) living patients; 80 of 150 (53%) patients reported improvement in symptoms after treatment [4]. There were significant differences in mOS with stage, performance status, and comorbidities [4]. One in 4 patients either did not complete the planned RT course or died within 30 days of treatment [4]. These patients were unlikely to have received maximal benefit from treatment but may have experienced side effects, making treatment futile [4]. Patients with good performance status and earlier stage disease survived longer [4].

Méry retrospectively reviewed radiotherapy for bladder cancer over the past decade and who were aged 90 years or older [5]. Ten patients (71%) had a general health status altered (PS 2–3) at the beginning of RT [5]. A total of 14 RT courses were delivered, including six treatments (43%) with curative intent and eight treatments (57%) with palliative intent [5]. Palliative intent mainly encompassed hemostatic RT (36%) [5]. At last follow-up, two patients (14%) experienced complete response, one patient (7%) experienced partial response, three patients (21%) had their disease stable, and three patients (21%) experienced tumor progression, of whom two patients with the progression of symptoms [5]. There was no reported high-grade acute local toxicity in 14 patients (100%) [5]. One patient experienced delayed grade 2 toxicity with pain and lower urinary tract symptoms [5]. At last follow-up, seven patients (50%) were deceased. Cancer was the cause of death for five patients [5].

Dirix evaluated haematuria-free survival as well as acute and late toxicity after hypofractionated palliative radiotherapy for bladder cancer [6]. After a mean follow-up of 10 months, 91% of patients were still hematuria free, with a mean hematuria-free survival of 13 months [6]. Severe ($\geq$grade 3) acute and late urinary toxicity was observed in 9% and 19% of patients, respectively [6].

Tey reviewed the outcomes of palliative radiotherapy (RT) for haematuria treated with modern RT techniques [7]. Sixty-seven percent of patients (39/58) responded to RT [7]. The median survival duration was 5.6 months (range = 0.02–47.6 months) [7]. One third (13/39) of responders had recurrence of haematuria [7]. Competing Risk regression with death as the competing risk showed that patients treated with low BED regimen (<36 Gy) had 5.76 times the hazard of recurrence compared to high BED regimen (>36 Gy) (p = 0.01) [7]. One patient (2%) developed grade 3 nausea and vomiting which required admission for intravenous hydration [7].

79.1.3 Palliative Chemotherapy in Muscle Invasive Bladder Cancer

Robinson reported the treatment delivery and survival associated with palliative chemotherapy in routine clinical practice [8]. The palliative chemotherapy regimen was identified for 710 patients with bladder cancer in Ontario during 1994 to 2008 [8]. Gemcitabine-cisplatin (Gem-Cis) was delivered to 37% (261 of 710), gemcitabine-carboplatin (Gem-Carbo) to 14% (96 of 710), and MVAC (methotrexate, vinblastine, Adriamycin, and cisplatin) to 8% (56 of 710) [8]. Other regimens were delivered to 42% of cases [8]. The proportion of cases treated with Gem-Cis increased during the study period: 3% in 1994–1999, 32% in 2000–2003, and 52% in 2004–2008 (p < 0.001) [8]. The median survival and 5-year OS by regimen was 10 months and 16% for Gem-Cis, 7 months and 6% for Gem-Carbo, and 10 months and 13% for MVAC, respectively [8]. Multivariate analysis controlling for age and comorbidity demonstrated improved survival for Gem-Cis and MVAC compared with Gem-Carbo (hazard ratio, 1.53; 95% confidence interval, 1.19–1.98) [8].

Kim conducted a retrospective analysis of the clinical features and chemotherapy outcomes of bladder adenocarcinoma [9]. Twelve patients were treated with 5-fluorouracil based chemotherapy, five were gemcitabine based, three were taxane and others [9]. Thirteen of them achieved complete response (10.3%) or partial response (34.5%) [9]. Median progression-free survival (PFS) and overall survival (OS) for all patients were 10.6 months (95% confidence interval [CI], 9.5–11.6) and 24.5 months (95% CI, 1.2–47.8), respectively [9]. The cases of urachal adenocarcinoma exhibited worse tendency in PFS and OS ($p = 0.024$ and $p = 0.046$, respectively) [9].

Bae compared the treatment outcomes of chemotherapy, surgery, and combination therapy in patients with lymph node-positive bladder cancer [10]. Treatment outcomes were retrospectively analyzed on the basis of clinical indices and survival time [10]. Out of 230 patients with bladder cancer, 44 (19.1%) were treated with palliative chemotherapy, 30 (13.0%) with neoadjuvant chemotherapy followed by cystectomy, 129 (56.1%) with cystectomy followed by adjuvant chemotherapy, and 27 (11.7%) with cystectomy alone [10]. For each group, median overall survival was 19.3, 49.1, 42.6, and 11.2 months, respectively [10].

Funakoshi conducted a nationwide survey using questionnaires on the clinical practice of chemotherapy for such patients [11]. Overall, 675 patients were registered and assessed for main primary cancer site involvement [11]. Of 507 patients with primary site involvement, 74 patients (15%) received chemotherapy (44 as palliative chemotherapy and 30 as perioperative chemotherapy) [11]. The most commonly used cytotoxic drugs were fluoropyrimidine (15 patients), platinum (8 patients) and taxane (8 patients), and the dosage and timing of these drugs differed between institutions; however, the dosage of molecular targeted drugs (24 patients) and hormone therapy drugs (15 patients) was consistent [11]. The median survival time of patients receiving palliative chemotherapy was 13.0 months (0.1–60.3 months) [11]. Three patients (6.8%) died from treatment-related causes and nine patients (20%) died of causes other than cancer [11]. Of the 30 patients who received perioperative chemotherapy, 6 (20%) died of causes other than cancer within 3 years after the initiation of chemotherapy [11].

References

1. Moher D, Liberati A, Tetzlaff J, Altman DG. "Preferred Reporting Items for Systematic Reviews and Meta-Analyses: The Prisma Statement." [In English]. BMJ (Online) 339, no. 7716 (08 Aug 2009):332–36.
2. Mays N, Pope C, Popay J. "Systematically Reviewing Qualitative and Quantitative Evidence to Inform Management and Policy-Making in the Health Field." [In English]. Journal of Health Services Research and Policy 10, no. SUPPL. 1 (July 2005):6–20.
3. Bianchi FM, Romagnoli D, D'Agostino D, et al. Is robotic approach useful to palliate advanced bladder cancer? A monocentric single surgeon experience. Cent Eur J Urol. 2019;72(2):113–20.
4. Ali A, Song YP, Mehta S, et al. Palliative radiation therapy in bladder cancer-importance of patient selection: a retrospective multicenter study. Int J Radiat Oncol Biol Phys. 2019;105(2):389–93.
5. Méry B, Falk AT, Assouline A, et al. Hypofractionated radiation therapy for treatment of bladder carcinoma in patients aged 90 years and more: a new paradigm to be explored? Int Urol Nephrol. 2015;47(7):1129–34.
6. Dirix P, Vingerhoedt S, Joniau S, Van Cleynenbreugel B, Haustermans K. Hypofractionated palliative radiotherapy for bladder cancer. Support Care Cancer. 2016;24(1):181–6.
7. Tey J, Soon YY, Cheo T, et al. Efficacy of palliative bladder radiotherapy for hematuria in advanced bladder cancer using contemporary radiotherapy techniques. In Vivo. 2019;33(6):2161–7.
8. Robinson AG, Wei X, Vera-Badillo FE, Mackillop WJ, Booth CM. Palliative chemotherapy for bladder cancer: treatment delivery and outcomes in the general population. Clin Genitourin Cancer. 2017;15(4):e535–41.
9. Kim MJ, Kim YS, Oh SY, et al. Retrospective analysis of palliative chemotherapy for the patients with bladder adenocarcinoma: Korean Cancer Study Group Genitourinary and Gynecology Cancer Committee. Korean J Intern Med. 2018;33(2):383–90.
10. Bae WK, Lee HJ, Park SH, et al. Comparative effectiveness of palliative chemotherapy versus neoadjuvant chemotherapy followed by radical cystectomy versus cystectomy followed by adjuvant chemotherapy versus cystectomy for regional node-positive bladder cancer: a retrospective analysis: KCSG GU 17-03. Cancer Med. 2019;8(12):5431–7.
11. Funakoshi T, Horimatsu T, Nakamura M, et al. Chemotherapy in cancer patients undergoing haemodialysis: a nationwide study in Japan. ESMO Open. 2018;3(2):e000301.

Index

Printed in the United States
by Baker & Taylor Publisher Services